FIRST
DO NO HARM

Drugs from the Ancients to Big Pharma

WALTER GRATZER

authorHOUSE®

AuthorHouse™ UK
1663 Liberty Drive
Bloomington, IN 47403 USA
www.authorhouse.co.uk
Phone: 0800.197.4150

Published by AuthorHouse 08/21/2017

ISBN: 978-1-5462-8105-4 (sc)
ISBN: 978-1-5462-8104-7 (e)

Print information available on the last page.

INTRODUCTION

So what is a drug? A cynical researcher defined it as a substance that, when injected into an animal, produces a publication. A more decorous definition might be 'a substance taken voluntarily with the object of engendering a benign effect'. By this measure alcohol and tobacco are drugs, as in a sense of course they are. Simpler perhaps just to settle for the more economical version in Doctor Johnson's Dictionary: 'An ingredient used in physick'. The great Canadian physician and pedagogue, Sir William Osler, writing at the end of the 19th century, contended that 'the desire to take medicines is perhaps the greatest feature which distinguishes man from animals'. Apes and other animals, it is true, seek out and chew medicinal plants when troubled by parasite infestations and some other afflictions, but they do not, so far as we know, invent illnesses for which to find a cure.

The history of drugs has its origin in the fog of antiquity. Their evolution was tortuous and slow, with many strange blind alleys along the way. For centuries, indeed millennia, the tale is one of superstition, obscurantism and stasis, interrupted by the rare probing beam of light. Only in the 19th century was the miasma gradually dispersed by the incursion of science, leading to a period of relatively sustained, and once in a while cataclysmic progress. Up to that time there were thousands of traditional remedies, nearly always useless, sometimes dangerous and often disgusting, but there were really only three preparations of proven value - digitalis (from foxglove) as a treatment for heart failure, citrus juice, as a cure and preventative of the dread disease of scurvy, and morphine in its various guises to ease pain. Mercury, arsenic and antimony and their compounds killed more often than they helped the sick: they were another route by which the Hippocratic Oath was regularly breached. Doctors thus had few curative resources at their disposal. 'The art of medicine', Voltaire wrote, 'consists in amusing the patient while nature cures the malady'.

The therapy for disease - any disease – rested for two millennia on the humoral theory, commonly linked in Europe with the name of Galen, the 2nd-century Greek physician. Galen's malign shadow hung over the healing profession through the epochs, although the theory actually has much older roots, and similar doctrines also stultified other ancient schools of medicine. Health amounted to an equipoise between the four bodily humours - blood, phlegm, black bile and yellow bile - which were associated respectively with sanguine, phlegmatic, melancholy and choleric temperaments. A disorder was cured by ingestion of remedies designated hot, dry, moist or cold, according to the nature of the imbalance identified with the disease. The most catastrophic consequence of the Galenic teaching was that practically all ills could be cured by blood-letting, which was generally aided by clysters (enemas), purges, and – in a later innovation – sweats to expel malign humours. Doctor Johnson's Dictionary gives 'purging' as one of the meanings of the verb, to 'physick'. (A secondary definition of 'pysick', the noun, is 'any thing without worth or value'.) An epigram making fun of a fashionable 18th-century London physician, Dr John Lettsome runs:

> Whenever patients come to I
> I physicks, bleeds and sweats 'em;
> If after that they choose to die,
> What's that to me – I let's 'em.

When patients who had been repeatedly bled, deprived of a great part of their blood, perversely 'chose to die', it was commonly considered as proof that they had not been bled enough. Thus was the ancient, supposedly Hippocratic, dictum, 'First, do no harm', perpetually, if unwittingly, violated.

The quest for therapeutic substances was subject to many absurd and enduring theories, such as 'the doctrine of signatures', which posits that evidence for the curative character of a plant or any part of it can be gleaned from its outward form. Thus to find a remedy for an ear complaint you must seek out an ear-shaped plant or leaf. These clues are scattered in man's path by divine providence. An analogy was the assertion by a19th-century English country parson that the white tails on rabbits were evidence of God's beneficence, for had the creatures not been equipped with this appendage they would have been impossible to shoot. The doctrine of signatures still lingers in some quarters, and has attached itself to homeopathy (itself an unaccountable survival from the dark age of medicine). In 1860 Oliver Wendell Holmes, the wise American doctor, poet and polymath laid this curse on the pharmacology of the day: 'If the whole *materia medica*, as now used, could be sunk to the bottom of the sea, it would be all the better for mankind – and the worse for the fishes'. Holmes also observed that 'no families take so little medicine as those of doctors, except those of apothecaries'. Young doctors, he thought, gave twenty drugs for one disease, while their older, time-worn confreres might give one drug for twenty diseases. The early to mid-19th century was indeed the golden age of public ignorance and credulity, on which mountebanks and charlatans fed. It was to be some decades after Holmes's pronouncements that the scourge began to recede, although of course it has never altogether disappeared.

As is often the case, progress depended more on the jettisoning of ingrained ideas than on the welcoming of new ones. Even with the growth of chemistry in the 18th and 19th centuries advances during most of this time in the study of drugs were remarkably sparse. The same period saw the rise of the synthetic dyestuff industry, notably in Germany, and also of natural-products chemistry, the isolation, analysis and synthesis, especially of plant substances. Yet drugs were still regarded as finished creations of nature, and the idea of an 'active principle' - the chemical compound embodying the curative property, which needed to be extracted and purified - was slow in coming. If there is one name forever associated with the genesis of rational drug discovery, it is that of Paul Ehrlich. It was mainly in response to Ehrlich's ideas and it was he who formulated the concept of a 'magic bullet' - that a new industry sprang up in Germany.

The first half of the 20th century saw synthetic chemistry gain preeminence in drug research with the emergence of several new products that alleviated much pain and misery. But despite all the new discoveries in human physiology, which were supposed to guide the design of new therapeutic compounds, the reality was in general startlingly unpredictable. An intended diabetes drug might turn out instead to control schizophrenia, a supposed antipsychotic to reduce hypertension, and so on. Genuinely rational drug design is of more recent origin, and has been based in large measure on the rise of molecular genetics, and of the powerful new techniques of cell biology, gene manipulation and immunology, unimaginable in their scope and sensitivity only two or three decades ago. All the same, the sheer complexity of living systems still repeatedly frustrates the best laid plans of the researchers. Along with a number of dramatic successes have come lurid failures and catastrophes. Some were unforeseeable, others the consequences of misjudgements, of overconfidence or simply of impatience and lust after quick profits. There have been spectacular scandals, followed occasionally by ferocious retribution.

Today the economic behemoth that is 'Big Pharma', made up of seven or so hugely bloated companies, dominates the world of drugs. These concerns were created out of cannibalistic takeovers and mergers. Their primacy in drug research and development is now challenged by smaller and more versatile organisations, in particular the many biotechnology companies. Much of the highest-quality research still also goes on in academic laboratories and independent research institutes, which however have grown ever closer to the industrial giants. Many researchers believe that the future lies increasingly in 'personalised medicine' – drugs and drug regimes matched to the genetic character of the patient, made accessible by discoveries in basic research. Drug research is at all events changing vertiginously, and in no less dramatic fashion than in the last century, governed as always by human ingenuity, persistence, obduracy, and dedication. These are opposed at times by self-aggrandisement and ruthless pursuit of profit. On display in this story, from the earliest recorded efforts to cure up to our own time, then, are all the human virtues, foibles and vices. It is shot though with the drama of discovery, of supreme achievement, of despair, and sometimes outrageous luck.

What follows is essentially a historical narrative. I have tried to keep the inescapable intrusions of science simple and accessible, with a minimum of formulae and jargon. I have included a glossary of technical terms that recur. Names of drugs are confusing. They are of two kinds, the distinction dating from the 20th century: the *generic name* is the one name officially given to the active ingredient of the product, whereas the *brand name* is the commercial designation invented for the drug by the company holding the patent rights. Once the patent has expired, the drug – then termed *generic* - can be copied and marketed under any name that the company doing the copying pleases. The generic product must have the same chemical structure, the same strength and safety characteristics, and be taken by the same route - whether by mouth, injection, enema, or skin-patch - as the original. So the same generic drug can appear under many names, but by convention the suffix reflects, whenever possible, the general nature of the drug. So, for example, if it is a monoclonal antibody – what that means is explained later – its generic name will end in *–mab*. Brand names are given a capital letter, generic names a lower-case. The number of drugs in the world, current and defunct, runs into tens of thousands, and so naming of a new drug requires imagination. There are many drug names so similar that confusion is almost unavoidable. This may become apparent even in relation to the very limited number appearing in the ensuing pages. I would like to thank, finally, helpful friends, and especially the, alas, late Peter Brown, who gave generously of his vast knowledge of chemical and pharmaceutical industry and of scientific publications; I am grateful also to the patient and knowledgeable staff of the indispensable Wellcome Library.

Chapter 1

MINDS WIDE OPEN

The fact is that there is scarcely any substance, whether animal, vegetable or mineral in character, which did not at some time have curative properties imputed to it. No sooner, for instance, had the potato reached Europe from the New World than the apothecaries discerned in it special medicinal virtues: they pronounced it to be a cure for sexual impotence and an aphrodisiac – but so, for that matter, were honey, onions, garlic (which one might have been supposed counter-erotic), truffles, a jackass's gall, menstrual blood, the placenta of a newborn foal, lodestone, and yet more. The early pharmacopoeias – the word comes from the Greek, to make drugs - were of huge scope. The most potent properties were assigned to the rarest, most costly remedies. Unicorn's horn (possibly the tusk of the 'Arctic whale', the narwhal, but probably more often beef bones) was a panacea and universal antidote, based probably on the legend that polluted waters were instantly made pure when the beast dipped its horn under the surface. Gold followed close behind, helped by the pronouncements of the alchemists. 'Potable gold', was known to the iatrochemists – the alchemical physicians – as 'tincture of the sun', for it was in the sun that gold was supposed to have originated. Gold, ingested in sufficient quantity, partaking, as the German iatrochemist, Glauber expressed it, of 'the fruit of the sun-tree', would banish any malady. So it was that in 1596 the English Queen Elizabeth's ailing ambassador to the French court, Sir Henry Winton, "was physicked with confectio alcarmas, which was composed of musk, amber, gold, pearl and unicorn's horn, and with a pidgeon applied to his side, and all other means that art could devise sufficient to expel the strongest poison, and he be not bewitched withal". The proviso was prudent, for the physick, unicorn's horn notwithstanding, did not avail. In truth, there was little that doctors or apothecaries could do for the sick, beyond easing pain with narcotics, which had been in use for millennia. Seeds of the opium poppy were found in European Neolithic burial sites, and the poppy was certainly known to the ancient Greeks; indeed, it was the tears of Aphrodite, lamenting the death of Adonis from which, according to legend, sprang the flower. In reality, the healing crafts changed remarkably little for close on two millennia.

In the beginning: ancient Chinese cures

Attempts to confront the effects of diseases and accidents probably began when, somewhere between 10 and 20 millennia ago, nomadic people settled and began to cultivate plants and later animals. The formation of communities of a kind would have led to exchange of knowledge and the growth of common superstitions. Many of the nostrums prescribed by the physicians (often also priests) who flourished in ancient civilisations would certainly have derived from such sources. The earliest compilation of medicinally useful substances is attributed to the legendary Chinese Yan Emperor, Shannong (Shen Nung), and is dated by tradition to the year 2737 B.C., but the written record stems from a much later period. The Emperor, whose name means 'the Divine Husbandman', supposedly introduced farming practices to China ('the five grains'). He was also said to have tested the effects of 365 herbs on himself, and to have succumbed eventually to an overdose. He had the advantage of a transparent body, which allowed him to observe the physiological effects of what he ingested. Shannong's pharmacopoeia, *The Herb Root Classic*, listed cures for a wide range of symptoms. One of his discoveries, allegedly, was that of tea, a brew of such potency that it could serve as an antidote against no less than 70 toxic plant substances. Among his plant extracts were opium, which was to become the scourge of China, hemp, ephedra, misused in our time by athletes and body-builders (p.), chaulmoogra, the oil which was practically the only treatment for leprosy until well into the 20th century, rhubarb, ginseng, and especially camphor. Ephedra was considered a remedy for poor circulation, for coughs and for fevers, and served also as a stimulant for slaves. There were also narcotics and analgesics, which were used in what little surgery was practised at the time, and special prescriptions were used to mitigate the pain suffered by the young boys destined to serve the imperial household as eunuchs.*

Treatments were commonly allied to religious ritual and forms of magic. A highly regarded Chinese remedy for painful conditions, such as rheumatoid arthritis, was (and still is) *moxa* from the mugwort, a root which was cured, pulverised and burned. It was applied to the skin, sometimes with needles, or was burned on the skin (moxibustion). To reduce the severity of the resulting wound, the moxa could be placed over a slice of fresh ginger. Around 500 B.C. the celebrated physician, Bian Que, dilated on the virtues of this treatment, which could relieve many conditions, and even turn round breach babies. Bian was credited with many other accomplishments, and may have been the first physician to realise that the pulse was a diagnostic indicator. He also recommended a treatment with a wine-based narcotic. One blessing above all for Chinese invalids, not granted to the sick in other cultures, was that they were spared the trauma of bloodletting, which was regarded as an insult to the body.

The drugs of the Pharaohs

The world's oldest surviving written document on medical practices comes not from China but from Mesopotamia. It is a Sumerian clay tablet, variously dated to about 2100 or 2500 B.C. It divulges that the Sumerians believed diseases to have supernatural causes, deployed by gods and demons, and that the physicians treated their patients with a

---

* In this brutal operation, penis and scrotum were severed as close as possible to the body, and the ureter was plugged until the wound had partly healed. The plug was then replaced by a tube. The genitalia, preserved in alcohol in a jar, were handed to the eunuch, who guarded them throughout his life so that they could be buried with him when he died; without them, the deities would see to it that, as an incomplete man, he was reincarnated as a she-mule.

3

repertoire of medicinal plants; some preparations were swallowed, others applied in the form of unguents or poultices. Medical wisdom from about the same period is also to be found, transcribed in Egyptian documents many centuries later. These give explicit advice on the treatment of many conditions. As early as 4000 B.C., in fact, the Egyptians used not only magic amulets but also plant products, to ward off or cure diseases, each caused, it was held, by one of an extended menagerie of demons. The apothecaries were apparently seen in ancient Egypt as the inheritors of the god, Horus, who had received the secrets of magic remedies from his mother, Isis. For this reason their symbol was the eye of Horus, which was transformed in European medicine into the Rx, still appended to doctors' prescriptions.

It is the famous Ebers Papyrus that casts most light on early Egyptian medicine. It is named after a German scholar, Georg Ebers, who bought it from a dealer in Luxor, the ancient Thebes, in 1872. The scroll was wrapped in mummy cloth, and was said to have reposed between the legs of a mummy in the necropolis of Thebes. Ebers took his find to his home base, the University of Leipzig, where a translation into German was quickly prepared. English translations followed some years later, and scholars still ponder the meanings of some of the ancient terms.

The Ebers Papyrus consists of 108 columns, numbered from 1 to 110 with two numbers unaccountably omitted; it is written in hieratic, a script based on hieroglyphs. The many separate sections have headings in red (rubrics) and the rest is black. At the end is a calendar, which indicates that the scroll dates from 1536 B.C. It is preceded by a remarkable picture of the state of anatomical and physiological knowledge of the physician-priests, who were learned in surgery, dissection, magic and embalming. They knew for instance that blood is driven around the body by the heart, and they mapped the connections to the other organs, but they also believed that the heart was the source of all other bodily fluids – sperm, urine and tears. The text leads off with a compendium of spells and incantations to drive off the various demons tormenting the patient. There follow sections on diseases of the stomach, with its main emphasis on intestinal parasites, such as tapeworms; the skin, treating separately irritant, exfoliating conditions and ulcers; the anus and digestive disorders; the head, notably migraines; urinary problems; coughs; injuries, such as burns and fractures; effects on the extremities; dentistry; eye, ear, nose and throat conditions; and gynaecology, including contraception. Some preparations were taken by mouth, others used in ointments, poultices, fumigants or inhalants. The fumigants were administered through the rectum or the vagina. Descriptions survive of inhalant devices consisting of a pot into which a hot stone was placed to vaporise the medicine. The fumes rose through a straw passing through a hole in the base of a second pot covering the first. The patient inhaled the health-giving vapours through the straw. Suppositories and enemas were well known to the physician-priests, and may have had a specially honoured place in their craft, for according to Egyptian myth, enemas were invented by the god, Thoth. There is mention at a later data of one Iri, 'the Shepherd (or Guardian) of the Anus', who may have served the Pharaoh himself in this capacity.

There are explicit instructions to the physician, beginning, 'When you examine a man and you find he has ... then shall you say ...', and the canonical treatment follows. There are numerous remedies, those devised and used by the gods treated separately. For a seriously ill patient, who apparently cannot take food, the physician should (having first pronounced a spell) prepare a concoction of ground 'bloodstone of Elephantine' (found presumably on the Elephantine Island in the Nile), red grain, carob boiled in oil, and honey. This should be administered for four days. A child with urinary incontinence should be dosed with beads of faïence (the glazed Egyptian ceramic), boiled until they formed a congealed mass; an older child should take this in one draught, while for a baby it should be mixed with its milk, and it should also be given to the mother or wet-nurse. Many of the concoctions contain large numbers of ingredients, among them seeds, resins and roots. A popular root extract is that from a Ricinus plant, which produced a form of castor oil. Castor oil, beer, and especially honey were all used as a base for many medicinal concoctions, and for treatment of wounds.

A long list of healing herbs enumerates their virtues. Some improve strength and vitality, some have an aperient effect, others the opposite, and some are diuretics; many ease flatulence (evidently a preoccupation at the time), assist digestion, relieve pain, suppress or prevent infections, or ease asthma and other forms of allergic distress. A number of these substances would have been effective, and probably none of them caused harm (in contrast to what came later, as we shall see). An example of an effective measure was the treatment of night-blindness with liver. There are several forms of the condition, all of them due to a deficiency of vitamin A, as a result of poor diet or of a hereditary metabolic defect. Liver is indeed a good source of the vitamin, and would have had a beneficial effect. On the other hand, one may doubt whether failing eyesight could have been much improved by a mixture of red ochre, honey and the vitreous humour from a pig's eyeball, poured into the ear. Even more inscrutable is the advice that an obstruction of the bowel is the result of stalled blood flow, and was to be treated with a concoction that included berries, wormwood and beer. This powerful medicine would cause congealed blood to issue from both orifices. Some herbs were used in unguents for massages, recommended for painful conditions, such as rheumatism. In one recipe herbs are mixed with honey, wine lees, bovine spleen and fat. Cosmetic blemishes were also to be treated with fatty salves, a balding pate, for instance with the fat of lions, hippopotami, crocodiles and other creatures. These also served for the treatment of other conditions, as did the gall of ox and tortoise, the uterus of a cat, bird lime, mother's milk (an enduring favourite through the next two millennia), and babies' faeces. There is great emphasis on emetics and laxatives (castor oil, senna, seeds of the colocynth, or bitter apple, and more), for the anus was considered a major seat of diseases, and a concern with intestinal worms, which were treated with pomegranate.

The Ebers is by no means the only medical papyrus. Among other notable finds there were the Brugsch Papyrus of about 1300 B.C., which takes its name from Heinrich Brugsch (known for his work on deciphering the Rosetta Stone), and the Kehun Gynaecological Papyrus of around 1825 B.C., discovered by the great Egyptologist, Sir Flinders Petrie in1889, which recommends such contraceptive measures as pessaries of crocodile dung. Above all there is the Edwin Smith Papyrus, which is primarily concerned with surgery. Edwin Smith was an American amateur, living in Cairo. He seems to have been a louche character, a dealer and money-lender with an interest in forgeries, some of which he may even have perpetrated. The papyrus came his way in 1862. It dates from about 1600 B.C., but is based mainly on surgical instructions compiled a millennium or so earlier. The surgeons of the time distinguished between conditions that they could mend, those worth a try, and a third category of hopeless cases. These last made up 14 of the 48 case histories described in the papyrus. Only in one case is there reference to magic. Particularly striking is the use of mouldy bread for treatment of infections, prefiguring the discovery of penicillin, some four millennia later. Honey was also recommended for the same purpose. Raw meat was used as a styptic for wounds, and would have worked by initiating clot formation.

Of course, many of the remedies appear to us now as no more than superstitions, based often on sympathetic magic. This principle endured through the millennia: it is typified in European lore by the supposed curative virtue of a hair of the dog by which one had been bitten, and later by homeopathy. By the same reasoning, ointments were smeared on the weapons (if they could be found) that had caused a patient's wound. The Egyptians made extensive use of the excrements of animals, common and rare, including the hippopotamus, pelican and flamingo, none of which are likely to have done the patients lasting good. It is likewise hard to know what to make of this test for pregnancy advised in the Brugsch Papyrus: the woman is to drink a mashed watermelon mixed with the milk of a mother who has borne a son. If she vomits, then she is pregnant, while if the draught engenders mere flatulence she will never again conceive. Nor does a roasted mouse seem the ideal teething ring for a distressed baby.

Mesopotamia

Like those of Egypt, the physicians of Babylon and Sumer cleaved to the principle that diseases were visited on the victims by gods and malign spirits, a different one for each part of the body. Accordingly, spells, prayers and incantations formed a large part of the physicians' art. Nevertheless, animal and vegetable remedies were also regarded as aids to the healing process. The great Law Code of Hammurabi, written in about 1770 B.C., alludes to medicinal plants, including licorice ("sweet root") – still sometimes used to disperse phlegm and ease sore throats, but believed by the ancients to cure disorders of the internal organs - and henbane, related to deadly nightshade; it also contains atropine, used by ophthalmologists today in drops to dilate the pupil; in small doses it has an agreeable soporific effect.

The traditions of Sumer, Babylon and Assyria were related, and much of what is known of their medicine comes from a cache of cuneiform clay tablets, 660 in all, which survived when, in 612 B.C., the Assyrian capital, Nineveh was destroyed, and King Asshurbanipal's library was burned. The oldest of the tablets are thought to date from about 1600 B.C., though some are of later origin. They encapsulate the medical knowledge accumulated over several centuries, and deal with many of the common diseases recognised today, with much acute observation. Treatment was in the hands of doctors, who could call on the services of members of an order of pharmaceutical healers, specialists in plant medicinals, and also in tending wounds. Some of the recipes developed by these healers combine many ingredients, especially in the plasters with which wounds were treated. The most interesting preparations involved treating animal fats and plant resins with alkali. The reaction between alkali and a fat is known to chemists as saponification, for it generates, as the name implies, a soap, so the plaster could well have had some antiseptic action.

Hindu healers

The Rig-Veda is thought to be the oldest of the four Vedas, the sacred Sanskrit texts of the Hindu religion, written somewhere between 1500 and 1200 B.C. In it are found the earliest allusions to the manner in which the Hindu sages dealt with disease. Like the Egyptians and the people of Mesopotamia, they relied equally on the supernatural, in the form of spells and incantations, as on drugs. Among the nostrums to receive a favourable mention is gold, which cures diseases and prolongs life. Frequently mentioned is soma, apparently an intoxicant or narcotic, perhaps even a hallucinogen, which plays such a prominent part in Aldous Huxley's novel, *Brave New World*. Scholars have long debated what it might have been – certainly a plant product, but beyond that there is as yet no agreement. Of later date, around 800-700 B.C. is the Ayur-veda – the veda of long life, a treatise in eight parts on all branches of medicine. Its teachings gave rise to a school of medicine, which evolved over the following centuries. Its most celebrated exponent was a Hindu surgeon, Susruta, whose masterwork, the *Susruta-Samhita*, contains a compendium of diseases and embraces surgery, pharmacology, toxicology and aphrodisiacs. The diseases, 1120 in number, include fevers, coughs, tumours and skin conditions. Procedures in which Susruta was evidently skilled include operations for cataracts and forms of plastic surgery.

Susruta lists no less than 760 plants considered to have medicinal value. Some preparations are taken as powders or potions, but many are used to generate unguents, inhalants or are even snorted as sneezing-powders. There are also substances of animal and inorganic provenance. One is an extract from the navel of a calf; the flesh of an owl was prized as an aphrodisiac (while also enfeebling the user's wits). Aromatic gums are favoured, and one product that remained in clinical use for nearly two millennia was the oil pressed from the seeds of the chaulmoogra plant, which was considered a sovereign – though in fact largely ineffective – remedy against leprosy (p.), and a variety of other conditions. Indian drugs are mentioned in Greek and Roman writings, by such authors as Xenophon and Strabo, so medical lore must have circulated rather freely through the ancient world.

The Greeks: origins of Western medicine

The Greek god of medicine, Asclepius, the son of Apollo, the sun god, surfaces in the Iliad and Odyssey, which are generally thought to date from around the 8th century B.C. Asclepius was supposed to have been born by posthumous Caesarean section, for his mother had died in childbirth and Apollo snatched her body from the funeral pyre and liberated the child, whence its name, meaning to cut open. The boy was raised by the wise and virtuous centaur, Chiron, who instructed him in the arts of healing. According to Homer, Asclepius killed a serpent that had coiled itself around his staff, whereupon a second serpent appeared, carrying a herb in its mouth, with which it restored its friend to life; hence of course the caduceus, which remained the symbol of the doctor ever after. Asclepius used the snake's herb to relieve pain, staunch bleeding, and even revive the dead, for which impiety Zeus smote him with a thunderbolt and turned him into a heavenly constellation. Through his two sons, who grew into doctors and warriors in the army of the Greeks, Asclepius became the founder of the ancient guild of doctors, the Asclepides. Asclepius, it seems, was highly regarded by the ancient Greeks, who built many temples in his honour, used as clinics for the sick.

The antiquity of certain medicinal plants is plain from their appearance in Greek mythology. Myrrh, for example, which is a brown resinous substance exuded by a class of trees and shrubs, and is commended in the early writings for the treatment of gynaecological and rheumatic complaints, takes its name from the nymph, Myrrha, who was transformed into a tree by the malign goddess, Aphrodite. Ovid relates in his *Metamorphosis* how the tree cracked open and "the sundered bark yielded its living load", the baby, Adonis, which the Nereid nymphs bathed in myrrh, the tears of its mother, the tree. Mint, which also found (presumably ineffectual) medicinal use, is also named after a nymph, Menthe, who had excited the lust of the god, Pluto, and was turned by his jealous wife, Proserpina, into the herb.

The first school of medicine sprang up in Cnidos, now in Aegean Turkey, in the 7th century B.C., but of much greater historical importance was the school founded by Hippocrates of Cos on the island of that name some 200 years later. Greek medicine of the classical age was based on the theory of humours, first formulated, it is thought, by Alcaemon, and later elaborated by Empedocles. The humours were four in number, each representing a bodily fluid, black bile, yellow bile, phlegm and blood. They were linked to the four elements of which, according to the Greeks, the world was composed, earth, air, fire and water, and to the four qualities recognised by Aristotle, dry, moist, cold and warm. Personality and the state of health were governed by the admixture of humours, which changed with age, from predominantly moist in childhood to dry in old age. Hippocrates (ca. 460-370 B.C.) adhered to the humoral theory, but is nevertheless regarded as the father of modern – in other words, scientific, or evidence-based – medicine. Illness, he asserted, had natural causes, which brought about an imbalance between the bodily humours, and the duty of the physician was to find means to promote the healing powers of nature. The vast body of writings, the Hippocratic Corpus, which was attributed to him, but was in reality the work of many hands over a period of two centuries, concerns itself more with dietary prescriptions than with drugs, but many – upwards of 200, depending on how a drug is defined – receive a mention. The great majority come from plants, though there were a few animal-derived remedies, such as snail mucus for skin conditions. Some were to be administered by mouth, others in the form of unguents, pessaries, inhalants, and so on. The emphasis was on purgatives, enemas and emetics, for a Hippocratic principle of medical practice was to purify the body through expulsion of noxious humours.

A more systematic comprehensive dissertation on medicinal plants is attributed to Aristotle's pupil, Theophrastus (ca. 371-287 B.C.), often called the 'father of botany'. He was a formidable polymath, whose most famous work (if indeed it was his) is a compendious encyclopaedia of plants, the *Historia Plantarum*, of which medicinal plants occupy book IX. It begins with the mandrake, the leaf of which, mixed with ground barley, is recommended as a poultice for wounds, while preparations from the root relieve erysipelas (a bacterial infection of the skin, also known as 'red fire' or 'holy fire', ignis sacer) and gout, and also yield a sleeping draught. Next comes hellebore, which is good for 'diseases of the spleen', the after-effects of miscarriages and more. Other plant extracts are recommended for epilepsy, leprosy and a host of other ills. Theophrastus mentions only a single nostrum of animal origin, namely seal's rennet - good for all manner of conditions.

Theophrastus probably relied for much of his botanical knowledge on a school of wandering scholars, the *rhizotomoi* (*rhizoma*, a tree root) or 'root-cutters', who collected and codified the plants of the region. Theophrastus was persuaded, for instance, that amber (which was held to possess medicinal properties, was no mere secretion of trees, but was the solidified urine of wild animals, which buried it. The name that survives from this period is Diocles of Caryustus (known to his contemporaries as Hippocrates II), who flourished in the 4th century B.C., and whose wisdom informed the medical world up to the time of Dioscorides, some four centuries later. By then the centres of medical learning in Greece had largely been supplanted by the famous School of Alexandria, established by Greek physicians in 331 B.C.

The Romans

Before the conquest of Greece in the 2nd century B.C. Roman medicine relied heavily on interpretation of dreams and divination, but when Greeks, trained mainly in the great school of Alexandria, began to arrive in Rome the Empiric tradition, based on careful observation, took root. The Empiricists took little for granted and were prepared to investigate the beliefs in which folk healing practices were rooted. Some of this wisdom found its way even into the famous manual of food and cooking by Apicius, who flourished in the early part of the first century (although the book was compiled a century of more after his death). He was, according to legend, a formidable gourmand who spent his fortune on extravagant feasts, and when the money ran out, committed suicide. The book contains, perhaps by another hand, various aids to digestion, with names like *oxyporum*, *pulmentarium ad ventrem* and *oxygarum digestibilem* (*garum*, a universally popular spice, mixed with vinegar). There is also a curious 'multipurpose' salt preparation to protect against chills, plague and other misfortunes. Several manuals for preservation of health, with recipes for cures which could be prepared in the home, were in circulation at this time, and generally urged that amateur physicians should practice on animals and slaves before trying their skills on the family.

The Romans, unlike the Greeks, did not greatly esteem their doctors: medicine was not a respectable calling, and most practising doctors in Rome were slaves or freedmen (until, at least, the time of Galen, whom we shall meet shortly). The most famous of the physicians who thrived during this early period was Aulus Cornelius Celsus (ca. 25 B.C. – 50 A.D.). Little is known of his origins, but he left for posterity a major work, *De Medicina*, dating from about 30 A.D. It ranges over all areas of medicine and surgery, and one of its books (Book V) enumerates the drugs and prescriptions that Celsus recommended. They are grouped according to the nature of their effects, by their capacity to staunch the flow of blood, clean wounds, soothe pain and irritation, induce sleep and so on. A special interest, to which we will shortly return, was antidotes. What is striking is how few of these remedies were for internal use: most were ointments, powders, plasters, pessaries and the like. Celsus did not much hold with purges and emetics, but he did list various pills or drinks to relieve pain, ease coughs and treat urinary disorders, nor did he neglect folk remedies, based on the sympathetic, or homeopathic principle.

This superstition, vestiges of which are still around today, is also called 'the doctrine of signatures', of features of the plant (or animal) that bear some resemblance to those of the disorder or of the afflicted organ. An example is the root of the celandine, which has nodules all too reminiscent of haemorrhoids, and is thereby marked as a cure for the condition. Similarly, the black hellebore - being black - will counter the imbalance of humours resulting from an excess of black bile, that is to say melancholia. The blood of a fallen gladiator is mentioned as a highly regarded treatment for the 'falling sickness', epilepsy – a belief that persisted at least into the next generation, as instanced by Pliny's description of epileptics surging into the arena to lap up the blood from gladiators' wounds.

These and many more examples can be found in *De Medicina* and in the works of other practitioners of the time, such as Scribonius Largus, a fashionable doctor, born and probably educated in Sicily. Largus became personal physician to the Emperor Claudius, whom he accompanied to Britain in 43 A.D. His fame rests largely on the *Compositiones*, written in 47 or 48, after his return to Rome. It contains 271 prescriptions, and is arranged in three sections. The first and much the longest considers disorders, working down from the cranium, with epilepsy and headaches, to the toes, with gout; the second is devoted to antidotes against insect and snake poisoning, and the third to external remedies – to plasters, dressings, unguents and the like. Largus is an enthusiast for drugs, which, he asserts, should always be preferred to surgery, but he is open to other measures too. Thus he suggests, as a treatment for gout, immersing the feet in water in which swim electric (torpedo) fish. The shocks would deaden the pain in the toes – a curious anticipation of the 18th-century preoccupation with the physiological effects of electricity.

Largus's materia medica are nearly all plant products, but he also mentions such folk remedies as blood of a turtle or dove for epilepsy; it must be from a male animal for a male patient and a female for a female. But he disapproves of drinking gladiator's blood, or blood out of the skull of a vanquished gladiator, or worse, a piece of the gladiator's liver, nor does he recommend a patient to drink his own blood from the vein. Gladiators clearly occupied a favoured niche in Roman folklore. Yet another epilepsy cure was to eat the brain of an infant deer, killed with a weapon that had killed a gladiator. Largus opined that such measures were incompatible with the doctor's calling, yet he conceded that they might have helped some sufferers. The placebo effect (of which much more later) is without doubt far-reaching. The *Compositiones* was later published in many European countries and widely consulted. After Celsus and Largus the study of plant-derived drugs became more systematised, most of all in the hands of Dioscorides.

Peianus Dioscorides ('Dioscorides the Greek'), born in about 40 A.D. near Tarsus in what is now Turkey, became a surgeon in the Roman army under the Emperor Nero. He took part in a series of campaigns, and spent time in Italy, Spain, Gaul and North Africa. In all these places he collected and catalogued plants, and recorded evidences of their medicinal properties. His great compendium of medicinal herbs, together with one book containing animal products, was published in Greek in about 70 A.D., some 20 years before its author's death, but has always been known by the title of its Latin translation, *De Materia Medica*. Dioscorides was put up to it by his friend and sometime teacher, Areius, whom he apostrophises in the prologue to each of the five books: 'and now, most loving Areius we will discuss ...' As the pharmaceutical bible, the *Materia Medica* held sway for the next millennium-and-a-half, though first rendered into English only in 1655. It meticulously describes each plant, as to appearance, smell and taste and habitat, with advice on selection and preservation, and on preparation of useful products. A magnificent modern-English translation by Tess Osbaldeston and Robert Wood, with beautiful engravings, from the 16th and 19th centuries, was published in 2000. A difficulty throughout was to link the plants from Dioscorides's description to a known species, and the translators have indicated where the identification is conjectural.

Here now is a taste of Dioscorides's scholarship:

The iris is the first plant in Book 1, which is dedicated mainly to aromatic plants. Dioscorides instructs his readers that it can combat coughs and reduce 'thick mucus'; both that and bile are to be treated by a draught of 7 spoonfuls of a decoction in honey water. The iris extract also induces sleep, engenders tears and eases bowel pains; taken in vinegar, it helps the victims of venomous creatures, and those taken with fits or chilled stiff; and drunk in wine draws out menstrual fluid, eases sciatica and heals sores, fistulas and wounds. It makes a good poultice and softens swellings, and if this were not enough, when applied to the skin in a mixture with hellebore and honey it clears away freckles and sunburn. In suppositories it even relieves fatigue.

Wormwood is recommended for disorders of the stomach, as a vermifuge (for worms were a common affliction until modern times, and are so still in developing countries) and for the treatment of jaundice; it is generally good for the health and favoured in the summer in Propontis and Thrace. (Wormwood is the bright green, bitter flavouring matter of absinthe, the *veuve glauque* of the 19th-century French bohemians. Its active ingredient is thujone which, taken in quantity, is a neurotoxin. Absinthe was banned in France and other western European countries at the beginning of the 20th century, as a danger to health, although this has been questioned. It is, at any rate, unlikely that wormwood is as beneficial as Dioscorides maintains.)

Cyclamen, says the sage, is of value as a purgative, when the extract is applied to belly, bladder and anus, an antidote to poisons, a cleanser of the skin and an aphrodisiac; and it will induce labour. *Physalis*, the 'Chinese lantern' berry, is both a sedative and a diuretic; when mixed with honey it will improve eyesight, and with wine will alleviate toothache. The *rose* has many virtues: a paste made from the petals will soothe the eyes, while an extract of the pollen, taken in wine, will relieve headaches, earaches and piles. *Arum*, or cuckoo-pint, is an antidote for snake-bite, and if spread on the hand will make it unpleasing to snakes. (This seems to be a piece of sympathetic magic, since Dioscorides notes that the stalk resembles a snake.) It is also an expectorant and is good for treating wounds. *Black nightshade* leaves are a remedy for diseases of the skin, while a decoction may be taken for indigestion, earache and internal bleeding. *Balsamon*, which is probably the biblical Balm of Gilead, is good for many things. Variously administered, it can be used to treat darkened pupils, and abrasions round the vulva; it expels menstrual fluid and the placenta, facilitates abortion, helps the flow of urine, breathlessness, cures snake-bites and combats pleurisy, pneumonia, coughs, sciatica, epilepsy, vertigo and asthma, assists conception, and added to a hip-bath, opens the vulva and expels moisture.

And so it continues for hundreds of plants. Curious additions are *Rupos, Rupos Palaistra* and *Gymnasion*. The first consists of scrapings from the public bathhouse, which is beneficial when rubbed on the joints, warms and softens the tissues and heals splits in the skin of the perineum. The second is dirt from the wrestling school, and the last is scrapings from walls or statues. All have healing qualities.

Not all of Dioscorides's prescriptions are absurd or credulous. At times there are hints of a doubt or two, and a few are certainly effective, as when he recommends a decoction of the willow as an analgesic, for this is indeed the precursor of aspirin (p.). The extract of the mandrake root – a plant about which myths and superstitions abound (p.) – would have contained hyoscyamine (p.) and was also recommended for the same purpose. This remained in use as a local anaesthetic until the introduction of ether in the mid-19th century.

Book 2 of the *Materia Medica* embraces animal products, as well as cereals and leguminous and some other plants. Many of the recipes have something of sympathetic magic about them. So the liver of a mad dog is 'thought to prevent' hydrophobia, that is rabies, while the skin of the hedgehog is good for alopecia. On the other hand, its dried flesh, taken as a drink in vinegar and honey, is good for 'inflamed kidneys' dropsy, convulsions, elephantiasis and cachexy, or malnutrition with the symptoms of starvation. The draught will also suppress discharges from bowel and liver (sic). There is a dissertation on the virtues of hippopotamus and beaver testicles, and on the lungs of the fox, which when dried and dispersed in a drink ease the distress of asthma, while the beast's grease soothes earache. Bedbugs, moreover, have much curative power: quartain fever (presumably malaria [p.]) crises can be averted by seven of the insects, swallowed with meat and beans, and even the smell will revive a woman who has fainted because of 'constriction of the vulva'. Chopped up, and introduced into the urethra bedbugs will ease painful evacuation. An infusion of seagull liver in honey water will expel the placenta, and stones found in the stomach of newly hatched swallows, taken from the nest at the time of the waxing moon, and wrapped in the skin of a heifer or deer before they reach the ground, can also encompass extraordinary cures.

Dioscorides then moves on to fats, with descriptions of, for instance, the preparation and applications of lanolin from wool. Rennets are contraceptives, that from the stomach of a young sea-calf (presumably seal) can be used to treat epilepsy and 'constriction of the womb'. Bodily fluids – blood, gall, urine - and even dung have their place. Menstrual blood is commended as a contraceptive and for alleviating the symptoms of gout and erysipelas, while the droppings of doves counter snake-bites, dissolve tumours (or, the translators speculate, goitre) and carbuncles, while those of mice, swallowed with frankincense and honeyed wine, will expel kidney stones. Even inhaling the smoke from the burning dung of male animals of the herd will restore a prolapsed womb. Leprosy may be treated with the urine of a dog, asthma and dim sight by that of an 'incorrupt boy', while that of the lynx (however that may be procured) is a specific for disorders of the stomach and intestines. Book 2 concludes with herbs of a sharp nature, such as leeks, garlic and onions, of which the text distinguishes elongated and round, red and white, fresh and dried and raw as against roasted. They purge the bowels, open the rear passage, ease haemorrhoids and angina pains, and properly applied, sharpen dull sight, eliminate white spots from the cornea and smallpox pustules, and more besides. Squill is a plant that acts on asthma, jaundice and other conditions, including dropsy, the retention of water. This was used as a medicine in Europe in later centuries, and famously, Dr Johnson, when dying of heart failure, dosed himself with massive quantities, despite the disagreeable side effects.

Book 3 treats of roots, which evidently includes stems of plants, so that rhubarb is recommended for a huge range of ailments, from 'gaseous weakness of the stomach', convulsions and inflammation of the kidneys to asthma, rickets, dysentery and the bites of poisonous creatures. Perhaps the most remarkable range of virtues enumerated here applies to a plant found in Crete, called *Diktamnos*, which the translators tentatively equate with dittany or candle plant. An extract swallowed, applied topically or inhaled as a smoke will 'expel dead embryos'. The Cretan goats that browse on the herb 'reject arrows' when shot, and so powerful is it that small doses drive away poisonous creatures, and the touch will kill them.

In Book 4, says Dioscorides, 'we will discuss herbs and roots not previously mentioned', and he kicks off with the *white opium poppy*, on the powers and dangers of which he discourses at some length, citing several authorities, who often disagree with one another. Among the most lurid properties are those of the *mandrake*. It comes, he asserts, in two forms, the black or female, and the white male. The roots have aphrodisiac powers, but the leaves of the female plant have a toxic, heavy scent. The apples of the mandrake are soporific and anaesthetic, and expel phlegm and black bile 'upwards'. Young leaves soften tumours, goitres and scrofula or glandular swellings, and ease painful joints. A decoction of the apples purges the womb, and staunches menstrual flow if applied with sulphur as a pessary. A root extract is an antidote to poisons, but in excess the products of the plant will deprive men of speech and may kill. The same, and worse, is true of the *yew tree*: even to rest in its shade can be fatal.

An extract of a plant called *Thapsin* must be consumed only in calm weather, for if one is standing against the wind it will cause the face to 'puff up' and blisters to appear on 'the naked parts', which should be protected by rubbing with a thick astringent ointment. But the juice purges both 'upwards and downwards', which is good for asthma, while applied externally it will suppress hair loss, sunburn and leprosy. And, most startlingly, it will restore the foreskin to the circumcised member by forming a 'tumour', which when washed and softened with a fatty unguent, fills in the missing area. The *Bryony* has almost equally prodigious powers, for its various products work against sunburn, varicose veins, freckles, scars, bruises and whitlocks. It will disperse inflammations, break abscesses and 'extract bones'. It will combat epilepsy, apoplexy and snakebite, obstinate pain in the side, urinary retention, hernia and convulsions, diseases of the skin and leprosy. And as if this were not enough, it will also induce an abortion.

The fifth and last book of *Materia Medica* encompasses 'wines and metallic things', or minerals. By wines Dioscorides means the fermented extracts of fruits and even vegetables generally, but the book begins with mere juices and other products of vines. So the juice of the grape is good for dysentery and gastritis and to restrain 'women that lust'; it is, therefore, an anaphrodisiac. The resin collected from the stem of the plant is also a good thing, for it heals skin diseases and leprosy, although the affected parts must first be rubbed with saltpetre (which we now know as potassium nitrate). The ashes of the branches and of the skins and seeds of the grapes are better yet, for they chase away among other ills glandular fevers and 'venereal warts'.

As to wines, Dioscorides distinguishes between aged and young, white and red, sweet and dry, and vintages from different regions. Old wines, he tells his readers, are bad for the nerves and the senses, and he warns against over-indulgence; 'yet they are pleasant to the taste' – as the oenophiles of the time might have discovered for themselves. Young wine has certain medicinal advantages, but is indigestible and a cause of nightmares. Something between old and young is recommended. White wine is healthier and more digestible than red, which is indigestible, heady and fattening. Dry wine encourages urinary flow, but leads to headaches and inebriation. Sweet wine is better in this respect, although it inflates the stomach and troubles both bowel and gut, but it is good for the bladder and kidneys. There is also a comparison between wines from grapes dried in the sun and on the vine (*Beerenauslese* in today's parlance), which, however, merit no special commendation.

The next section is on the effects of wines (rather loosely interpreted). The wine from the island of Lesbos is evidently famous, and is used to treat queasy stomachs, 'plague symptoms' (possibly smallpox), and lustful women. 'Black wine' from the wild grape has different merits, and then there are mixtures – old wine with honey or with mead (fermented from honey), mead and water, honey and sea-water, and so on. There are wines made from quince, from pears, pomegranates, rose, myrtle, palms, the turpentine tree, figs (best avoided, for it causes elephantiasis), pine cones, lavender, parsnips, mandrake, and more. Vinegar is of special interest. It acts on wounds, bleeding gums, ulcers, erysipelas, and properly applied, for instance with sulphur, eases gout and fevers. It is an antidote to poisons, expels leeches lodged in the throat, and, when dropped in the ear, kills worms. When its fumes are inhaled it puts an end to 'hissing in the ears'. This is by no means all that vinegar can do, especially when mixtures with honey, with salt, with sea-water and other additives, are included.

To conclude, there is a long section on *Metallic Stones*. These encompass a variety of inorganic substances, many of which can be identified with some confidence. There are several metallic oxides, such as rust, litharge (lead oxide) scales from brass, 'white flowers of brass' (which when blown into the ear will cure deafness) and verdigris. There are ores of lead, iron, mercury, copper, antimony and arsenic, many of them highly toxic. Arsenic, in the form of various of its compounds, is one that has featured in traditional Chinese medicine for three millennia, and also in Hindu medicine. Dioscorides appears to have been largely unaware of the dangers, although he does note that orpiment, a sulphide of arsenic, makes the hair fall out, and he at least warns against the dangers of drinking metallic mercury (*hydrargyrum*, or liquid silver, which was already well-known at the time), because, he thought, it would destroy the internal organs by reason of its weight. The known salts, sodium chloride, or common salt, and ammonium salts, had many medicinal uses, as did alum (a mixed aluminium and potassium sulphate, familiar as a styptic, used to staunch bleeding, especially in the days of cutthroat razors).

Superstition and magic rear their heads, however, as the book draws to a close. *Magnetite* is the magnetic iron oxide (Fe_3O_4), and a source of wonder to the ancients. It draws out 'thick fluids', says Dioscorides, and 'they say' – the locution may reflect a trace of scepticism – that it can distinguish a faithful from an adulterous woman. Placed secretly in the bed, it exerts 'a certain natural strength', which causes the faithful woman, once overcome by sleep, to extend her hands to her husband and lie close to him. But the adulteress, 'troubled in dreams with foul labours', falls out of bed. When, moreover, two men carry a piece of the stone, 'it frees them from all strife and causes harmony'; and when worn on the chest it soothes.

The *Eagle Stone* is another mineral to which magical properties have been imputed since the earliest times, and it was even prized by the Druids. It is also called aetitis, aquilaeus, rattle stone, and pregnant stone. Pliny (p.) wrote about it, and perpetuated the belief that the rattling stones were to be found in the nests and stomachs of eagles, whence the name. The eagle stone is in fact a small geode – a hollow ball of rock – containing small fragments of mineral, which rattle when it is shaken; it was said, therefore, to be pregnant with baby stones. The stone consists of an iron oxide (not the magnetic variety), together with flint, alumina and other matter. It is no surprise that on the sympathetic principle the stone should be endowed with magical properties relating to pregnancy and birth. Thus Dioscorides instructs us that it prevents miscarriages, and that it should be tied to the left arm of a woman before, and around her thighs during delivery, 'and she shall bring forth without pain'. But the eagle stone has yet another magic property: it can be used to expose a thief, for if he is offered bread in which the stone has been secreted, he can chew but not swallow it, nor will he be able to swallow food with which the stone has been boiled. And with that remarkable assertion, and a final greeting to his 'most loving Areius', Dioscorides the Greek leaves us. He imposed his mark on generations of apothecaries and physicians over many centuries. As late as the mid-18th century, Voltaire has his hero, Candide beaten almost to death by a regiment of Bulgarian soldiers, and then cured by a skilful surgeon with the aid of 'an ointment prescribed by Dioscorides'. And even in the mid-20th century some 100 products of plants that occur in his great opus still found a place in the pharmacopoeias.

A collector and encyclopaedist even more wide-ranging than Dioscorides, if less discriminating, was Pliny the Elder, Gaius Plinius Secundus, who lived from 23 to 79 A.D. Pliny sprang from the Roman establishment, a soldier as much as scholar, whose limitless curiosity eventually killed him. His nephew, Pliny the Younger, left a heart-warming picture of his uncle. Pliny regarded time spent away from his books as time sinfully wasted. His waking hours were consumed with reading and writing. His opinion was that no book was so bad that something could not be learned from it. The only time he took off from reading or writing, according to his nephew, was for his bath, but only during actual immersion, for he would arrange that while he was being towelled down and massaged, a minion would be on hand to read to him or to take dictation. He even scolded his nephew for choosing to walk when he could take a Sedan chair and use the time for study.

Only a part of Pliny's abundant output has survived, but this includes his magnum opus, the *Historia Naturalis.* The title, *Natural History,* does not imply that it is a work of history as we would now understand it, but a comprehensive treatise on contemporary knowledge of the natural world. Pliny completed this immense labour in A.D. 77, and dedicated it to the Emperor Titus. Two years later he was dead. As a civil servant, he had been made responsible for the Roman fleet stationed in the Bay of Naples. While he was attending to his duties there Vesuvius erupted, burying the towns of Pompeii and Herculaneum. Pliny's curiosity about this manifestation of nature's power overcame him: disregarding the entreaties of his nephew, he headed into the inferno to get a closer look, and was overcome by the fumes. When his body was found, his nephew relates, there was not a mark on it.

The *Natural History* occupies 37 books, and mentions no less than 900 drugs – 300 or so more than Dioscorides. Book 1 is a description of the contents of the remainding books, and a bibliography, Book 2 comprehends cosmology, astronomy and meteorology; Books 3 to 6 are about the geography of the parts of the known world; Book 7 is anthropology and human physiology; Books 8 to 11 contain zoology, each dedicated to a separate class of living creatures; Books 12 to 17 are about the classes of flora of the world; Book 18 about farming, and Book 19 horticulture; and then the next ten books, from 20 to 29 – the ones with which we are concerned - are about drugs and diseases; Book 30 concerns magic, and Book 31 water; Book 32 reverts to zoology, being about creatures of the sea; Books 33 and 34 are about the known metals, and Book 35 about earth, while book 36 is about stone and 37, the last, about precious stones.

Pliny tried to distance himself from the Greek tradition of biology and medicine, and his disdain for the Greeks often surfaces. Nor did he have any great love of doctors, whom he regarded as for the most part overpaid unscrupulous incompetents: 'Only doctors', he wrote, 'can kill a man with impunity'. He was, at the same time, far ahead of his time in his concern for the preservation of nature and distress at man's despoliation of his environment. But for all his engaging curiosity, reason was not always at the forefront of Pliny's thinking, nor was he punctilious in eliminating errors. This, and perhaps his intemperate observations on the medical profession, may have caused the obloquy thrown at him by later scholars, such as the 15th-century Italian, Leoncino, who published a work entitled *De Erroribus Plinii*.

Many of Pliny's favoured nostrums for common maladies were wholly or partly based on magic. He identified roots which relieved fevers, but only if the patient's name was spoken while they were dug up. This kind of belief was entirely in tune with the superstitions that thrived among the plebeians, who traded amulets and sympathetic objects to counter disease. For fever a bag of cat's skin containing emeralds would be worn around the neck; other stones were also held to have powers for countering diseases, and excrescences resembling the warts on the skin of toads and other animals were applied to growths. The practice of rubbing toads on the skin in fact persisted in some rural populations until almost our own time. Snails, Pliny thought, had great curative powers, probably because they were soft. A pulp of snails would ease wounds, while snails (especially of the African variety), boiled then grilled, and taken with wine cure stomach ache, and in one form or another are good for people with fainting fits or mania. Like many other Romans, Pliny set great store by amber**,

---

* Amber was also called *electron*, and the word, electricity is derived from it, because of the electric charge it acquires when rubbed.

and did not dissent from the view (p.) that it was excreted by animals. (That of the lynx was best.). A ball of amber, or *pomum ambrae*, worn as an amulet, would ward off the plague. Amber was used as a cleansing fumigant and also taken internally. It was supposed to combat digestive problems, dysentery and other conditions. (Ambergris, the waxy solid regurgitated by sperm whales and found on beaches, was often used interchangeably with amber, although the two substances are unrelated. Ambergris today has a high market value on account of its use in perfumery: it has a faint, generally agreeable smell, but it acts as a 'fixative', which retards the fading of expensive scents. It also features in the gastronomy of some cultures.)

Here now, in John Healy's translation, are some choice examples, taken from the huge number of the curative properties that Pliny relates:

Onions 'provide a cure for poor vision through the tears caused by their very smell. Even more effective is the application of some onion-juice to the eye' [ouch!]. They are good for health generally if consumed on an empty stomach, 'they ease the bowels by moving gas along; when used as a suppository they disperse haemorrhoids'. Moreover, 'added to that from fennel, onion-juice is marvellously efficacious when used in the early stages of dropsy'.

Lettuce is 'soporific, and can check sexual appetite, cool a feverish body, the stomach and increase the volume of blood. Lettuces disperse flatulence, suppress belches and aid digestion'. And, bafflingly, 'no food is more effective in stimulating or diminishing the appetite'. At the same time, while too much loosens the bowels, a little less will make you costive.

As to *cabbage*, one can barely scratch the surface of its virtues, since 'Chrysippus the doctor [five centuries before] devotes a volume exclusively to this vegetable'; and Cato the Elder, nearly three centuries before Pliny, had averred that it surpasses all other vegetables, for when applied as a poultice it will cleanse and heal suppurating wounds and tumours, 'which no other medicine can do'. Mixed with other plants, says Pliny, 'it is good for headaches, impaired vision, spots before the eyes, for the spleen and stomach, and for hypochondria' – and much else. *Walnuts* too are remarkable, for they will expel tapeworms, and when very old will heal gangrene, carbuncles and bruises.

Acorns, ground and mixed with axle-grease (composition unstated) do away with callouses, and a list of worse conditions.

The *juniper* tree produces an exudates which is good for toothache, and the hard berry is even better, for biting on it breaks the tooth, causing it to fall out, 'thus relieving the pain'. Juniper oil preserves dead bodies but rots living ones. Pliny is cautious about the juice, which he suspects is corrosive, and then sounds an unaccustomed sceptical note. A tall story has it, he tells his readers, that it acts as a contraceptive if applied to the penis before intercourse.

Pliny warns, with the help of some chilling anecdotes, against misuse of the opium poppy, hemlock, and mandrake (the mere smell of which can rob you of speech, and worse [p.]). On the other hand, Pliny commends *erigeron* (a large genus of flowering plants, commonly known as fleabane) for treating toothache. But its application is no simple matter, for one must first draw a line around the plant with an iron implement, then dig it up and touch it to the afflicted tooth three times, spitting in between, and finally replace it where it was so that it remains alive. And then, Pliny assures the reader, that tooth will never ache again. There is much more in the same vein. Some of Pliny's remedies have survived, even into our own time. To take just one example, aconite, 'the queen of poisons', from the highly toxic root of a plant imported into Rome, so Pliny states, from Aconis on the Black Sea, was used for centuries by assassins. It came into use later for treatment of heart ailments, and later still to lower blood pressure, for which it still finds application in some quarters.

After Pliny, in the first half of the 2nd century, another treatise on drugs, in four books, appeared. Its author was a Greek doctor, Soranus of Ephesus, whose fame derives mainly from his enlightened precepts on obstetrics and gynaecology. He concentrated on pregnancy, fertility, contraception, childbirth and abortion. He urged that pregnant women should avoid taking drugs, and his prescriptions for contraception and difficulties in pregnancy were for concoctions for external application. A typical example of a contraceptive preparation in the form of a pessary runs as follows: unripe oak galls are ground with ginger and the inner layer of the skin of a pomegranate; the mixture is made into a paste with wine and formed into small balls, which are then dried. These are inserted into the vagina before coitus. There are several variations on this theme. Sorianus's works were translated into European languages at later dates and acquired high repute.

Galen and his influence

Claudius Galenus, or Galen, was the dominant figure in medicine in the Roman Empire, and for the next millennium-and-a-half throughout the western world. He was a Greek, born, probably in 129 A.D. in Pergamum in Asia Minor (now Bergama in present-day Turkey, but then an outlying part of the Roman imperium), and died at an uncertain date, 200 according to some scholars, and as late as 217 to others. His family was rich and he grew up in an intellectual milieu, underwent the customary education in rhetoric, grammar and philosophy, and turned to medicine after, it was said, the god, Asclepius appeared to his father in a dream. In Pergamum and Smyrna he was instructed in the Hippocratic tradition, and in his writings he later referred to 'the divine Hippocrates'. For some years the young Galen travelled widely and in 152 arrived in Alexandria, the pre-eminent centre of medical learning and hub of the ancient world. There he learned about drugs from the Egyptian, Indian and African traders who brought them to the city. In 157 he returned to Pergamum and finally began to practise as a physician and surgeon in his position as doctor to the local gladiators. In this he was reputedly highly successful in that most of his patients lived. His next move, in 162, was to Rome itself, where he soon became celebrated as doctor, savant, philosopher and man on the make. His lectures and anatomical demonstrations, based on what must now seem remarkably callous vivisections on a variety of animals, attracted large audiences. One of his most celebrated demonstrations was to cut the nerves in the neck of a living pig one by one, leaving until last the one to the larynx, when the squealing instantly ceased. Galen apparently was garrulous and insufferable. He evidently made little effort to conceal his superior intelligence and erudition, and his success, mingled with his arrogance and intolerance of dissenting opinions, brought him many enemies. Whether, in 166, they hounded him out, or whether his departure was provoked by the outbreak of an epidemic of cholera or smallpox in the city is unclear, but two years later he was invited to enter the service of the Emperor. After a year with the army under the Emperor's son, Commodus, Galen became physician to Marcus Aurelius himself. By the end of his life he had served in this capacity under four Emperors.

Such was Galen's authority that his doctrines were scarcely ever questioned. He brought many innovations to the healing art, and rejected astrology, magic and divination, which permeated much of medical practice. He sniffed, for instance, at an Egyptian remedy, which consisted of laying on a disordered stomach a carving of a legendary Pharaoh on a piece of jasper. (The jasper, he insisted, worked just as well without the carving.) He taught that the character of the pulse reflected the state of the patient, he distinguished between veins and arteries, noted the difference in colour between venous and arterial blood, and showed that urine was secreted by the kidneys. He developed new and daring surgical procedures, and he introduced bloodletting as a treatment for a wide range of disorders, leaving thereby a pernicious legacy that endured into the 19th century. It had its origins in the concept of the humours and the four qualities, moist, dry, hot and cold, to which Galen was firmly wedded. Disease was a consequence of an imbalance between the qualities, and should be countered by diet, by drugs if this failed, and by surgery as a last resort.

Galen encapsulated his principle of treatment in the adage, *contraria contrarii curantur* – the noxious element causing the disorder is driven out by foods or drugs of the contrary nature (the very opposite doctrine to homeopathy, which we will encounter later). So, for example, a cold in the head stemmed from phlegm, which was moist and cold, therefore the cure had to be dry and warm – something perhaps on the lines of a pungent herb. Galen assimilated the botanical wisdom of Dioscorides and other of his predecessors, and compiled a list of what became known as *simples* (p.). To these he allocated degrees of potency from 1 to 12, with indications of side-effects. The work, however, remained unfinished. Galen's classifications diverged from those of Dioscorides in that he based them only on their actions on the humours, and in some cases the two sages assigned them quite different properties.

Galen also devised complex mixtures of simples, and the approved remedies came to be called *galenicals*. (The use of such mixtures, of which some schools of later practitioners disapproved, was termed *polypharmacy*.) As the number of drugs available to the apothecaries grew with the expansion of trade, increasingly complex mixtures were invented, and the rarer and more expensive the ingredients, the more potent they were held to be. *Mithridate*, or *mithridatum*, was a famous nostrum, an antidote against snakebites and poisons in general, taken also as an all-purpose restorative. In its original form it was accredited to the famous King Mithridates VI of Pontus two centuries earlier (although his court physician, Crateuas the Herbalist could also have had something to do with it). Mithridates was by repute a scholar, possessed, so Pliny relates, of limitless erudition, who spoke 22 languages and could address any of his subjects in their own tongue throughout his rule of 56 years. Yet he had reason to fear assassination by treacherous courtiers and relations, as well as his enemies, the Romans. He was said to have habituated himself to all known poisons by taking small amounts of each for much of his life. A.E. Houseman commemorated the King's ruse in a poem, which concludes:

They put arsenic in his meat
And stared aghast to watch him eat;
They poured strychnine in his cup
And shook to see him drink it up;
They shook, they stared as white's their shirt:
Them it was their poisons hurt,
- I tell the tale that I heard told –
Mithridates he died old.

In the end, so it was said, his cunning worked against him: old, enfeebled, and cornered by a Roman army, his attempts at suicide by poison failed, while two faithful daughters found it easy. Mithridates had to ask a vassal to kill him.

There were many recipes for *mithridate*, and their complexity grew with time. According to Pliny, Pompey the Great, having defeated Mithridates, found a notebook inscribed in the King's own hand with a mithridate recipe, consisting of two dried walnuts, two figs and twenty leaves of rue, pounded together with a little salt. 'Anyone taking this on an empty stomach,' Pliny declares, will be 'immune to all poisons for the whole day'. This is simple enough, although Pliny adds that Mithridates additionally drank the blood of the local ducks, which (he says) fed on poisons. But the version in Celsus's *De Medicina* contained 35 ingredients, and by the time Galen, who had his own name for the brew (*Theriac*), took it up, there were 77. Another elder of the Roman medical fraternity, the Cretan, Andromachus the Elder, who became personal physician to the infamous emperor, Nero, had a mithridate of his own, which he called *Galene*. It was also later referred to as Venice Treacle. The composition, set out in a verse of 87 couplets, differed little from earlier versions, but was strong on narcotics, and generous amounts of viper flesh, where Mithridates had specified lizard. There is no reason to suppose that any of these witches' brews did any good, but *Theriac* remained in vogue as a remedy for snakebite and other venoms, and in time became popular as an all-purpose tonic.

Of the many doctors who followed in the footsteps of Celsus and Galen before the end of Roman dominance, the most famous and fashionable was Alexander of Tralles, whose dates are generally given as 525 – 605, and it is certainly on record that he lived into old age. He was born in Lydia, now the western Anatolian part of Turkey, the youngest of five sons of a physician, all of whom rose to fame: the oldest was the architect of Santa (now Hagia) Sophia in Constantinople, another the leading Byzantine jurist of the time, while a third achieved distinction as a doctor. Alexander was probably trained by his father and absorbed the Byzantine teaching of medicine. He travelled widely, assimilating diverse knowledge and collecting medicinal plants, and eventually found his way to Rome, where he acquired a high reputation as physician, surgeon and scholar. Of his many writings, the most influential and expansive was his *Twelve Books on Medicine*, which he compiled towards the end of his life, and which dealt with all aspects of his calling. Alexander developed a number of new surgical procedures, and laid down rules of medical practice, but his fame rests above all on his pioneering work in helminthology, the study of parasitic worms, contained in one of the twelve books. He distinguished between different species and found effective treatments, by mouth and by enema. Such scientific leanings co-existed in his mind with a firm faith in amulets and charms. He did not doubt that stomach disorders would yield to a stone engraved with the figure of Hercules overcoming the Nemean lion; an infallible analgesic was a piece of umbilical cord from a baby, encased with a little salt in silver or gold; epilepsy was best treated by wrapping the patient in the skin of a goat and immersing him in the sea (a treatment resembling that meted out to King George III of England when he was overtaken by his fits of madness). Nor did he deviate from the doctrine of the four humours, which informed his therapeutic reasoning. He was nevertheless a man of considerable independence of mind, willing to contradict even the venerated Galen when necessary.

More than 600 medicinal substances appear in the *Twelve Books*. First comes the description of the malady, with a discussion of the progress of symptoms and the outcome, and then follows the treatment, including a list of the materia medica available to the physician. The remedies are based almost entirely on the simples listed by Dioscorides and again by Galen and others. But the prescriptions are largely of mixtures, permutations of simples in carefully defined proportions, usually different from those laid down by Galen. There are several innovations that would have been effective. Perhaps the most notable is the autumn crocus, which Alexander prescribed for gout. This plant contains the toxic alkaloid (p.), colchicine, still prescribed today (though in cautious doses) for the same affliction. For full effect an incantation was also required, however. Alexander, who was probably a Christian, died in Rome soon after completion of his greatest work.

Chapter 2

THE MIDDLE AGES

The 'Golden Age' of Islam

By the 8th century Graeco-Roman civilisation had succumbed to barbarian conquests, Europe had entered the Dark Ages, and new centres of learning had sprung up elsewhere. In India and China indigenous traditions of medicine thrived, but it was in the Islamic world that a new dawn broke. It coincided with the foundation in 750 of the Abbasid Caliphate, which established its base in Baghdad twelve years later, and endured for two centuries. This was the Islamic 'Golden Age' when philosophy, poetry, mathematics, science and medicine flourished. In the 9th century it is estimated that there were more than 800 hospitals in Baghdad, and pharmacy had become a respectable profession alongside medicine and surgery. Hospitals and pharmacies were supervised by inspectors appointed by the Caliphate - a prototype national health service. The shadow of Galen hung over everything. Hunayn ibn Ishaq (ca. 809-873), who became known in the West at Johannitius, was a Christian, born in what is now Iraq, a linguist and physician, who travelled around the Byzantine empire collecting the works of Galen and the Greeks. These he translated in great number into Arabic and Syriac, and thus gave the local physicians access to the Galenic precepts.

The first of the great physicians of the Islamic world was al-Razi, known as Rhazes, born in about 850 in the Persian city of Rayy, the ruins of which lie near the modern Shar-e-Rey, not far from Tehran. Rhazes, known to his countrymen as 'the Persian Galen' was a polymath, learned in many disciplines. Of some 250 published works his huge encyclopaedic survey of medicine – Greek, Roman and Syriac, as well as Arabic – was the most famous. It is thought to have filled 22 volumes, but only parts of it survive. The first Latin translation appeared in 1297, under the title *Liber Continens*, and remained the principal textbook of the medical schools of Europe until the 17th century. Another influential work was *The Secret of Secrets*, a treatise on chemical processes, many relating to pharmaceutical preparations. It was his belief in the powers of alchemy to encompass transmutation of the elements that is supposed to have brought about Rhazes's downfall, for he undertook to demonstrate this prodigy before the Prince of Khorassan. The Prince, in the expectation of a rich harvest of gold, paid for the apparatus and materials so, when the experiment failed, vented his displeasure on its author; Rhazes was disgraced and died poor.

Rhazes practised first in a hospital in his home town, and then moved to Baghdad as head of one of the city's great hospitals. Towards the end of his life he returned to Rayy, and died there in about 930. Rhazes was famous for the acuity of his clinical observation. He gave probably the first full descriptions of measles, smallpox and chickenpox, and left meticulous case notes on his patients. He introduced opium as an anaesthetic for surgery, and many herbal and mineral drugs, as well apparently as apparatus used for the next millennium in pharmacies, such as pestle and mortar, spatulas and glassware. For the most part he cleaved to the galenic method, including the extensive use of bleeding. Rhazes laid great emphasis on a good diet, one that would restore the balance of the patient's humours. He wrote a self-medication guide to diets and remedies for common ailments, and warned against overdosing, especially on wines.

Among the herbal remedies that appear in Rhazes's case notes and his pharmacopoeia are extracts of vegetable marrow, rose, deadly nightshade, spikenard, endive and cucumber seeds; 'remedy of musk' and of turmeric; barley water features frequently, as does 'dragon's blood', a gummy secretion from a species of palm, and pulp of colocynth, the toxic medicinal plant already mentioned (p.). There are mixtures, simple and complex, among which is theriac. The influence of alchemy makes itself felt in Arabic medicine, for purified chemical substances appear in its materia medica for the first time. Thus it was that inorganic substances found uses in Rhazes's system, among them sulphuric acid (which it is thought he was the first to isolate in the laboratory), sal ammoniac (ammonium chloride, or smelling salts), compounds of mercury, copper, gold, arsenic and antimony, and earths, clays, corral, tars and so on. Many of these were applied externally in ointments and in suppositories, while others were taken as pills or draughts, and there were also inhalants. A patient with pains in the hip was treated with mustard paste, which it seems engendered blisters on the skin, and thereby (says Rhazes) effected a cure. Sympathetic precepts, linked to the humours, also surface in the writings. So, for example, he taught that a patient with nosebleed must not look at a bright red surface, nor expose himself to red light, for this would agitate 'the sanguineous humour', while blue light would suppress it.

A remarkable dissertation in Rhazes's writings concerns the wandering quacks who preyed on the sick at the time. They all promised magical cures, and offered ingenious demonstrations of their efficacy. Some purported to concentrate the noxious fluids responsible for the disease in one spot, proving that they had done so by rubbing a concealed inflammatory substance on the designated area; then they would 'draw out the poison' by simply neutralising the burning sensation with an oily solvent. Others would extract alien objects or creatures from where they had previously secreted them - small shreds of fabric drawn with a flourish from the eye, a piece of liver, resembling a worm, dug with a probe out of a wound made in the patient's nose, or glass splinters painfully extracted from an intimate orifice. Styles of quackery have changed, but the practice has never ceased.

Rhazes's mantle fell after his death on the shoulders of the most illustrious name in the Islamic canon, that of Ibn Sina, more commonly known as Avicenna (ca. 980 – 1037). A hallowed name to this day, the 'Prince of Physicians', 'the Aristotle of the Arabians' was not in fact an Arab, but another Persian. Born in Afshana near Bokhara, in what is now

Uzbekistan, he was a polymath of intimidating scope – the leading doctor of his day, a philosopher (famous for his exegesis of Aristotle's works), astronomer, mathematician and poet, soldier and statesman. He was largely self-educated, having as a boy quickly surpassed in knowledge and intelligence the tutors engaged to teach him. Medicine, he found 'not difficult', and at the age of 17 he was already physician to the Emir of Bokhara. He later settled near Tehran, or possibly Isfahan, and founded a highly regarded school. He corresponded with philosophers, pondered the physics of heat, light, motion and gravity, and made astronomical observations. He invented instruments, including something akin to the vernier scale, and made appreciable contributions to alchemy. Avicenna is thought to have died in the Persian city of Hamadan.

Some 240 of Avicenna's estimated 450 works survive, of which 40 relate to medicine. The most famous are a sweeping philosophical overview of the entire field, *The Book of Healing*, and a practical text, *The Canon of Medicine*, known simply as the *Canon*. A work of eclectic compass, it was translated into Latin by one Gerard of Cremona somewhere between 1150 and 1187, and made an immediate impact in the major medical schools of Europe. It remained in circulation into the 17th century, and is reputed to be an inspiration still to doctors in the Muslim countries. However, Avicenna's medical philosophy remained anchored to Aristotle's four humours On the other hand, he did in some sense prefigure the notion of clinical trials, and laid down precepts for determining the efficacy of a remedy. He taught that drugs should be tested for side-effects on animals and only then tried on patients, and he compiled a materia medica, which is included in the *Canon*. It comprises some 760 substances, mainly plant-derived, with indications of the maladies that they are meant to alleviate. Among them were cannabis, opium, black henbane (*Hyoscyamus niger*), and nearly 40 other products with supposed anaesthetic or analgesic properties. Avicenna laid stress on accurate observation - of the pulse, the urine and other indicators. He identified many diseases, and described the symptoms, for instance, of diabetes, including the sweet taste of the urine and the liability to gangrene of the extremities, and he treated it with lupin, fenugreek and zedoary (a kind of turmeric). He made extravagant claims for some of his remedies, which include such oddities as the application of amber, iron and particularly magnets to cure everything from diseases of the chest or spleen and dropsy to hair loss. But Avicenna appeared also to have grasped the nature of contagions and epidemics, to have recognised that tuberculosis is a contagious disease, and to have conceived the stratagem of quarantine. His is a hallowed name in the east, and there are allegedly scholars still living who believe that he discovered the *elixir vitae*, the elixir of eternal life, and is living somewhere still.*

A near-contemporary of Avicenna's was the Andalusian Arab, Abu al-Qasim al-Zahrawi, known as Abucasis (936-1013). He grew up and practised in Cordoba, and became most celebrated as a pioneering and innovative surgeon. His famous work of medical scholarship, *at-Tasrif,* was published around the year 1000 in 30 volumes. The part pertaining to drugs, mainly simples, was translated into Latin in 1288 under the title, *Liber Servitoris*, and became a standard source for medieval physicians and pharmacists. A century later another Islamic physician and sage rose to fame. Ibn Rushid, known as Averroes, was born in about 1125 in Cordoba, which was then at its apogee as a centre of Andalusian Islamic culture, and died in Marrakesh in Morocco in about 1198. He, like his predecessors, was a follower of Galen, indissolubly wedded to the theory of the four humours. His massive medical treatise, entitled *Generalities*, or in its Latin form, the *Collyget*, is suffused with the influence of Avicenna's *Canon*. It too contained a long list of plant remedies, and had early observations on problems of kidneys and bladder, and of sexual malfunctions. The many translations of the *Collyget* found their place in the libraries of medical schools in the east and west.

---

* The notion of an elixir had been around for some centuries, and perhaps longer. Alchemy seems to have originated in China, and its practice received the imperial sanction in 133 B.C. A leading practitioner, Wei Powei-Yang, who lived from about 100 to 150 A.D., wrote humbly that more than 10,000 formulations were required to concoct the 'pill of immortality', and so deep a problem could be confronted only by an exceedingly wise man. Wei believed in fact that he had arrived at a solution, but would not give out his formula until he had shown that it worked on a dog. Since no more seems to have been heard of the matter, one can only suppose that the either dog had died, or perhaps Wei before he could convince himself that the animal was indeed immortal.

By the following century the medical and pharmacological wisdom of the Arabs had been disseminated through most of Europe by travellers, and especially returning Crusaders. Arabian pharmacies stocked a huge range of medicaments, drawing on Greek, Roman and far-Eastern remedies, all assimilated into their own tradition. European physicians benefited from these riches, and in the mid-13th century a new comet appeared on the Spanish horizon: Arnold of Villanova, otherwise Arnaldus de Villa Nova or Villanueva, was a Catalan, born around 1235 in Valencia. He rose to fame as a doctor, alchemist, philosopher, lawyer and occultist, and author of a prodigious number of works of medicine and other subjects. He was schooled by the Dominicans and studied medicine in Paris and at the great medical school in Montpellier, where he afterwards taught. He was physician to three popes and two monarchs – the King of Aragon and later the King of The Two Sicilies. His prestige was established after he (apparently successfully) ministered to Pope Boniface VIII, a martyr to the stone.

Arnold adhered mainly to the Arabic school, which was inseparable from the doctrine of the humours. He promoted astrology and other superstitions, including the value of amulets for a host of conditions, from sore throats to mania and possession by demons. (A maniac, when such measures failed, was to be treated by drilling a hole in his cranium to allow the poisonous vapours engulfing his brain to escape.) Arnold sought not only the philosopher's stone but also the secret of eternal youth. This, or at least the assurance of longevity, he evidently thought, could be attained by repeated application to the breast of a curious plaster containing saffron, rose petals (only red would do), sandalwood, aloes and amber, emulsified with rose oil and wax.

Yet, Arnold was clearly also a thoughtful and adroit doctor. He taught that the imagination could have an important influence on the healing process, foreshadowing therefore the discovery centuries later of the placebo effect. He stressed the importance for health of diet, and he prescribed a mixture of extract of opium poppies, mandragora and henbane for surgical anaesthesia, to be administered through a sponge, the *spongia somnifera*. Arnold's greatest contribution to pharmacology stemmed from his alchemical studies (which, it is said, resulted in, among other discoveries, that of carbon monoxide): he found (ahead of Paracelsus (whom we will encounter shortly), that active principles of medicinal plants could often be extracted in concentrated form by alcohol, which he purified by distillation. Such extracts, or tinctures, have remained in use ever since. Arnold was supposed to have cured Pope Innocent V of the plague with a tincture of gold. Arnold was also probably the first European savant to extol the virtues of alcohol. Distillation of wine, he wrote, would yield the 'true water of life' in precious drops. 'We call it aqua vitae, and this name is remarkably apt, for it is really a water of immortality. It prolongs life, expels ill-humours, revives the heart, and preserves youth'. Arnold's near-contemporary, Ramon Lull (p.) was of the same mind: the essence came as an emanation from God. (Alcohol, it has to be said, found medicinal applications in Ayurvedic medicine, and in the Arabic lands and elsewhere in the East. When Sir Wilfull Witwould in William Congreve's comedy, *The Way of the World* boasts that 'To drink is a Christian diversion Unknown to the Turk or the Persian', he was wide of the mark.)

Arnold seems to have been an intolerant and arrogant man, who alienated his colleagues. He was accused of heresy, thereby attracting the attention of the Inquisition, and evidently found it prudent to seek shelter in Sicily. But the reigning pontiff, Clement V, admired and patronised Arnold, and even circulated his clergy with the demand that they search for a lost book by his protégé, *De Praxi Medica* (*The Practice of Medicine*). It was never found, and its author died on his way to call on the pope in Avignon in about 1311.

The many Jewish communities in the Islamic lands were famous for their physicians, pharmacists and travelling herbalists. Evidence of their activities can be found in document collections, of which the most famous is the Cairo Genizah. A Genizah is a store-room, formerly built into some synagogues, containing a cache of scrolls and other writings. These were preserved because it was not permitted to destroy or throw away writings in which the name of God occurs. The Cairo Genizah, uncovered in the 19th century, contains some 200,000 manuscript fragments, dating from about the 5th to the early 19th century. Four languages in use in the Islamic world occur – Arabic, Judaeo-Arabic, Judaeo-Persian and Hebrew. Among them are early treatises on medicine and drugs. In all, 242 medicinal substances are discussed, of which 195 are plant-derived, 20 are of animal origin, and the remaining 27 mineral. The recipes are detailed, and interspersed with pious asides. A typical one begins, 'In the name of God, the Merciful, the Compassionate', and then lists ingredients: 'Chicory seeds and liquorice stems, of each three *dirhams*. barberry seeds, tamarisk, and pistachio shells, of each two ....'. [A *dirham* was a unit of weight – about 3.2 grams.] And it concludes with the instruction to boil it all. The physicians seem to have their feet on the ground, judging by such observations as 'Beneficial if God wills'. Much of the material clearly derives from Graeco-Roman practices.

Medieval Europe

The common view of early medieval medicine has been that it was a period of stasis, if not regress. The Greek tradition still held sway in the Byzantine regions and certain western European enclaves, where the value of bloodletting was not questioned, and the complex galenicals were prescribed. Elsewhere Galen's grip was loosened a little, and the practice of bloodletting dwindled, which must have spared many lives. On the other hand, ancient and obscurantist practices endured, even here and there such absurd treatments as castration for leprosy, epilepsy and other, especially mental, diseases. As to drugs, the emphasis was heavily on folk remedies, a few of which would (as recent research has shown) have been effective. The pharmacopoeia was also rationalised: the 900 or so herbs listed by Dioscorides were pruned down to 71 in the widely circulated compendium, *Ex herbis feminis* – the significance of the title is elusive – prepared by an unknown hand in the 6th century, and periodically updated over a millennium. There were also new substances, stemming from various parts of Europe, including the German and Hispanic territories. Thanks no doubt to the thriving trade in commodities, centred on the Mediterranean, such novelties as ambergris (p.) and camphor came into use. Ambergris, spewed out by sperm whales, was held at the time to cure or mitigate a variety of ailments, and lumps of it were carried to ward off the plague. Camphor is a secretion from a species of laurel tree; it has mild analgesic properties, has been used since its discovery as a rub, and is still to be found in some proprietary cough medicines.

Numerous other books of herbs and recipes (*receptoria*), issuing generally from monasteries, were in circulation throughout the medieval years. For the most part they were eclectic Latin translations of Greek works, intermingled with local folk wisdom. Most of the medicinal herbs available to the poor came in fact from the gardens of monasteries and convents, whose inmates also treated the sick. The Benedictines were famous in this regard, and above all, the revered Abbess Hildegard of Bingen (1098-1179), otherwise Saint Hildegard, and sometimes also called the Sybil of the Rhine. Hildegard was a scholar of prodigious scope. She was a theologian, poet, playwright (author of the first extant morality play), a composer, whose sacred music is still performed, a botanist and physician. One of ten siblings, she was donated, as was customary, to the church, and so formidable were her learning and her personality that she was elected *magistra* by the nuns of Rupertsberg on the Rhine. She did not take kindly to authority and quarrelled persistently with the Church hierarchy and was sacked but later reinstated.

From early childhood Hildegard was subject to visions, in one of which God enjoined her to record all that she saw and heard. From her description of these moments of ecstatic insight neurologists, notably Oliver Sacks, have concluded that she suffered from migraines. These attacks would have been accompanied by a flashing visual aura, also called a scintillating scotoma, and a feeling of disorientation, followed by intense lassitude. Hildegard's two major works of medical wisdom were *Physica* and *Causae et Curae*, which were afterwards brought together under the rubric, *Liber Subtilatum* – the book of the subtlety of the divine nature of things. *Physica* is a herbal, in which most of the entries are common plants, such as aloes, apples, raspberries and so on. Their uses have a strong admixture of folklore and sympathetic magic; you are to treat sore eyes, for instance, with a topaz dunked in wine. Dietary and other prescriptions were more rational. Her dietetic precepts still have followers, especially in Germany, and her name is enshrined in the widely available Hildegard bread.

In general diseases were treated by the medieval healers according to their symptoms by simples, one herbal ingredient, often chosen on the basis of sympathetic magic, for each symptom; there would be one remedy, for instance, to treat a fever, another for the accompanying cough, and so on. In addition treatment was expected to take into account the sex, age and disposition of the patient and the instructions implicit in his horoscope. The treatments were often therefore very complicated, as physicians sought to cover all the options. And because not all of the materials could have been available to any one pharmacist, the *quid pro quo* system came into use, probably in around the 12th century: for every herb others were listed that might have similar qualities and could be substituted.

In the 13th century the first attempts were made to regulate the sale and use of drugs. In Paris a royal edict, promulgated in 1271, instructed the Faculty of Medicine to ensure that apothecaries administered remedies only in the presence of a doctor, making an exception only for commonplace (presumably peasant) remedies. Forty years on regulations concerning weights and measures were introduced, and this was followed in 1328 by a ruling that dangerous substances, laxatives and abortifacients could be provided only on the order of a doctor - in effect a prescription system. The apothecaries were, moreover, expected to offer a comprehensive range of remedies, and were told what they must stock, although *quid-pro-quo* substitutes were permitted, thus bears' fat for foxes' fat, sugar for honey, and so on. There were also now punishments for the sale of contaminated or adulterated medicaments. In time the authorities in other European countries followed suit, but progress was slow.

The medical school at Salerno

A rational and often effective approach, remarkable for its time, to the treatment of sick and wounded people had meanwhile emerged at Salerno in the south of Italy. The Medical School, probably founded in the 10th century, became the pre-eminent centre of medical learning in the West, and is often described as the first university. Its rise is associated with the name of a Benedictine monk, Alphanus, a doctor and scholar, who rose to become Bishop of Salerno. Alphanus left a record of the School's early years, which revealed that its founding faculty consisted of four doctors, a local man, a Greek, an Arab and a Jew, who all taught in their own language.

The rigorous course of study was much like that of today's medical students, in that it comprised three years of college education, followed by four years of clinical training. The emphasis was on hygiene and diet, as set out in its canon, written in Latin verse, the *Regimen sanitatis Salernitatum*. The teaching adhered to the Hippocratic method, based on the humours, and urged caution in the use of drugs. There was a repertoire of simples, and some innovations, such as the use of sponges for goitre, which would have been effective because they collect iodine from sea-water (p.), and iron for an enlarged spleen. The School owed most of its prescriptions to a travelling monk, Constantinus Africanus, or Constantine the African, born around 1020 in Carthage in modern Tunisia. He was a tireless savant, who took up residence in the hilltop Monastery of Monte Cassino, not far from Salerno, where he dedicated himself to rendering Greek and Arabic texts, including those of Galen, into Latin. His name was evidently familiar to the intellectuals of the time, for he makes an appearance in Chaucer as the 'cursed monk' in The Merchant's Tale, by reason evidently of a dissertation on aphrodisiacs in one of his works. One of Constantine's most important labours was to edit and translate a work by Hunayn (p.), *Medical Questions*; this, under its new title of *Liber Ysagogarum*, became a standard work of instruction in Salerno and the other early European medical schools. Later, in 1140, another scholar, Nicolas of Salerno, compiled a pharmacopoeia of his own, made up of 273 simples. This was the first such collection to appear in print in the 15th century. The School of Salerno reached its zenith in the 12th century, but its influence persisted for several centuries more. The *Regimen* was rendered into English in 1608 in a famous verse translation by Sir John Harington, poet and courtier, who placed modern man in his debt with his invention of the water-closet. A couplet, often quoted, which appears in the introduction, encapsulates the principal teaching of the school:

> Use three doctors still, first Dr. Quiet,
> Next Dr. Merry-man and Dr. Dyet.

Here is a sample of the more specific kind of advice that the *Regimen* dispenses:

> 'If unto Choller men be much inclin'd
> 'Tis thought that Onyons are not good for those,
> But if a man be flegmatique (by kind)
> It does his stomack good, as some suppose:
> For Oyntment iuyce of Onyons is assign'd
> To heads whose haire fals faster than it growes;
> If Onyons cannot helpe in such mishap,
> A man must get him a Gregorian cap.
> And if your hound by hap should bite his master,
> With Hony, Rew, and Onyons make a plaster.'

Astrological influence is in evidence:

> 'Three Speciall Months (September, April, May)
> There are, in which 'tis good to ope a veine;
> In these 3 months the Moone bears greatest sway,
> Then old or yong that store of bloud contain ....'

Moreover,

> 'In Spring and Summer let the right arme bloud,
> The Fall and Winter for the left are good.'

It is striking how medical science, such as it was, permeated European learning in late medieval and renaissance Europe. Geoffrey Chaucer was an educated man, a civil servant, diplomat and of course writer, whose *Canterbury Tales* appeared in 1380 or soon after. In the Prologue the narrator tells his readers: 'With us ther was a DOCTOUR OF PHYSIK', whose prowess he then describes. In Nevill Coghill's translation into modern English, it goes like this:

> Well could he calculate the planetary position
> To improve the state his patient is in.
> He knows the cause of every sickness,
> Whether it brings heat or cold, moisture or dryness.
> And where engendered, and of what humour;
> He was a very good practitioner.
>
> Well he knew old Esculapius,

And Deiscorides, and also Rufus,
Old Hippocrates, Hali and Galen,
Serapion, Rhazes, and Avicen,
Averroes, Gilbertus, and Constantine,
Bernard and Gatisden, and John Damascene.

Here Chaucer shows off his knowledge: Rufus of Ephesus (p.) and Haly Abbas were physicians familiar to historians, as were Bernard de Gordon, who practised in France but may or may not have been Scottish, Gilbertus Anglicus, or Gilbert of England, John of Gaddesden, whom we will shortly meet, and St John Damascene. (The others have already made an appearance above.) Chaucer's doctor conspires with the apothecaries to dun his patients, and turns out to be a despicable hypocrite. It is conjectured that Chaucer's model was this same John of Gaddesden. Chaucer was learned in science, and arsenic and a long list of other chemical substances crop up in *The Canon's Yeoman's Tale* ('arsenyk, sal armonyak, and brymestoon'), but not in a medicinal context. His physician, though, knows that in medicine 'gold is the best cordial', even if this is not the reason he likes it.

The Luther of Medicine

Philipp – who later re-invented himself as Theophrastus Philippus Aureolus Bombastus – von Hohenheim, and later still as Paracelsus (greater than Celsus), is said to have bequeathed us the word, bombastic. He was also probably Goethe's model for Doctor Faustus. Paracelsus was born in 1493 in the Swiss village of Einsiedeln to a Swiss mother and a Swabian father, Wilhelm Bombast von Hohenheim, a doctor. The boy was evidently something of a prodigy: he was sent to work as a chemist in the local metal mines, but at sixteen was studying medicine at the University of Basel, and three years later entered into a nomadic existence, which took him around nearly all the countries of Europe in search of new knowledge. His longest sojourn was in Ferrara, where he may have remained three years, emerging, by his own account, with a doctoral degree. He served for a time as a military surgeon, and acquired some fame, or notoriety, through his subversive writings on medicine and astrology. His reputation, at all events, sufficed to win him the position of City Physician in Basel, and soon also a Professorial Chair at the University there. Paracelsus almost at once proceeded to make himself hugely unpopular with his medical confrères and with the local apothecaries, whom he denounced for their greed and incompetence.

Paracelsus had strong and heterodox opinions in medicine, philosophy and science. He was undoubtedly a man of principle, and his unyielding character earned him the sobriquet of 'The Luther of Physicians'. Nature, he conceded, had not made him biddable. He had been raised, not like his opponents, 'on figs and white bread', but 'on cheese, milk and oat bread'. He rejected, in particular, the teachings of Galen, which held sway throughout the western world, and argued for empirically based medicine, relying on observation. Although he did not altogether dismiss the medicinal virtues of herbs, he held that inorganic substances had far greater potency. His lectures, delivered in German, not in Latin as custom decreed, attracted wide attention and scandalised the faculty. His public assertions were so strident and contemptuous of dissenting opinions, and his ministrations to the sick apparently so successful as to attract almost universal hatred. This came to a head when he staged a public burning of the works of Galen, Theophrastus, Avicenna and Dioscorides in a brass vessel, it was said with sulphur and nitre (sodium nitrate). He also had the misfortune to kill, or more probably just fail to cure, a prominent citizen of the town, Johannes Froben, known as Frobenius, a famous publisher and printer, an intimate of Holbein and Erasmus, who had brought much business and renown to Basel. Added to this Paracelsus took a cleric to court for not paying his fee for treatment. Paracelsus lost his case, was adjudged to have grossly overcharged his patient, and was threatened with a prison sentence. A quick departure by night was the only option, and Paracelsus returned to his itinerant life-style, which again took him all round Europe and then into Egypt and Asia Minor. He wrote books and many pamphlets, which brought him renewed fame. He was eventually welcomed by the burghers of Salzburg, where he settled and soon afterwards, in 1541, died, aged 48, fittingly, it was said, in a tavern brawl. It was only after his death that Basel claimed him as one of its foremost citizens, and saw the publication of his collected works in 11 volumes: the project was completed in 1591.

Paracelsus is mainly remembered for introducing such substances as mercury, sulphur and arsenic – though also laudanum, an alcoholic solution of opium – into medical practice, and for his insistence on the empirical method of gathering knowledge. Some of his treatments did not in fact greatly diverge from the conventions of the time. Indeed, arsenic and also the irritant zinc chloride were used in medieval times, and their merits for treating sores and even cancers were urged by the leading surgeons and physicians of the time, notably the French royal physician, Henri de Mondeville, who died in about 1320, and his near-contemporary, Guy de Chauliac, personal physician to three popes. Paracelsus, though, preferred plant remedies where possible. He described for instance treating a syphilitic patient for a nasal ulcer by injecting into the nostril a decoction made from carefully specified amounts of honey, salt, aloes and juice of celandine, after which he administered a mercurial purge. But he also held that therapies could not be divorced from astrology, and he found room for such superstitious nonsense as powdered mummy and human skulls, as well as amulets. He taught that besides the gross material body man was possessed of an *archaeus*, the principle of life, enveloped in an elusive, invisible substance, the *mumia*. The mumia represented the benign, life-giving power of nature and exerted a kind of magnetic healing force, but in excess it could engender disease in any organ in which it was concentrated. Hair, blood, nail clippings and bodily effluvia all contained a dose of mumia. If faeces were dried and baked their mumia was lost, and they would then acquire an affinity for mumia, like a sponge for water. Applied to the ailing body they would then draw out the surplus mumia and effect a cure. There is more: the extracted mumia and the mumia remaining in the body interact.* If now the urine, faeces or anything else derived from the body is mixed with earth, then a plant allowed to grow in it will absorb the mumia and release it. The liberated mumia will exercise its magnetic influence on the mumia in the body and cure the disease or prevent it from worsening. But this will only work if the plant bears the signature of the disease. Properly performed, then, the procedure will transfer the fever, cancer or any other disorder to the plant or to a properly chosen animal. Paracelsus gives many examples of this practice, which was widely followed in folk medicine (p.).

---

* This somewhat creepily prefigures Einstein's 'spooky action at a distance', his description of the phenomenon of quantum entanglement, the coupling of the quantum states of two particles far removed from each other in space.

Paracelsus was no mere physician and proto-pharmacologist, for he achieved fame as an alchemist, although he did not concern himself with the philosopher's stone for the transmutation of base metals into gold – in his view a sordid preoccupation. He upheld the ancient principle of the four elements, but he also propounded the theory that the world was made up of three primal constituents, the *tria prima*. These were represented by mercury, sulphur and salt, which were associated with the properties of matter and spirit. In relation to plants, mercury was the essence of life, while the volatile materials, especially what are now called the essential oils, to which the plants owes its smell and taste, are represented by sulphur, the element of fire; this leaves salt, the residue remaining when the volatiles have been eliminated. But Paracelsus's therapeutic philosophy was based on the seven known metals, each connected with one of the seven heavenly bodies recognised at the time, and the seven major organs of the human body. The metals were gold, silver, tin, copper, lead, iron and mercury. Oddly enough zinc, which Paracelsus had named, was not included, perhaps because it would have spoiled the numerical unity. The heavenly bodies corresponding to these elements were the Sun, the Moon, Jupiter, Venus, Saturn, Mars and Mercury, and to these were linked the organs in the following order: heart, brain, liver, kidney, spleen, gall bladder, lungs. There must, according to Paracelsus, be harmony between the body (the microcosm) and the universe (the macrocosm), and the physician's task was to restore to the sick the proper balance of the elements that prevail in the cosmos. Curative substances contained an active essence, or *arcanum*, a hidden remedy, which he attempted to extract in the form of a tincture – a solution in alcohol. This very modern idea ran counter to the teaching of the time, and derived from Paracelsus's alchemical approach to the study of matter. The alchemist's craft was based on the purification of essences by distillation and extraction with solvents. Paracelsus had a name for the application of such techniques to the preparation of medicaments *spagyrics*, from two Greek words, meaning to open up and to collect. He prepared alcohol extracts (tinctures) with medicinal or toxic properties from hellebore, camphor and other plants. Tinctures were not new, but Paracelsus refined the concept with a caveat: the extraction, he insisted, left behind a complementary curative principle. This could be concentrated by burning what remained after extraction, and reducing it to ash. Therefore reuniting the ash with the tincture would result in a more effective medicine.

The metals and their compounds were to be used in treating disorders of their cognate organs, but everything depended on the dose. For all substances were both toxic (*venona*) and beneficent (*essentia*), and sickness derived from an excess of one of the principles, which reached the patient in the form of cosmic exhalations. The physician's task was to identify the seat of the disease, and determine whether the organ in question had too much or too little of the vital essence. Now, since everything was in principle a poison, it followed that a poison could be used to cure a condition caused by an insufficiency of the same poison. Here perhaps were the seeds of homoeopathy (considered later). Paracelsus was denounced by the medical profession for his use of known poisons, and for other kinds of heterodoxy. He published a rebuttal, of which the gravamen was his 'Third Defence' (out of seven). This argued that since all substances were intrinsically poisonous if taken in sufficient amount, it was only the dose which determined whether they did good or harm. This was rational, and appears uncontroversial to us now. But Paracelsus had an Achilles heel, for he also cleaved to the doctrine of signatures, which he called *signa naturae*. These applied as much to minerals as to plants. So yellow topaz was a cure for jaundice, and anything red for diseases of the blood. Moreover, a divine providence had seen to it that there lurked somewhere a cure for any disease or group of related diseases. The task, therefore, was to bring these substances to light. Paracelsus also proposed classifying maladies according to the remedies that could cure them, giving them new names, such as *Morbus terpentinus* (sickness cured by turpentine), but he apparently did not persist with this curious scheme.

The principle that diseases, and therefore also the substances that would cure them, had a specific target in the body was original. Paracelsus was also not far off the mark in his belief that such diseases as gout and the stone were caused by deposits of poisons. He called these states 'tartaric' and treated them with alkali, which could have done the patients little good. His inorganic nostrums included all the then-known metals. He had great faith in mercury, arsenic and antimony and their compounds, all in greater or lesser degree toxic, and he introduced tartar emetic (potassium antimony tartrate) as a treatment for a variety of conditions, a nonpareil. It became known, in fact, as *panacea antimonica*. This highly toxic compound remained in the pharmacopoeia for centuries. (Its only practical use now is as a mordant in dyeing.) Another compound of antimony, an oxychloride, was held by Paracelsus to possess rejuvenating properties. (It became known later as powder of Algaroth, or simply Algarot, after Vittorio Algarotti, an Italian alchemist and follower of Paracelsus. Pure elemental antimony also had its uses: constipation was treated with the aid of a large pill of the metal, enough of which dissolved in the acid stomach juice to produce the desired effect. The pill was then recovered, and cleaned, ready for use by the next patient. Even in modern times, peasant families in France, and no doubt elsewhere, kept to hand such a pill, which would have passed through the gastrointestinal tracts of previous generations. (Another treatment was to swallow a pound or two of mercury, which could no doubt be recovered in the same way.) Antimony and its compounds became the main focus of contention between Paracelsus and his enemies. In Paris, the stronghold of the Galenist doctors, its use was proscribed in 1566, and the ban remained in force for a century. Paracelsus detested the French savants, and a great deal of the text of his *Nine Books - Of the Nature of Things* is devoted to scurrilous abuse of them.[*]

The disease that occasioned the greatest dread in Paracelsus's day was the Great Pox, also called the French Malady, the Neapolitan Boneache, the Castillian Disease, the English Disease, or in Turkey, the Christian

---

[*] Antimony remained a source of intermittent, but angry debate for another three centuries. It has a comprehensive entry in Samuel Johnson's dictionary, but the etymology is elusive, rooted probably in Arabic alchemical writings. A fanciful, but widely held conjecture is that it derives from the French *antimoine*, a killer of monks (*moines*), from a legend that Basil Valentine, a 15th-century German monk, who dabbled in alchemy, dosed his colleagues with it to fatten them, as it had done the monastry's pigs, with lethal effect. Basil Valentine in fact produced a strange work, mingling theology and the science of the time, with the title in the English translation, *The triumphal Chariot of Antimony*. Antimony was used from the third millennium B.C., or even before, as a cosmetic and medicine. It appears in the Bible: Jezebel, the temptress painted her eyes with stibium, the word for antimony in Latin and other languages. The chemical symbol for the element is Sb.

Disease, that is to say syphilis. (The name is a euphemism derived from a poem about a syphilitic shepherd, but more of this later.) The contagion is thought to have first emerged in Naples, during a prolonged siege in 1493, the year after Paracelsus's birth. Within a few years it had engulfed the whole of Europe. It was far more virulent in its early manifestation than in its (relatively) attenuated form two centuries on, when its prospect so frightened the likes of Pepys and Boswell. All that the 16th-century physicians could offer as a remedy was guaiac, an extract of lignum vitae or similar wood. Applied to the skin or inhaled as a choking vapour in a closed chamber, it was both expensive and ineffective, and Paracelsus railed against its use, thereby precipitating a ferocious quarrel between those of his persuasion, the 'metalists', and the 'herbalists', who defended the use of guaiac. Bloodletting, purging, enemas and sweating were other popular measures, and there were learned physicians who treated sufferers by whipping, by starvation, and trepanning – drilling a hole in the skull to let out evil humours – was recommended. All manner of lethal and ineffective remedies were deployed, and indeed the disease gave sustenance to generation upon generation of quacks. Paracelsus wrote three works on syphilis, the symptoms and course of which he described in meticulous detail, and he was also among the fist to recognise that it was transmitted sexually.

Paracelsus favoured immersion in sulphurous springs and especially treatment with mercury and its compounds. The use of mercury was not actually new. The so-called 'greasers of pox' were active in Europe, anointing their patients with 'saracenic ointment', an unguent invented in earlier centuries for the treatment of leprosy, and consisting of mercury mixed with herbs and oils or fats. Paracelsus used mercury, calomel (mercurous chloride, Hg_2Cl_2) and probably cinnabar (mercuric sulphide), both externally and internally, but in much smaller doses (in accordance with the principle of his Third Defence) than administered by his successors. (Others, among them the great anatomist, Fallopius, warned against excessive use of mercury, but to little avail, and many syphilitics would certainly have died of mercury poisoning before the disease could run its course.) It is hard now to determine how much benefit his patients derived from Paracelsus's ministrations, but his teachings were certainly absorbed by a school of followers, and influenced pharmacological thinking for the next two centuries. His Third Defence is also regarded by some historians as foreshadowing the concepts of a dose-response relationship of drugs and of a threshold concentration of drug action. If this is valid, it is no mean part of his legacy.

Among Paracelsus's medical contemporaries and near-contemporaries, Hieronymus Braunschwig (1450 – ca. 1512) is perhaps the most interesting. He was a chemist, physician and surgeon, remembered mainly for several widely used books. The most important was 'The true art of distillation', written in German and published in 1500. This is a manual, remarkably advanced for its time, of the apparatus and techniques of distillation of products such as plant oils and of course alcohol. This was allied to a compendium of medicinal plants and plant products, with particular emphasis on the value of distilled remedies. Brandy, Brunschweig believed, would cure baldness, deafness, toothache, mouth ulcers, bad breath, swellings of the breast, shortness of breath, indigestion, flatulence, dropsy, gout, fevers, the stone, the torments of fleas and lice, and many more trials.

Paracelsus's doctrines attracted numerous followers, but his most illustrious successor was the Flemish doctor, theologian and chemist, Johannes Baptista van Helmont (1577-1644). He was, besides, an intrepid polemicist, whose writings brought him into conflict with the Spanish Inquisition, menacingly active at the time in the Low Countries, and it was only highly-placed connections which enabled him to avoid a prison sentence or worse. It was van Helmont who invented the word 'gas', having discovered that the 'gas sylvestris', issuing from burnt charcoal, was identical to that generated by fermentation, that is to say carbon dioxide. His most famous experiment was to plant a willow tree in a pot, water and tend it for five years, and at intervals weigh the tree and the soil. Since the soil scarcely changed weight over this period, van Helmont inferred that the tree was made up only of water. He rejected the doctrine of humours, and based his physiological thinking on a concept of bodily fluids, pancreatic juice, saliva, and lymph, which governed the digestion. From Paracelsus he took his belief in the presence in the body of *arcana*, though he saw their function as nourishing the *archeus*, which resided in the stomach and controlled all the body's activities. Van Helmont was an iatrochemist, who favoured chemical remedies, notably tartar emetic, but was not above prescribing the patients who came to his practice in Antwerp, more or less repulsive animal substances.

Van Helmont's famous younger contemporary was the German-born Franz de la Boë (1614-1675) of Leiden, better known as Sylvius (a transliteration of his name). He too was an ardent iatrochemist, who adhered to van Helmont's theory of bodily fluids, and was much given to prescribing antimony derivatives. He also regarded stomach acidity as a critical measure of health, and regulated it with acids or alkalis, according to whether his patient was short of acid or had too much. He did, on the other hand, repose much faith in the efficacy of opium, which earned him the sobriquet of *Doctor Opiatus*.

Treasures from the New World

In the wake of the conquistadors monks and other learned men arrived in American Indian lands, and took note of the local flora and of the use to which they were put by the indigenous peoples. Several Spanish and Portuguese doctors and scientists collected the information and published compendia of useful plants and their medicinal applications. The most influential of these men was probably Nicolás Monardes (1493-1588), a physician from Seville, author of a medical text, widely used in the European centres of learning. Between 1565 and 1574 he published in a series of instalments his *Historia medicinalde las cosas que se traen de nuestras Indias Occidentales* – the medicaments coming from 'our West Indies'. It contains many products that were quickly assimilated into medical practice, and in its English translation by John Frampton it had the snappy title, *Joyfull newes out of the new-found worlde. Wherein are declared, the rare and singular virtues of divers herbs, trees, plantes, oyles & stones, with their applications to the use of phisicke and chirurgery.* This flood of riches from across the Atlantic caused, or at least coincided with a great ebullition of interest in botany, and during around the same time plants and plant products also appeared from the East, especially India. A noted Portuguese physician and scholar, Garcia da Orta, acquired an encyclopaedic knowledge of the plants of the western region of the subcontinent, and of their medicinal properties. He had accompanied the viceroy to Goa in 1538, and worked there as the personal doctor to the local ruler and to a succession of viceroys. Garcia was a marrano, a Christian from a Jewish family, who apparently held clandestinely to the faith of his ancestors. (In 1680, twelve years after his death, the Inquisition got wind of his apostasy, and had him exhumed and burned.) Garcia was also a polyglot, master of five or more languages, which helped him to collect information from traders in plants and medicaments, on which he drew for his magnum opus, *Colóquios dos simples e drogas e cousas medicinas da India* – Conversations on plants, drugs and medicaments of India.

The book was translated from the Portuguese into Latin by one of the great figures in the history of botany, the Flemish doctor and scientist, Charles de l'Écluse (1526-1609), better known as Carolus Clusius. He is remembered now for creating the medical garden of the University of Leiden, where he was a professor, and before that a similar garden in Vienna. It was also Clusius's studies in Leiden on tulips that launched the Dutch tulip industry. Clusius produced a huge output of books on plants and their medicinal applications, culminating in 1605 with his *Exoticorum libri decem*, for he had cultivated a network of correspondents, especially among travellers in the New World. Among his many works was a dissertation on cannabis (which had excited much interest when it first appeared in Europe) and opium. Guaiac, already mentioned, and sarsaparilla, extracted from a type of vine, were quickly put to ineffectual use in the treatment of syphilis. Sassafras was another wholly inert new-world product to gain an extravagant reputation as a cure for syphilis, the plague and much else, and traded at grossly inflated price. Balsam of copaiba from an Amazonian tree was used mainly to treat venereal diseases.

A plethora of new medicinal substances quickly followed, among them ipecacuanha, a ferocious emetic and a supposed antidote to strychnine. It was administered as 'ipecac syrup', prepared from the root of the plant. The root features in *The Natural History of Brazil*, published in 1684 by Wilhelm Piso, a Dutch physician. It soon found its way to Europe, and a young Dutch doctor, Johann Adrian Helvetius perceived its pecuniary possibilities. In Paris he disseminated advertisements in the streets for a great new 'secret remedy'. The Dauphin, who was apparently a martyr to intestinal disorders came to hear of it, tried it, was pleased with the result and bought the 'secret' from Helvetius for the huge sum of 1000 louis d'or. Other treasures from across the ocean were Peru balsam, a soothing ointment; *cascara sagrada*, the sacred bark; a powerful laxative derived from a species of blackthorn; cocaine from coca leaves, valued by the Central American Indians as a narcotic, and hyoscyamine, the active constituent of an extract from a number of plants; it has hallucinogenic and local anaesthetic properties, and is still sometimes used to treat gastrointestinal complaints. But much the most important of the new plant products was cinchona bark, containing quinine, and for centuries the only useful treatment for malaria. There were more, for Francisco Hernández, personal physician to King Philip II of Spain, sent by his master to report on what could be learned about remedies in the New World, reported that the Mexican Indians knew the properties of some 3000 plants.

Yet the most exciting new arrival was tobacco. From the beginning, all manner of therapeutic virtues were imputed to it, for its medicinal use by the Indians had been noted by the Hispanic missionaries and explorers, such as the Portuguese, Pedro Alvarez Cabral, as early as 1500 or so. In the latter part of the 16th century learned works on tobacco flowed from the pens of the Swiss, Conrad Gessner, and the Italian, Pietro Mattioli, following on from reports, starting in 1560, by the French ambassador in Lisbon, Jean Nicot, whose name is commemorated in that of the plant, and its addictive constituent, nicotine. Nicot was not a doctor, but a keen observer, who followed up reports of cures effected by such measures as application of mashed tobacco leaves. He so informed the doctors to the King in Lisbon, and word quickly spread. Physicians began recommending tobacco as a cure for gout, scrofula (the 'King's Evil'), cancer, ulcers chilblains, intestinal parasites, of course syphilis, and any number of other scourges, and it was praised for its analgesic properties. Tobacco was proclaimed by some as a panacea – 'the holy herb', or *sana sancta*, and God's remedy – capable of banishing any ailments: Monardes listed 48 diseases that it would cure. There were claims that it could arrest the progress of the plague, although its failure to do so must have quickly become apparent. Tobacco was applied internally in the form of a decoction or a syrup, in ointments and in poultices, and it could also be given in the form of an enema. (The practice of administering enemas of a tobacco infusion for stomach and other complaints continued in many places until the 19th century; infusions and smoke blown into the rectum were also tried as a last resort for reviving the recently deceased.) John Frampton's *Joyfull newes* introduced tobacco to the medical men of England, who latched on to it eagerly. For the next two decades it was imported and prescribed for everything, and of course it was smoked for pleasure.

In time dissenting voices were heard. In one of the many books about tobacco, which appeared in the 16th and 17th centuries, a (presumably) English doctor, writing under the pseudonym, Philaretes, discoursed on the dangers of tobacco. Its purgative effects were too violent, it sapped the sperm, procreation would cease and the population would decline; it impaired the blood, stupefied the senses like opium, and engendered melancholy. In 1602 William Vaughan, a Doctor of Civil Law published in London the first of seven editions of a book, *Naturall and artificial Directions for Health, derived from the best philosophers, as well moderne as auncien*. The author admits that he is not 'a Practitioner of that noble Science [of medicine], yet my chiefest pleasure ever since my childhood, hath been to read more books on Physicke than of any other ...' On tobacco he cautiously suggests that 'well dried and taken in a cleane Pipe fasting, in a moist morning, during the Spring, cureth the megrim, the toothache, obstructions proceeding of cold, and helpeth the fits of the mother'. Yet it should be avoided by lean, choleric and melancholy persons and by young people, women with child, husbands who desire to have children, and especially all such under 50 years of age whose brains were hot and dry. Tobacco, Vaughan thought, was as violent as quicksilver, in bringing fear and dullness to the understanding, will and memory. That same year, King James the Sixth of Scotland and First of England weighed in with his famous polemic, *Counterblast against tobacco*. This was aimed at smokers, but the King shows himself well schooled in Galenic philosophy: 'First, it is thought you say a sure Aphorisme in the Physickes, That the braines of all men, being naturally colde and wet, all dry and hote things should be good for them; of which nature this stinking suffumigation is, and therefore of good use to them ....' This argument is demolished by some neat logic-chopping: Man, the King reminds his readers, is 'composed of the foure Complexions (whose fathers are the foure Elements) .... ', but 'must the diverse parts of our Microcosme or little world within ourselves be diversly more inclined, some to the one, some to another complexion, according to the diversity of their uses'. In any case, the evil effects of tobacco become clear from the autopsies of smokers, for 'Surely smoke becomes a kitchen oftimes in the inward parts of man, fouling and infecting them with an unctuous and oily kind of soot'. In sum, the King concludes, smoking tobacco is 'a custom lothsome to the eye, hatefull to the Nose, harmfull to the braine, dangerous to the lungs and in the blacke stinking fume thereof, nearest resembling the horrible Stigian smoke of the pit that is bottomlesse'. And soon after this majestic admonition came a proclamation introducing import duty on tobacco. Despite King James's best denunciation tobacco remained not only in the shops (and a source of income to the exchequer), but also in the pharmacopoeia. It will surface again from time to time later. Meanwhile, we must return to the emergence of systematic compilations of herbs and drugs in Europe, and how such materials were used by the impoverished masses in town and country.

The origins of the European pharmacopoeias

A treatise in two volumes is the only record that remains of medicine in Saxon England. It was translated in the 10th century from a Latin version compiled a century before, and is known as the *Leechbook of Bald*. Leech here does not refer to the worm but to a physician, from the Nordic word *laekere*. It contains, amongst other things, a recipe for a theriac, but is chiefly famous for referring to a plea to the Patriarch of Jerusalem for a reputedly effective medicine to succour Alfred the Great. It was evidently of little avail, for the King died soon after. Botanical knowledge in early medieval Europe resided in the monasteries, with their extensive gardens, rich in medicinal plants. The great Benedictine monastery of Monte Cassino in Italy was, as already mentioned, one of the most prominent.

The German monk, Walafried Strabo, published a compendium of plants in the form of a poem, his *Hortulus*, in the ninth century, but of far greater scope was the collection made by the formidable Hildegard of Bingen (p.).

In the ensuing centuries many practitioners wrote down their thoughts and prescriptions. In England, John of Gaddesden (the spelling varies) was perhaps the most interesting, if only because his compilation of about 1314, called *Rosa Anglica*, the English Rose, or *Rosa Medicinae*, and subtitled, 'The Practice of Medicine from the Head to the Feet', was reputedly the first printed medical work by an English writer. It did not, however, appear in this form until 1492, long after its author's death in 1361 or earlier. John of Gaddesden, born around 1280, was a prominent practitioner, a court doctor to King Edward II, and a priest. In his reliance on sympathetic magic and other superstition he appears entirely at one with his contemporaries. So, for the treatment of tuberculosis he assures his readers, the milk of a young woman with brown hair suckling her first baby (which must be a boy) is the best nourishment. If such a one is not to hand, then at a pinch animal milk, preferably from an ass, will serve. But if not drunk from the udder, it must first be boiled with salt and honey to prevent it from coagulating in the stomach, for that could be fatal.

Amulets and charms are also given prominence. A cuckoo's head worn round the neck is used to banish epilepsy. To combat toothache, the physician, or primal dentist, must write on the patient's jaw the words, 'In the name of the Father, the Son and the Holy Ghost, Amen, +Rex +Pax +Nax +in Christo filio', and the pain will leave at once, 'as I have often seen'. The book is replete with advice in the same vein.

The coming of the printing-press towards the end of the 15th century saw the dissemination of many therapeutic treatises, such as the *Clavis Sanationis* from Padua, and *L'Arbolayre* from Paris, and many translations of classical texts by Avicenna, Rhazes, Constantine the African and others. Soon thereafter came what was probably the first genuine pharmacopoeia published in the West, bearing the stamp of official approval. This was the *Antidotarium Florentinum*, produced in Florence in 1498, with the blessing of the local medical school. In general, though, the European apothecaries and doctors still cleaved to the compilations of simples by Avicenna and other earlier writers, and the prescriptions from the School of Salerno. A much more comprehensive pharmacopoeia, the *Dispensatorium valerii Cordis*, came out in 1542 in Nuremberg, with the approval of the local senate. It contained medicinal formulations collected from a wide range of sources by a peripatetic German scholar, Valerius Cordus (1515-1544), who in his brief life made advances in medicine, chemistry and especially botany. (In chemistry he achieved the first synthesis of ether, which he called *oleum dulci vitrioli*, sweet oil of vitriol, since it was formed by the action of sulphuric acid, or vitriol, on alcohol.).

The 16th century was, as will by now be clear, a golden age for botany in Europe, and several notable scholars devoted their efforts to the search for drugs in common plants, which the bulk of the population would be able to afford. Among them were Otto Brunfels (1488-1534), philosopher, theologian and physician, often called 'the father of botany' (although botany seems to have had many fathers), and Leonhart Fuchs (1501-1566), who identified 488 species of plants, wrote some 50 books and established the first botanical garden in Germany. But the most important figure was probably Conrad Gessner (1516-1565), a Swiss doctor, linguist, botanist and chemist, who made it a practise to try new plant extracts on himself, and published not only a vast compendium in six volumes of zoology, his *Historiae animalium*, but also two mighty and greatly esteemed botanical works, published only after his death, the *Enchiridon historiae plantarum*, and the *Catalogus plantarum*.

Other cities and states gradually followed Nuremberg's example, for there was wide concern that ineffective or dangerous drugs and treatments were being peddled by unqualified entrepreneurs. In England an attempt had been made in 1512 to regulate the chaotic situation by an Act of Parliament, which proclaimed that 'the science and cunning of physic and surgery' was being practised by 'a great multitude of ignorant persons, of whom the greater part have no manner of insight into the same, nor in any other kind of learning'. These reprobates were offering spurious cures for diseases, 'to the high displeasure of God, great infamy to the Faculty, and the grievous Hurt, Damage, and Destruction of many of the King's liege People, most especially of them that cannot discern the cunning from the uncunning.' And therefore those wanting to practice physic in London must first satisfy a panel of examiners consisting of the Bishop of London or the Dean of St. Paul's, assisted by four learned doctors of physic, whom he could co-opt.

In 1518 a group of doctors got together and petitioned the King, Henry VIII, to grant a royal charter for a College. This body would have sole authority to license practitioners in London and its environs. The College of Physicians had as its primary aim to 'curb the audacity of those wicked men who shall profess medicine more for the sake of their avarice than from assurance of any good conscience, whereby many inconveniences may ensue to the rude and credulous populace'. Five years later an Act of Parliament enlarged the College's rule to cover the whole country. (It acquired its Royal prefix much later, in 1674.) Then in 1540 the College was charged by statute with responsibility for inspecting the premises of apothecaries for adulterated or decayed medicinal substances and receptacles, and ensuring that any such that their inspectors discovered were destroyed. Not only that, but the Pharmacy Wares, Drugs and Stuffs Act made a special proviso for the oversight of theriac and mithridate production, which was later entrusted to one apothecary in his shop in Poultry, close to where the Bank of England now stands.

The College had from the outset an uneasy relationship with the apothecaries, among whom there were indeed many unscrupulous, fraudulent, or at best ignorant, operators. The apothecaries were in fact allied to the Grocers' Company, and drugs were widely sold in grocers' shops. They strove to separate themselves from the Grocers, and in 1617 they finally achieved their independence, and were awarded the coveted charter, and the Worshipful Society of the Art and Mystery of Apothecaries was born. It was to have authority over the sale of drugs, and to allocate apprentices to masters of the trade. It was to act, however, under the supervision of the College of Physicians, a source of enduring rancour. The College had been making feeble attempts for some years to compile a pharmacopoeia, but the plan eventually came to fruition: in 1618 the official product appeared, partly in English and partly in Latin, with the title, *Pharmacopoeia Londinensis*. A royal proclamation instructed all apothecaries to acquire this book. A year later a second, enlarged and much altered edition appeared, in which, amongst other things, a list of new 'chemical' medicines had been added to the traditional 'galenicals' (not to mention such ancient and repellent substances as mummy flesh). Several of these were actually dangerous, none more so than compounds of antimony and mercury, and under the direction of the most famous and influential doctor of the day, William Harvey, who had discovered the circulation of the blood, the College took control of the distribution of a number of substances, designated as toxic. It was another affront to the apothecaries. The relationship was to deteriorate further.

The *Pharmacopoeia Londinensis* was an imposing production. Its title page proclaimed (in Latin) that it detailed ancient and new medicaments, painstakingly collected and examined with the utmost accuracy, confirmed by daily experience. It was an opus of the College of Physicians of London by mandate of the most Serene Highness, the Monarch. The text launched first into a directory of 'simples' – roots, herbs and flowers - 1190 in number, most of them traceable to Galen and Dioscorides, and their various extracts. Then came a list of outlandish animal sources of medicinal materials – crayfish, ants, 'intestines of the earth', that is to say earthworms, millipedes, grasshoppers, lizards, leeches, spayed dogs and many more. Organs and other parts of animals, variously prepared - some dried or powdered, others chopped, sliced or roasted – followed; there were eyes, testicles, horns (especially of the non-existent unicorn, although narwhal was a permissible substitute), even the magical bezoar stone from the intestines of goats (preferably the Persian wild variety). In Paris, at least, the famous surgeon, Ambroise Paré (ca. 1510 – 1590), more intelligent and rational by far than the run of physicians, mocked the use of fashionable remedies, such as unicorn's horn and mummy flesh, by the rich, as superstition. Nevertheless, the Parisian doctor, Jean de Renou, born some 50 years after Paré, published a pharmacopoeia in 1608, alluding to the value of animals (centipedes, worms, leeches, scorpions, snakes, birds and others) and animal parts (antelope brain, elephant tusk, frogs' hearts, foxes' lungs, and many more), and human residues. These included fat, blood, fragments of skull (before burial) and bones. In Paris, human grease could, in fact, be harvested from executed felons, and later sold by the hangman; it was much prized and was often compounded with other arcane substances for treating rheumatic and other conditions.

In England, too, bodily fluids were not disregarded: blood, bile, saliva, sweat, even 'excrements'. 'Spirit of blood', prepared by distillation of human blood mixed with aromatics, was considered excellent for asthma among other conditions. The London pharmacopoeia listed (in additions to all the simples) many such preparations designed for the treatment of particular conditions. Expensive ingredients, such as gold leaf, lapis lazuli, amber and pearls featured prominently. Some recipes were enormously complex, and would have taxed the resources of the apothecaries, none more so than a theriac (p.), made up of 50 ingredients, many from remote corners of the known world. Theriacs, or treacles, were held to be cures for all bodily woes, and if such a preparation failed to do the trick, the fault, it was surmised, lay with an incompetent or dishonest apothecary, who could sometimes be punished. The Rolls Royce form of theriac was far beyond the means of the ordinary citizenry, and a simpler compound, the famous London Treacle, made up of more accessible materials including a little opium, was widely sold instead, especially during the plague years. The 'plague water', which as he relates in his diary, Samuel Pepys took during the great epidemic of 1665-6, was probably a version.

'Plague water of Mathis' was a formulation dreamed up by the College of Physicians, and this is how it was to be made: 'Take the roots of Tormentil, Angelica, Peony, Zedoarie, Liquorish, Elacampane of each half an ounce, the leaves of Sage, Scordium, Celandine, Rue ... [and 13 other plants] ..., leaves and flowers of each a handful. Let them be cut, bruised, and infused three days in eight pints of White wine in the monthe of May, and distilled. Take of London Treacle two ounces, of Conserve of Wood-sorrel three ounces, of the temperate Cordiall species half an ounce, of Syrup of Limons enough to make all an electuary [a paste]. Of this may be taken a dram and a half for prevention, and the double quantity for cure.' Plague water could be taken by mouth, as indicated, or could be smeared on the buboes – the painful swellings in the groin and armpits, from which bubonic plague takes its name. One of many doctors who had a high opinion of theriac as a sovereign cure for plague was John Woodall, who during his career did more good than most. He was a naval surgeon, who rose to be surgeon-general of the East India Company. He had written a remarkable book entitled *The Surgeon's Mate* (1617), full of wise advice to doctors entering the navy, and urging, in particular, the merits of citrus fruit to combat the dreaded scurvy. Many more sailors in the Royal Navy died of this disease than were killed in battle, and had the Admiralty taken note of Woodall's advice thousands of lives would have been saved. But Woodall was far from the mark when he observed that 'no Medicine can be generally so safe, for the first intention and entrance upon this cure of the Plague, as is a true Diaphoretick or sweat-provoking Cordiall medicine ...', or that 'London Treacle is a very good Antidote or preservative well-approved, and *Electuar De Ovo*, or the Electuary of the Egge is also a very good Cordiall: also *Theriac. Diaressar*. By the ancient writers, called the poore mans Treacle, by myself much experienced, and all approved to be good.' The *Pharmacopoeia Londinensis*, with its theriacs and mithridates, endured through a succession of editions into the second half of the 19th century.

European folk remedies

The line between the medicines of the scholars and the unlettered multitude during this period is blurred. The popularity of folk remedies, based on ancient, often local lore, resisted the incursion of purportedly scientific medical teaching. They were without number, especially outside the towns, and the vast majority useless - except of course as placebos (see Chapter) – and some were actually harmful. Certain of the treatments were not, properly speaking, medicines at all. Lapidary medicine – the use of stones of various kinds and organic materials to effect cures or prevent disease – traces its origins to very ancient times. Amulets were much favoured in Egyptian and Roman medicine (pp). A source of medieval folk beliefs is a work by Erasmus Francisci, written much later, in the mid-17th century. This is a huge compilation, which betrays the occasional hint of scepticism. To take just a few examples, Francisci states that *agate* is very effective against snake and scorpion bites; the *emerald* was good for poisons, 'the bloody flux', ruptures and much else; lapis lazuli, perhaps because it was expensive, had a great range of curative properties – against quartan ague (malaria) and gout, poor eyesight and insomnia among others; *sapphire* is good for many things: some claim, Francisci cautiously observes, that it will stop the spread of malignant tumours, if a circle is drawn round the growth, and others hold that, when carried by a lecher, it will lose its power; and *soapstone* eases the agonies of gout. Many, if not most of the minerals and stones have inscrutable names, which now convey nothing. What, for instance, is this *bone stone*, which, by reason of its shape, was believed to possess the power to heal a broken limb?

The doctrine of signatures (p.) prevailed, as also did the conviction that a benign deity had provided in nature an antidote for every ill, a remedy for every disease. There was also the homeopathic wisdom that a minute quantity of a noxious substance will counteract a condition caused by a larger amount of the same or a related source of corruption. Shakespeare's Friar Laurence evidently held to this belief:

> Oh, mickle is the powerful grace that lies
> In herbs, plants, stones and their true qualities.
> For naught so vile that on the earth doth live,
> But to the earth some special good doth give.

Sympathetic magic pervaded folklore, and the notion that an affliction could be shed by passing it on to an animal or inanimate object. To take away warts, for instance, you were to cut off the head of an eel, and rub it over the skin so as to coat it with blood. The head was then to be buried in the earth, and as it rotted, the warts would recede. Another surefire method was to rub the warts with a slug or snail, then impale it on a thorn, and as it dried out the warts would gradually vanish. This, though, had to be performed on nine successive nights for the full effect to be felt. A remedy for cancer, which is said to have survived into the early 20th century in rural parts of France was based on the medicinal properties attributed to frogs. William Bainbridge, a New York surgeon, cites in his book, *The Cancer Problem* (published in 1914) an account of a woman with breast cancer cured by perforating the breast with eight holes, and then attaching to it a muslin bag containing eight green frogs. The frogs sucked on the wounds like leeches until they were fully gorged, and they were then seized

First Do No Harm

with hideous convulsions and died. After twenty frogs the tumour had gone and the breast recovered its pristine form

No less a savant than the Honorable Robert Boyle ('son of the Earl of Cork and father of modern chemistry') described in his book of 1692, *Medical Experiments: a Collection of Choice and Safe Remedies*, which went into several editions, a cure for tuberculosis, tested allegedly by a doctor on himself. He boiled an egg in his own urine, made holes in the shell to allow the liquid to permeate, and buried it in an ant-hill. The insects consumed the egg, thereby absorbing the disease, although whether the ants caught tuberculosis is not recorded. Moreover, the recipe seems to date back to Paracelsus, if not even earlier. Other tricks with urine for curing tuberculosis were also tried, such as burying a bottle of it under an ant-hill, or drinking a solution of sugar in the urine in a copper pot.

The doctrine of signatures was at least rational, if one believed that God had salted his creation with therapeutic clues. The following examples come from Thiselton Dyer's book, *The Folk-lore of Plants* (1888): red roses were linked to blood, and could be used to staunch a bleeding wound, or to bring colour to the cheeks: a drop of blood left under a rose-tree would do the trick. The plant, tutsan, the seed-pods of which contain a red fluid, cured conditions associated with bleeding, and was known as heal-all. The spotted leaves of the lugwort were thought to have an affinity with the lungs, and would accordingly heal lung diseases. The walnut was nothing more than a botanical head, complete with cranium and brain, and was used to treat head wounds and mental disturbances. The leaf of the clover, being heart-shaped, 'defendeth the heart against the noisome vapours of the spleen', while the pith of the elder, when squeezed with the fingers, 'doth pit and receive the impress of them thereon, as the legs and feet of dropsical persons do' - a sure cure therefore for oedema. The scales of pine cones were held to 'resemble the fore-teeth', and therefore an infusion of pine leaves, boiled in vinegar, was given for toothache. Plants with quivering leaves, like the aspen, were thought remedies for the ague, or malarial fever, which caused violent trembling. Moss scraped from a human skull ('usnea') was much prized for its medicinal powers, for diseases of the head in particular. Yellow plant extracts, like turmeric, were used to treat jaundice.

The thinking behind many treatments was altogether inscrutable: why should gout be eased by a paste concocted from pig's marrow, earthworms, a selection of herbs and the hair of a red dog? How should nine lice, taken in ale for seven days on end, combat jaundice, and how might an earful of the fat of a fox and gall of a hare restore hearing to the deaf? A treatment for the 'falling sickness', or epilepsy, which can be traced back to John of Arderne, the most famous and innovative surgeon in 14th-century England, was to blow the ash powdered remains of a roasted cuckoo into the patient's nostrils. No rationale for such proceedings was ever offered, although a theory occasionally surfaced that the ingestion of disgusting substances would ensure that evil invaders of the body, responsible for disease, were put to flight.

Two especially influential compendia of drugs emerged during the latter part of the 17th century from France. The first was the *Traité de la Chymie*, published in 1660 by Nicaise (or Nicolas) Le Febvre (or Le Fèvre), trained in Sedan as a pharmacist, and after a period as assistant to one of the King's physicians in Paris, Professor at the Jardin royale. The Treatise attracted attention in England, and Le Febvre was invited to come to London as pharmacist to the court of Charles II. There he thrived, becoming in due course a Fellow of the Royal Society. Among his other publications was his *Discours sur le grand cordial de Sr Walter Rawleigh* (1665). Raleigh was a scholar, soldier, adventurer, poet and socialite, now especially remembered for introducing tobacco into England. His cordial was a vaunted tonic, although he did not make the extravagant claims of some of his adherents for its health-giving properties. It contained saffron, zedoary (an Indian herb credited with many medicinal virtues), cinnamon, cloves, nutmeg, cardamon, sugar and powdered crabs' claws, and was supposed to have cured Queen Anne of a deadly illness. Le Febvre died in London in 1669, Raleigh having lost his head for political indiscretions half a century before, in 1617.

Two more influential French treatises appeared in the course of the following decades. One was the *Pharmacopée universelle* of 1697 by the chemist, Nicolas Leméry, already famous for his *Cours de chimie*, a standard text for many decades, which ran to 13 editions. His *Pharmacopée* recommended many preparations derived from animals, such as cow's urine and a distillate of cows' regurgitate collected in the month of May. This was called *eau de millefleurs* and was considered a cure for many grave afflictions, including dropsy, asthma and gout. Cow's urine was regarded as a suitable substitute. The other substantial work to appear at about the same time was by Pierre Pomet, a Parisian apothecary, learned and widely travelled. The fame of his fashionable pharmacy brought him to the attention of the Court, and he was appointed pharmacist to the King. In 1694 Pomet published the most comprehensive account, lavishly illustrated, of the nature, effects and histories of drugs. It kept its place for more than a century with the aid of translations into many languages, appearing in England under the title, *A compleat history of druggs*, in 1712. The text is pleasantly discursive, with digressions into natural history, agriculture, industry and anthropology.

Cannibal drugs

Pomet was clearly fascinated, among other things, with remedies derived from human materials. In one section, entitled, *Of Mummies* he dilates on the provenance, the embalming and preparative processes and uses of the material. He warns against counterfeit mummy products (most commonly the powder) and tells how they can be distinguished from the real thing. He is also in no doubt about the value of human skulls, recovered from the cadavers of executed criminals. 'The Sculls of Criminals newly hang'd', he tells his readers in the English translation, 'strip'd of the fleshy Membrane, and the Brains taken out, being well wash'd and dry'd, and separated with a Saw from the lower Part, is what Druggists sell by the name of *Human Scull*'. But, alas, these are scarce in the Parisian apothecaries' shops, for they can be bought directly from the public hangman, who also sells samples of human fat – excellent for rheumatic conditions. Highly prized also was the 'moss', or 'usnea', presumably mould, that in time grew on the cranium. It was, among other things, a sovereign remedy for nosebleeds when drawn into the nostrils like snuff.

There were many other dissertations besides Pomet's on the value of human effluvia and body parts, which featured prominently in the materia medica of practically all cultures. Urine was used both externally and internally, and is a special feature of Ayurvedic medicine. It was drunk, and matured and concentrated preparations were massaged into the skin. In European folk medicine it was recommended for a great variety of conditions from fevers and melancholy to toothache and gout. Pliny recommended the urine of a virginal male child. Six centuries on, Robert Boyle, the rigorous man of science, relates in a letter to a friend that a 'gentlewoman', sick of 'diverse chronical distempers' whose life had been despaired of, was prescribed, instead of 'more costly physick', 'morning draughts of her own water; by the use of which she strangely recovered, and is, for aught I know, still well. And the same remedy', he continues, 'is not disdained by a person of great quality and beauty, that you know; and that too after she had travelled as far as the *Spaw* [the spa] for her health's sake.'*

Saliva is even today held to possess remarkable curative properties in many cultures, and for that matter in modern 'alternative medicine'. Christ deployed his saliva to effect miracle cures, and Pliny was not far behind with equally improbable accounts. Nicolas Leméry recommends mother's milk as a cure for sore eyes, and many other human items to treat particular conditions. Even faeces were smeared on sores. When outbreaks of the Black Death struck the cities of Europe the cesspits were opened in the hope that their exhalations would ward off the contagion.

Cannibalism, in the form of remedies consisting of human body parts, was practised throughout Europe by those who could afford such indulgence. Long before Pomet wrote his treatise the importation of powdered mummy flesh from Egypt had become a sizeable industry. But although it had been acknowledged as a potent medicine centuries earlier, its origins were curious and confused. The story was disentangled nearly a hundred years ago by a medical historian, Warren Dawson. *Mumia*, whence mummy, is a Persian word, which referred to a bituminous material, found around the

---

* Twentieth-century Europeans were fascinated to learn the prescription of Morarji Desai (prime-minister of India from 1977 to 1979) for a long and healthy life: it was to not waste one's urine and drink every drop, he told the world when he turned ninety-nine. Urine therapy' (or 'urinotherapy') still has a following, which is by no means confined to India.

Dead Sea and in some other parts, and known as Lake Asphaltite. It was valued for its supposed curative properties by the Egyptian physicians, and commended by, among others, Pliny. It was also at the same time wrongly believed to be the embalming material favoured by the Egyptians, who in reality used a resin. In time mumia, the bitumen, became conflated with the mummy, and it grew into an article of medieval; medical lore that the vital spirit of the embalming substance – the supposed mumia – transferred itself to the flesh of the body that it permeated. The dried and powdered mummy flesh became by this route the substance that any self-respecting apothecary would display on his shelf. It was regarded as an indispensable medicine, most of all apparently in Germany and in France. Ambroise Paré (p.) attested to that and complained about it. ('This wicked kind of drug does nothing to help the disease ....'). And of course progressively, as the supply of Egyptian mummies dried up, bodies were increasingly procured from the gallows and from burial grounds. Paré was particularly disgusted by the practice of the Parisian apothecaries of preserving the corpses of executed criminals in salt and herbs, and baking them to simulate mummy flesh. Oswald Croll, the German doctor, known as Crollius (1580-1609) thought that a young felon, aged about 24 years and of ruddy aspect, would yield the best medicine. The high demand in the 16th and 17th centuries brought in bodies from many sources, from Africa, and even pretreated, from places where embalming was the custom. Many of the corpses entering England were imported from Ireland. No doubt, though, many of the bottles in the pharmacies contained dried animal flesh. Later in the 17th century, indeed, the mummy concept was extended to animals, and many recipes exist, in Culpeper [p.] for example) for medicines made out of mummified birds especially. What now seems most surprising is the seemingly unquestioning regard that even such rational men as Francis Bacon and Robert Boyle had for mummy medicine.

Fluid exuded from embalmed bodies was also held to possess curative properties, and so also was the sweat of a dying man – not easily come by, except perhaps on the gallows. Blood was more easily obtained, and would often be donated to treat sick relatives. The story goes that when Pope Innocent VIII (one of the less attractive pontiffs) was dying in 1492 his doctors exsanguinated three young boys to provide the Pope with the best-quality life-giving blood, but to no avail, for all four, boys and pontiff, died. From the 16th century onwards blood, fresh and warm, from a decapitated criminal, was commonly collected and drunk at the foot of the scaffold by ailing citizens, or given to children, especially those suffering from epilepsy.* But a soverign remedy for that malady, as for many others, was an extract from a human skull, or even better, of a brain, preferably that of a young man who had died a violent death. There are several recipes by eminent doctors and scholars, such as Sir Kenelm Digby, Elizabethan courtier, man of science and adventurer. They generally involved making a pulp in wine with various additives, and distilling it. It is said (see p.) that King Charles II of England, who took a keen interest in science, himself concocted a preparation that contained human skull and brain, and dosed himself with it during his final illness.

In equally eager demand was human body fat, which was considered the best treatment for joint and muscle pains from arthritis or rheumatism and gout. It was common practice in European countries to allow the town executioner to retain the bodies, as a perk of his profession. Little would be wasted. The fat would be stripped and rendered, and the grease sold to apothecaries or directly to the public. Porcelain jars labelled *Axungia hominis* (human fat) were to be found in the pharmacies. Bones were also ground up and the powder applied to painful limbs and joints. The hand of an executed felon would also be sought after, for its tough was believed to eliminate warts and other excrescences. One can of course argue that the use of human blood and body parts in the 16th and 17th centuries, and on occasion much later, is no different in kind, if assuredly less effective, than

---

* The consumption of human blood had ceased in Western Europe by the 19th century, but in France it remained a common custom until the beginning of the 20th century for people, especially young women of fashion, to visit abattoirs for a drink of fresh blood. This was held to promote vigour and a healthy complexion. In Britain during the Second World War blood donors came forward in great numbers to ensure that there were sufficient reserves to treat the wounded in bombing raids. When it became known that huge volumes of outdated blood were regularly thrown away, there was some indignation, and the Ministry of Food received frequent suggestions that, in this time of shortages, the surplus blood might be turned into black pudding. This proposal was evidently rejected as cannibalistic and un-English: tastes had clearly changed since the previous century.

blood transfusion and organ transplants today (nor are criminal practices associated with them entirely unknown in some parts of the world).

The great Chinese collection of materia medica, the *Bencao Gangmu*, compiled by a noted scholar, Li Shizen, was published in several editions during the latter part of the Ming dynasty, starting in 1578. One of its constituent books has the title in the English translation of 'Man as Medicine'. The strangest entry concerns the possibly apocryphal *mellified man*, or human mummy confection. Honey (*mel* in Latin) was always prized for its health-giving properties, which are here taken to an extraordinary extreme. The substance was said to originate in 12th-century Arabia, where some farmers, reaching the end of life, supposedly offered up their bodies to the common good. They would eat no food except honey, and would also immerse themselves in it. In time their excreta would be converted into honey, and presently they would die (presumably of malnutrition). The body would be laid into a coffin of stone filled with honey and sealed. There the corpse would macerate for 100 years, after which the seals would be broken, and the contents of the coffin dispensed as a cure for all ills when swallowed, and to heal fractures and wounds when applied externally. Mummy confection, presumably fake, was even to be purchased in the bazaars. Li Shizen concedes that the veracity of this tale is unconfirmed. It is worth remarking finally that strange superstitions survive in indigenous cultures, none more so than in traditional Chinese medicine, which is responsible for the near-extinction of rare animals, and the infliction of great cruelty, through its insistence on the unique therapeutic virtues of such materials as powdered rhinoceros horn, tiger bones and other parts, and bear bile.

The English herbals – Nicholas Culpeper

Anglo-Saxon medicine relied heavily on charms, prayers and chants, and such remedies for broken limbs as the application of warm bull's droppings, but there were many herbal remedies. An Anglo-Saxon herbal, the first ever produced in England, appeared at the very beginning of the 11th century; it is referred to as the 'Herbarium of Apuleius Patonicus', and was a translation of an original work in Latin, dating from about

600 A.D. Similar compilations appeared elsewhere in the West, notably *De Viribus Herbarum* – Of the Properties of Plants, attributed to Bishop Odo of Meung in France. Then, after a long interval, and following the invention of movable type in about 1440, herbals in the vernacular, rather than just Latin, began to proliferate in the European lands (as well as reprints and translations of ancient texts, such as the highly regarded *Compendium of Medicine*, written around 1250 by Gilbertus Anglicus – Gilbert the Englishman). All leaned heavily on Dioscorides, being mainly compiled by learned men who travelled in Eastern Europe and beyond in search of plants listed in *De Materia Medica*. The best-known from this period appeared in Germany, among them the *Buch der Natur* by Konrad von Megenberg, of 1475, and ten years later, the *Herbarium zu Teutsch* by Johann von Cube. In England another century passed before herbals of any significance emerged. William Turner's *Newe Herball* saw the light in 1551. In 1578 a work in Dutch, the *Nievve Herbal*, was translated into English, by way of French, by Henry Lyte, and then in 1597 came a more substantial compilation, John Gerard's *Herball*. The same year saw the publication of William Langham's formidable *The Garden of Health: containing the sundry rare and hidden virtues and properties of all kinds of Simples and Plants. Together with the manner how they are to be used and applied in medicine for the health of mans body, against diuers diseases and infirmities common among men.* The commendation continues: *Gathered by the long experience and industry of William Langhan, Practitioner in Physicke.* All these added their own enthusiasms and many local traditional remedies to the wisdom of Galen and Dioscorides. Here, for instance, is Langham on the merits of black hellebore: 'the root steeped in wine, and made into pouder, and drunke, helpeth those that be mad, melancholy, and witless, the falling sicknesse, swimming in the head, giddinesse, gout, dropsie, fevers, quarten, leprosy, cramps, torments of the intralls'.

Gerard's compendium, though, achieved the greatest popularity. Gerard, trained as a barber-surgeon evidently became interested in plants, and the College of Physicians of London set him up as curator of its Physic Garden, from which later grew the Chelsea Physic Garden, which thrives to this day. Gerard's great work, which ran to nearly 1400 pages, with many illustrations, bore as its full title, *The Herball, or General Natural*

History of Plants. He drew of course on earlier knowledge, but his work is suffused with his passion for botany, and he lists in meticulous detail the medical uses of the plants.

Other notable additions to the genre sprang from the pen of William Coles (1626-1662), *The Art of Simpling* and *Adam in Eden*. Coles laid particular stress on the 'doctrine of signatures' – the principle, already discussed (p.) that a benevolent deity had left clues to where men should look for cures for their ailments. Some of the signatures described by Coles were more obvious than others. Walnuts, as already mentioned, were unmistakable images of the head, for 'The Kernel hath the very figure of the Brain, and therefore it is very profitable for the Brain, and resists poisons; for if the Kerne; be bruised, and moistened with quintessence of Wine, and laid upon a Crown of the Head, it comforts the brain and head mightily.' Or again, *Hypericum*, or St John's wort, he observes, is good for wounds or diseases of the skin, for 'the little holes whereof the leaves of Saint Johns wort are full, doe resemble all the pores of the skin'. A belief in signatures was very prevalent, which is why many common plants still have names such as lousewort, liverwort, toothwort, and the like. A special mystique adhered to the mandrake, with its divided root, which in the fancy of the time resembled the lower limbs of a man. It was said to scream when pulled up, and the belief was that whoever heard it would shortly die. The lore in some regions dictated that it must be pulled out by a dog inside a magic circle. It was believed to have the power to cure a range of conditions, and was therefore worth collecting, notwithstanding the danger to life. It could be collected only by night and at specified periods, and to evade the fatal scream the gatherer would stop his ears with wax and blow a trumpet at the critical moment.

All these early herbals were overshadowed by the celebrated *magnum opus* of Nicholas Culpeper, a man of broader learning. (For a compelling account of Culpeper's life and its historical setting see Benjamin Woolley's book, *Heal Thyself.*) He was born in a village in Kent in 1616, within days of the death of his father. His education was supervised by his maternal grandfather, vicar of a country living. At the age of 16 the lad, destined for the Church, was sent to Cambridge, where he entered into an amorous liaison and took to the fashion of the day, tobacco. An ill-fated elopement ended Culpeper's formal education, and his grandfather promptly disinherited him. Culpeper now headed for London, where he fell into raffish, if not riotous company, but also settled on the vocation of an apothecary. He probably around this time developed a passionate interest in astrology, a subject not far separated from his chosen profession. The young man had an independent, rebellious nature, and embraced an extreme version of nonconformism, which repudiated the authority of both Church and State. This later led him also to rally to the Roundhead cause in the Civil War, and as a member of the Trained Bands of citizens, he sustained a serious wound at the bloody Battle of Newbury in 1643, from which he never fully recovered.

The young Culpeper signed up to an apprenticeship under a master with a shop by the Temple Bar, the gateway separating the Cities of London and Westminster. Apprentices were bound to their masters for seven arduous years, during which they undertook not to marry, but Culpeper's master went bust and fled. A second master died two years after Culpeper joined. When he found his third master to be unsatisfactory, he decided finally to break his bond and establish himself as an independent healer. He married, set up a practice at the lodgings he and his wife took outside the City, and also entered into an agreement which allowed him to use the premises of a former colleague from his apprentice days, and who now had an apothecary shop of his own. Culpeper evidently inspired confidence and did not want for patients, although his career did not always run smooth: he was once accused of witchcraft by a woman whose health had deteriorated after taking his medicines, and was imprisoned, but later adjudged innocent and released.

Culpeper was a man of immense botanical learning, and dedicated himself to the collection, and often rediscovery, of traditional remedies. His contrary nature revealed itself in his unconcealed loathing of the medical profession, with its fine airs and predilection for rare and expensive medicaments. His preference was for common plant materials, available free in fields and gardens. He also promoted what is today referred to as 'holistic' healing – treating the patient, not just the condition. He paid attention to cleanliness and healthy living, and he recognised that patients who came to him in distress often had no organic illness, but were in want of sympathy and advice. Treatments had to be suited to the age, character and sex of the patient, and had also to be related to astrological exigencies. This last was by no means a new idea: for example the celebrated surgeon, John of Arderne (ca. 1307 – 1392), had recommended as a cure for a lady's red face (regarded evidently as a serious blemish) the blood of a virgin, to be drawn at full moon at a time when the moon was in Virgo and the sun in Pisces.

But Culpeper adhered to a system called 'decumbiture'. Whereas conventional astrology took into account nothing but the state of the zodiac at the time and place, decumbiture focussed on the moment when the disorder had first manifested itself. This was when the forces of the cosmos had smitten the patient, and the positions of the planets at that instant indicated to the wise astrologer (Culpeper) the nature of the malady. The gathering and application of the plants had also to adhere to astrological precepts. Culpeper spoke to the Society of Astrologers on the astrological basis of diseases, and published his lectures as *Semeiotica Uranica, or An astrological judgement of diseases*. Yet Culpeper's professional success seems to have been based primarily on his evident acuity of diagnosis, and reliance on common sense, rather than tradition and mystique. Whether his herbal remedies cured any diseases is another matter.

In 1649 Culpeper made his first big splash: in that year there appeared under his name a volume with the title, *A Physicall Directory*. It was nothing less than an English translation from the Latin of the *Pharmacopoeia Londinensis*, and indeed more than that, for Culpeper had added a large number of simples, and more than doubled the length. But his most inflammatory move was to specify the conditions against which the cures were meant to act, and to set out instructions for their preparation and use, something the authors of the original had been careful to omit. The reader could now be his own physician. Culpeper also threw in gratuitous aspersions on the motives and competence of the physicians, and corrected errors, with many sarcastic observations. In his introduction to the book he declared that 'the Liberty of our *Common-Wealth* ... is most infringed by three sorts of men, *Priests, Physitians, Lawyers*'. In a fine turn of phrase, he explained: 'The one deceives men in matters belonging to their Souls, the other in matters belonging to their Bodies, the third in matters belonging to their Estates'. The 'company of proud, insulting, domineering Doctors', Culpeper instructed his readers, did nothing but lead the public by the nose with their obfuscations.

Culpeper had already quarrelled with the Society of Apothecaries, and now he incurred the fury of the College of Physicians, who, along with anonymous allies in the public prints, poured ordure on his head. He was variously branded a cheat, a drunk, a lecher, a poisoner and an atheist. But neither he nor his publisher, who was to profit mightily from the publication, were intimidated, and two new and enlarged editions soon appeared, as well as many cheap pirated versions from small publishers hoping to cash in on popular demand. There was now an all-out war between Culpeper and the College. Accusations against him and his publisher of transgressions of the law came to nothing, and it was not long before a second, enlarged and yet more vituperative edition of the *Physical Directory* appeared, and then a third. Culpeper, now in full spate and at the height of his popularity, was already working on what was to become the magnum opus for which he is now chiefly remembered. In 1652 appeared *The English Physitian – or An Astrologo-Physical Discourse on the Vulgar Herbs of this Nation*, with the grandiose subtitle: *Being a Compleat Method of Physick, whereby a man may preserve his Body in Health; or cure himself, being sick, for three pence charge, with such things only as grow in England, they being most fit for English Bodies* – By *Nich. Culpeper*, Gent. Student in *Physick* and *Astrologie*. Its seven sections comprised methods for preparing plasters, ointments, decoctions and so on; a compendium of all medicinally useful plants to be found in England; the times they were to be gathered, based on both botany and astrology; how best to store the materials; how to preserve juices, so as to have them ready for use when needed; preparation of compound remedies; and guidance on how to match the remedy to the cause and nature of the disease and the part of the body affected. *The English Physitian*, more commonly known now as *Culpeper's Complete Herbal*, was thus a practical household manual of self-medication. It was written in a manner 'whereby you may find the very Ground and Foundation of Physick, you may know what you do, and wherefore you do it, and this shal call me Father, it being (that I know of) never done in the world before'. Small wonder the physicians were dismayed.

Culpeper instructs the reader that everything in creation is governed by the stars. 'Here', he asserts, 'is the right way to begin the study of Physick if thou art minded to begin at the right end, for here thou hast the Reason of the whol Art. I wrote before in certain Astrological Lectures which I read, and printed, intitulated Semeiotica Uranica what Planet caused (as a secondary Cause) every Disease, and how it might be found out what Planet caused it; here thou hast what Planet cures it by Sympathy and Antipathy', following which is a series of instructions on how to get the best out of the book. Then we arrive at the medicinal plants themselves, arranged alphabetically, from Adder's Tongue to Yarrow. Here is a typical description of a plant and its uses:

THE PEACH TREE …. 'The Fruit round, and sometimes as big as a reasonable Pippin, others are smaller, as also differing in colours and taste, as russet, red, or yellow, waterish or firm, with a frieze or Cotton all over, with a cleft therein like an Apricock, and a rugged furrowed great Stone within it, and a bitter Kernel within the stone. It sooner waxeth old, and decayeth, than the Apricock, by much.' The description leads on to the value of the plant, for example: 'The Kernels of the Stones do wonderfully eas the pains and urgings of the Belly through wind or sharp Humors, and help make an excellent Medicine for the Stone upon all occasions, in this manner: Take fifty Kernels of peach Stones, and one hundred of the Kernels of Cherry Stones, a handful of Elder Flowers, fresh or dried, and three pints of Muscadine, set them in a closed pot into a bed of Horse dung for ten daies, which after distill in Glass with a gentle fire, and keep for your use.' Various preparations come next, and then some astrological explanation and advice: 'Lady Venus owns this Tree, and by it opposeth the ill effects of Mars, and indeed for Children and young people, nothing is better to purge Choller, and the Jaundice, than the Leavs and Flowers of this Tree, being made into a Syrup or Conserve, let such as delight to please their lust regard this Fruit, but such as love the health of their Children, let them regard what I say, they may safely give two spoonfuls of the Syrup at a time, 'tis as gentle as Venus her self.'

Astrological asides abound. Of rosemary, for instance, Culpeper states: 'The Sun claims Priviledg in it and 'tis under the Celestial Ram'. Some of the entries are long. Of roses - white are better than red – Culpeper observes: 'To write at large about everyone of these [preparations from roses] would make my Book swell too big, it being sufficient for a Volum by itself to speak fully of them. But briefly ...' (the term is relative). There are also echoes of Galen, as when adder's tongue is classed as 'temperate, in respect of heat, but dry in the Second Degree'. The text is interspersed with barbs aimed at various targets of his scorn, most often the doctors and their accursed College. Here is how he begins his dissertation on *Angelica*: 'In times of Heathenism when men found out any excellent Herb &c, they dedicated it to their gods, As the Bay-tree to Apollo, the Oak to Jupiter, the Vine to Bacchus, the Poplar to Hercules. These the Papists, following their Patriarchs, they dedicate them to their Saints, as our Ladies Thistle to the Blessed Virgin, St Johns Wort to St John, and another Wort to St Peter &c. Our Physitians must imitate like Apes, (though they cannot come off half so cleverly) for they Blasphemously call Pansies, or Hartseas, an Herb of the Trinity, because of its three colours: and a certain Oyntment, an Oyntment of the Apostles, because it consisteth of twelve Ingredients. Alas poor Fools, I am sorry for their folly, as grieved at their Blasphemy. God send them the rest of their Age, for they have their share of Ignorance already', and a good deal more in this vein before he discloses what the weed is actually good for: 'It resisteth Poysons, by defending and comforting the Heart, Blood, and Spirits, it doth the like against the Plague ....'

Wormwood is a favourite: Culpeper launches into it with a long homily regarding its strong and weak forms, the weak being 'common commanded by Doctors and sold by Apothecaries', for 'the one must keep his Credit and the other get Money, and that's the key of the work'. But '[t]he Herb is good for something, because God, he reminds the reader, made nothing in vain'. Culpeper can never resist a poke at the physicians when opportunity offers: 'If the liver be weak and cannot make Blood [its supposed function at the time] enough (I would have said Sanguified if I had written only to Schollers) …'. Or, 'I would willingly teach Astrologers, and make them Physicians (if I knew how) for they are most fitting for the Calling, if you will not believe me, ask Dr Hippocrates, and Dr Galen, a couple of Gentlemen that our Colledg of Physicians keep to vapor with, not to follow'. Culpeper evidently felt that he had an unrivalled insight into God's dispositions. Thus for example, 'The tender Mercies of God being over all his Works, hath by his eternal Providence planted Scriphium by the Sea side, as a fit Medicine for the Bodies of those that live near it'. Culpeper certainly had predecessors with similar views concerning the divine origin of healing plants. A prominent scholar whose work he would have encountered was Andrew Boorde (1490 – 1549, a Carthusian monk, who renounced his vows to study medicine in Glasgow. He visited the leading universities of Europe, while engaging on the side in espionage for Henry VIII's chancellor, Thomas Cromwell. Glasgow. Boorde anticipated Culpeper in his belief that 'There is no Herbe, nor weede, but God hath given vertue to them, to helpe man'). But no-one had Culpeper absolute assurance concerning the innumerable virtues of so many plants. We leave him with his characteristically oracular comments on the common weed, *agrimony*: 'It openeth and clenseth the Liver, helpeth the Jaundice, and is very beneficial to the Bowels, healing all inward Wounds, Bruises, Hurts, and other distempers. The Decoction of the Herb made with Wine and drunk is good against the stinging and biting of Serpents, and helps them that have foul, troubled or bloody waters, and makes them piss cleer spedily; It also helpeth the Chollick, clenseth the Breast, and rids away the Cough. A draught of the Decoction taken warm before the fit, first removes, and in time rids away the Tertian or Quartan Agues [probably malaria]; The Leaves and Seed taken in Wine, stayeth the Bloody Flux [dysentery]. Outwardly applied, being stamped with old Swines grease, it helpeth old sores, Cancers, and inveterate Ulcers; and draweth forth Thorns, Splinters or Wood, Nails, or many other such things gotten into the Flesh; it helpeth to strengthen the Members that be out of joynt; and being bruised and applied, or the Juyce dropped in, it helpeth foul and imposthumed Ears.' (It is, in short, a complete medicine chest.)

The English Physitian gave a huge boost to Culpeper's already considerable fame, but he did not live long to enjoy it. He continued to write, urged on by his publisher and friends, but his health grew progressively worse and in 1654 he died, almost certainly of tuberculosis. This did not staunch the flow of publications bearing his name. His wife, Alice, and the charlatan who was to become her second husband were mainly responsible, and amongst other activities, started a lucrative trade in a quack nostrum called *aurum potabile*, potable gold, or gold liquor. This, like the philosopher's stone, was a universal cure for all diseases, and its magical virtues were also proclaimed by Paracelsus and other alchemists. How it was prepared is unclear: gold can exist in an effectively water-soluble (colloidal) form, but whether this could have been produced at the time is uncertain. It was known, on the other hand, that the metal could be dissolved in aqua regia, a mixture of nitric and hydrochloric acid. Alice Culpeper claimed that that her product was devoid of 'corrosive medicine', but this seems unlikely, since aqua regia is ferociously corrosive, and not easily neutralised. But then, of course, her potable gold may not have contained gold at all. The efficacy of *aurum potabile* was powerfully promoted in a pamphlet portentously headed: *Virtues, Use, and Variety of Operations of the True and Philosophical AURUM POTABILE, Attained by the Studies of Doctor Freeman* [an associate of the Widow Culpeper], *and Doctor* [a title he never pretended to] *Culpeper, and left with his Widow, and administered by a Physician in her House near London*. This shameless imposture was denounced, most effectively in a pamphlet by an unknown hand, headed: 'Culpeper revived from the grave, to discover the cheats of that grand impostor call'd Aurum potabile: Wherein is declared the grand falsities thereof, and abuses thereby. Published to undeceive the people, and to stop the violent current of such mischievous designe'.

This was by no means the end of poor Culpeper's posthumous effusions, for his infamous widow declared that she had in her possession no less than 79 books, written or translated by her late husband. She, her second husband and Culpeper's two publishers were also busy creating new material, and in time fell to squabbling among themselves. The most notorious forgery was *Culpeper's School of Physick*, new editions of which appeared even long after Alice's death. It was subtitled, *Or The experimental practice of the whole art.* The title page goes on, *Wherein are contained all inward diseases from the head to the foot, with their proper and effectuall cures; such diet set down as ought to be observed in sickness or in health. With other safe waies for preserving of life, in excellent aphorisms, and approved medicines, so plainly and easily treated of, that the free-born student rightly understanding this method, may judg of the practice of physick, so far as it concerns himself or the cure of others, &c.....* The book consists of a collection of oddities, including various outré recipes, involving baked head of cat and penis of hare; elsewhere the reader is told that 'An excellent cure for the Gout, is to take a Puppy, all of one colour, if you can get such a one, and cut him in two pieces through the back alive'. You must then apply the warm, reeking fragments to the affected part. Culpeper at least was not forgotten, nor, in herbal medicine, is he yet. Whether any of his vast number of cures did any good at all is open to doubt. Even foxglove, one of the first truly useful medicinal substances to be discovered (p.) – though this had to wait more than 100 years after his death – was recommended by Culpeper as a treatment (illusory) for epilepsy, rather than heart disease; 'Myself', he further noted, 'am confident that an Oyntment of it is one of the best remedies for a Scabby Head that is'. Another English herbalist, John Gerard had done no worse half a century previously: 'Foxe gloue boiled in water or wine, and drunken, doth cut and consume the thicke toughness of grosse and slimie flegme and naughtie humours; it openeth also the stopping of the liver, spleene and milt and of other inward parts'.

Rudyard Kipling summed up this melancholy history in his poem, *Our Fathers of Old*:

Excellent herbs had our fathers of old -
Excellent herbs to ease their pain –
Alexanders and Marigold,
Eyebright, Orris, and Elecampane –

Wonderful tales had our fathers of old,
Wonderful tales of the herbs and the stars –
The Sun was the Lord of the Marigold,
Basil and Rocket belonged to Mars.

Pat as a sum in division it goes –
(Every herb had a planet bespoke) –
Who but Venus should govern the Rose?
Who but Jupiter own the Oak?
Simply and gravely the facts are told
In the wonderful books of our fathers of old.

Wonderful little, when all is said,
Wonderful little our fathers knew.
Half their remedies cured you dead –
Most of their teaching was quite untrue –
"Look at the stars when a patient is ill.
(Dirt has nothing to do with disease),
Bleed and blister as much as you will,
Blister and bleed him as oft as you please.
Whence enormous and manifold
Errors were made by our fathers of old.

At least, unlike so many of his contemporaries and successors, doctors as well as apothecaries, Culpeper probably never poisoned anyone, nor hastened a death by blood letting.

Chapter 3

REASON CONFRONTS TRADITION

For close on two millennia the sovereign weapons that doctors wielded when confronted with a disease, no matter what, were the lancet and the clyster, or enema, and later that dismal instrument, the cupping glass. The necessity of blood-letting was never questioned ('let out the blood, let out the disease' the old saw went), and even barbers were entitled to open a vein. Wet cupping, though, was a later refinement, performed by physicians. It allowed blood to be taken from an inflamed or otherwise affected part; deep scars were made in the skin, and a glass cup, heated in a flame, was then pressed over them. The resulting vacuum generated as the glass cooled was sufficient to draw up as much as 10 fluid ounces (nearly one-third of a litre) of blood into the cup. For some purposes dry cupping was used: here the noxious humours were drawn into a large blister, formed under the hot cup. It was a long time before the value of these painful and debilitating procedures was questioned. Other treatments, in particular the administration of drugs, were also taken on trust, handed down from teachers to pupils. There are many appalling tales of torments inflicted by doctors on the sick and dying, especially the wealthy sick, by their ministrations. A well-documented example is the death in 1685 of Charles II. Taken ill with an uncertain ailment, possibly a mild stroke, he treated himself with a nostrum then much in vogue, known as Dr Goddard's Drops, or English Drops (*Guttae Anglicanae*). The King had supposedly bought the recipe from the eponymous doctor, a famous physician and surgeon, professor at Gresham College in London, who had ministered to Oliver Cromwell. Goddard had received a stupendous sum, reported by a later writer to have been £6000, a fortune at the time. The King intended, it was said, to make the marvel widely available to his subjects, whence it became known as 'the King's Drops'. A number of formulations have been handed down, although no authentic recipe was ever divulged. It was commonly thought to have contained a distillate of human bones, or of the cranium of a hanged criminal, with vipers' flesh and hellebore. According to other accounts, it was a preparation derived from the *Bates Dispensatory*, a respectable work, originally printed in Latin as the *Pharmacopoeia Bateana*, comprising a mixture of 'flegm, spirit, oyle, and volatile salt'; this brew was fermented, and the evil-smelling oil was collected. It could be improved – elixirated - and rendered less noxious by addition of nitric acid ('spirit of nitre') and diluting with alcohol ('spirit of wine'). Whatever it was, taken in a glass of 'Canary' wine, it was 'a medicine beyond comparison'. For a human bone preparation best results, for gout, say, would result if it was made from bones that came from a limb corresponding to the one affected in the patient.

At all events, the drops did nothing for the King, who went into convulsions. The doctors were summoned and went to work in the customary manner. A large quantity of blood was drawn by lancet and by deep scarifying and cupping. Next, violent and highly toxic antimony purgatives and zinc sulphate were administered, and also emetics and a one-pint enema: these measures all failed to drive out the malign humours. And so the King's head was shaved and red-hot metal was applied to his scalp to raise blisters. Hellebore powder was blown into his nose to provoke sneezing, and plasters of pitch and pigeon guano were applied to his feet. Over the next two days the invalid, fed with various liquids, rallied from time to time, then relapsed. Peruvian bark (already known as a treatment for malaria, which the King did not have) was administered, and also a mysterious brew, known as Raleigh's antidote. Then, as a final desperate measure, the King was made to swallow an extract from the skull of a recently deceased man and crushed bezoar stone. He faced all these tortures stoically, and made his famous apology to the doctors: 'Gentlemen, I fear I am an unconscionable time a-dying'. His death soon after, at the age of 53, must have come to him as a friend.

Such was the up-market medicine of the late 17ᵗʰ century. Yet from time to time a muted voice of scepticism would make itself heard. In the mid-16ᵗʰ century the great Ambroise Paré was questioning orthodox beliefs. The introduction of gunpowder into warfare gave rise to new kinds of battlefield injuries, and the belief arose that gunpowder in a wound caused poisoning. The military surgeons of the time therefore treated wounds by cauterisation with boiling oil. Paré, surgeon to four French monarchs, also served time with the army, and used the same treatment, until one day his supply of oil gave out, and he discovered that, far from dying of poison, the men with untreated wounds did better than those subjected to the agonising treatment. He thereupon developed his own medication, an ointment made up of egg yolk, oil of roses and turpentine, which had antiseptic properties. Paré was also sceptical of the efficacy of fashionable drugs, as a famous story of a pharmacological experiment attests. He doubted the validity of the belief that the bezoar – the stone occasionally found in the entrails of goats and other ruminants – really was an infallible cure for poisoning. The King of France, Charles II, possessed and cherished a bezoar, and agreed to an experimental test of its efficacy. A cook, condemned to death for stealing silver plate, was offered and accepted a deal: he would be freed if he survived a lethal dose of a poison followed by a flake of the bezoar. The nature of the poison was not revealed, but it was said to be corrosive, so possibly oil of vitriol (sulphuric acid). The cook died after hours of agony, and the King threw away his bezoar in disgust. (Paré did, though, take note of the advice of an old woman who recommended a folk remedy for burns, consisting of the application of raw onion juice; this was apparently successful when used to treat a kitchen boy who had been extensively scalded with boiling water. This treatment seems to have its adherents in Europe still.)

Haematophobia and filth

The late 17ᵗʰ and 18ᵗʰ centuries saw some rationalisation of the pharmacopoeias, with elimination of magic-based, poisonous and useless simples and mixtures. Notable examples of the more critical attitude were the two famous publications by the Parisian apothecary and chemist,

Nicolas Leméry (1645-1715). Born in Rouen and educated in Montpellier, where he lectured in chemistry, he produced his highly successful *Cours de chimie* in 1675, and then, after 24 years during which he collected 'all the descriptions of 'old and modern pharmacy', came the *Pharmacopée universelle,* and the year after that his *Traité universel des drogues simple.* The *Pharmacopée* in particular was a notable advance on all that had gone before, and remained a source book for generations of European druggists. There were still, to be sure, some fairly outlandish prescriptions; for example, Leméry recommends for the skin, as well as for tuberculosis and nephritis, a snail preparation, which involves washing the gastropods, grinding them, shells and all, in a marble mortar, mixed with fresh donkey's milk, leaving the mess to ferment in a glass vessel for twelve hours and finally distilling it. The bottled distillate was to be kept in the sun for some days, and was then ready for use.

Worse by far than this were the prescriptions contained in a work, widely circulated and repeatedly reprinted for at least a century, with the unappealing title, *Heilsame Dreckapotheke,* the healing filth-pharmacy. Its author was the distinguished court physician of the German city of Eisenach, Christian Franz Paullini (1643-1712). Paullini was a man of great learning, who had studied in many countries, first at the University of Leiden, then in Germany, Scandinavia and England, at both Oxford and Cambridge. He was a respected historian and philosopher, corresponded with the likes of Gottfried Wilhelm Leibniz, and wrote many books. The *Dreckapotheke* was evidently based on the perceived need to guide the poor of Europe towards remedies that they could afford, in fact in general cost nothing at all, but it also followed a course that led back to the Middle Ages, especially in Germany.

The belief that bodily waste and physiological fluids possessed unique curative properties can be found in the writings of the Egyptians, and also of Galen, to whose philosophy Paullini steadfastly adhered. Ingestion of malodorous and generally disgusting substances would cause evil spirits to depart and seek more congenial lodgings. Paullini's prescriptions were also shot through with sympathetic magic. Thus falcon droppings were recommended for weak eyes, those of a squirrel for dizziness, and pieces of skull for epilepsy. Consumption could be cured by drinking the foam from the mouth of a horse – but the horse would die. For sore or watering eyes, there was nothing better than application of still-warm cowpat, mixed with salt and vinegar, although earwax or the urine of a young boy would also serve. In general, excrement, human and from specified animals, deployed in the form of draughts, pills, salves, poultices, enemas (but see p.) and suppositories, would cure any condition – gout, dropsy, syphilis, warts, itch, failure to conceive and so on. Paullini also gives abundant cosmetic advice; thus, skin will benefit from distillates of white roses and other aromatic flowers, but also from cow manure, which, Paullini thinks, diffuses a musky odour, applied morning and evening, but the distillate of human ordure is also good, for it imparts a fine colour. Teeth are best cleaned with urine, that of a virgin being especially effective, but for healthy gums an outlandish mixture, in which dog faeces feature, is recommended. There are equally strange ways to improve, retain or change the colour of the hair, requiring such aids as a mole's grease, ox gall or specified animal faeces.

Because of his attachment to the Galenic doctrine, Paullini's treatments lean heavily on bloodletting, purgatives, enemas and sweats to rebalance the humours – although he was also an enthusiastic proponent of therapeutic whipping for some conditions, a practice that, for the mentally ill at least, was retained for another two centuries. Yet from Paracelsus Paullini took mineral remedies, such as calomel and compounds of the other known metals, also saltpetre (potassium nitrate), verdigris, soil, ground stones of various kinds, and commonplace substances, such as vinegar. For both therapeutic and cosmetic purposes, the *Dreckapotheke* makes copious use of menstrual blood, while semen, sweat and placenta also have their place. One of the strangest cures, though not new (p.) – for warts and birth marks – is to apply the sweat of a dying person, or failing that and if the sufferer failed to get there in time, the water with which the cadaver has been washed. Another option was to press the hand of the corpse against the warts, so that the coldness would pass into the body, and deprive the wart of its sustenance. Paullini, then, was a throwback, and the esteem in which he was held illustrated the confused state of medical practice in a time of transition.

The light and the dark

The most important development during this period was indeed the emergence of scepticism, and especially about the value of bloodletting. The physicians who opposed the practice became known as haematophobes - blood-haters. Early in the 17th century the celebrated physician, Santorio Santorio, also known as Sanctorius of Padua (1561-1636), reported that during the outbreaks of plague in Venice, where he worked and grew rich, the poor, who were not blessed by the ministrations of doctors, were more likely to recover than the rich, who could afford to pay for bleeding and purging. A fierce dispute raged for the next two centuries between the more enlightened and the traditional school of physicians. In Paris, the good work of Ambroise Paré was set at nought by the Dean of the Medical School, probably the most influential physician in the country, Guy Patin (1601-1672). Patin was a true obscurantist who rejected Harvey's discovery of the circulation, and who asserted that 'one can cure any sickness with the clyster [enema] syringe, the lancet, cassia, senna and rose and peach blossom syrup [laxatives]'. He did not record how many patients died under his rigorous care, but he railed against the iatrochemists and the apothecaries, on the grounds that they dosed patients with poisons, especially mercury and antimony (the ban on the use of the latter in Paris having been lifted in 1666). He gloated over Van Helmont's death – a man he said 'who never did anything of value: I have seen everything he did. This man thought only about a medicine of chemical secrets and empirical'; the expression is revealing, for 'empirical' meant what we would now call evidence-based medicine, as opposed to the theory-based, Galenic practices to which Patin was wedded. It was a famous 20th-century physicist who said that one should never believe an experimental result until it has been verified by theory – but this was spoken in jest. Patin's more specific barb against Van Helmont was that 'he was fixedly against bloodletting, for want of which he died in a frenzy'.

Patin in fact regarded those who abjured bloodletting as a cure-all, the haematophobes, as deranged. He writes in a letter: 'Haematophobia is a dangerous heresy, and one that allows many people to die when they might have recovered. I am astonished that the Germans [among whom the iatrochemists were in the ascendant] do not repent of this so strange abuse, which is so injurious to them'. Records reveal the extent of Patin's single-mindedness. Thus for instance, he bled a boy of seven with pleurisy thirteen times in fourteen days, and his own consumptive son twenty times for 'a fever'. He bled his wife twelve times for a 'chest congestion' and himself seven times for a common cold, and he made no exception even for his eighty-year-old father-in-law. Prophylactic bleeding, too, was recommended; so King Louis XIII bared his arm to the lancet 47 times in six months, his fundament to the clyster syringe 212 times and his digestive tract to powerful purges 215 times*. '*Qui bene purgat, bene curat*' (he who purges well cures well), went the physician's saw.

Patin was, at the same time, a man of wide culture and an indefatigable letter-writer. His voluminous correspondence with doctor friends, touching on politics and Parisian life and manners, makes pleasant reading, when not interspersed with frothing abuse of confrères, less learned and less skilful, in his unwavering opinion, than himself. There are also many asides about his professional prowess and the gratitude of the patients he

---

* Such procedures were attended by much ceremony. In France enemas were administered by apothecaries, who attracted much mockery for profiting from this activity, although it may indeed have demanded special skill. (The proper design of cannulas was debated by learned physicians, and one of them, Régnier de Graaf even published a treatise on the subject, *De Clysteribus* in 1668). An account of an episode that enlivened the attempt at such an operation on the person of Louis XV (in the next century) was provided by the grand master of the royal wardrobe. The king was 'with much difficulty dragged to the edge of the bed', placed in 'the appropriate position, his face buried in the pillow, his rear exposed and in position'. The doctors of the Paris faculty entered and arranged themselves around the bed; then came the master-apothecary, cannula in hand, followed by the apothecary's assistant, 'respectfully bearing the body of the syringe, and the servant of the bed-chamber, carrying a light, intended naturally to illuminate the scene. The master-apothecary was advantageously positioned to put the cannula in place, when suddenly the servant of the bed-chamber, seeing the light fall on the royal posterior and imagining it might be a danger to the health, or at least comfort, of His Majesty, snatched a hat from under the arm of a doctor and interposed it between the candle and the place on which M. Forgeau was directing all his attention. I could scarcely portray the servile and scornful rage of the apothecary, when the eclipse caused him to miss his aim, and the urge to laugh on the part of the assembly, happily placed to witness the scene.

has saved. Here he goes on a despised colleague, Dr Vautier: 'He was first physician to the King and the last in the kingdom in capability, and so that you should know that he has not died without cause, he took antimony three times that he might die by his method, with the consent and advice of Guénault. Had he died seven years earlier he would have saved the lives of many honest men who were killed by his antimony. Finally he has died himself at the age of fifty-three. Because he was reputed even at Court to be very ignorant, he wanted the reputation of possessing chemical secrets and of excelling in the preparation of antimony. The importance of his patient sustained his credit. He said among other things that the doctors of Paris were correct in saying that antimony was a poison, but that as prepared by him it was not; nevertheless, this good preparation failed him.' Elsewhere Patin quotes the words he claims a patient, the Superintendent of Finances of the royal household, addressed to Vautier: 'Here were three Inspectors of Finances killed by antimony this year, monsieur; I beg you that I may not be the third.'

There is much more in the same spirit, and repeated exhortations to bleed and purge: 'There is no remedy in the world that works as many miracles as bleeding. Our Parisians generally take little exercise, drink and eat much and become very plethoric. In this state they are hardly ever relieved of whatever illness comes on them if bleeding does not proceed powerfully and abundantly.' Even children of 2 –3 months are to be bled, and, Patin proudly tells his correspondent, he even bled a three-day-old baby, thereby curing it of erysipelas: it thrived and was grown up and a captain at Dunkirk. In another letter Patin relates that he had cured himself of a severe toothache by taking blood from the same side as the pain; the toothache returned the next day, when he bled himself from the other arm, and the relief was now complete. (Whether to bleed from arm or foot, and on the same side as a disorder or the opposite were matters of hot learned debate. The Eastern way, as laid down by Avicenna and his followers, was to bleed from the opposing side; this was called 'revulsive bleeding', while in Europe the converse, or 'derivative bleeding', was the general rule.) There was yet more to bloodletting. Here is Patin again: 'The fools who do not understand our profession imagine that there is nothing to do but to purge, but they are mistaken, for if copious bleeding has not preceded it, so as to suppress the impetuosity of the vagabond humour or to empty the great vessels, and to tame the intemperance of the liver which produces the serum, the purgation would be useless.' A measure of Patin's ample store of scorn is also discharged at the apothecaries, ignoramuses and rogues one and all. He has no time for their nostrums, even for the one remedy that really works – the Peruvian or Jesuit's bark from the New World. He refers to it as 'Loyolitic powder': 'the madmen run after it, because of its high price, but now that it has proved ineffective, it is mocked'.

One of the victims of Patin's vendettas was an eminent doctor and writer, Théophraste Renaudon, a product of the hated (and much more enlightened) school of medicine in Montpellier. Renaudon had powerful patronage, notably from Cardinal Richelieu, and became court physician to Louis XIII. He did good works in the city, especially in establishing and financing a free dispensary for the poor, much to the fury of the local medical establishment. Patin exerted himself to have Renaudon barred from practising in Paris, and succeeded only after Richelieu's death (hastened by the doctors, who left him, as his protégé, Cardinal Mazarin put it, 'quasi deprived of blood' on his deathbed after eight bleedings). Patin had published a pamphlet denouncing Renaudon, who retaliated with a witty verse:

Nos docteurs de la Faculté,
Aux malades s'ils rendaient la santé
Ont besoin de l'apothecaire,
Mais Patin, plus adroit, par la charité,
Avec les « 3S » les enterre.

(that is to say, 'our doctors of the Faculty, if they are to give health to the sick, have need of the apothecary. But Patin, cleverer, charitably buries them with his "3S"'.) Patin had in fact become known in disrespectful circles as 'the doctor of the 3S'. They are *seignée, son, séné* – bleeding, bran and senna. Patin would have added to these the flower and fruit syrups, notably those of the highly prized 'pale rose' of Damascus, chicory and also rhubarb, which had been introduced from China: all these were regarded as purgatives.

It has been conjectured that Molière used Patin as one of his models for the doctors whom he mocked in his plays, *L'amour médecin*, *Le médecin malgré lui*, and *Le malade imaginaire*. He also wrote an epigram on the death of Henrietta Maria, sister of Louis XIII and Queen of England:

Le croiriez vous, race future
Que la fille du grand Henri
Eut en mourant même aventure
Que fut son père et son mari ?
Tous trois sont mort par assassin,
Ravaillac, Cromwell, médecin;
Henri, d'un coup de baionette,
Charles fini sur son billot,
Et maintenant meure Henriette,
Par ignorance de Valot.

(Would you believe, people of the future, that the daughter of great Henri would have the same experience of dying as her father and her husband? All three died by an assassin's hand, Ravailllac [the notorious anarchist and murderer], Cromwell and doctor; Henri by a dagger thrust, Charles on the block; and now dies Henrietta by the ignorance of Valot.) Valot was the royal physician, and the libel laws were then more lax.

In *Le malade imaginaire* Beralde, tries to separate his hypochondriacal brother from M. Purgon, the rapacious doctor, by explaining that when a doctor 'speaks of purifying the blood, of refreshing the bowels and the brain, of correcting the spleen, of rebuilding the lungs, of renovating the liver, of fortifying the heart, of re-establishing and maintaining the natural heat, and of possessing secrets with which to lengthen the life by many years, he repeats to you the romance of physic. But when you test the truth of what he has promised you, you find that it all ends in nothing'. And when Dr Purgon confronts his now hesitant patient, he sounds off: 'I must tell you that I give you up to your bad constitution, to the intemperance of your intestines, to the corruption of your blood, to the acrimony of your bile, and to the feculence of your humours' – and so on. The patient is ultimately terrified by the chants of the apprentices, with their refrain,

'*Clysterum donare, Postes seignare, Ensuite purgare*'. Small wonder then that the King asked Molière, whose health was fragile, about his relations with his doctor. He was rewarded with the reply, 'Sire, we talk together, he prescribes remedies for me, I do not take them, and I recover'.

While Patin certainly represented an extreme position, most sceptics, and even iatrochemists, did not by any means abandon the practice of bloodletting, but at least they used it with much greater restraint. Thomas Sydenham, who towered over medicine in England for several decades of the 17th century, was a pragmatist. He had no time for theory, and believed that the science would advance only through punctilious observation of the development of symptoms and of the course of the disease. He was much admired – 'the English Hippocrates' - and the great Hermann Boerhaave in Leiden, it was said, would always raise his hat when Sydenham's name was mentioned. Sydenham was born in 1624 into a landed family in Dorset, and had begun on his studies in Oxford when the Civil War erupted. He enrolled in Cromwell's army, and fought through the entire war, in which his two brothers were killed. He then returned to his studies, moved to Cambridge, and then established himself as a highly successful practitioner in London. There he became a member of an elite intellectual circle, which included John Locke, Robert Boyle, Robert Hooke and Christopher Wren.

For most of his life Sydenham was a martyr to gout, and he also suffered severely from kidney stones. His most famous written contribution was on fevers, but he also wrote about gout, his nemesis. He was an elegant stylist, and his description of the ravages of the disease has been much quoted. (This is how he describes the pain which comes in the night: 'Now it is a violent stretching and tearing at the ligaments – now it is a gnawing pain, and now a pressure and tightening. So exquisite and lively meanwhile is the feeling of the part affected, that it can not bear the weight of the bedclothes, nor the jar of a person walking in the room. The night is passed in torture.') There was little to be done, and indeed Sydenham, the sceptic, wrote, 'I confidently affirm that the greater part of those who are supposed to have died of gout, have died of the medicine, rather than the disease'. Yet he did not lose his sense of humour: 'For humble individuals like myself, there is one poor comfort, which is this, viz that gout, unlike any other disease, kills more rich men than poor, and wise men than simple.' Not for nothing was it known as 'the royal malady'. For all his scorn of theory, Sydenham cherished one of his own, namely that in acute conditions the accompanying fever or inflammation was part of nature's healing process; chronic illnesses, on the other hand, were the result of a derangement of humoral equilibrium, caused by unsuitable food or life-style. These were to be treated by diet, fresh air and exercise, most of all by riding, in which Sydenham, the old cavalryman, had excessive faith. He also recommended warming the sick by packing them with young children or kittens. Bloodletting was practised in moderation, and as for drugs, Sydenham favoured almost exclusively laudanum (opium in an alcoholic solution), Peruvian bark, which he helped to get into the London pharmacopoeia, against malaria, ground dear horn for dysentery, iron preparations for anaemia, and mercurials for syphilis.

Syphilis was then and would remain for another two centuries an insurmountable problem for the hospitals of Europe. According to William Clowes (1544-1604), a surgeon at St. Bartholomew's Hospital in London, fifteen out of every twenty admissions to his institution were infected with the *morbus gallicus*, the French pox. Clowes knew how little could be done for them. He wrote of 'the filthye life of many lewd and idell persons, both men and women, about the citye of London and the great number of lewd alehouses, which are the very nests and harbourers of such filthye creatures: by which disordered persons and some other of better disposition are many tymes infected and many more lyke to be, except there be some speedy remedy provided for the same'. The only remedies available to the doctors were guaiac and mercury. Guaiac, or guaiacum, the resin from the bark of a tropical tree, being far less toxic, enjoyed a long vogue, but it did little more than provoke profuse sweating, which was also one of the effects of mercury poisoning. Mercury and its compounds remained the only effective treatment – twenty minutes with Venus, twenty years with mercury, was the quip - and Sydenham made this one of the few exceptions to his principle of moderation, for he believed in the merit of salivation, which mercury engendered in intolerable abundance. So he inflicted on his syphilitic patients massive doses that produced an effusion of up to 4 litres of saliva per day. Soon also the gums rotted and the teeth loosened.* Little wonder therefore that many syphilitics preferred to die of the disease – an unpleasant end with the decay of the nose as only the most visible manifestation - than of the treatment. Sydenham, who was a caring and conscientious doctor, died in his house in Pall Mall in London in 1689 at the age of 65.

An older contemporary of Sydenham's was Théodore Turquet de Mayerne (1573-1655), one of many Huguenot doctors who fled from persecution in France. He was born the year after the St. Bartholomew's Day massacre of Protestants in 1572. In 1593, when the pseudo-Catholic Henri IV entered Paris (remarking that 'Paris is worth a Mass') and eased the worst of the restrictions on the Protestants, many exiles surged back. Soon the great majority of Parisian doctors were Huguenots, and almost to a man were followers of Paracelsus. Thus, after passionate debate, the Galenic doctrine in the medical schools was largely supplanted by the principles of chemical therapeutics. Turquet established himself as one of the leaders of the new physic, together with Joseph Duchesne, or du Chesne (ca. 1544-1609), who was appointed personal physician to the king. Duchesne, who had studied medicine in Montpellier and Basel, took root in Geneva, the centre of Calvinism, where he became a prominent citizen and diplomat. A chemist, or at least alchemist, as well as a doctor, he published his works under his Latinised name of Josephus Quercetanus (the Latin, *quercus*, for an oak replacing the French, *chêne*). In the most famous of his writings, with the title in its English translation, *The Practise of Chymicall and Hermetycall*

---

* A surgeons' assistant at St. Thomas's Hospital in London left a graphic account in about 1725 of the treatment. 'A salivation', he recorder, 'is caus'd by some of ye preparat of Mercury and tis the saline particles of calomel that vellicates [agitates] ye fibres of ye Stomack so as to discharge its contents, and thereby part of ye salts fixes upon ye glands of ye mouth and causes a salivat'. This means that the stomach goes into painful spasms. To encourage more salivation and sweating the patient was kept hot before a fire and clothed in thick flannel. The chancres - the hard growths depicted in prints by Hogarth and Gillray on the faces of the ladies of easy virtue as a mark of syphilis - were cut off with scissors, and other sores could be treated surgically or by caustic (sodium hydroxide). At least one doctor at St. Thomas's offered a less painful, though wholly ineffective remedy: snail water was a mixture of many components – 6 gallons garden snails, bruised, 3 gallons earthworms, bruised, an assortment of plants, wine and spring water, incubated for 24 hours and decanted.

Physicke for the Preseruation of Health, Duchesne set out his stall: the pure chemical remedies of the Paracelsian school would supplant 'filth of eares, sweates of the body, the dung of man and other beasts, spittle, urine, flyes, the ashes of Owles head', and other such 'filthy' medicines.

Turquet, who was born in Geneva and was a follower of Duchesne, became physician successively to three kings, the first time as Duchesne's successor at the Parisian court. But after Henri IV's murder he decamped to England, where he became a society doctor, and was soon appointed physician to the Queen, and in due course to James I, and then to his son, Charles I. One of his patients was Oliver Cromwell, which may have helped to spare him embarrassment after the Civil War. In any event, Sir Théodore, as he was by then, kept his head down, and continued unmolested in his profession. Turquet adhered to the teachings of Paracelsus but also prescribed plant-derived medicines. His biggest contribution may have been to promote the preparation and publication of the London Phamacopoeia, to which he contributed the dedication to the King, and the insertion of mercurous chloride - calomel. He also introduced the widely used 'black lotion', or *lotio nigra*, which kept its place in the materia medica for two centuries. This was a suspension of an oxide of mercury, prepared by oxidation of calomel, and was used mainly to treat skin diseases.

A more important figure was Thomas Willis (1621-1675), who overcame his humble origins as a west-country farm boy, and an unprepossessing presence – for he was short and a stammerer, and had 'hair like a dark red pigge' – to reach the pinnacle of his calling, as Professor of Medicine at Oxford. He was a royalist, and, like Turquet de Mayerne, a court physician to Charles I, and was stripped of his material inheritance by the Cromwellians after the Civil War. His publications, *De Fermentatione* and *De Febribus* elevated his professional standing, and he was able to attach himself to the group of intellectuals of which Sydenham was a member. Willis was primarily an anatomist and physiologist, whose fame rested largely on his studies of the brain. 'I addicted myself', he admitted, 'to the cutting open of heads'. He also, however, recommended and performed tests on animals of medicaments. Willis was a true scientist, a keen observer, and it seems to have been he who first recorded that the urine of diabetics contained sugar. A diabetic patient, he found, excreted 'wonderful sweet water, that tasted as if it had been mixed with Honey'. His greatest achievement as a doctor was to press successfully for the use of Peruvian bark against malaria. At the same time, having left Oxford and entered into full-time medical practice in London, he was not above prescribing such remedies as ground millipedes (which always had a place in the materia medica), and wolf's liver, and was all for bloodletting on a frightening scale. His interest in th brain also led him to recommend a medicine composed of ground human skull with chocolate to cure fits.

Another addict of the lancet was Willis's contemporary, Richard Morton (1637-1698), physician and divine, a parliamentarian, who was ejected from his living after the Restoration but restored to favour by William of Orange. Morton also recommended cures of many odd varieties, such as milk in which a hot iron had been repeatedly quenched. But his considerable reputation rests on his studies of tuberculosis. He performed many autopsies and established that tuberculosis of the lungs was invariably accompanied by the formation of tubercles, the small granular growths that gave the disease its name. Morton wrote a book on the subject, which appeared in its original Latin form in 1689, and five years later in an English translation with the title *Phthisiologia, or A treatise on consumption* (phthisis being the name for the disease preferred by the physicians). The topic was important enough, for modern estimates suggest that some 20 percent of deaths in London at the time were caused by tuberculosis. Here, though, is Morton's treatment regime: in the first stage of the disease 6-8 ounces of blood are let at intervals, followed by emetics, and then by regular administration of laxatives. Opiates are given continuously, and the unfortunate sufferer is subjected to cupping on the arm or between the shoulder blades. Many other supposed remedies are inflicted on the patient, the regime becoming ever more elaborate as the illness progresses. Morton also held that a milky diet was desirable, as well as water from chalybeate (that is iron-containing) springs. Shellfish were supposed to help, such as parts of crabs – eyes, claws, coral and so on.

A prominent figure on the medical scene of London was George Cheyne (1671-1743), trained in Edinburgh and a man of broad culture (and physique). He was a friend of Isaac Newton, and was captivated by the great man's mathematical work. He even published some cogitations of his own on the theory of fluxions, that is to say calculus. Cheyne established himself as doctor to the quality, a genial man and *bon vivant*, whose insistent craving for good food and drink worked on his health and was responsible for his legendary bulk. Cheyne eventually resolved to amend his ruinous lifestyle, and renounced both dinners and alcohol. The diet worked, although he lamented that it lost him all his friends, and he published a tract on the conquest of obesity. But as time passed he gradually reverted to his earlier habits and again became monstrously fat. (At his peak, he claimed with apparent pride, to have reached a weight of 32 stone – more than 200 kilograms.) He again repented and went on a milk diet, with satisfactory results. By then he had established a new practice in Bath, England's premier watering place, and proclaimed the benefits of its sulphurous waters.

Cheyne wrote many learned works on medicine and health, of which the best-known was probably *The English Malady, or A Treatise on Nervous Diseases of all kinds, as Spleen, Vapours, Lowness of Spirits and Hysterical Distempers*. A major theme of his discourse is the sovereign virtue of sweating, on the grounds that any nervous disorder was 'principally owing to a partial or total obstruction of the *Perspiration*'. He then offers a list of diaphoretics (sweat-inducing medicines), starting with 'Gascoign Powder', and including *Confectio Alkermes*, Venice Treacle and Sir Walter Raleigh's Cordial (all already mentioned); all these could with advantage be combined with '*Volatiles* and *foetid Gums*, and appropriated *Juleps*'. Gascoigne's Powder, like Venice Treacle, was strictly for the rich: it supposedly contained 'crabs' eyes' (in reality the black tips of the claw), ground 'pearls of Orient, bezoar (see p.), and coral, shaped into a ball with a gelatinous plant extract. Cheyne favoured in addition asafoetida pills as a remedy of broad application.

Another well-regarded treatise of Cheyne's concerned gout. He also expatiated on nervous conditions in *The Natural Method of Curing Disorders of the Body and Disorders of the Mind Depending on the Body*. Here he also goes into his own besetting vice of gluttony. 'Many a gross Glutton', he writes, 'has been cured by a Ring of Changes of *Coral, Crabs-Eyes* and *Pearl*, with *Asses Milk*, to damp his *voracious* Appetite, who could not have borne the word *Abstinence*'. Nevertheless, Cheyne reflects the predilection of the time for mercurials in several forms: metallic mercury, calomel, *æthiops*, which appears often in his writings, and is the black mercurous oxide, or possibly the sulphide, and *alcalisatus*, an ill-defined mixture, probably mainly the carbonate. Cheyne does, though, warn against their excessive or unsupervised use. His medicine chest also contained Peruvian bark, lime, sulphur, calcined egg shells, millipedes, rhubarb, valerian and other plant preparations. Leaving aside his unfounded preoccupation with sweating, Cheyne was no great innovator, and his prescriptions probably reflect fairly faithfully the common medical practices of his time.

In France the religious orders were still the most abundant providers of medicinal substances, and learned monks constantly developed new preparations. The most highly regarded were the Capuchins, who had set up, by royal edict, what amounted to a factory in the grounds of the Louvre. Their endeavours were led during their most productive period in the latter part of the 17th century by the abbé Rousseau. The laudanum preparation and the 'tranquil balm' (*Baume Tranquille*) of the Capuchins du Louvre were particularly sought-after. Another of Rousseau's inventions was Essence of Rosemary, also called Water of the Queen of Hungary because it was said to have relieved the lady's rheumatism; it was said to relieve a variety of other ailments besides, and illustrious figures of the *haut monde*, such as Madame de Sévigné, swore by it. Recipes for this and the other products of the Capuchins were published as 'Secrets and proven remedies', and many imitations and fakes flooded the market. Many of the Capuchins' formulations contained a large number of ingredients and a succession of elaborate steps were involved in their preparation. A large proportion were based on earlier recipes, dating back to medieval times, and it can be safely assumed that practically all (making an exception for laudanum) were wholly ineffective.

The royal malady

The prevalence of gout – 'the disease of kings and the king of diseases' - among the prosperous classes during Sydenham's time and later has long been a subject of debate. It has been traditionally associated with excess, especially in consumption of wine. George Cheyne, writing forty-five years after Sydenham's death, fulminated in *The English Malady* (see above), 'Since our Wealth has increas'd, and our Navigation has been extended, we have ransack'd all the Parts of the *Globe* to bring together the whole Stock of Materials for *Riot*, *Luxury*, and to provoke *Excess*'. Abstinence was the best cure. This, though, is certainly not the whole story. We now know that the accretion of uric acid (p.) - the material of the tophi, the needle-like crystals deposited in the joints, and also of the kidney stones commonly formed as an accompaniment – is promoted by lead. Lead was a common contaminant of wine at the time, and also leached out of the lead crystal glass favoured by rich.* Lead compounds inhibit one of the enzymes in the metabolic pathway that generates urea as the terminal waste-product excreted in the urine. An intermediate in urea formation is uric acid, which consequently accumulates in the blood.

Gout has always been surrounded by curious myths and superstitions. A traditional belief, for which there is some, albeit sketchy, evidence is that the amount of uric acid naturally produced by individuals (and therefore

---

* In the mid-20th century a researcher at the University of Alabama, Gene V. Ball assembled quantitative evidence to link the gout epidemic to the ingestion of lead. In the 18th century fortified wines - port and madeira – became fashionable in England among those who could afford such luxuries, and to an extent supplanted the more expensive French wines. Ball analysed samples of fortified wines of the period, and found that their lead content was much higher (by a factor of ten or so) than those now produced. The lead probably came from the tubing used in the stills that yielded the fortifying brandy. The lead glass decanters of the rich also released surprising amounts of lead into wine kept in such vessels for any length of time. Ball also gathered evidence from his own time: he analysed moonshine liquor, popular among the poor local population in Alabama, and distilled through home-made condensers, held together with lead solder. He found that 40% of the moonshine thus produced in the 1960s had a high lead content. Moreover, almost the same proportion of patients with gout treated in a hospital in Birmingham, Alabama had lead poisoning, and had been comforting themselves with the local moonshine.

perhaps their liability to gout) is correlated with intelligence (however one chooses to define this). Yet another commonly articulated theory, allegedly supported by a loose correlation, was that the disease is, or was, often accompanied by psychotic disturbances, beyond what might be explained by the effects of continuous pain. A French physician, François Boissière Sauvage de Lacroix (1706-1767) among others, viewed this as a syndrome of its own, and gave it the name, *goutte mélancholique* in a famous compendium of nosology (the categorisation of diseases). In England it became known as 'gouty mania'. Also unexplained is why gout seldom afflicts women.

It was one of the founders of modern chemistry, Carl Wilhelm Scheele (1742-1786), the Swedish apothecary, who besides discovering a multitude of new elements and compounds, and isolating oxygen, analysed kidney stones and found that they consisted of uric acid,* like the crystalline needles in gouty joints (p.). A German chemist determined that the insoluble uric acid could dissolve in lithium chloride solutions – about which more later – an observation rediscovered not long after by Jean-Martin Charcot (1825-1893), whose clinic at the Sâlpetrière hospital in Paris was for more than thirty years the world's foremost centre of neurology. Charcot stated that lithium carbonate had a remarkable capacity to dissolve uric acid, and an equally remarkable curative effect on gout. Here he was deceiving himself, and so equally was a respected English doctor, Alfred Baring Garrod (1819-1907), an authority on the disease. Both he and Charcot convinced themselves that lithium carbonate could dissolve kidney stones *in situ*, but this is not so. All the same, the notion persisted that lithium salts were beneficial for kidney and bladder complaints. Whether they alleviated the 'gouty melancholia', and whether that condition is anything more than a figment of the distinguished physicians' imaginations remains unresolved. Lithium was, however to come into its own in the mid-20th century, as we shall see, while as for gout, a fully satisfactory treatment had to wait for an intervention by the science of biochemistry (p.).

---

* This is actually true in only a minority of cases, in which there is generally a disposition to gout. Most kidney stones are composed mainly of calcium oxalate.

The clash of theories

As the 18th century dawned, rival schools of thought arose. In the hierarchy of European medical schools Leiden had pride of place, mainly because of its revered professor, Hermann Boerhaave. He was born in 1668, when the Low Countries were at the height of their intellectual and cultural pre-eminence. He rose to fame as a botanist, chemist and physician, and a charismatic teacher, adulated by students and visiting scholars, who came to sit at his feet. Dr Johnson was one who admired him, and indeed wrote his biography. The Leiden Medical School represented the mechanistic view of physiology: the body was a chemical machine, and diseases were treated globally rather than by symptom. After Boerhaave's death in 1738, it was said that his students discovered the notebook in which they expected to find his precepts and recipes, but it was empty, except for an inscription on the first page: 'Keep the feet warm, the head cool and the bowels open'.

Boerhaave had not altogether turned his back on bloodletting, nor on such remedies as goat's blood and mother's milk. The current materia medica comprised 44 recipes, but Boerhaave's favourite medicines were opium, which was used in abundance, tartar emetic and mercurials. At the other end of the spectrum was the rival school of Georg Ernst Stahl (1660-1734) in Halle in Germany. Stahl's place in history derives above all from his chemical studies, for he was the principal begetter of the erroneous but productive phlogiston theory of combustion, which dominated the thinking of chemists for more than a century. (Phlogiston was a weightless fluid, a kind of essence of fire or energy, which permeated combustible or reactive substances. When such a substance burned, the phlogiston was released in a swirling motion, which we call flame. When oxygen was discovered, with its remarkable property of reigniting dying embers, it was presumed to be drawing the phlogiston out of the coal or wood, and because it was clearly in want of phlogiston it was called 'dephlogisticated air'.) But when it came to physiology and medicine, Stahl, who was a society doctor, and ended up court physician to the Prussian King, Frederick William I, was a vitalist. He taught that living organisms contained a tangible substance that prevented disaggregation and decay, and escaped at death. This type of belief had considerable traction in the minds of doctors and biologists well into the 19th century. Stahl's influence extended even into the illustrious medical school of Montpellier. He recommended bathing in the healthful waters of the European spas as a cure for disease generally, and perhaps related to this was his emphasis on the psychological influence on illnesses. Stahl did not favour many medicaments, and especially abjured inorganic substances. Thus he opposed the use of iron and opium, and even Peruvian bark, the efficacy of which against malaria (prevalent in parts of Germany) was already well established. He did prescribe laxatives, but his general philosophy was to allow nature to do the healing.

Yet, for the most part, the influence of Boerhaave predominated in Europe, even if after his death the great school of Leiden underwent an eclipse. The second half of the 18th century saw instead the rise of Edinburgh and Vienna as centres of teaching and research, their faculties heavily populated by products of the Leiden school. In Edinburgh William Cullen held court. He was a much-loved teacher and patron, whose lectures – given, against all tradition, in English instead of Latin – were legendary. He was born in 1710 in Lanarkshire, attended the local school and the University of Glasgow. He took the conventional route into medical practice by way of an apprenticeship with a local surgeon, but then he travelled to London and took a position as a ship's surgeon on a voyage to the Caribbean. Following that, he found work with an apothecary, wishing evidently to gain knowledge of drugs. He returned to Scotland for three years of further study in Edinburgh, and a period in practice in his home-town of Hamilton. But Cullen was clearly cut out for an academic career, and so in 1746 he was entrusted with the responsibility of lecturing in chemistry, materia medica, botany and physic at Glasgow University, where in the course of time he was appointed Professor of Medicine. When the Professor of Chemistry at the University of Edinburgh died, Cullen was elected to succeed him, and he also undertook a course of clinical lectures at the Royal Infirmary in the city. Such was his renown as a lecturer that the medical students petitioned the University governors to invite him also to teach the materia medica course. In the end, Cullen achieved what he had probably always desired: he was appointed Professor of Medicine in Edinburgh, the most illustrious position in academic medicine in Britain, which he retained until shortly before his death in 1790.

William Cullen was a man of immense authority and learning and it was largely thanks to him that the medical school in Edinburgh became a magnet for young and ambitious physicians from around Europe and even America. Yet the fact is that Cullen's name is not associated with any great innovation or discovery. His philosophy was close to that of Boerhaave, who is also indeed remembered more for the influence he exercised through his teaching than for any major advances in clinical practice. Like Boerhaave, Cullen did not altogether reject bloodletting for some types of illness, but he relied mainly on the well-tried remedies of laudanum, wine and camphor, and to a lesser extent on mercurials. Hydropathy (in essence cold baths) was also considered beneficial. The treatments were fitted to the character of the disorder, according to Cullen's classification of the known diseases into four major groups. Wine and other alcoholic drink was forbidden to sufferers from gout for example, a disease on which Cullen's word was sacrosanct. And that word was "[g]out is manifestly an affection of the nervous system". Therefore blood-letting and "the antiphlogistic regimen" - a depletion of the body's excess energy - must be the treatment, being based on purges, emetics, cupping and enemas, a true throwback.

A source of grief to the benevolent Cullen was the apostasy of a disloyal pupil, John Brown, which brought about a philosophical schism. Brown's theory amounted to a distortion of Cullen's doctrine of physiology, which was in essence that the nervous system, and through it the major organs, were energised by an essence issuing from the brain; they were kept by this means in an 'excited' state, and disease resulted when the level of excitement diminished. Brown's version, which became known as the Brunonian System, posited that the brain, the emotions, and external input in the form of heat and nutrition, maintained the body in a perpetual state of stimulation, or 'excitability', perceived as life. Diseases were of two kinds, those in which stimulation was in excess of normal levels, and those in which it was deficient. These Brown named sthenic and asthenic. Diseases of the first kind were to be treated with sedatives, which generally meant the great cure-all, laudanum, the second with stimulants, most often generous quantities of Scotch. Besides those medicines there was only occasionally calomel. Sthenic diseases also demanded 'debilitating' measures, especially bloodletting and emetics. In the English translation of Brown's infamous book, *Elementa Medicinae Brunonis*, is set out the belief that opium 'banishes melancholy, begets confidence, converts fear to boldness, makes the silent eloquent' and more. Brown, who was known as the 'Excitability Doctor', followed his own precepts to their logical conclusion, for it seems that he sought to keep his system in balance by dosing himself liberally with laudanum and whisky. He also suffered from gout, which he classed as an asthenic condition. Before lecturing he would take 40 or 50 drops of laudanum in a glass of whisky, repeating the dose several times in the course of the lecture. In time he became hopelessly addicted, got into debt, was forced to lecture to his devoted students in the debtors' prison, and died in 1788 at the age of 53. Brown collected a number of faithful adherents, but his absurd doctrine never caught on in Britain. In Germany and Italy, on the other hand, it unaccountably acquired a huge following, which persisted well into the 19th century. Its practitioners were given to prescribing dangerous and ineffective substances, such as hydrocyanic acid (of which more later) for 'sthenic' conditions.

The most prominent English Brunonian was a doctor and chemist, Thomas Beddoes (1760-1808). He studied chemistry in Oxford and medicine in Edinburgh, where he was inspired by the teachings of the eminent chemist, Joseph Black, a protégé of William Cullen. Back in Oxford, Beddoes was appointed Reader in Chemistry, but incurred the disapproval of both faculty and students because of his political opinions, which he did not conceal, and most of all by his celebration of the French Revolution. (The irony of this was that he admired, and had visited the great Antoine Lavoisier, the pre-eminent chemist of his, indeed arguably any other, time, who overturned the phlogiston theory, and died on the scaffold.) Beddoes's special interest lay in the 'factitious airs' – the gases which had recently been discovered, among them oxygen, hydrogen, nitrogen, carbon dioxide and nitrous oxide. He believed, since oxygen and carbon dioxide were implicated in fermentation and animal respiration, that gases must possess medicinal virtues, and in particular that oxygen would work as a stimulant, and could therefore be used to treat asthenic patients in accordance with the Brunonian system. Sthenic patients, conversely, would benefit from oxygen deprivation. Oxygen is indeed a stimulant, and Beddoes was persuaded that breathing air enriched with oxygen had improved the condition of consumptive patients. In 1793 he published a pamphlet on the treatment of consumption by his factitious airs.

Joseph Priestley, who with Lavoisier and arguably the Swedich apothecary, Scheele, could lay claim to the discovery of oxygen, was one of several other savants who believed for reasons of their own that this and carbon dioxide (then known as 'fixed air') would prove to be effective drugs. Carbonated water (soda water), invented by Priestley, was touted as a method of dissolving kidney stones (in addition to its brief vogue as a cure for scurvy [p.]). Beddoes was well-connected. The celebrated socialite and *salonnière*, Georgina, Duchess of Devonshire, was a patron, the fashionable novelist, Maria Edgeworth, was his sister-in-law, and his father-in-law was a member of the Lunar Society, the group of intellectuals, based in Birmingham, who met monthly when the moon was full. Also of their number were Priestley and James Watt of the steam-engine. Because his family was afflicted with tuberculosis Watt was at once captivated by the curative prospects of Beddoes's oxygen, and together they published, in five volumes, *Considerations on the Medicinal Powers and the Production of Factitious Airs.* Watts did more: he lent his formidable engineering skills to the development of machines for preparing and delivering factitious airs. Full of optimism, Beddoes resolved to devote his life to the project, and with the financial assistance of the Lunar men, led by the prosperous Josiah Wedgwood, set up his Pneumatic Institution for Relieving Diseases by Medical Airs. The site he chose was Clifton in Bristol, and he engaged a young westcountryman, to manage the operation. This was none other than Humphry Davy, soon to emerge as one of the dominant figures in the history of chemistry. The sick converged on Beddoes's Institution, and the conditions of some may have been somewhat mitigated by inhaling oxygen.

At the same time Davy was experimenting with nitrous oxide ('laughing gas'), first on animals and then on himself, with gratifying results. It engendered in him, as in several of his friends, including the poet, Samuel Taylor Coleridge, who gave a vivid description, a wild euphoria. It remained a curiosity and an intoxicant for enlivening the parties of the bohemian rich – an early 'recreational drug' - until its first use as an anaesthetic, nearly fifty years later. Another probable offshoot of Brunonian thinking was the notion that exhaled breath of cattle would prove beneficial to the Pneumatic Institution's patients, and an arrangement was contrived for introducing the exhalations into the wards. In the end Beddoes's enterprise foundered, for it became apparent that the factitious airs did not cure the patients of their complaints. Beddoes, for all his intelligence and good intentions, died a disillusioned man. On his deathbed he penned a poignant (and ungrammatical) note to his protégé, Humphry Davy: 'Greetings from Dr Beddoes, one who has scattered abroad the Avola Fatua [wild oats] of knowledge, from which neither branch, nor blossom, nor fruit has resulted'.

The American Vampire

We can at least conclude with some confidence that Thomas Beddoes adhered to the dominant principle of the Hippocratic Oath: 'First do no harm'. That could never be said of his near contemporary, the highly esteemed American doctor, Benjamin Rush (1745-1813), after whom a medical school was named, and still thrives in Philadelphia. Rush was an austere man, a Presbyterian, intelligent, high-minded, prodigiously active, and humourless. He was born near the city, and entered the College of New Jersey, which became Princeton University, graduating at the age of 14 (still a record for this famous seat of learning. He learned the principles of his profession from eminent professors, and continued his studies at the feet of William Cullen in Edinburgh, where he was awarded a doctoral degree. Rush had powerful patronage from, among many others, his fellow-Philadelphian, Benjamin Franklin. He was a signatory – one of four working doctors - of the Declaration of Independence, was a Congressman during the War of Independence, and surgeon-general of the army, and he also served in the field. He lent his name to a series of good causes, such as the campaign against slavery – he was president of the Abolition Society – and women's education. He had, Oliver Wendell Holmes thought, 'a messianic mission to correct all the world's evils'. He established a highly successful medical practice, which in time attracted much of the aristocracy of Philadelphia, and grew rich (which was as well, since his young wife had borne him 13 children), though he was also generous in treating the poor. To his many admirers he was the 'Philadelphia Hippocrates', or the 'American Sydenham'.

Rush cleaved to the Galenic tradition of treatment. His weapons for combating disease – any disease – were emetics ('pukes', as they were called in America), purges, enemas, sweats, and calomel, but above all the lancet. He bled his patients with frightening zeal. His diagnoses were simple: the enemy was fever, and all fevers were the same, diseases began, nearly always, with inflammation, progressed to 'excitation of the blood', and had to be treated by bloodletting, or as he preferred to call it, 'depletion therapy'. As the old adage has it, to the man whose only tool is a hammer, every problem is a nail. Rush believed that in serious cases sthe patient could profitably be deprived of 80% of their blood. His finest hour came during the yellow fever epidemic, which ravaged Philadelphia in 1793. He and his devoted students went to work, bleeding many hundreds of citizens in the front garden of his house. It was said that the grass was encrusted with dried blood, which rotted and was soon black with flies. Many of the patients were bled repeatedly. A volume of one U.S. pint or 20 fluid ounces (of the order of a half-litre) at a time was routine, and often the patient would yield up such amounts on four, five or even seven successive days. It is uncertain how many survived such an assault: one estimate suggests that about half died (many of whom would of course have died of the disease, which left to itself probably killed about one-third of those it infected). There is indeed evidence that the death rate leapt when Rush hit his stride. He, though, saw matters quite otherwise. At the height of the epidemic he wrote to his wife (for he had sent his family out of the city for their safety, having no regard to his own), 'Yesterday was a day of triumph to mercury, jalap, and bleeding. I am satisfied that they saved, in my hands only, nearly one hundred lives'.

Residing in Philadelphia at the time was the great English polemicist, political agitator and reactionary, William Cobbett. Cobbett, a merciless critic, detested Rush's libertarian principles, and was appalled by his clinical practices, which were also beginning to offend much of the city's medical establishment. Cobbett ridiculed his victim in the style that would have been familiar to the readers of his newspaper, *Porcupine's Gazette*. He liked sometimes to impale his victims with hurtful little darts in verse:

The times are ominous indeed
When quack to quack cries purge and bleed.

He accused Rush of exaggerating his successes, failing to keep proper records and suppressing his abundant failures. His methods, Cobbett opined, could be counted among 'those great discoveries which have contributed to the depopulation of the earth'. More, 'The patients accustom themselves to live without blood, but the moment the process is completed they expire'. As for calomel, which Rush had notoriously dubbed 'the Samson of medicine', '[I]n his hands and those of his partisans it may indeed justly be compared to Samson: for I verily believe they have slain more Americans with it than Samson ever slew the Philistines. The Israelite slew his thousands, but the Rushites have slain their tens of thousands.' There was more in the same spirit, and the vain, humourless Rush, who undoubtedly believed that he had saved, not slain tens of thousands, was not a man to turn the other cheek. He took Cobbett to court for libel, and won his case: Cobbett was fined the ruinous sum in those days of £5000, reduced on appeal to £4250.

Cobbett departed for New York and somehow survived, and indeed hit back with more philippics against Rush and his disciples. One opportunity in particular was too good to miss, for in December of 1799 George Washington expired with the assistance of his doctors. It is generally thought now that his final illness was a respiratory infection. He had been surveying his plantation on horseback in cold and rain, and two days later began to feel exceedingly unwell. He summoned his factor, who had been schooled in bloodletting, and who let about a pint of blood from the president's arm. Doctors were summoned, all unfortunately of Rush's persuasion. They bled and cupped their patient, administered calomel and tartar emetic and applied a poultice of sugar and bran to his throat. The weaker Washington became the more they bled him. In all, according to Cobbett, he was deprived of some 9 pints (U.S.) of blood – well over 4 litres – though other estimates ranged between that and a mere 5 pints. Not surprisingly, he died before the day was out. Cobbett observed that Washington had expired on the very day that he, Cobbett, had been found guilty of defaming Rush. He had been punished for condemning the practice that had done for the president.

With the aid of friends and well-wishers Cobbett eventually paid off the damages (which Rush apparently donated to charity), and would have taken satisfaction in the damage the affair did to Rush's career; for his prospects of an eagerly anticipated professorial chair at Columbia University in New York vanished under the weight of ridicule that the Cobbett affair had heaped upon him. He continued to teach medical student in Philadelphia with widely admired élan, but Holmes thought him shallow, and 'imbued with the idea that even Nature itself had been under the control of the American Revolution, and of course by his own success in the practice of medicine'. His friend, John Adams, the second President of the United States secured for him a sinecure as Treasurer of the Mint.

Like most of his medical contemporaries, Rush prescribed only a handful of drugs to supplement his bloodletting therapy. Chief, of course, was calomel, given in such huge doses that the recipient might lose teeth and sometimes even the jawbone. For the rest there were jalap, a ferocious laxative, and the emetic, ipecacuanha, there was tartar emetic, which was nearly as toxic as calomel, and there was – almost as bad - lead acetate. Calomel did not take as many lives as bleeding, but its effects were invariably worse than the disease it was meant to cure (except perhaps in the case of syphilis, although, as we have seen, many sufferers opted for the disease in preference to the cure). But Rush also had a notion of his own: he had come to believe that various unpleasant manifestations were caused by an inadequate flow of bile. This led, he maintained to constipation (dreaded by many patients and doctors over the centuries, as will appear), 'sick headaches', general enfeeblement and lassitude. 'was the cure for 'bilious' patients. (The designation, a 'bilious attack', still sometimes used to describe a bout of indigestion, entered the vocabulary later.) Rush concocted his famous Bilious Pills, commonly known at the time as Rush's Thunderbolts, to suit the purpose. They delivered a massive dose of two powerful aperients, calomel and jalap, and from the description must have been the size of a horse pill.

Paris: vampirism resurgent

As a bloodletting zealot on the other side of the Atlantic, François-Jean-Victor Broussais must have run Benjamin Rush close. Broussais (1772-1838, and thus a younger contemporary of Rush's) blazed like a comet for two decades or more, and then faded as abruptly as he had risen. He even makes an appearance as a guiding light of Dr Lydgate's in George Eliot's novel, *Middlemarch*. The son of a provincial doctor, he embraced the Revolution, as did his parents, who were murdered by Royalists on Christmas Eve 1795. The son joined up as a naval surgeon and then, having gained his doctorate in Paris, as medical officer in Napoleon's army. He served in the Spanish campaign as head of the imperial army's medical service, and was evidently noted for his imperious manner and hair-trigger temper. An anecdote attesting to these traits is related in the memoirs of Antoine Fée, an apothecary with the army. At Jerez Broussais visited an ailing officer, on whom he had imposed an intolerably strict dietary regime. The patient's resolve had broken, and Broussais

"stopped at the threshold, his face inflamed with rage, and striding up to the bed cried out in his loudest voice, 'You have brought it on yourself, wretched man! Very well, you will die', and turning to those in attendance added, 'We will dissect him, Gentlemen'. The patient shuddered, stammered out a few words and promised to be good, unhappily too late. He died a few days later, and when Broussais saw him in the post-mortem room he addressed the corpse with the words, 'I told you so', followed by a deep sigh."

After the Emperor's defeat Broussais returned to Paris with a position at the Val-de-Grâce military hospital. There he began to formulate his eccentric theory of disease, which he called 'physiological medicine', and which set him against his contemporaries on the Faculty of the Paris Medical School, which boasted at the time some of the most celebrated names in the history of medicine. Broussais's theory in brief was that diseases were not associated with a disorder in any one organ or tissue, but resulted from an imbalance in one of the normal processes in the body, which might be operating too strongly or too weakly. Moreover, the seat of the problem was almost always excessive 'gastrointestinal irritation', or inflammation, which could manifest itself in a secondary inflammation elsewhere in the body. And how was this problem to be overcome? Why, by bleeding, so as to draw out the inflammation. As to drugs, Broussais prescribed only the so-called antiphlogistics – the traditional remedies for fevers, but he also placed much emphasis on a frugal, near-starvation diet to aid recovery. Purgatives, emetics, calomel and alcohol were denounced as irritants. He explained his system in a book with the sonorous title, *Examen des doctrines médicales et des systèmes de nosologie, renfermant la substance de la médecine physiologique.* (Nosology is the categorisation of diseases.) Broussais produced several other books, including one on 'Irritation and Insanity'.

The bloodletting method of choice, Broussais proclaimed, was the leech – first apparently introduced into medical practice by Nicander of Colophon, a Greek physician of the 2nd centure B.C., but never before embraced with a fanaticism akin to Broussais's. This worm, *Hirudo medicinalis*, swells up when engorged from about one inch to six inches, and some fifty of them, when applied according to Broussais's directions, could rapidly deprive the patient of three litres of blood. And the application was repeated at frequent intervals, so that Broussais's patients must have collectively surrendered hundreds of barrelsworth of blood. The leeches were to be placed on the part of the body most obviously affected – the chest, for instance, in cases of pneumonia – but failing that, they might be applied all over. At the height of Broussais's influence, when the rich and famous came to him for treatment, around 1835, France was importing some 40 million leeches each year. The saying went that Napoleon had decimated France, and now Broussais was bleeding it white. Broussais was by then Professor of Pathology and Therapeutics on the Paris Medical Faculty, for by reason of ambition, a fiery personality and bravura performances on the lecture podium, he had acquired powerful patronage and a considerable, often passionate, following among the younger members of the profession. The great American doctor and writer, Oliver Wendell Holmes, had studied in Paris, and in one of his *Medical Essays*, based on his retirement address to the Harvard Medical Faculty in 1882, he reminisced about his encounters with Broussais:

"Broussais was in those days like an old volcano which has pretty nearly used up its fire and brimstone, but is still boiling and bubbling in its interior and now and then sends up a spirt of lava and a volley of pebbles. His theories of irritation and inflammation as the cause of disease, and the practice which sprang from them, ran over the fields of medicine like flame over the grass of the prairies. The way in which that knotty-featured, savage old man would bring out the word *irritation* with rattling and rolling reduplication of the resonant letter *r-* might have taught a lesson in articulation to Salvini [a celebrated Italian actor, much admired in America]. But Broussais' theories languished and well-nigh became obsolete, and this no doubt added vehemence to his defence of his cherished dogmas".

By this time Broussais's eccentricity had extended to a fervent espousal of phrenology, the interpretation of personality through the study of bumps on the cranium.

Gradually Broussais's preposterous theories lost ground, thanks to the opposition of many distinguished contemporaries in France. Data collected from the Val-de-Grâce hospital showed that his own claims of exceptionally low death rates among his patients were grossly distorted. Evidence accumulated that in reality his methods had done little but weaken the already sick. The medical students, ever fickle, turned their backs, which must have been hard for a man of such immense vanity to bear. Here is Holmes again describing the scene when Broussais was followed in the lecture-hall by a now more favoured professor:

As his lecture drew to a close, the benches, thinly sprinkled with students, began to fill up; the doors creaked open and banged back oftener and oftener, until at last the sound grew almost continuous, and the voice of the lecturer became a leonine growl as he strove in vain to be heard above the noise of the doors and the footsteps.

A band of disciples nevertheless kept the faith, and took Broussais's methods to even greater extremes. A new edition of his *Examen* ran to 2200 pages, of which one-third were devoted to the denunciation and abuse of his adversaries. When he was dying, apparently from rectal carcinoma, Broussais perversely turned to homeopathic remedies in search of a cure. At his death the eulogies and the obituaries in France and beyond were fulsome. When *Middlemarch* was published in 1873, 35 years after he had been laid to rest in the cemetery of Père Lachaise, Broussais was evidently still a name to conjure with. Another ten years on he was dug up and re-buried at the Val-de-Grâce beneath the monument erected in his honour.

The use of leeches was of course by no means confined to France. Wordsworth in his long poem, *Resolution and Independence*, pictures an encounter on a wild moor with an aged leech-collector:

> He told that to these waters had he come
> To gather leeches, being old and poor:
> Employment hazardous and wearisome!
> And he had many hardships to endure,
> And in this way he gained an honest maintenance.

The old man complains,
> "Once could I meet with them on every side;
> But they have dwindled long by slow decay;
> But still I persevere and find them where I may."

And indeed it is thought that the almost complete disappearance of leeches from British bogs and marshes was the result of the continuing demand from hospitals. Leeches did not entirely fall out of favour with Broussais's death. It was even reported that leeches were applied to Stalin when he was close to death. In recent years, in fact, they have found new applications in ensuring blood-flow to grafts in plastic surgery, and in reducing swellings after local operations, especially of the eye. The leech injects a protein, hirudin (after the Latin name of the worm) with powerful anticoagulant activity. This is of advantage to the leech for it prevents the blood from clotting as it enters. The hirudin remains in the minute wound made by the leech and causes the blood to continue to flow (and ooze from the puncture for some hours). An extract of leeches, containing hirudin, was first tried out in surgery as far back as 1909, but it is only with the advent of recombinant DNA technology, which allows hirudin to be prepared in pure form in bacterial cultures, that it has become widely available for the elimination or prevention of blood clots.

Bloodletting in one form or another, though widely denounced by responsible doctors in the 19th century, seems never to have quite disappeared. It was certainly still practised on the remoter fringes of medicine well into the 20th century. Some theories were put forward in perfectly reputable circles that led to supposedly therapeutic bleeding in some lung conditions, including chlorine poisoning on the First World War battlefields. These futile measures were soon abandoned.*

Calomel, the Samson of medicines

Calomel, mercurous chloride, entered into medical practice around 1600, most of all, as we have seen, through the advocacy of Paracelsus, and it remained in currency for three centuries. To Sylvius in the late 17th century it was *mercurius dulcis*, and Leméry referred to it as *sublimé doux*, the sweet sublimate (a substance condensed from the vapour when the parent solid is heated). These names imply that it tasted sweet, but calomel is in fact quite tasteless, so the powder offered to patients must have been contaminated, probably with a lead compound. Its effects were frightful, as some doctors (such as Sydenham) were well aware. Yet in all too many cases the sickness and deaths that it caused were not attributed to its action. A popular form was 'white panacea of mercury', which was a suspension of the calomel in brandy. It was also made into a paste with jalap to enhance therapeutic efficacy by way of a volcanic laxative effect. William Cullen promoted the use of calomel, which he regarded essentially as a purgative, but he was aware that it carried dangers, and was one of the first to apply it externally to the genitals of syphilitics. Used in this manner it had modest effects in healing the sores.

---

* Today bleeding is only used to treat patients with a genetic over-production of red blood cells, which would otherwise cause a dangerous increase in blood viscosity.

The effect of calomel in provoking torrential salivation was held to be to be the outward sign that it was working. Sydenham, who prescribed it in abundance, nevertheless warned against the dangers of excessive doses, but Benjamin Rush would keep administering more and more until it engendered the required output of saliva. The redoubtable surgeon and anatomist, John Hunter (1728-1793) had already, as was his custom, experimented on himself with calomel, and reported that it had induced sore gums, loosening of teeth, and a disagreeable metallic taste in the mouth. Rush disregarded the evidence, the unease of much of the lay public, and the objections of more cautious doctors. He cleaved instead to the conviction that mercurials had the power to sweep out of the body the undefined toxins responsible for disease. In doing this, they substituted for the sickness a 'mercurial disease', which was transitory. Such was Rush's reputation before his exposure that opposition to his brand of 'heroic medicine' was scarcely heard, and even the most important organ of the dissemination of medical information, the *Boston Medical and Surgical Journal*, allowed no critical discussion of the matter. So it was that calomel treatment for almost anything remained in use in the United States long after it had declined (though by no means disappeared) in Europe.

The evidence of what calomel treatment could do was not far to seek. Reports appeared in the same *Boston Medical and Surgical Journal* and elsewhere. In 1827 a Boston physician described the condition of a young woman who had been treated by another doctor. Her 'gums, submaxillary glands, cheeks and tongue were greatly swollen; the latter was covered with a dense, hard, black secretion, the jaws could scarce be separated, the utterance was inarticulate, the flow of saliva was constant'. From the characteristic 'fetor of the breath' the doctor diagnosed mercury poisoning. His patient evidently recovered, but a little girl 'of about ten years old', seen by another New England doctor, was not so fortunate. She 'had taken, in the course of ten days, four cathartic doses of calomel, repeated once in two or three days ..... When I first saw her, the swelling of the parts about the mouth were called canker. The swelling of the parts about the mouth progressed uninterruptedly to gangrene and sphacelation [decay?] of both lips, and the greater part of the right cheek, before her death, had left such a hideous spectacle in the countenance of the child, as made it desirable she might not survive. Our wishes were realized.' There were many more such gruesome accounts, and yet many doctors regarded such symptoms as suppurating gums as a sign that they were on the right track – that the mercury was taking effect. During the American cholera epidemics in the early 19th century children were dosed with amounts of calomel regarded even in foregoing decades as 'fit for a horse'.

Calomel and nostrums containing it were available over the counter, and remained so for another century and more. Ching's Yellow Worm Lozenges and his Brown worm Lozenges were given to children to expel intestinal worms. Directions for preparing them at home were even to be found in a popular manual, *The Complete Confectioner, Pastry Cook, and Baker*, by Eleanor Parkinson, published in Philadelphia in 1844. Here is the recipe for Ching's Yellow Worm Lozenges: fine sugar, 28 pounds, calomel washed in spirits of wine, 1 pound, saffron, 4 drachms; all this to be mixed with gum tragacanth (a viscous plant sap preparation), sufficient to make a paste, and formed into lozenges, each containing one grain of calomel. (A drachm is about 1.8 grams, and a grain about 65 milligrams, amounting to a hefty dose). Ching's Brown Worm Lozenges are not very different, but there follows another recipe, this one for 'Panacea'. This is made up of one ounce of calomel ('panacea of mercury'), 2 ounces 'resin of jalap' and 2 pounds of sugar, all made into a paste with gum tragacanth in rose-water. The lozenges should contain a quarter grain of calomel and a half grain of jalap. How many victims these confections claimed is not known.

The disappearance of mercury compounds from the pharmacopoeias towards the end of the 19th century did not altogether eliminate mercury poisoning from the western world. The origin of a terrible affliction of babies, known as Pink Disease (also sometimes called Feer's Disease, Swift's Disease, or acrodynia) was resolved only in 1948 by a doctor in Cincinnati. The condition took its name from the bright pink extremities of the little victims. The colour spread into the palms and soles, skin would peel, and pus-filled blisters would erupt. Babies in more advanced stages sweated and salivated profusely, their hair, nails and teeth would loosen and fall out, and the muscles would become slack. Further distressing symptoms would develop and deaths were frequent. Survivors were often plagued by ill-health throughout their lives. The cause was of course mercury, in the form again of calomel, an ingredient of commonly used teething powders. Since that time there have been occasional epidemics of mercury poisoning. The most notorious occurred in Japan in the 1950s, when mercury compounds in industrial effluent polluted the seas and contaminated fish. This was called Minamata Disease.

Powder of Saturn and related poisons

Although it did not attract as much attention in the healing arts as mercury, lead also did great damage. It was used for two millennia by physicians and surgeons in China, in India and in Europe, even when the terrible toll in exacted on the lives of lead miners was already clear to all. Dioscorides expatiates on the virtues of lead, as does Pliny. Lead was associated with the planet Saturn, whence the French name, *sucre de Saturne* for lead acetate. Powder of Saturn was an impure form of 'white lead', lead carbonate, and was commonly prescribed for chest complaints, especially asthma and tuberculosis. Lead shot was also sometimes swallowed in the hope of mitigating the symptoms of twisted bowel syndrome, a deformation of the gut. The respected 16th-century physician, Turquet de Mayerne (p.) thought sugar of lead was a safe medicine, which would 'sweeten the humours, as its taste doth witness'. A century later Pierre Pomet (p.) asserted in his great compendium of drugs that lead acetate was a sure cure, even when all else had failed, for internal haemorrhages and gut complaints. The recommended dose was 3 - 4 grains (a hefty 180 - 240 milligrams).

Lead and its compounds, then, are highly toxic. Some historians have suggested that lead poisoning was responsible for the fall of the Roman Empire, for the rich governing classes drank their wine from lead vessels, and would even sweeten their drinks with lead acetate, or 'sugar of lead' as it was often called. Another manifestation of lead poisoning was the 'great colic', which afflicted the citizens of Amsterdam each autumn in medieval times. This was caused by the plane trees bordering the canals that shed their leaves into the lead vessels in which rain water was collected. The rotting leaves made the water acid enough to dissolve some of the lead. In the same way, acidity in wine would have attacked leaden goblets (and, as related above, may have contributed to the rise of gout by leaching lead salts out of lead crystal glass [p.]). Lead oxide was used for centuries in much of Europe to neutralise the increased acidity of wine that was turning to vinegar. (Twentieth-century medical students were also taught about the plight of the London cabman who was always first into the pub in the mornings, and so received the liquid that had stood overnight in the lead pipe, which conveyed the beer from cellar to pump.)

The great champion of lead treatments in the 18th century was a professor of surgery in the medical school at Montpellier, Thomas Goulard. His most famous work was published in 1766, and in English translation as *Treatise on Lead*, seven year later. Goulard despises mercury but rates lead the greatest of remedies, unaccountably neglected during the foregoing years, even though it was well-known to the ancients. He invented a nostrum called Extract of Saturn, prepared by grinding up litharge, boiling it with vinegar (preferably from French wine), letting the sediment settle and collecting the supernatant liquid. In small doses, he specified, it could be given internally, but its chief virtues were expressed in external applications. Mixed with brandy, it was to be used against all manner of inflammations, especially of the eye. Goulard used it for ear problems, including deafness, against wounds, bruises, burns, ulcers, fistulas, haemorrhoids and ruptures, and against cancers and all skin conditions. For many of these, and a variety of other complaints, the Extract could be applied in the form of plasters or ointments. Such pastes had been known since Roman times as *diachylon*, and there were many formulations, the simplest of which consisted of litharge stewed with olive oil and water and used to impregnate a fabric, which could then be applied to sores and wounds as a poultice. More up-market versions incorporated oils, waxes, fragrant resins and other additives. Such concoctions were not without their dangers: applied to wounds, lead compounds could seep into the bloodstream and cause lead poisoning, or plumbism as doctors learned to call it. There were also reports, well into the 19th century even, of lethal diachylon pills, used as abortifacients, but most doctors from the late 18th century onwards opposed ingestion of lead compounds. An exception was Benjamin Rush, sure as ever of his own opinions, who used lead acetate to treat childhood epilepsy (and no doubt also adults). 'I was', he noted, 'first led to prescribe sugar of lead in epilepsy by hearing that a man had been cured of it by swallowing part of a table spoonful by mistake, instead of a table spoonful of loaf sugar'.

No conflicts in Rush's mind, then, between anecdote and a controlled trial, which as we shall see the more discerning physicians were by then espousing. Mostly, by the late 18th century, the use of lead compounds was being restricted to external applications. Even so, lead acetate, the lead oxide, litharge, and the mixture of oxides known as red lead, retained their place in the dispensaries long after knowledge about lead poisoning had become widely disseminated. Indeed, recommendations for the use of lead compounds in the British Pharmacopoeia were already restricted to lotions. They retained their place until the mid-20th century in this form, and may in some cases even have done some good. Lead ointments can still in fact be bought.

One disease, one cure: malaria and the Jesuit's bark

Malaria was endemic and commonly lethal through much of Europe up to modern times. The Pontine marshes in the Lazio province, southeast of Rome, were the most notorious region. Each year as summer approached much of the population of Rome fled. The Vatican, on low land and uncomfortably close to the Tiber, was especially vulnerable, and even the cardinals were reluctant to assemble for their conclave when the pope inopportunely died. In the 16th and 17th centuries, in fact, a succession of popes succumbed to the fever, and in the conclave of 1623, following the death of Gregory XV, ten or more of the 55 assembled cardinals fell ill, of whom several died then or later from malaria. The disease was known in England as tertian or quartan fever (according as the crises seized the sufferer every second or every fourth day), or more commonly as the ague. In Italy it was called malaria, or bad air, for it was thought to arise from the miasma that settled on the marshy land during the season. The Roman scholar, soldier and writer, Marcus Terentius Varro, who lived in the 1st century B.C., suggested in his agricultural treatise, *De Rerum Rusticarum*, that the miasma was composed of microscopic animalculae, which entered the body through the mouth and nose and caused the disease; this was an inspired conjecture. Bleeding was the most common treatment for malaria, but there were many folk remedies, involving animals, whose breath was supposed to carry beneficial properties, and the ingestion of various fruits and herbs, to the accompaniment of ritual incantations.

But by the mid-17th century an effective treatment was at hand, the first drug with a defined target in the history of medicine. Peruvian bark seems first to have been mentioned in Europe around 1630 in the writings of a monk, apothecary to the main hospital in Rome. An apocryphal story had spread around Europe that the wife of the Spanish Viceroy in Lima, Doña Francisca Henriquez be Ribero, having been copiously bled to no effect, was miraculously brought back from the brink of death by an infusion of a mysterious tree bark, brought from the rain forest by a Jesuit missionary. (In reality the lady had apparently been in good health throughout her stay in Peru, and died on the voyage home to Spain.) It was evidently, in fact, an Augustinian Friar, Antonio de la Calancha, who drew the miraculous substance to the attention of the Europeans. Calancha was born and grew up on the Bolivian Altiplano among the local Indians. He reported that a tree found at high altitudes in the district of Loja in Peru was known as the tree of fevers, and a drink prepared from its bark had worked marvellous cures on sufferers from tertian fevers in Lima. Debate continues still on whether the medicinal virtues of the tree were known to the Indians long before the Europeans came, or were discovered by missionaries. In 1639, at all events, a Jesuit, Father Bernabé Cobó published a History of the New World, in which he alluded to 'a tree for the ague', from which was derived a powder, already celebrated in Europe, and in high demand in Rome. Yet the European physicians viewed it for the most part with mistrust, and some, like Guy Patin, with outright derision. The remedy was variously described as Peruvian bark, Jesuit's bark or quinquina, from the local Indian expression. In England suspicion fell on it because of its Jesuit connection: was it perhaps a papist plot to foist an insidious poison on the Protestant land? There was also some confusion between the prodigious bark and that of the Peruvian balsam tree, which was therapeutically useless. Nevertheless, the apothecaries realised that the genuine article was a powerful specific for malarial fevers. Unfortunately, though, the distinction between this condition and fevers of other origins was not clearly defined, and consequently the treatment was not always effective. This, indeed, set a pattern for the misuse of the few useful drugs available to doctors, ever in search of a panacea: a substance that had proved its efficacy against one condition would then be prescribed for a myriad of unrelated illnesses, and would accordingly fall out of favour. Also, since cinchona bark had to be imported into Europe at great expense, some physicians and apothecaries tried to make do with the bark of indigenous trees, such as the cherry, a cause of further obfuscation. But worst of all, the concept of a cure applicable to a single disease was incompatible with the dogma of the humours, and the bark was therefore rejected by practitioners who adhered to the traditional teachings.

In Italy, though, the bark caught on. Pope Urban VIII, beneficiary of the deaths of his predecessor and rival candidates for the top job, became a patron of one of the great centres of medicine in Europe, the Ospedale Santo Spirito in Rome. The pope appointed as director of the hospital pharmacy a Spaniard, Juan de Lugo, a Jesuit and academic lawyer, later created Cardinal. De Lugo and his chief apothecary promoted the Peruvian bark, and received shipments from the Jesuits in Peru, especially through the good offices of a monk, Agustino Salumbrino, who had established a great pharmacy in Lima. Thanks to their efforts the terrors of the Roman fevers receded. But elsewhere in Europe there was still resistance. In 1653 the Archduke Leopold Wilhelm of Austria, Governor of Belgium, caught the fever. His personal physician, Jean-Jacques Chiflet, a true reactionary, was reluctantly persuaded to treat his master with the bark. The fever abated, but a month later it returned, and the Archduke, incensed by the failure of the promised cure, refused a second course. More, he instructed Chiflet to issue a denunciation of the Jesuit's bark. His pamphlet on the 'exposure of the febrifuge as a fraud, inferior to myrrh and other older febrifuges and liable to putrefy the humours, drew a powerful response from a pseudonymous Jesuit scholar in Rome. Strident exchanges continued, and the Protestants, especially in England, continued to oppose the use of the bark.

By the time the Lord Protector Cromwell, who had spent much of his life in the malarial Essex marshes, had been struck down by the ague and treated with the Peruvian bark, many of the country's physicians had, however reluctantly, acknowledged its value. In 1658 advertisements for 'that excellent powder known by the name of the Jesuits Powder, which cureth all manner of Agues, Quotidian, Tertian, or Quartan' appeared in London. It was to be had 'at the Black-Spred-Eagle over against Black and White Court in the Old Baily, or at the shop of Mr John Crook, at the sign of the ship in St Pauls Churchyard, a bookseller, with directions for using the same'. The very mention of Jesuits was imprudent and undoubtedly roused suspicions, but then the powder found a much cleverer champion. Robert Talbor (sometimes Tabor and also Talbot) was a precocious entrepreneur, who, like Cromwell, hailed from Cambridgeshire. He had entered St John's College, Cambridge but left without graduating, and then served an apprenticeship in an apothecary's shop, where he must have encountered the miracle drug. For in 1670, at the age of 28, he set himself up as a pyretiatro, or fever specialist – a profession he invented for himself. He advertised his skills in a book with the audacious title, *Pyretologia, or A Rational Account of the Cause of Agues*. Talbor was evidently a man of wit and ingenuity. To avert Protestant suspicions he warned against incautious use of the Jesuits' powder, which could destroy health. He himself had formulated a sure cure for the ague, which consisted of four ingredients, one of which was of course Peruvian bark, but he would disclose only that it was 'a preparation of four vegetables, whereof two are foreign and the other domestick'. Talbor started his book with a sprightly verse:

> The Learned Author in a generous Fit
> T'oblige his Country hath of Agues Writ.
> Physicians now shall be reproacht no more
> Nor Essex shake with Agues as before
> Since certain health salutes her sickly shoar.

The remedy came to the ears of King Charles II, apparently through a French officer at court, whom Talbor had cured. The King, ever fascinated by new discoveries, was impressed with Talbor and in due course appointed him one of his physicians (no matter that he had no medical qualifications), then in 1678 bestowed a knighthood on him. It may have been the King who sent him to France to treat the daughter of the Duke of Orléans, brother to Louis VIII, but in any event Talbor turned up in Paris and proceeded to effect startling cures with what became known as his *remède anglais*. He became the personal physician to King Louis's niece, by now the Queen of Spain. Talbor's name appears frequently in the famous letters of Madame de Sévigné. The Chevalier Talbor had brought back from the brink of death a succession of the French nobility: 'son remède a fait des merveilles cette année'. One friend 'en a été guéri comme par miracle, et milles autres'. Then the Dauphin caught the fever, and Talbor promised the King on his life that he would perform cure. This sealed Talbor's reputation and secured him a reward of 2000 *louis-d'or*. The King persuaded Talbor to part with the recipe of his remedy, but on condition that it would not be published until after its author's death. That ensued all too soon: Talbor returned to England in 1681 and died in Cambridge, adorned with many honours, a few months later. It took five years for an account of the remède anglais to appear in print in France – where in due course it was even celebrated in a poem by La Fontaine - and later the same year in translation in England. It emerged that the main ingredient, besides cinchona bark, was wine, and Talbor had also thrown in some lemon juice and rose leaves.

Talbor's success infuriated the medical establishment, who reviled him as an 'empiric', a mere 'debauched apothecary's apprentice', a quack, and in the main refused to countenance the use of his fever remedy, or for that matter the Jesuit's powder. But Talbor's nostrum was reputed to have saved the King's life. John Evelyn, writing albeit more than a decade after the event, recorded in his diary a conversation which featured 'much discourse concerning the Quinquean which the Physitians would not give the King, at a time when in a dangerous Ague it was the onely thing could ever cure him, out of envy, because it has been brought into vogue by Mr. Tabore an Apothecary; Til Dr. Short (to whom the K. sent to have his opinion of it privately, he being reputed a papist, but was in troth a very honest good Chrristian): he sent him word, it was the onely thing could save his life, and then the King, injoyn'd his physitians to give it him, and was recovered: Being asked by this Lord why they would not prescribe it: Dr. Lower [the

King's doctor] said, it would spoil their practise or some such expression: and at last confessed it was a Remedy fit onely for Kings.' The moguls of the College of Physicians must have been even more discomfited when the most respected of them all, Thomas Sydenham convinced himself that the Peruvian bark, and come to that Talbor's remedy, did indeed work. In 1676 he commended its use in his magisterial textbook, *Observationes medicae*. Even ten years earlier, in his first book, *Methodus curandi fibres*, he had made cautious reference to the drug. Sydenham's endorsement dealt a heavy blow to the old tradition of medicine, based on the four humours and bloodletting, and could be said to have begun a new and more enlightened movement.

The wide recognition of the value of the Peruvian bark initiated a search for the tree throughout South America. Related species were found in several locations, and the different values of the white (useless), yellow (better) and red (best) types of bark were properly recorded. A depot was established by the Spanish at Cartagena in Colombia for the processing and export of bark, although it became clear that the product of the Colombian species was less effective. We owe to the founder of taxonomy, Linnaeus the modern name for the *quinquina* tree of the Indians: he coined for the genus the systematic term, *Cinchona*, in honour of the legendary Countess of Chinchón (who had had nothing to do with it). Attempts were made to create plantations of the trees in India and the Dutch East Indies with only modest success. It was only in the early 19th century that the active principle, quinine, was isolated, as we shall see.

Meanwhile malaria continued to take its toll of Europeans venturing into alien climes. The military were the most conspicuous victims. A famous debacle, attributed to malaria occurred in 1809, when the Government in London decided to strike a blow against Napoleon's rampant forces in the Low Countries, which were said to be 'pointing a pistol' at the head of England. The campaign was slow in preparation and incompetent in execution. In July a force of 40,000 soldiers was landed by ships of the Royal Navy on the island of Walcheren in the Scheldt estuary. By August the men were being tormented by mosquitoes, which thrived in the marshy reclaimed land. The provisions of Peruvian bark and other medicines were minimal, and within weeks the Army medical services were overwhelmed by the needs of sick and dying men. More than 40% of the force fell victim to fevers, from which some 4000 died (compared to about 100 killed by the enemy). The military physicians and surgeons, few enough in number, mostly cleaved to the ancient doctrine that fevers were generated by a miasma – toxic vapours from the decaying vegetation of the marshes – and demanded purification of the victims' contaminated blood, in other words bleeding, purging and emetics. Tobacco was also considered a help. The expeditionary force was withdrawn after four calamitous months amidst much acrimony and many recriminations. Recent research on the symptoms of Walcheren fever, as it became known (or sometimes Flushing sickness from the name of the town on the island), has indicated that malaria, then termed intermittent fever, was only a part of the problem. The most lethal form of malaria, caused by the parasite, *Plasmodium falciparum*, had not reached northern Europe, nor did other symptoms always conform to those of malaria. It is thought nonetheless that malaria, compounded by dysentery, typhus and other infections, may have wrought much of the damage, but those conditions alone probably also caused many deaths. It was in Africa that malaria decimated the European, as well as African populations, as it still does.

From panaceas to specifics

The 18th century Enlightenment was accompanied by the rise of empirical – evidence-based – medicine. Reliance on what is now referred to as 'anecdotal evidence' was gradually replaced by the concept of controlled trials. A more cautious and sceptical approach to therapy was now in evidence, and with it a new attitude towards secret remedies, which now provoked the disapproval of the more respectable elements of the medical profession. Another sign of progress was the gradual decline of the panacea concept, which led to the discovery of only the second specific remedy for a single more or less well-defined condition. Remedies that were later identified with a single disease were still used indiscriminately. One such was cod (or other fish) liver oil, which had been known as a folk remedy for centuries, and in China much longer. Pliny refers to the use of dolphin liver oil, both externally and internally, for skin conditions, while in European fishing communities it was held to be generally good for health. The medical profession took little notice until the 18th century, when Dr Thomas Percival of Manchester began to broadcast its virtues, and in 1771 introduced it into the *British Pharmacopoeia*. He urged its use in cases of 'obstinate chronic rheumatism, sciatica, 'premature decrepitude, which originates in immoderate labour, repeated strains and bruises, or exposure to continuous dampness and cold'. He wished, he said, to see it introduced into hospitals and workhouses. Some 50 years later fish oils were coming into use in France and Germany for the treatment of 'scrofular affections'. Percival proudly asserted: 'This medicine is dispensed so largely in the hospital here, that near a hogshead is annually consumed'. (A hogshead is 239 litres, or 48 gallons.) And according to a letter in the *Association Medical Journal* (precursor of the *British Medical Journal*) by another Manchester doctor, his hospital got through 50-60 gallons per year. It is remarkable that the patients were willing to put up with the taste of the oil, which was made by squeezing out rotting fish livers, on such a scale. After the discovery of iodine and its curative capacity (p.), for goitre in particular, the theory took hold that cod liver oil owed its efficacy to its iodine content. But when analyses showed that it in general contained very little iodine, the oil went out of fashion, to be rediscovered half a century later.

Misapprehensions about how therapeutic substances might act were allied to loose definitions of the conditions they were purported to cure or alleviate. The appellations, rheumatism for instance, might serve to describe any of a variety of debilitating states. Arsenic compounds were commonly recommended for such ailments during the 18th century and even later, most often in the form of an oxide, 'white arsenic'. It had featured in Chinese medicine for centuries, and the iatrochemists had used it in addition to mercury. Despite its known toxicity, and the part it played in many notorious murders and accidental poisonings*, many European physicians continued to prescribe it in alarming doses even in the early 19th century. There were many arsenical medicines to be had during this period, some in the pharmacopoeias, such as the deadly Donovan's solution, prepared from mercury and arsenic iodides, and Lanfranc's collyrium for treatment of eye complaints, a mixture containing, among other ingredients, white wine, verdigris (copper carbonate), and orpiment (arsenic trisulphide). But the most famous arsenical nostrum was Fowler's solution, initially sold under the innocuous-sounding name, *Solutio mineralis*, and later more candidly as *Liquor arsenicalis*. It was composed of arsenious oxide dissolved in a potassium carbonate solution (forming potassium arsenite) and an extract of lavender. It was devised by Thomas Fowler (1736-1801), a doctor and apothecary in rural Staffordshire. Fowler was well aware of its alarming toxicity, but also convinced that in controlled dosed it had powerful curative properties. His treatise, *Medical Reports of the Effects of Arsenic*, published in 1786, convinced many of his confrères of the validity of this proposition. The concoction appeared in the pharmacopoeias and was prescribed for fevers (especially the malarial 'ague'), asthma, epilepsy, goitre, pernicious anaemia and such conditions as loss of libido. Many doctors apparently came to consider it a panacea. Fowler himself was in no doubt about its exceptional virtues. He tried it on many patients and persuaded himself that it had wrought prodigious cures. 'I flatter myself', he wrote, 'its Reputation will soon be established on so firm a Basis as to render it highly useful, not only to the present, but future Generations.' Fowler's solution retained its high reputation for many years, during which doctors discovered a long succession of applications for everything from asthma to rheumatism, and the suffering of many patients was compounded by its use. Several offered it as a tonic.

---

* Arsenical pigments were responsible for many such, especially the infamous Scheele's Green (copper hydrogen arsenite, first prepared by the great Swedish chemist, Karl Wilhelm Scheele). It was used to colour wallpapers and women's dresses, and most scandalously cakes and sweets. Exposure to the skin and inhalation of the dust from decaying wallpaper caused poisoning and sometimes cancer. It has been conjectured that one victim was Napoleon in exile on St. Helena.

Some arsenic compounds could be absorbed through the skin, and much damage must have been done through their use in treating skin diseases, including cancers. Marsden's arsenical mucilage was another dangerous brew. It was invented by William Marsden, a noted surgeon who in 1851 founded the Brompton Cancer Hospital in west London, now the Royal Marsden Hospital. The mucilage consisted of arsenious oxide and gum acacia, made into a paste with water and applied to the skin excrescences, which were supposed to fall off as a crust some hours after the paste had dried. This treatment would probably have ensured that the cancer grew. Many lethal patent medicines containing arsenic were peddled by quacks. A popular (and ineffective) antidote to snakebites, favoured by the British military in India, was the Tanjore pill, which contained arsenic and black pepper with some mercury added for good measure, and root extracts

One of the most curious applications of arsenic was in 'arsenophagy', a practice followed during the 19th century in the Alpine province of Styria in Austria. Arsenic in the form of mineral deposits was apparently consumed in remarkable quantities by the local people to give a bloom to the complexion (probably an early symptom of poisoning), render the skin softer and make the female figure provokingly plump. It was also believed to strengthen the breathing and therefore endurance when climbing. The reported quantities of arsenic ingested by these people would suggest that a mithridating effect – development of tolerance - brought about by gradually increasing the dose from an initial low level, was in play. Arsenicals were gradually expunged from the pharmacopoeias over the next hundred years, but came selectively into use again in the first half of the 20th century.

Less harmful but wholly ineffective were powders and pills of various earths and stones, favoured as antidotes against poisons and snakebites. They were generally imported from remote climes and were correspondingly costly. The best were held to come from the Mediterranean, from islands, such as Lemnos and especially Malta, the *Terra Melitlosis*, which would come with a certificate of provenance, probably most often forged.

A major 18th-century innovation was the introduction of animal experiments to evaluate the effects of drugs and their safety. Up to then it was generally thought that nothing an experimenter might learn from the effects of drugs or poisons on animals could have any bearing on how a human would react. An early example of the lessons that could be drawn from animal experiments concerned the medicinal use of hydrocyanic acid, also known as prussic acid. This notorious poison was encountered most commonly in the form of cherry-laurel water. The cherry laurel is a shrub, which was long held to have medicinal properties. The leaves contain a compound, prulaurasin, chemically related to amygdalin, the bitter-almond essence in apricot kernels, which acquired notoriety in the 20th century as a spurious cancer cure (p.). When the cherry-laurel leaves were steeped in water and distilled the prulaurasin was partly decomposed by the heat, giving rise to a small amount of hydrocyanic acid and benzaldehyde, a compound with a fragrance and taste of bitter almonds. The hydrocyanic acid itself is often wrongly said to taste of bitter almonds, but those who can detect it experience an almond-like odour. (Whether one is or is not capable of detecting it is genetically determined.) At all events, cherry-laurel water was used in the past as a flavouring for drinks and puddings.

In 1731 the dangers of this practice became apparent. A surgeon and anatomist at Trinity College, Dublin submitted a letter to a learned journal, the *Philosophical Transactions of the Royal Society* in London, which began: 'A very extraordinary Accident that fell out some Months ago has discovered to us a most dangerous Poison, which was never before known to be so, though it has been in frequent Use among us.' It was evidently a custom in Dublin to add a shot of cherry-laurel water to brandy, but the concentration of hydrocyanic acid would have varied widely between one preparation and another, depending on the amount of leaves, probably their age, and the amount of water used to prepare the extract. On this occasion a shopkeeper who sold the water gave a bottle to her servant, Martha Boyse, who passed it on to her mother, Anne, 'as a very rich Cordial'. Mrs Boyse gave it to her sister, also a shopkeeper, who in turn sold some of the contents to Mary Whaley. The sister and Mary Whaley shared two ounces (nearly 60 ml), presumably in brandy, of which the latter took two-thirds. After 15 minutes she was seized with 'violent Disorders of the stomach', was carried home and died an hour later. Her dismayed companion sent word to her sister, Anne Boyse, who insisted that the laurel-cherry water could not possibly have been the cause of her sister's friend's death, and to prove it drank three spoonfuls, and then another two. And, 'She was hardly well seated in her Chair, when she died, without the least Groan or Convulsion'. Dr Maddern, the author of the letter, went on to describe a series of experiments on dogs, which he undertook to demonstrate the toxic properties of the water. Many animals were sacrificed to make the point. Small doses, given by mouth or enema, led to convulsions, from which the dog might recover, larger doses to desperate attempts to breathe and paralysis of the limbs, and death soon followed.

This early attempt to relate an effect to the magnitude of the dose was pursued by many subsequent experimenters on many kinds of animals. The belief grew that any substance with such potent physiological effects as the laurel-cherry water must, in carefully controlled doses, have some therapeutic potential also. The best-known exponent of the theory was Browne Langrish, an English country doctor, remembered now for some wide-ranging physiological studies. Langrish was apparently persuaded that cherry-laurel water might turn out to have useful curative properties. He satisfied himself of its high toxicity by killing a dog, and thereupon decided that to test the effects of small doses reproducible preparations were essential – a considerable conceptual advance. He weighed the laurel leaves and extracted them with a defined volume of water. He gave a small daily dose to a dog for a month with no discernible ill-effect, then twice that dose, again with no sign of any distress. The dog put on weight and Langrish also thought that its arterial blood was of a fine bright colour, so the treatment, he concluded, must be doing the animal good. He carried out a series of measurements on the blood, and took its impaired clot formation to imply that the blood was being beneficially 'thinned'. Langrish published his results (*Physical Experiments upon Brutes*) in 1746, and urged the use of the laurel water as a general-purpose tonic.

This does not seem to have caught on at the time, but not long after the great Swedish apothecary, Carl Wilhelm Scheele, commemorated as the co-discoverer of oxygen and much else (p.), isolated hydrocyanic acid from an inorganic precursor. This meant that the active principle of cherry-laurel water was now available in its pure, therefore reproducible state, and with proper care could be administered with only a small risk of killing the patient. It accordingly came into use for the treatment of a range of conditions, especially after its espousal by the great French physiologist, François Magendie – the chief target of the Victorian anti-vivisection movement. ('Tais-toi, pauvre bête' he would tell the shrieking, writhing creature under his knife.) Magendie, in a paper in 1817, recommended the use of hydrocyanic acid for the treatment of tuberculosis and other lung conditions. His reasoning was based on a careful study of its physiological effects, and the treatment was probably quite often beneficial. It also came into use for the easing of throat spasms and as a sedative, and retained its place in the French, British and American pharmacopoeias for close on a century, in the company of other poisons. The widely consulted 4th edition of J. Moore Neligan's *Medicines – Uses and Mode of Administration* pronounced hydrocyanic acid helpful for a range of conditions, as well as various arsenic, antimony and mercury compounds, and it even recommended ergot – the fungus of rye responsible for outbreaks of the deadly ergotism, or St. Anthony's Fire - to stimulate contractions during childbirth. The last mention of hydrocyanic acid in English pharmacopoeias seems to have been in 1909. More effective, and certainly safer, remedies for the conditions it was purported to alleviate became available in the first two decades of the 20th century.

Hydrocyanic acid was of course by no means the only deadly medicine deployed by 18th-century physicians. Hemlock, forever commemorated as the lethal draught downed by Socrates, was another that enjoyed a considerable vogue, enhanced by an enthusiastic commendation from a rising Viennese doctor, Anton Storck (1731-1803) in 1760. He was aware of its reputation as a poison, but as all the world knew, he insisted, there was nothing that a benevolent deity had not created to be of some use to his creatures. And so Storck prepared a sample from the hemlock plant, *Cicuta vulgaris*, and having noted its unpleasant odour, tried some on a dog. The dog made no objection, and thus encouraged Storck took a grain (about 50 milligrams) twice a day. When, after eight days, he felt no reaction he doubled the dose, again without effect. When he applied some of the solid to his tongue there was indeed a reaction: the tongue swelled painfully and stiffened, and for some time he was unable to speak. This was apparently enough to persuade him and his confrères in Vienna of hemlock's potency, and it became a favoured treatment for cancer, ulcers and a number of other disorders. Its use spread when Storck's treatise on the plant was published and translated into several languages. He also tried other toxic plants, such as henbane and used them as remedies. Storck prospered and became dean of the Medical School, Rector of the University, and after treating the Empress Maria Theresa for smallpox, from which she recovered, was created a Baron and her personal physician. How many patients died of hemlock poisoning is not recorded.

The irrepressible quacks

Despite the animus of the professional bodies against patent medicines and secret remedies the quacks still flourished, and secret formulae were of course the basis of their success. If the 18th century is its golden age, quackery did not greatly decline for at least another hundred years. Even now there is enough gullibility in the population to ensure that the practice will endure, for as Voltaire put it, quackery was born when the first knave met the first fool. Look in Dr Johnson's Dictionary and you will find the following definitions of a quack: '1. A boastful pretender to the arts which he does not understand. 2. A vain boastful pretender to physic, one who proclaims his own Medical abilities in public places. 3. An artful tricking practitioner in physic.' Yet even many of the most notorious quacks in the 18th century had some experience of medicine; some had been apprenticed to physicians or surgeons, others had attended medical schools for a few years, and some were trained as apothecaries. There was therefore a broad spectrum from those who honestly believed in the nostrums that they offered (like the homeopaths today) to the out-and-out mountebanks. Joshua ('Spot') Ward, of the infamous 'Pill and Drop' (of which it was said that 'their action was rough upwards and downwards') was one of the latter. He was a malefactor, who had served time in the pillory and in prison, and apparently devised, or had more likely stolen his recipe in France, where he fled to escape justice. A contemporary London physician observed that Ward's activities were 'too well known among the undertakers and coffin makers and sextons of this City', for it was only Ward who had acquired the 'art to kill with one Drop only, while others must fill phials and sometimes quart bottles so to do'. Or, as a doggerel of the day had it,

> Before you take his Drop and Pill
> Take leave of Friends and make your will.

Ward nevertheless treated the King (George II), who apparently took a liking to him. In the words of Pope's tart couplet

> Of late, without the least pretence to skill,
> Ward's grown a famed physician by his pill.

Many of the longest-enduring quack medicines profited from endorsements by the nobility or even the monarch. Queen Anne seems to have been one of the most credulous of all. William Read began as a tailor or possibly a cobbler, and then went into practice as an oculist. His comprehensive ignorance of the anatomy and physiology of the eye is exposed in his book (possibly, however, written by a paid hack), *Account of all the Diseases incidental to the Eye*, of which the intelligible parts were found to have been plagiarised. A large section of the book is shrewdly devoted to 'Some errors committed by the pretended Practitioners for the Eyes', in which he denounces ancient folk remedies, such as the application of 'the juice of goose dung', and 'the white part of hen's dung'. On the strength apparently of a few dubious operations and his 'styptic water', he rose to the position of oculist to the Queen and after her death to George I. Read was knighted by Queen Anne for his services. He was succeeded by a most notorious quack, oculist to the quality, including George II, the bombastic 'Chevalier' John Taylor, who Dr Johnson said, was an exemplar of 'how far impudence will carry ignorance'.

Many of the quacks of the period made fortunes from their trade. Joanna Stephens was one who advertised widely and guaranteed to eliminate 'the stone', an affliction that, like gout, was the source of much agony. Operations, conducted without anaesthetic, were hazardous with a high mortality rate, due to infection. Samuel Pepys was successfully operated for a bladder stone, which had blighted his life in the foregoing years; it was the size, he noted, of a tennis ball (even if the royal-tennis ball was smaller than the modern lawn-tennis kind). Sufferers were therefore easy prey. Joanna Stephens, at all events, was widely believed, and demanded extravagant fees for her services. Then in 1738 she placed an advertisement in the *Gentlemen's Magazine*, offering to sell the secret of her remedy for what was then the enormous sum of £5000. A public subscription, with contributions from the nobility and from churchmen, raised only £1365. This did not satisfy Joanna, and a public uproar ensued: the secret of the wonderful remedy must not be lost. A petition to Parliament led to the creation of a commission of archbishops, the Lord Chancellor, Government functionaries and a collection of physicians and surgeons to consider the evidence for the efficacy of the medicine. Four witnesses, all martyrs to the stone, were summoned, having been examined by doctors before and after a course of the treatment. The commission found that 'the utility, efficiency and resolving power thereof' were beyond doubt and stumped up. When the magic formula was disclosed it turned out to contain dried herbs, snail shells, a great deal of soap and lime water, and as time went on there were fewer and fewer reports of successful treatments. There then began the excuses, familiar to all who have come up against a retreat from a firmly held position: did it, the learned men of science asked, matter whether the source of the lime water was limestone of shells, and what of the provenance of the soap? One of them, Robert Whytt, President of the Edinburgh Royal College of Medicine, published *An Essay on the Virtues of Lime Water in the Cure of the Stone*, in which he expatiated on the necessity of ingesting soap, which has 'Power of dissolving the Stone but likewise will destroy all acid Humours of the Stomach and the Guts and contribute greatly to keep the Belly easy and prevent Costiveness that might otherwise be occasioned by the Lime Water'. Sufferers, of whom the Prime Minister, Sir Robert Walpole was one, were already consuming vast quantities of soap to no effect.

In time Joanna Stephens and the £5000 were forgotten, and other quacks came to the fore. There was Baron Schwanberg's 'Liquid Shell', which in 1749 was 'Daily confirmed by Experience not only to be a sure Dissolvent for the Stone and Gravel but a most powerful and efficacious Medicine in the Spasmodic and windy Cholic, Pains in the Breast, Hypochondriacal

Diseases [!], and all kinds of Flatulence, Diarrhaea or Looseness, Cardialgia, or Heart-burn, acid Eructation, or sour Belching...' and more. None of the concoctions were any more effective than the sympathetic medicine procured by killing a cock, taking the stones out of its gizzard and pounding them to a powder. In the United States the quacks thrived at least as well as in Britain. Mrs. Sybilla Masters from Philadelphia (remembered also as an inventor) produced the first patented medicine in 1711 and brought it to England (where it did not catch on) the following year. It was called Tuscarura Rice, was supposed to cure consumption and other conditions, and was nothing more than finely ground maize (cornmeal). Philadelphia was the centre of the fake medicine business, and where Mrs Masters led many enterprising operators followed, with Dr Bateman's Pectoral Drops, Daffy's Elixir Salutis and many more.

A famous case, perhaps of delusion more than outright quackery, for the perpetrator probably cherished a belief in his method, occurred in French Canada in the late 18th century. A learned divine, who was also a qualified surgeon, the Abbé Pierre-Joseph Compain advertised his remedy for skin tumours (which may have been cancerous, or merely canker sores) in Quebec and Montreal. It was to be applied as a poultice and would quickly cause the growths to fall off. In 1794 the Abbé induced a number of doctors to purchase samples, some of whom reported remarkable cures. The Abbé finally gave the recipe to the nuns who nursed the patients in the Hôtel-Dieu hospital in Quebec and to the sisters of an Ursuline convent. The deal was that they would all pray for its inventor's health, and not divulge the formula before his death.* When the composition was eventually revealed, it turned out to consist of compacted oats, moistened with water, and wrapped in cobwebs.

The horrors of mercury therapy encouraged quacks to tout an endless variety of supposed treatments for syphilis. Various roots and barks were in fact thought to have a beneficial effect, including sarsaparilla and

---

* The use of nuns as praying machines capable of precipitating amounts of divine favour had a long history. Cardinal Richelieu was one of the princes of the Church who founded orders of nuns specially for the purpose during the Thirty Years War in the previous century.

guaiacum. One of the most enduring potions was Zittmann's Decoction, which came in two strengths, of which the more potent actually contained mercurial compounds. It was devised early in the 18th century by a Saxon army doctor, Johann Friedrich Zittmann and was still in occasional use two centuries later. The choice then was between the weak form, which was wholly inert, and the other, which would give the innocent user an expensive bout of mercury poisoning. It comprised a large measure of calomel, some cinnabar (mercuric sulphide), and alum (the less toxic potassium aluminium sulphate), sugar, sarsaparilla root and fennel, cinnamon, anis and other spices. The fate of syphilitics of the period is summed up in this epitaph to one Thomas Bamford:

> No Marble Monument shall cover
> The Grave of this poor Martyr's Lover,
> Here lie no Bones nor Flesh, but rather
> *Guaiacum*, and *Sassaphras*,
> And *Turpentine*, the Quacks' disgrace,
> Have sent Tom Bamford God knows whither.

One of the most egregious of all the shifty personalities who inhabit the long chronicles of quackery flourished in the early years of the 19th century. John St John Long was born in Limerick in 1797, and became a tolerably successful portrait painter. He somehow acquired some exiguous medical knowledge and moved to London, having evidently decided on a career as a medical confidence trickster. He let it be known that he could infallibly diagnose and then cure tuberculosis, a prevalent and much-feared disease. His technique was to drop a little sulphuric acid on the victim's skin to generate an unpleasant sore, to which he then applied an ointment of undivulged composition, which was in reality an irritant to prevent the sore from healing. The suppurating wound, he explained to his patients was drawing out of the body the evil humour of the disease, which the poor patient undoubtedly had. By this means, Long, who extracted large sums from his victims, got rich. But in 1829, John Wakley, the crusading founder and editor of the medical journal, the *Lancet*, decided that Long must not be allowed to continue to get away with these shameful activities. He wrote a strong editorial, accusing Long of imposture and exploitation of the public's ignorance. Long reacted with a letter proclaiming his noble campaign of saving lives, and quoting testimonials from his many patients. Wakley merely commented in reply: 'Mr. The Lancet Long should not write thus when he talks of "my mode of treatment", and while he keeps that treatment a profound secret. Had Mr. St. John Long any means of curing consumption, he should not hesitate to make it known. Concealment in such cases is a bad feature, and to the well informed a sufficient proof of HUMBUG.'

This exchange in the *Lancet* did not impede Long's progress, but the following year nemesis of a kind overtook him: a 24-year-old woman died, it was presumed from his ministrations. Long was arraigned on a charge of manslaughter and found guilty, Wakley himself having appeared for the woman's family. The judge, evidently disagreeing with the jury's view, imposed a fine of £250 (equivalent to several thousands in today's money), which Long, who was rich, paid on the spot. (It was said, however, that the court was besieged by Long's female admirers - of whom there were many, for he was handsome and charming – and that they organised a collection to pay off the debt.) Long continued on his course until, not long after, a second patient died. This time, despite much public indignation, he was acquitted for want of sufficient evidence. Long's infamous career was brought to an end only by his death, ironically from consumption, at the age of 37. Wakley composed a fitting epitaph in the *Lancet*: 'As that archimpostor JOHN LONG has ceased to live, a worthy votary of his living in Camden-town has advertised that he is in possession of Long's "secret". If the nobility should nibble at a bait like this, they are lost past redemption. It is our duty to tell this simple advertiser that the "secret" of every knave is *dishonesty*'. Long is buried in Kensal Green Cemetery in London beneath an ostentatious marble monument with a long inscription, adverting to 'the benefits derived from his remedial discovery'. Thomas Wakely lies within shouting distance, beneath a modest memorial.

The public prints all carried an endless succession of quack medicines guaranteed to cure any condition. An editorial in the *Lancet* in 1905 surveys the advertisements for quack medicines in the *Times* of London and the *Observer* of 100 year before. In those days (and up to the mid-20th century) the front page of the *Times* carried only advertisements, and on a typical day near the end of the 18th century nearly half were for quack nostrums. They bore such names as Dr. James's Analeptic Pills, Dr. Solomon's Balm of Gilead Cordial, Madden's Vegetable Essence for asthma, coughs, consumption &c., Robbards' improved Balsamic Elixir – the litany continues. Most were accompanied by affidavits from purported satisfied patients, endorsements from bishops, Members of Parliament and peers of the realm, and such modest promises as 'The following remarkable cures of Cancers, without incision, by Mrs. Plunket Edgcumbe of Bath, may be depended on, as the Cancers are preserved in Spirits'. Again, Howley's Invaluable Fever Pills, of which a mere two had 'Cured Mr. John Sartin, a shoe-maker, supposed to be on his death-bed, of a violent Fever, of which his Wife had died, and he never ailed anything for 20 years after.' Then there was 'that excellent Pill of the late eminent and worthy Dr. Trigg of Tower Wharf', the Golden Vatican Pill, 'famous for the Cure of most Diseases of either sex', of which there is a long and spine-chilling list. In some cases there was the address at which the pills or potions might be bought, but in most cases it was a postal address at which application could be made, enclosing an invariably hefty sum of money. Perhaps the most abundant and enduring quack medicine was Dr James's Fever Powder, already mentioned. Dr Robert James took out a patent on his formula in 1746, and over a twenty-year period almost 2 million of his pills were bought; they were still being bought in the early part of the 20th century. The politician, man of letters, and champion hypochondriac, Horace Walpole declared that James's fraudulent remedy could 'cure most complaints that are not mortal or chronical'. The precise composition seems never to have been established, but the active, and lethal, ingredient was an antimony compound. A surprising number of quacks, as also reported in the *Lancet*, were associated with religious organisations. The *Methodist Times* was one paper that carried many advertisements and puffs, such as a full page (as noted by the *Lancet*) on the miraculous successes of one 'Professor Hern', specialist 'in the cure of "hopeless" cases and so-called "incurable diseases"'. The Professor had achieved 'astounding cures' of unfortunates afflicted by dire maladies, 46 of which are listed, together with their symptoms, followed by testimonials from ministers of the Methodist Church.

Some of the leading quacks advertised their wares through posters and handbills distributed around the towns. Many were made memorable by verses. Well-known around London was Dr Case, who offered to cure venereal diseases:

> All ye that are of Venus' race
> Apply yourself to Dr. Case –
> Who with a box or two of pills
> Will soon remove your painful ills.

Quackery was of course equally prevalent in other countries. Useless and dangerous nostrums were abundantly peddled in the United States, and in France and Italy. Fioraventi's balm (*baume de Fioraventi*), devised by an Italian, was one of the most long-lived, and consisted largely of alcohol with a dash of turpentine and various aromatics. And from Palermo emerged, in Thomas Carlyle's words, 'the quack of quacks', 'Count' Cagliostro (born Giuseppe Balsamo in 1743). Cagliostro was a many-sided confidence trickster and libertine, who insinuated himself into the French aristocracy and cut a swathe through a succession of countries, including England, He had some knowledge of drugs, which he employed profitably, but he saw the interiors of several prisons and died in one of them at the age of 52.

In France there appeared in the middle of the 19th century a mysterious and other-worldly figure, with the *nom de guerre* of Doctor Noir. He hailed, it was said from the French Antilles in the Carribbean, and he brought with him an infallible cure for cancer, widely advertised on posters around Paris. Many desperate sufferers paid up for 'Dr Noir's pills', but the incident which made him famous occurred in 1856. Adolphe Sax, the Belgian-born Parisian instrument-maker, who invented the saxophone, the bass-clarinet and several other wind instruments, developed a distressing tumour on his lip, which doctors pronounced incurable. Dr Noir had been publicly praised as a benefactor of humanity by prominent personalities, and when Sax's plight became known a galaxy of prominent musicians, including Vieuxtemps, Halévy, Meyerbeer and Berlioz (who, having once trained as a doctor, should have known better), raised a subscription to enable him to take advantage of the infallible cure. Sax was cured, and lived to a good age. (He believed that playing wind instruments promoted longevity by averting disorders of the lungs.) Sax was a famous man, and Dr Noir was lauded in the press for saving his life and those of many others. But the brouhaha attracted the attention of Professor Alfred Velpeau, a celebrated surgeon, based at the Hôpital de la Charité. Veloeau (hose name is commemorated in the Velpeau bandage) examined the pills and the evidence, and declared them useless. His conclusions were published, but did not entirely put an end to Dr Noir's activities, for several of his customers believed themselves cured, or at least better. There were however several accusations of quackery and lawsuits, and Dr Noir, whose real name was Vries, seems to have departed in some haste.

Here, to conclude this brief tour of a territory that has inspired many books, is a gem of the advertising genre, spotted by a doctor, who felt it should be shared with the readers of the *Lancet*. 'Delighted', he writes, 'with the information disclosed to me by the annexed advertisement taken from the Supplement to the *Times* of Nov. 24th [1846], I beg to offer you the same means of increasing your store of scientific knowledge', and then follows the text:

VEGETABLE-OXYDE of BEES'-WAX for PURIFICATION of the BONES, as liquifying the chilled marrow through flame-light electricity, causing reflow of joint-oil lubrication, for stiffened joints, ossific gout-rheumatism, cancer'os' and ulcer'os' contractions, without confinement or alteration of diet. Sun-like opening, as in plant animal physiology, the nervous fibrils, these respirative tubes, being intercorporeal for arial circulation, giving cartilegen'os' expansion for sleep at will. Consultations 6 to 8 a.m., and 11 to 12, at 5, Swallow-street, Quadrant.

It has to be said that descriptions of cures, couched perhaps in less fulsome prose but just as devoid of meaning, can still be found in advertising for 'alternative' medicines today.

Chapter 4

PROGRESS AND REGRESS

William Withering and digitalis

Dropsy, swelling of the body through accumulation of water, would now be diagnosed as a probable case of congestive heart failure. It was (as it still is) treated with diuretics from ancient times, although many physicians before the late 18th century recommended instead a rigorous diet, sometimes surgery and all too commonly bloodletting. Celsus in the 1st century A.D. (p.) listed 25 plants with diuretic properties. The most effective was probably squill (from the Latin *scilla*), the bulb of *Urginea maritima*, the 'sea onion', which is most abundantly found round the Mediterranean. It was mentioned in dispensatories from the time of Galen or before as a treatment for many diseases; Galen had in fact suggested that dropsical patients might gain relief by sucking the dried plant, but squill was never widely used. It became at least somewhat better known in Europe in the early 18th century. From the first edition of the London Pharmacopoeia onwards it was recommended in many forms of preparation as a diuretic for dropsy and an expectorant in asthma, but its use was sparse, probably because of its limited efficacy and unpleasant side-effects, for after taking it for a few days patients would experience vomiting and violent stomach pains. A vivid picture of the ordeals that dropsy inflicted on its victims comes from descriptions of Dr Samuel Johnson's suffering during his last years. Johnson had a dread of death and was willing to try anything to keep it at bay. He even attempted in his desperation to relieve the swelling in his legs with a knife, and he dosed himself liberally with squill, which had some effect: 'Last week', he wrote to Boswell, 'I emitted in about twenty hours, full twenty pints of urine, and the tumour [swelling] of my body is very much lessened'. It did not last, and Johnson died at the age of 75 in 1784. Had he but known of the researches by his younger contemporary, Dr William Withering!

The most important event in 18th-century medicine came about through the astuteness and persistence of this English doctor. William Withering was born in 1741 in Wellington in Shropshire. His father, a surgeon and apothecary, apprenticed his son to another surgeon, but William had wider ambitions, and in 1762 he enrolled in the medical school in Edinburgh. There he came under the influence of William Cullen (p.), then at the height of his fame, and of a noted botanist, John Hope, who was a pioneer in the application of Linnaean systematics to the study of British plants. Carl von Linné, otherwise known as Carolus Linnaeus, was producing, between 1735 and 1767, a succession of ever more comprehensive editions of his famous system of taxonomy of plants and animals, *Systema Naturae*. It was based on physical characteristics, and classified living organisms according to kingdoms, classes, orders, genera and species. The interest in the medical school was of course in the used of plant-derived medicines. Withering was well aware of this, and had botanised from his early years, although after he graduated in 1766 he lost interest. His thesis for the M.D. degree bore the title, *De Angina Gangraenosa* (Of the putrid throat).

In 1767 Withering moved south to Stafford, where he worked both in private practice and in the local infirmary. He married one of his patients, and his wife, who made pictures of plants, reanimated his pleasure in botany, to the extent that he published a two-volume treatise, *Botanical Arrangement of Vegetables*. A second edition occupied four volumes, and the work ran in all to eleven editions (the last few posthumous and edited by his son). His botanical work secured for Withering the Fellowship of the Linnaean Society, and commemoration of his name in that of the shrub, *Witheringia solanacea*. He also pursued other interests. He studied chemistry and published several papers in the subject, and he was astute enough to reject Priestley's phlogiston theory (p.). He had a broad knowledge of minerals, and one was named in his honour – witheringite. By the time such recognition of his manifold achievements, crowned by a Fellowship of the Royal Society, came to him he had long forsaken the backwater of Stafford; for after eight years in the town he had received a communication from the illustrious Erasmus Darwin, grandfather of Charles, a doctor in the bustling city of Birmingham, inviting him to take over the practice of a local doctor who had died. Withering accepted with probably some eagerness, for not only was Birmingham a lively intellectual centre, but the practice, allied to a position at the General Hospital, afforded him a generous income. Erasmus Darwin was, moreover, a member of the Lunar Society, a club of high-minded, free-thinking and brilliant men, and they welcomed the polymathic Withering into their circle. Yet Withering was not a clubbable man: he was taciturn and prickly and suspicious, but he did form a number of close friendships, and in a bitter dispute with Erasmus Darwin it was Withering who was the injured party.

Withering's health was never robust, and by 1792 and not yet 50, he resigned his hospital appointment, abandoned his private practice and travelled to Lisbon, where he wintered that year and the next. The warmer climate must have cheered him, for he kept busy with such projects as analysing the hot sulphurous waters from a resort near the capital, and was elected to the Portuguese Academy of Sciences. But back home there was trouble. Withering's friend, near-neighbour and fellow-member of the Lunar Society, the great chemist, Joseph Priestly, had become a target of the 'Church and King' party by reason of his non-conformism and support for the French Revolution. His house was attacked by a mob, and his library and laboratory were destroyed. Withering was of the same general persuasion (as were most of the members of the Society), and his house too came under siege, but the attackers were beaten off and little damage was done. These trials and the illness of his wife probably undermined Withering's fragile health. He clung on for another seven years and died at the age of 58 from what may have been tuberculosis. A friend sadly wrote that the flower of English botany was Withering. The funeral was attended by great crowds of admirers.

So much then for his life and career, but Withering's well-merited fame rests on his discovery of a drug for heart disease. It came about by chance. He did not, following his move to Birmingham, neglect his patients in Stafford. Once every week he would make the 30-mile journey in his coach, stopping halfway to change horses. During such a break on one occasion in 1775, he was summoned to call on an old woman with severe dropsy (congestive heart failure). The outlook was unpromising, but when he next saw the woman he was astonished to find her apparently restored to health. Withering had no faith in herbal remedies, which he thought mere superstitions, but when his patient told him that she had been cured by a plant infusion, he took note. The 'secret recipe' derived from another old woman, living in Shropshire who had, it was said, cured many apparently dying people. The medicine contained some 20 herbs, and having contemplated the recipe, he arrived at a conclusion, for 'it was not very difficult for one conversant with these subjects to perceive that the active herb could be none other than the foxglove', *Digitalis purpurea*. Why this should have been so obvious was never made clear. There had indeed been accounts in earlier times of medicinal applications of foxglove for various conditions, including epilepsy and tuberculosis. Dioscorides had an entry for foxglove, and Leonhart Fuchs actually recommended its use against dropsy. On the other hand, John Gerard (p.) in his herbal had firmly written off the foxglove, of which he recognised two species, as a source of useful remedies. They were, in Galenic terms, 'hot and drie, with a certaine kinde of cleansing qualitie joined therewith; yet are they of no use, neither have they any place amongst medicines, according to the Antients'. But perhaps Withering's inference, given his antipathy to folk remedies, rested more on the known poisonous nature of the plant. In his book, *Account of the Foxglove*, published a decade later, he described the symptoms: 'The Foxglove, when given in very large and quickly repeated doses, occasions sickness, vomiting, purging, giddiness, confused vision, objects appearing green or yellow, increased secretion of urine, with frequent motions to part with it, and sometimes inability to retain it, slow pulse, even as slow as 35 in a minute, cold sweats, convulsions, syncope [fainting due to a drop in blood pressure], death'. It was, then, clearly a physiologically active agent. Withering made a long and careful study of dosages and effects, and means of administration as a diuretic and treatment for heart failure. Dried and ground-up leaves of the plant, he found, gave the most consistent results. He conducted his research mainly on the poor of Birmingham, of whom he treated, by his own estimate, between 2000 and 3000 free of charge each year. In return they evidently offered themselves up as guinea-pigs.

Withering was a true clinical scientist, arguably the first in the long history of medicine. He spurned what we would now call anecdotal evidence: only a statistical evaluation of successes and failures would do. To publish on the basis of one or two successful outcomes was a dereliction, and failing to record the failures was worse. He was appalled to hear that, when word about the medicine got around, many doctors had seizes on it as a cure for all manner of diseases, which there was no reason to suppose it would ameliorate. In his *Account of the Foxglove*, published in 1785, he set out this stern principle: 'It would have been an easy task to have given select cases, whose successful treatment would have spoken strongly in favour of the medicine, and perhaps have been flattering to my own reputation. But Truth and Science would condemn me for the procedure.' Withering had meticulously recorded the results of treating 156 patients in his private practice, and another seven in the hospital. He had also received reports from brother physicians around the country, but he would not include these in making his conclusions, not, he said because he doubted their competence and veracity, but because he feared that they would have laid more emphasis on the successful cases than on the failures.

It was an early and spectacular success that brought about the rift with Erasmus Darwin. Withering described the event, which occurred in 1780. The subject, a middle-aged woman, a patient of Darwin's, was in extremis. Her body was grossly swollen and she had almost ceased to urinate. Darwin sought advice from Withering, who was initially reluctant to administer his digitalis, for he judged that the woman was almost certainly beyond help and feared that a failure would 'discredit a medicine which promised to be of great benefit to mankind, and I might be censured for a prescription which could not be countenanced by any experienced practitioner'. But finally he yielded and suggested to Darwin that they should try it. Darwin acceded and Withering prepared the draught. The results were dramatic: 'Within the first twenty four hours she made upwards of eight quarts [9 litres] of water' and the swelling subsided. Relations between the two men had become strained, apparently over unwanted advice from the polymathic Darwin when Withering was compiling his edition of *An Arrangement of British Plants*. Withering may have annoyed Darwin by his quickness to take offence, but in 1785 Darwin gave him cause. Knowing full well that Withering had been working for the last decade on the properties of digitalis, Darwin submitted a paper to the College of Physicians with the title, "An account of the successful use of foxglove in some dropsies and in pulmonary consumption". Withering's name did not appear, but when the paper was published some months later in the College's Transactions, it bore a postscript, stating that while "the last pages of this volume were in press", 'Dr Withering of Birmingham' had published "a numerous collection of cases in which foxglove had been given, and frequently with good success". The effect on Withering of what seems to have been a wantonly treacherous act can well be imagined, especially since his book on foxglove was approaching completion. The breach was irreparable and was further widened by a later accusation of Darwin's that Withering had been poaching his patients. Darwin, well known as a poet, not only a scientist and physician, published a long botanical poem in two parts, the *Botanic Garden*, in which appear the following, not at all bad, lines:

> Bolster'd with down, amid a thousand wants,
> Pale Dropsy rears his bloated form. and pants,
> "Quench me ye cool pellucid rills!" he cries,
> Wets his parch'd tongue and rolls his hollow eyes.
> So bends tormented TANTALUS to drink,
> While from his lips the refluent waters shrink;
> Again the rising stream his bosom laves,
> And thirst consumes him 'mid circumfluent waves,
> -Divine HYGEIA from the bending sky
> Descending, listens to his piercing cry;
> Assumes bright Digitalis dress and air;
> Her ruby cheek, white neck, and raven hair;
> *Four* youths protect her from the circling throng,
> And like the Nymph the Goddess steps along -
> O'er him she waves her serpent-wreathèd wand,

Cheers with her voice, and raises with her hand,
Warms with rekindling bloom his visage wan,
And charms the shapeless monster into man.

The overdue idea: a controlled trial

A doctor has a number of patients suffering from a malady with a name. He doses them all throughout some period with a drug of which he has high expectations; and indeed many of them get better, and shower him with thanks and also with more bankable rewards. The drug is clearly effective, and the doctor, vindicated in his belief, publishes a paper to this effect. This was the way of things until, some say, James Lind showed his medical confrères in 1746 that they were in error. For how many patients with those symptoms will recover without the help of the drug? Is it a greater or a smaller number? And what part is played by the comfort the patient receives from his faith in the skill of his doctor, or in the money the treatment is costing him? Or could it be that what is now known as the psychosomatic effect of merely taking a pill that the patient is assured will cure him (the placebo phenomenon) will make him feel better? And how can we be confident of the doctor's objectivity in judging whether the patient's condition has improved, given that he is persuaded from the outset of his favourite drug's merit? It was the slow incubation of these insights that gave rise to the concept of the randomised placebo-controlled trial. A sufficiently large number of patients, matched for the seriousness of their condition and for other factors that could affect their health - age, weight, diet and so on - are divided into two groups. Each participant is allocated to one or the other group at random. One group is given the drug, the other – the control group – something that looks like the drug, a placebo, sometimes referred to as a 'sugar pill' (a bad description, for neither its appearance nor its taste must give away its identity). The patients are not told which they are to receive, and at the end of the course of treatment the states of the patients in the two groups are evaluated. Much later, the double-blind principle was added: the doctors examining the patients before and after the trial are also kept ignorant of which patient has the drug and which the placebo, so that their judgement cannot be biased by preconceptions. This innovation, though, had to wait until the 20th century.

The concept of a controlled trial does not, after all, seem to us now a hard one to grasp or even to think up, yet although it surfaced from time to time over the years, it was hardly ever put into practice. It is often said that the first such attempt was the scurvy trial by the navy surgeon, James Lind in 1743, although there were some credible earlier and contemporaneous suggestions about how a trial should be conducted, but which all came to nothing. A remarkably prescient plan for a critical comparison of two different medical procedures was outlined by van Helmont, whom we have already met (p.). Sceptical of the merits of bloodletting, and an adherent of the iatrochemical school, he suggested dividing into two groups 200 or even 500 victims of fevers, bleeding and purging half of them, and treating the remainder with inorganic substances, such as mercury compounds. A century later, while Lind was already engaged in his study of possible cures and prophylactics for scurvy, George Berkeley (1685-1753), Bishop of Cloyne in Ireland, was a philosopher, who conceived the doctrine of subjective idealism, and also a mathematician of note and a poet. Berkeley formulated a test for a nostrum of his own. He had in fact a bee in his bonnet: when young he had been cured of a colic attack by a draught of tar water, and he had become persuaded that it would cure many other ills, and was indeed perhaps a panacea. Tar-water was made by stirring up powdered tar with water, letting it stand for two days and settle, and decanting the clear liquid. Berkeley used this not only as a medicine but as a prophylactic, which required him to drink a half pint twice a day. The extract would have contained several chemicals, some of them carcinogenic, chief of which was probably phenol, also known as carbolic, and used until recently as a disinfectant. Berkeley wanted it tested on victims of smallpox, with a control group, given the treatments of the time; both groups were to receive an identical diet and to be similarly housed. The experiment was never performed, but tar-water had considerable vogue. A friend of Berkeley's wrote that it had 'become as common to call for a glass of tar-water in a coffee-house, as a dish of tea or coffee'. The aesthete and hypochondriac, Horace Walpole, who was a devotee of tar-water, quoted with approval the following doggerel, published anonymously in a news-sheet:

Who dares deride what pious Cloyne has done?
The Church shall rise and vindicate her son;
She tells us all her bishops shepherds are,
And Shepherds heal their rotten sheep with tar.

Lind, as will appear, did a lot better than Bishop Berkeley.

The question remains: why did the rather obvious notion of a controlled trial find so little favour for so many years? One reason, which troubled some physicians, and still sometimes does even today, was ethical, for if a doctor believed that a drug could save a patient's life, what right had he to deny it to that patient in favour of a placebo? The question was debated as long ago as 1760 at a session of the *Académie des Sciences* in Paris. Daniel Bernoulli (1700-1782), scion of a great dynasty of Swiss mathematicians, was a pioneer of probability theory, and one of many problems to which he applied it was the efficacy of inoculation against smallpox, which had probably first been brought to the west in 1721 by Lady Mary Wortley Montagu. She had witnessed the process in Constantinople, where her husband had been sent as His Majesty's Ambassador to the Sublime Porte. In a letter to a friend back home she described 'inoculation parties, to which mothers brought their children, and old women came with nutshells 'full of the best kind of smallpox' A woman would poke into an arm vein 'as much as can lie on the head of her needle'. These women must have been very skilful in judging both the quality of the smallpox fluid and the amount to be injected. On her return to England in 1721 Lady Mary had had her two children inoculated.

The epidemic, which struck not long after that, caused many deaths, but inoculation was not without its dangers, and undoubtedly killed some of the recipients because of the uncertain volume injected and the variable virulence of the material. Bernoulli collected statistics on deaths from inoculation and from the disease as normally transmitted during epidemics, and concluded from his analysis that, taking into account the probability of deaths from inoculation, the process offered an average increase in a recipient's longevity of about 3 years. It seemed clear that a programme of mass inoculation should be undertaken. In the debate in Paris Bernoulli was opposed by another great mathematician, one of the *Encyclopédistes*, Jean Le Rond d'Alembert. D'Alembert argued that probabilities were not a consideration for parents concerned to safeguard their children: what might happen years in the future was irrelevant to the possibility of a death inflicted by an inessential intervention. This argument seems, for the time being, to have prevailed. We will return later (Chapter) to the problems that still beset clinical trials.

Captain Lind and scurvy

Whether vitamins, which after all come unbidden in our food, or are made in our bodies, can be regarded as drugs is a moot question. All the same, James Lind's controlled experiments on a group of British sailors to test a possible cure for one of the most dreaded maladies of the age stands as an early model for today's clinical drug trials, and a landmark in man's struggle against disease. Lind was born in Edinburgh in 1716, 25 years before Withering, who outlived him by only five years. In 1739, having served his apprenticeship with a local surgeon, he joined the Royal Navy, and soon encountered scurvy, which engaged his interest for the rest of his working life. The experiment on which his fame rests was conducted in 1746, and that year he set out his credo, very much like that of Withering: 'I shall propose nothing dictated from theory, but shall confirm all by experience and facts, the surest and most unerring guides'. In short, evidence-based medicine, as today's mantra runs.

Scurvy was the scourge of seamen, of soldiers, of convicts and the poor, who endured life in institutions. It was a distressing condition, marked by severe pains in the joints, softened muscles, such that a finger pressed into the arm would leave an imprint for minutes, constipation so refractory that it could be relieved only by surgery, loosened teeth and rotting gums that made eating a torment, and a putrid breath. Many more sailors died of scurvy than by shot. When Commodore George Anson returned in 1744 from his voyage of circumnavigation (which had begun in 1740 with an attack on the Spanish fleet off South America), his complement of 2000 men and boys had dwindled to about 600. Of those who did not return, four had been killed in battle, and nearly all the rest had died of scurvy. This was by no means atypical at the time, and an endless' source of concern to the Navy Board. Anson was more perceptive than most of his colleagues, and he used his prestige to support Lind's efforts to get to the bottom of the problem. At the time the widely accepted view was that scurvy was caused by foul air below decks, and the unhealthy living conditions in general, allied to the perceived constitutional indolence of sailors. Many other theories were in circulation, but there had also been intermittent reports from many quarters, even from officers in the navy and from the masters of the East India Company's ships, that fruit, and especially citrus juice, had wrought miraculous recoveries. In 1612 a Royal Navy surgeon, John Woodall had published a widely consulted book, *The Chirurgeon's Mate*, in which he asserted the value of citrus fruits and tamarind as antiscorbutic agents; lemon juice, he insisted, was 'the most precious helpe that ever was discovered against the "Scurvie"'. But the Navy Board and most ships' captains and surgeons paid no attention. Instead, their favoured remedies were the fraudulent Doctor James's Fever Powder, and Joshua Ward's Pill and Drop (p.), and also Sir William Cockburn's 'Electuary', or paste. The first was regarded by many throughout the country as a panacea, while the Pill and Drop, also popular, was peddled by Ward, who as related above, was widely recognised (though not by the Admiralty) as a charlatan. Cockburn was a fashionable physician, with an unrivalled record of being wrong, as when he continued to heap scorn on the use of citrus juice. His electuary was a mixture of inert, but at least harmless, herbs and oils, whereas both Dr James's Powder and the Pill and Drop contained predominantly antimony, and must have been responsible for many deaths. A few captains were nevertheless persuaded of the value of citrus fruit, and did their best to ensure that their ships were properly provisioned, or could stop whenever possible to take on fresh fruit. Admiral Vernon, known to his men as 'Old Grog' after the grosgrain cape he affected in bad weather, ordered in 1740 that lemon juice should henceforth be added to the daily rum ration (whence of course the name, grog for this energising mixture).

In 1746 Lind was posted to HMS Salisbury, a fourth rate ship of the line with a complement of 350, under the command of George Edgcumbe, a well-connected and enlightened commander, who encouraged Lind's efforts. Lind was by no means wedded to the view that citrus juice really was the answer to the problem of prevention. He thought rather that scurvy was brought on through bad air, inattention to hygiene and apathy, and he evidently regarded prevention and cure as separate issues. The very possibility that a disorder could result from the lack of something rather than the presence of a noxious substance or influence was beyond imagining, and a violation of the Galenic principles that still held most physicians in thrall. But were any of the numerous medicines claimed at one time or another to alleviate the symptoms of scurvy actually effective? Lind devised a way to investigate. He divided his small group of a dozen sailors into six pairs, the trial to last fourteen days. The men had been carefully selected, being all in a fairly advanced scorbutic state. They were housed together and given the same shipboard diet, but the six pairs all received different treatments, as follows: *pair 1* – one quart of cider daily; *pair 2* – 25 drops of 'elixir of vitriol', that is sulphuric acid diluted in water; *pair 3* – two spoonfuls of vinegar before and after meals, with more added to the food; *pair 4* – a half-pint of sea-water daily; *pair 5* – two oranges and a lemon daily, but the supply ran out after only 6 days; *pair 6* – an electuary 'the size of a nutmeg', containing Peru balsam (p.), mustard seeds, garlic, and 'gum myrrh'. (There was an additional and larger group, offered only laxative and cough syrup, but for some reason the fate of those was not included in Lind's report.)

The results could scarcely have been more dramatic: at the end of six days group 5 were totally cured and fit for duty. Of the rest the two men of group 1 were adjudged slightly improved, and all the rest had deteriorated further. Lind soon after left the navy and returned to Edinburgh, where he wrote a thesis on syphilis for his doctoral degree and his 400-page work, *A Treatise on Scurvy*, in which he clung to his unreconstructed theories about the cause of the disease, but emphasised that citrus fruits were the infallible cure. The point, it might be thought, was proved, yet the Admiralty remained obdurate. The essence of citrus fruit was its acidity, so why then should vinegar or 'elixir of vitriol', which were cheaper and did not rot, be any less effective? These were recommended as antiscorbutics, as were many other useless substances - malted barley, sauerkraut, sugar and many more. There was even a brief interest in soda water, recently invented by

Joseph Priestley, who had bubbled carbon dioxide (fixed air) into water, for fermentation was held to be life-giving and curative, and carbon dioxide was one of its products. The saddest attempts to find a suitable prophylactic for scurvy, suitable for long voyages, during which lemons and limes rotted and lost their activity, was that of Lind. He had the perfectly rational idea of preparing a concentrate of orange and lemon juice by separating it from the pulp and heating it in vats of boiling water until it was reduced to a syrup, to be bottled and sealed to keep it sterile. This was called a 'rob', and was wholly ineffective, because the heating destroyed the active component – vitamin C, or ascorbic acid. Lind had become supervisor of the naval hospital at Haslar on the south coast, but was disappointed not only in his rob but also by the scorn with which his great discovery was treated, and in having an invention – a shipboard pump to circulate warm clean air through the living quarters of the sailors – stolen from him. He died impoverished and forgotten.

Another controlled trial was performed by a young surgeon who went to sea on a slave ship: in 1783 Thomas Trotter observed that when the slaves, who suffered appallingly from scurvy and other diseases of malnutrition and bad hygiene, were given guavas to eat, they always opted for under-ripe, sour fruit. This led him to wonder whether the preference might not stem from folk wisdom. He put this conjecture to the test by giving three groups of slaves, all suffering from scurvy, ripe guavas, unripe guavas and lime juice. All except one of his experimental subjects in the second and third groups, but none of those in the first, quickly recovered. Trotter was disgusted by the conditions on the slaver, and on his return from the Caribbean he immediately signed off and departed for the medical school in Edinburgh. He published a treatise on scurvy, later joined the Royal Navy and sought to ensure that there would always be a good supply of fresh citrus fruit on his ship. Yet another enlightened ship's doctor, who distinguished himself in battle, and was to achieve high distinction in his profession was a Scotsman and protégé of William Cullen, Gilbert Blane. He estimated that of the 1600 casualties in Admiral Rodney's squadron, fighting the French on the West India station in 1781, 60 had died in battle, the rest from scurvy. Despite his powerful patronage and his eloquence, and the success of his 'lemon and lime cure' during the campaign, his exertions to impress the Sea Lords came to nothing, for had not the citrus rob been found ineffective?

Scurvy was to claim many more victims. A poignant and wholly purposeless act of self-sacrifice deprived England of a dedicated young doctor, William Stark. Stark was a protégé of Sir John Pringle, physician to the royal family, later President of the Royal Society and the recipient of many high honours, including a memorial in Westminster Abbey. Pringle had done good work improving the medical services of the British army, but he held obdurately to the view that scurvy could be cured only by encouraging the processes of fermentation in the gut, and would not consider that fresh fruit might have some virtues. In 1769 Stark decided to try for himself the effects of various diets on the human frame, each regime lasting 30 days. It was said that one of these was inspired by Benjamin Franklin, whom Stark had met, and who claimed to have subsisted for weeks at a time on bread and water during his indigent youth. The diet which did for Stark in 1770 consisted of cheese and honey. Despite the onset of scurvy, Stark persisted, and his patron, Pringle could think of nothing better to alleviate his condition than bleeding, which could only have hastened his end, which resulted probably from an infection that commonly carried off sufferers from scurvy.

In the end it was Gilbert Blane who gained sufficient influence through his various connexions - which included Admiral Rodney, the First Sea Lord under whom he had sailed, and the Duke of Clarence, later William IV, whom he had known as a midshipman - to ensure that His Majesty's ships were provisioned with an abundance of lemon juice. By the early years of the 19th century, the British Navy and also the merchant fleet were more or less free of scurvy. The disease nevertheless reappeared from time to time, when the fruit was of poor quality, and especially during long voyages of exploration in the Arctic and Antarctic, and also at times in the army. Outbreaks of scurvy occurred as late as the Crimean War (1853-1856) and even in World War I. A final resolution came in 1918, when a group of women scientists at the Lister Institute in London, led by Harriette Chick, found that West Indian limes had a low content of the antiscorbutic factor, and what they did contain was rapidly degraded. This ex[;ained why consignments of limes delivered to the navy were so often ineffectual. By this time the company founded in Edinburgh by Lauchlan Rose during the previous century was producing Rose's Lime Juice Cordial in huge amounts, as it still does.

Suffer the little children

In 1721, as we have seen, inoculation against smallpox was introduced in England. The process was simple enough: fluid from a pustule on the arm of a smallpox patient was applied to a scratch in the recipient's arm to provoke a mild smallpox infection. (This was not vaccination, which came into use only in 1796, when Edward Jenner showed that infection with cowpox gave almost complete protection.) It was quickly established, first by another English doctor, James Jurin, that inoculation was very effective: whereas smallpox was fatal to 1 in 6 of the uninoculated children, only about 1 in 50 of those who had been inoculated succumbed. (Bear in mind that in the 18th century an estimated 30% or so of all children in London caught the disease.) With the passage of time the skills of the practitioners improved, the methods were refined, and the failure rate dropped further. The success, though, was widely attributed to the practice adopted by most English doctors of dosing the children beforehand with strong purgatives, and often also administering calomel and antimony with the inoculum to neutralise its supposed toxins. What, then, was the reality? In 1767, when such practices had already been in use some 40 years, William Watson (1715-1787), resident doctor at the Foundling Hospital in London (or to give it its proper name, the Hospital for the Maintenance and Education of Exposed and Deserted Children) decided to find out. It was probably no coincidence that Watson was a deeply-read scholar with wide interests in science. His study, if less dramatic than that of Lind on scurvy, was better conceived and more comprehensive, and stands as a monument in the history of clinical trials.

Dr Watson selected 31 children, matched for age and circumstances. He divided them into three groups and inoculated them all. The first group of five boys and five girls were dosed with calomel and the savage laxative, jalap, the second, similarly matched, with the milder agents, senna and rose syrup, and the remaining eleven were spared all medicines. To determine the extent of the resulting illness, Watson and his assistants counted the number of pustules that each child developed, for the greater the number the worse the prospects of recovery in the uninoculated victim. Watson did not stop there. For one thing, he wondered whether the laxative might have nullified any effect the calomel could have had, supposing it it to have been instantly voided. He therefore dosed a group of children three times with calomel, but no laxative, alongside the control group, which received only senna and rose syrup. Finally, Watson determined to answer another long-debated question: was it better to inoculate with the fluid from a mature than from an early pustule? The total pustule count from all 74 children in the trials was 2,353, but almost half belonged to five of the children, in whom the inoculation had clearly failed. As to the other 69, with an average pustule count of 17, Watson was able to conclude that the calomel had served no useful purpose, nor did the source of the inoculum, whether from young or mature pustules, make any difference.

A large part of the medical profession, it has to be said, continued to take little notice of the evidence on this or any other such matters. As the great German physicist, Max Planck observed, new truths seldom gain acceptance by convincing the sceptics. Once, he said, scientists believed in the corpuscular theory of light; now they believe it is a wave, and that is because those who adhered to the corpuscular view have died off[*]. The survival of homeopathy is perhaps the best example of this principle. Yet it must also be recognised that there are many pitfalls in the design of controlled trials, as we shall see later.

The early 19ᵗʰ century: tradition challenged

Despite the accumulation of physiological knowledge and the evidence of more or less scientifically devised trials of medicines and treatments, the majority of doctors clung obstinately to their old habits. The baleful shadow of Galen and his humours still hung over the profession. In some ways doctors were now an even greater danger to the sick than ever, for

---

[*] It was later revealed, partly through Planck's own work, that it is both at once.

the favoured purgatives and emetics - still the customary therapeutic measures, were based on highly toxic mercurials and arsenicals. It has been conjectured that an epidemic, which gripped parts of Paris in 1828, was the result of mercury poisoning. The disease, never before encountered by the Parisian doctors, was given the name of acrodynia, and revealed itself in acute pains in the hands and feet, and paralysis of the limbs leading in some cases to death. It was accompanied by a reddening of the affected parts, reminiscent of 'pink disease' in babies (p.), but the retrospective diagnosis is uncertain, and some authorities have suggested pellagra, a vitamin deficiency disease, as the cause.

The passion for bloodletting had not abated. The most famous physician in Germany, and one of the most respected of his time in the world was Christoph Wilhelm Friedrich Hufeland (1762-1836). Son of a court doctor in Göttingen, he rose rapidly to positions of eminence as professor, court physician, director of the famous medical school, the Charité in Berlin and a Councillor of State under the Prussian Kaiser Friedrich Wilhelm III. Hufeland was well-connected: he was a friend and doctor to Goethe and to other of the great German intellectuals of the day. He was a special intimate of the polymath – physicist, philosopher, satirist and aphorist, Georg Lichtenberg - to whom he dedicated his *magnum opus, Makrobiotik*, subtitled, 'the Art of Human Life', and with whom he shared an enthusiasm for electricity as a life force. (This was the fad that animated Mary Shelley in writing her novel, *Frankenstein*.) Hufeland was socially progressive, with enlightened views on the care of children, public hygiene, inoculation against smallpox and on medical education, yet in his profession he was a reactionary of the darkest hue. He abjured all systems and theories, and regarded himself as an 'eclectic', but his treatments were primarily based on his 'three heroes' – bleeding, vomiting and opium. His pharmacopoeia for the poor, compiled early in his career, nevertheless contained no less than 550 remedies (reduced in a later work to 275).

The awe in which Hufeland was held undoubtedly contributed to the unremitting enthusiasm for bloodletting, which continued to take its toll of the sick and injured. It was widely inflicted on patients in the cholera epidemics that erupted around Europe and the East - the worst treatment that could have been devised for a disease which kills by dehydration. Here, as late as 1849, is the view proffered by a supposed specialist, Dr William Robertson, Physician to the Edinburgh Cholera Hospital: 'Of the practice of *blood-letting* in the early stages of the disease, I have now had considerable experience, and am confirmed in my opinion of its efficacy in preventing or modifying the more formidable symptoms of the disease'. After describing the effects of taking small and large quantities of blood from 30 patients (some of whom, he admits, may have been misdiagnosed in the first place) he concludes, 'The remedy is, I think, most efficacious when cramps and oppression of the chest are prominent symptoms; at least the immediate relief to the patient has, in such circumstances, been most remarkable; and when venesection [bloodletting] has been followed by the administration of opium in full doses, the progress of the disease has sometimes been apparently arrested'. Dr Robertson may have been more restrained than many of his contemporaries, who would continue to bleed until no more blood would come, on account of the dehydrated condition of the patient. A hefty dose of calomel might then help to finish them off. In New York similarly, the Special Medical Council advised bleeding 'to mitigate the spasms and render the system more susceptible to the action of the grand remedy, Mercury'. Opium in the form of laudanum was used in conjunction with bleeding, as in some quarters was tobacco smoke introduced through the nether passage. (Some doctors even gave jalap, the most powerful available laxative, which would have ensured more rapid and probably fatal dehydration. The more enlightened President of the New York Medical Society took the opposite route by closing the rectum with beeswax.)

Bloodletting was even used for conditions associated with blood loss, including surgery. It was long the normal practice to bleed women before parturition, and to bleed before an amputation to extract the blood that the limb was thought to contain. There is an account by a Colonel of the Coldstream Guards (which can be found in Thomas Dormandy's outstanding book, *The White Death*) that affords an extreme illustration. The Colonel was impressed, while riding across the battlefield at Waterloo in 1815, of the cool devotion of an army surgeon crouched over the body of a wounded guardsman from whose leg blood was spurting. It was clearly a case of a severed artery, and the Colonel dismounted and tore off his belt to use as a tourniquet when he observed that the surgeon was attempting to take blood from the soldier's arm on the other side. Before the Colonel could act the bleeding stopped: the soldier was dead. (The rationale would have been that withdrawing blood from one side would have sucked back the blood from the other, and so staunched the haemorrhage.)

Another medical bugbear of the period was the brunonian system (p.), which still prevailed in some corners of medical learning in its original or one or other modified form. Hufeland railed against brunonianism, but appropriated some of its tenets all the same, for he taught that diseases were of two kinds, corresponding to Brown's sthenic and asthenic. An additional and widespread belief, amounting to a superstition, had it that certain common diseases, including fevers and gout, were better not treated at all because any intervention could result in the release of noxious humours from the affected areas, which could then infect the vital organs. At least practitioners who adhered to this doctrine might do less harm than the massive doses of calomel that were still forced on luckless patients. Hufeland also flirted with the principle enunciated by Hahnemann, the founder of homeopathy, that like drives out like, so that every medicinal intervention amounted to the introduction of a (presumably benign) disease (a so-called *morbus salutaris*). Certain natural diseases were also believed to expel others: if, for example, you had leprosy you would not catch bubonic plague or syphilis (or of course might be denied the opportunity), whereas bubonic plague would mercifully protect you against scurvy.

The homeopathic aberration

The most enduring superstition in the recent history of medicine is homeopathy. The curious notion that a poison with effects thought to simulate the symptoms of a disease might, when administered in minuscule quantities, cure that disease cropped up at intervals over the centuries. An early example occurs in the writings of Paracelsus, who conjectured that small amounts of something capable of causing a malign condition might be useful for treating that same condition. But a comprehensive therapeutic system along these lines was not formulated until three centuries later. Its begetter was a German physician, Christoph Friedrich Samuel Hahnemann, born in Meissen in 1755, who coined the neologism, homœopathy, from the Greek, *homoios* meaning like, and *pathos*, or pain. The great epiphany came to him in about 1807, as he was preparing his German translation of William Cullen's *Materia medica* (p.). He was excited especially by Cullen's views on the mode of action of cinchona bark, which he found unconvincing. Hahnemann thought its activity might be centred on the stomach, and he tried some on himself to see what would happen. The results were gratifying: Hahnemann was seized with a fit of shivering, fever and joint pains, which all felt much like a bout of malaria. He thereupon made a bold intellectual leap: *any* diseases, he decided, must be curable by a substance that mimics in its effects the symptoms of that disease. The principle was summed up in the adage, *similia similibus curantur* – like is cures by like, so burns are healed by heat, dysentery by purgatives, and so on.

This, though, was only the beginning, for Hahnemann now elaborated his theory. Diseases were caused by external agents, called miasms, three in number (though added to later). Each miasm was responsible for a broad class of maladies, of which the most important, embracing everything from gout and rheumatism to cancer, were called *psora*, meaning itch. The mischief begins in the skin, is internalised, and eventually attacks a vital organ. Remedies are chosen according to the Doctrine of Signatures, a regression to medieval medicine (p.), and again to Paracelsus. A benevolent deity has provided clues, which can take the form of a shape, a colour or a smell. A plant with liver-shaped leaves is used to treat conditions of the liver, a meadow flower with leaves penetrated by stems, and indeed called 'boneset', will heal fractures, and so on. Remedies are supposed to act by stimulating the 'vital force' of nature, which pervades the body (known also by other names, such as *élan vital*), and thus the state of the patient's mind is an important factor in combating the miasm surging into the body. Most important, though, are considerations of toxicity. Clearly, an agent that has the effects of the disease – almost by definition a poison – is not something a caring physician would want to inflict on his patient. Hahnemann's answer is simple: merely dilute the substance to the level at which it is no longer toxic. Indeed, dilute it until none is left, for it is not the substance itself, but its healing essence, that effects the cure. And so a drop of the agent in a 'mother tincture' – a solution in alcohol or distilled water - is diluted 1 to 100 with distilled water, then 1 to 100 again, and so on commonly 30 times. (Some homeopaths varied the successive dilution factors.) A preparation resulting from 30 successive dilutions is called 30C (C for 100). After each dilution the solution had to be agitated to release its power, and the process was (and is) in fact called 'potentiation', or sometimes 'dynamisation'. It was accomplished by 'succusion', which means beating the vessel against an elastic surface, generally something hard, covered with leather. If the curative substance was an insoluble solid, such as snail or oyster shells, it would be ground up with lactose (milk sugar), and treated as before; this was called 'trituration'.

The enormous dilution meant of course that a small amount of a drug could be used for many millions of prescriptions, which struck fear into the local apothecaries, who joined together to drive Hahnemann out of the town. His confrères, at the same time, greeted his theories with derision, and it was some time before his system caught on. That it eventually did so was largely a consequence of the growing disillusionment in the profession with murderous treatments, especially bloodletting and dosing with huge amounts of calomel and other poisons. The patient, it was said, could choose between homeopathy and allopathy (conventional treatments with alien substances), between, that is to say, dying of the disease or of the remedy. But homeopathy had one great virtue: it could do no harm, and so conformed to the first article of the Hippocratic oath. (There were, though, variants of the homeopathic principle that may not have been quite so innocuous. One such was isopathy, devised by one Johann Joseph Wilhelm Lux, a veterinarian at Leipzig University, which made use of diseased matter as the supposed therapeutic agent. Pus or urine, or worse, from a sick person would be treated in the same manner as the more usual homeopathic remedies. In time such matter as saliva of dogs with rabies and testicle extracts, not to mention woodlice, cockroaches and many more, entered the homeopathic pharmacopoeia. If a pathological effluvium or other insanitary material was sticky it might not have dispersed fully during dilution, adhering instead to the walls of the vessel, and been ingested.)

Homeopathy reached its zenith in the first half of the 19th century, and it was probably the remarkable Boston physician and sage, Oliver Wendell Holmes, who contributed most strongly to its decline. Holmes was a polymath- doctor, legendary lecturer, both in the medical school and at large, reformer, essayist and poet. His most famous collection of essays, still an American classic, is *The Autocrat at the Breakfast Table* (published in 1858). Born in 1809, he studied first jurisprudence and then medicine at Harvard, where he eventually became Dean of the Medical School. As Dean, he sought to have women admitted to the study of medicine – one of his few failures, for the measure was adopted only in 1945. It was Holmes who gave us the word, anaesthesia, and who urged its use, despite prevailing opposition. He did much more. He revolutionised clinical teaching, introduced the use of the stethoscope (invented in France by René Laënnec), and convinced himself that puerperal (childbed) fever, which killed so many women in the maternity wards of Europe and America, was a contagious disease, spread mainly by the attendant doctors.[**]

As a freshly qualified doctor, Holmes had taken the unusual step of continuing his training in Paris under Pierre Louis (p.). From Louis he absorbed the *méthode expectante*, which posits patience, continuous observation of the patient's condition, a concern with the natural process of recovery and avoiding interventions that might impede it. As a professor, Holmes enjoined his students to follow these precepts. His studies in Paris, he wrote, had taught him 'at least three principles'. These were, 'not to take authority when I can have facts; not to guess when I can know; not to think a man must take physic because he is sick'. Such thinking was rare

---

[*] Holmes's paper, *The Contagiousness of Puerperal Fever*, delivered to the Boston Society for Medical Improvement in 1843, four years before Ignaz Semmelweiss reported his own observations on the matter to the medical establishment of Vienna, provoked an equally hostile response from the Boston obstetricians. One of the moguls of the profession responded in fact with a paper entitled, *The Non-Contagiousness of Puerperal Fever*.

in medicine. Holmes enlarged on the last of his three maxims some years later, indeed, he told his audience at the Massachusetts Medical Society:

'Throw out opium, which the Creator himself seems to prescribe, for we often see the scarlet poppy growing in the cornfields .... throw out a few specifics, which our art did not discover and it is hardly needed to apply; throw out wine, which is a food, and the vapors which produce the miracle of anaesthesia and I firmly believe that if the whole materia medica, as now used, could be sunk to the bottom of the sea, it would be all the better for mankind, - and all the worse for the fishes.'

Holmes had, at the same time, no patience with homeopathy. In 1842 he published a work with the title, *Homeopathy and its Kindred Delusions*, based on an influential lecture he delivered at the Boston Society for the Diffusion of Useful Knowledge, in which appears the following passage:

[Homeopathy] is lucrative and so long as it continues to be will surely survive, - as surely as astrology, palmistry and other methods of getting a living out of the weakness and credulity of mankind and womankind.'

This is perhaps less than fair, for many, perhaps most homeopaths undoubtedly believed fervently that they were curing their patients. But the cult went out of fashion, and remained largely dormant until its resurgence in the 20th century, when some of the ruling houses of Europe, such as the British Royal Family, led the way.

The absurdity of homeopathy should have become clear to all with the emergence around Hahnemann's time of the atomic theory of matter. The evidence was accumulated by several chemists, most notably John Dalton in Manchester and Amadeo Avogadro in Turin. In short, an atom of every element has a characteristic weight. If the lightest, hydrogen, is arbitrarily allocated a weight of unity (one-sixteenth the weight of an oxygen atom), then the very heavy element, uranium, has a weight of about 238. The weight of a molecule is the sum of the weights of its constituent atoms, so water, H_2O, with two hydrogen atoms and one oxygen, has a molecular weight of 18. A gram-molecule (or in modern parlance a mole) of water then weighs 18 grams, a gram-molecule of common salt, NaCl, with one sodium and one chlorine atom, 78.5 grams, and one of common cane or beet sugar 344 grams. It now follows that a gram-molecule of any substance contains the same number of molecules as a gram-molecule of any other substance. This number is accurately known, and is called the Avogadro number, and amounts to about 6×10^{23}, in other words 6 followed by 23 zeros. Suppose now, for the sake of argument, that your homeopath wishes to prepare a 30C solution of sugar. If he starts from 3.4 grams, that is a hundredth of a gram-molecule, he will have in his flask 6×10^{21} atoms of the substance. If he dissolves it in 10 millilitres of water, then each millilitre will contain 6×10^{20} atoms, and if he now dilutes 1 millilitre of this 'mother solution' into 100 millilitres of water, and continues to perform the same operation 30 times, succussion and all, the therapeutic medicine that results would contain, if this number had any physical meaning, 6×10^{-40} atoms per millilitre, or 6 divided by 1 followed by 40 zeros. A 1-millilitre dose of this medicine has therefore about one chance in 100000000000000000000000000000000000000 00 of containing a single atom, or on average there would be one atom in that number of millilitres of water. This would be about a million billion times as much water as is contained in all the Earth's oceans. The patient's medicine, in short, will be water and nothing else (except of course the impurities it contains). Ben Goldacre in his book *Bad Science* has made an even more striking calculation: the volume of water of a 30C dilution that would on average contain a single molecule of the substance in question would correspond to a sphere with a diameter of 150 million kilometres, the distance from the Earth to the Sun. Indeed, a glass of water taken from any of the Earth's oceans or rivers will contain an unimaginable number of doses of a myriad of homeopathic remedies concocted over the centuries.

Modern-day homeopaths are apt to retort that the health-giving substance does not actually need to be there at all to do you good. They will no longer talk, like Hahnemann, of its vital essences but of the memory of its presence that is retained by the water.** Now water (the most intensively studied of all substances), with its molecules in constant rapid motion, is intrinsically incapable of retaining any kind of footprint; moreover, water has been in continuous agitation since the newly formed Earth began to cool, so that the molecules in any glassful taken at random will have encountered millions upon millions of therapeutic measures of any homeopathic nostrums ever produced and excreted many times over by

---

* Another favourite trope of homeopaths, now less often heard, is that of an 'energy' yet to be defined. In 1923 Albert Abrams, a 60-year-old doctor in San Francisco published a book on what he called Spondylotherapy, but it was only after the end of the First World War that it attracted wide attention. Abrams was a fraud, who laid claim, for instance, to a degree in medicine from Heidelberg University, but he may have believed the nonsense that he promulgated. He seems to have been inspired by the discovery of new forms of radiation during the first decade of the 20th century – X-rays and the three forms of radiation emitted by radioactive elements – and so conceived the idea that the living body also emitted some elusive 'electronic' energy. This was finely tuned, and changed its magnitude (however defined) only in disease. Different diseases caused their own signature shifts in the radiation. Abrams invented a rudimentary electric circuit which he advertised as a unique means of identifying the seat of an undiagnosed illness from a tissue sample, such as a drop of blood. The gadget, which Abrams dubbed the Dynamizer, became more widely known as the Abrams Box, or just 'The Box'. The malady being identified, it was but a short step to a cure by homeopathic remedies, devised to match the aberrant radiation characteristic. Many members of the medical profession swallowed the story, and boxes manufactured in Abrams's Electromedical Institute were sold around the world. Tests made by doctors on their patients' blood were adjudged a triumphant success. Arthur Conan Doyle, the begetter of Sherlock Holmes, was a doctor and a believer in the occult, as also in the existence of fairies, and the Box convinced him entirely. He hailed Abrams as a genius, and he was not alone. Many patients, among them a British Member of Parliament, declared that they had been cured by Abrams's procedures, and a former President of the British Medical Association and knight of the realm, became its most fervent advocate. A Scottish entrepreneur marketed his own, supposedly improved version of the Box and became rich, as did many doctors who espoused it. The tests of the Box's efficacy were not of course properly designed or controlled. Some American doctors easily made fools of the adherents by sending drops of chicken blood or a healthy specimen of their own to Abrams, when, of course, they received a diagnosis (in the case of one doctor of congenital syphilis). Excuses were made: Abrams was being traduced by antisemites, for he was Jewish, and so on. The hoax, if it was that rather than honest self-deception, took years to fade into medical history. Abrams died rich in 1924.

all the patients who have lived since Hahnemann started diluting and succussing. All properly conducted trials of homeopathic remedies have delivered the same result - that they are ineffective, no better, at all events, than a placebo, yet 4 million Americans spend yearly about $1 billion on them, while in France and in Germany the industry brings in about €400 million per year, and £40 million in the U.K. The government health services of most advanced countries still scandalise the mainstream medical profession by providing funding for homeopathic treatments. This strange aberration, then, still retains its unaccountable resilience.

The White Plague

The scourge of tuberculosis was familiar to the ancients, and the symptoms of the disease were faithfully recorded by Roman physicians. Scrofula, or the King's Evil, so-called because from early times the touch of the monarch was commonly held to be the only cure, is tuberculosis of the lymph nodes. But it is pulmonary tuberculosis, formerly known as consumption or phthisis, that was the dreaded killer, and indeed still is, for a million or so people die of it every year, most of them in the poor countries of the south. In 19th-century literature the disease is commonly associated with tragic, premature and poignant death. The heroines of those unsinkable opera house favourites, *La Traviata* and *La Bohème*, and of course of the French novels on which they were based, both expire on a soft note in the final scene. John Keats was perhaps the most famous of the literary figures who died young - he was 26 - of tuberculosis. Chopin was thought to have been another romantic victim: a drawing in a French journal showed a weeping fashionably clad figure, captioned: 'The only countess in whose arms Chopin did not die'.

Tuberculosis is infectious – a fact not recognised for many centuries – and therefore a particu;ar hazard for doctors; Keats was one such, and Laënnec (p.) another. Few of its victims ever recovered from the disease. Keats's friend, John Arbuthnot Brown gave a harrowing account of the first manifestation of the infection. It was winter and Keats, who had been out riding, returned to the house he and Brown shared in London, shivering with cold. Put to bed, Keats coughed, murmured, 'this is blood' and asked for a candle to examine the stain on the bedclothes more closely. Brown recalled: 'he looked up into my face with a calmness I can never forget and said: "This is arterial blood: I cannot be deceived by its colour. It is my death warrant."'. (Keats was right, though as a doctor he might have known better in at least one respect: venous blood, which has a bluish tinge, would instantly take up oxygen when exposed to the air, and acquire the colour of arterial blood.) The treatments offered by doctors to their tuberculous patients did no more than compound their agonies. Keats was put on a starvation diet, as commonly recommended by the experts, savagely bled every time he coughed up blood, and poisoned with antimony, probably in the form of tartar emetic. Another medical colleague decided that the patient's lungs were in fine shape, and prescribed an ample diet, which brought about a temporary improvement, allowing him to travel to Rome. Yet another favoured fresh air and exercise on horseback, but more haemorrhages ensued, followed each time by bloodletting and often antimony, until death supervened. Keats was at least spared hydrotherapy, which consisted of repeated immersion in cold water.

In earlier years consumptives were dosed with asses' milk, which could have done them no harm (or good). Folk remedies for consumption were plentiful. Many parts of many animals were used, such as lungs, especially of foxes, or best of all, of young men who had come to a violent end, preferably on the gallows. Not only asses', but also human milk was was highly valued as a treatment in many countries. Dormandy (ref) mentions an entry in a popular manual of 1824, *The Family Oracle of Health*, for a home-made substitute for asses' milk based on an extract of snails. Raw meat, urine, dung, and burnt horns of various animals all had their adherents, as did a vast variety of plants. Water from certain wells was considered a cure. For the literate classes a superstition existed, it seems, that Book IV of Homer's Iliad placed under the pillow at night would expel the disease.

Many medical practitioners and the armies of quacks had their own cures consisting of antimony, arsenic, gold and mercury compounds, various complex formulations from the pharmacopoeia, and poultices of animal fat and the like. An ancient remedy for leprosy, stemming from India, and mentioned in legends, was sometimes adopted for treating tuberculosis; this was an extract of the seeds of the chaulmoogra tree, a particularly repugnant oil, which could be applied externally if found too intolerable to swallow. (It is still to be found in present-day 'alternative medicine' advertisements.) Cod liver oil in massive amounts was also favoured, as was creosote from charred wood or the soot from chimney flues. Soot, dignified by the name, *fuligo ligni*, was itself considered a valuable medicine, though mainly for treating skin conditions. The creosote preparations preceded the coal-tar distillate, used as a sealant for wood; all contained phenolic and other toxic and especially carcinogenic compounds, and were prescribed for many ailments. Preparations from seaweed or sponges were often administered, particularly to sufferers from scrofula, which was commonly confused with goitre: eight centuries earlier, the monks of Salerno (p.) recognised the value of these iodine-containing materials (to which we will return later) in curing goitre. Dormandy cites a 19th-century English doctor who, for obscure reasons, recommended boa constrictor excrement. Drinking fresh blood of animals or humans was another remedy espoused by some. The enormously toxic hydrocyanic (prussic) acid, as proposed by Magendie for combatting tuberculosis (p.), had a modest vogue.

The estimable Dr Beddoes at his Pneumatic Institution in Bristol tried, as we have seen, to cure consumptives with the newly discovered gases and with the exhalations of cattle in stalls at the back of the wards housing his patients. This measure derived in fact from a time-honoured superstition in many countries; even the effluvium from ripe sewage was often thought to have broadly healthful properties, which was why, during plague epidemics, the municipal cesspits would often be opened (p.). Beddoes, though, was too honest a doctor and scientist to fool himself for long about the efficacy of cattle breath. Some enterprising but less informed practitioners made their patients inhale other gases, and a vogue for such therapies developed in the latter part of the 19th century. Dormandy in his definitive history of the subject, gives some hair-raising examples: such dangerous gases as hydrogen sulphide (sulphuretted hydrogen), and coal gas, a favoured means of suicide and homicide, were pumped into the hapless patients' lungs. Even odder was the treatment based on the discovery by the German bacteriologists that their organisms were killed by exposure to high temperature. Accordingly, air heated to 150 degrees was pumped into the recipient's rectum. It was reputed, says Dormandy, to have given good results. Tobacco smoke by the same route would surely have been less painful, though of course useless. It was in fact only with the discovery of 'the germ theory' of disease in the late 19th century, and the simultaneous flowering of organic chemistry that a dim vision of rational therapies began to take shape in the enveloping fog.

Chapter 5

THE GLIMMER OF SCIENCE

Making the pain go away

The greatest benefit that 18th-century science brought to the sick was analgesia. The records of the agonies that they had to endure before the age of anaesthetics make harrowing reading – the account by Samuel Pepys of his operation for his bladder stone (the size of a tennis ball) and Fanny Burney's of her mastectomy are among the most vivid. The surgeons' primary recourses were to brandy and to speed. The specialists at 'cutting for the stone' prided themselves on the despatch with which the job was done. 'Time me, gentlemen', an English surgeon invited his colleagues standing by, and in the course of the two-minute procedure he not only extracted the stone from the patient, but also sliced the tails from the frock-coat of one observer, and struck such fear in another that he dropped dead of a heart attack. (The chances would have been that the patient also died, so the surgeon probably achieved a mortality rate of 200%.) Weak analgesics were in fact known and occasionally used, notably an alcoholic extract of mandragora (mandrake) root, a soporific familiar to Shakespeare:

> Give me mandragora, [says Cleopatra]
> That I might sleep out this great gap of time
> My Antony is away.

It was indeed known to the early Egyptians and is discussed by Dioscorides. And then there were opium preparations, such as laudanum (p.), and in India hashish, or hemp. Imports of opium into Britain from Turkey, Egypt and Persia (Iran) increased fivefold in the first half of the 19th century, and it was the universal painkiller at the time, and was thought also to be an effective treatment for a variety of distressing conditions. There were many other opium-based medicines on the market, especially the 'paregoric [soothing or comforting] elixirs'. The *London Pharmacopoeia* of 1721 listed an *Elixir Asthmaticum*, which was replaced in the 1746 edition by *Elixir Paregoricum*. In these preparations the opium was enriched with camphor, honey and a variety of other ingredients. But the first really effective counter-measure, more or less free of side-effects, against severe pain was nitrous oxide, or 'laughing gas' (p.).

It was first prepared in 1772 by Joseph Priestley (p.), who called it 'phlogisticated nitrous air', and as we have already seen, its effects when inhaled provoked entertainment and much mirth (p.). In 1799 Humphry Davy described all that in a book, *Researches, Chemical and Philosophical* (philosophical meaning physical), but he went further, for he also noted that the gas was an analgesic and even speculated that it might find uses in hospitals. Nobody took any notice, and it was to be another 44 years before the analgesic effect was explored any further. The hero of the story was Horace Wells, an American dentist, practising in Hartford, Connecticut. Nitrous oxide was enjoying a certain popularity in America as a comic turn (the 'gas frolics'), and it was a lapsed medical student, performing on the stage under the name of 'Professor' Gardner Quincy Colston, who exploited it with the greatest exuberance and success. The occasion in December of 1844 at which the great idea came to Horace Wells was graphically narrated in 1933 by Dr H.W. Erving, who had it directly from a surviving member of the audience.

Colton took a dose of the gas himself from a rubber bag with a crude tap, and then called for volunteers in the crowd, who reacted, upon inhalation, in the usual grotesque manner. 'Some danced, some sang, others made impassioned orations, or indulged in serious arguments with imaginary opponents .....'. Among them was a young pharmacist's assistant, Sam

Cooley. He breathed the gas, and at once careered about the stage in a most extraordinary manner, when suddenly he espied in the audience an imaginary enemy, and sprung over the ropes and after him. The innocent spectator, frightened out of his seven wits, summarily abandoned his seat and fled, running like a deer around the hall with Cooley in hot pursuit, the audience on its feet applauding in delight. The terrified victim finally dodged, vaulted over a settee and rushed down the aisle, Cooley a close second. Half way to the front the pursuer came to himself, looked about foolishly, and amid shouts of laughter and applause slid into his seat near to Dr. Wells. Presently he was seen to roll up his trousers and gaze in a puzzled sort of way at an excoriated and bloody leg.

"How did that happen, Sam?2 exclaimed the doctor.

"I've no idea." Cooley replied. "it's the first I knew of it."

He had scraped his shin on the sharp back of the settee when he sprung over it.

"Didn't you feel it at all?" exclaimed Dr. Wells.

"Not at all," said Sam, "I just felt a little smarting on my shin and looked." And there and then was the great discovery made!

Dr. Wells was tremendously excited, and on the very next morning, Dr. Riggs in his office, with Dr. Colton giving the gas, - a larger quantity than anyone else had ever before inhaled – extracted, after insensibility had been effected, a molar from Dr. Wells' jaw, with no pain whatever on the part of the patient. A great event had taken place – it was a momentous occasion.

Wells and Riggs proceeded to use nitrous oxide routinely in their practices, earning the widely proclaimed gratitude of their patients. But for Wells the story had no happy outcome. Elated by his discovery, he arranged to demonstrate his gas at the Massachusetts General Hospital in Boston before an audience of medical students and doctors, and in particular the doyen of the profession, the acerbic and highly sceptical John Collins Warren. Wells had brought along a patient and administered the gas.

But he was nervous, and by his own account fumbled the operation and withdrew the bag too soon. In any case, at the first yank on the forceps the fully sentient patient made his displeasure known to all in earshot, the student booed and jeered, and Wells departed in ignominy. It was a humiliation from which he never recovered.

The sweet oil

The message, though, was not lost on William Morton, a young dentist who had learned his trade from Wells, and afterwards entered Harvard medical school. He did not, however, stay the course, and it also later transpired that his supposed qualification in dentistry from Baltimore was fraudulent. But Morton made up for these shortcomings by an excess of impudence. Another actor now entered the drama. This was Charles Jackson, a chemist, doctor and entrepreneur, who had grown rich by conducting geological surveys for the state, having apparently persuaded the authorities that great wealth lay under the earth. Jackson was an unscrupulous individual with a record of stealing other men's discoveries (including Samuel Morse's electric telegraph, which he claimed to have invented). Morton, who had tried out nitrous oxide for himself, applied to Jackson for stocks of the gas, and Jackson, who derided the very idea of anaesthesia, told him that he might just as well try ether, which, just like nitrous oxide, induced euphoria and engendered extravagant behaviour ('ether frolics').

The discovery of ether is generally attributed to the German alchemist, Valerius Cordus, who made his 'sweet oil of vitriol' by distilling a mixture of alcohol and sulphuric acid (p.). The result was published posthumously in 1562 (although the alchemist, philosopher, theologian and mathematician, Ramon Lull (Raimundus Lullius) may have anticipated him by some three centuries). Because of its mode of preparation it was known in Morton's day as sulphuric ether, and in earlier times as *spiritus aetherus*. Another name, current up to the end of the 19th century, was Hoffman's Anodyne, after the 18th-centure German chemist, Friedrich Hoffmann, who recommended its use as a sedative. Ether (properly called diethyl ether, since the ethers form an entire class of organic compounds) is a highly volatile liquid – certainly not an oil as Valerius's designation implied - with a boiling point below blood temperature and an unmistakable smell. It is used as a solvent for organic substances, including fats and greases, and is highly inflammable. By the time of Morton's visit to Jackson it was already widely available, and Jackson in fact referred Morton to the local pharmacy.

Morton, in thrall now to the vision of fame and riches, did as Jackson advised, and soon an opportunity presented itself. Morton had set himself up in a practice in Boston with two apprentices, and one night a young man in agonies from a rotten tooth appeared at his door. He reluctantly submitted to the ether, which was applied on a cloth over his nose, and the tooth was extracted before the patient awoke. Morton also extracted a stiff fee and a testimonial, and the following day exhibited the grateful patient at the office of a local newspaper. This duly reported the historic event, and commented in words sounding suspiciously as if penned by Morton himself that a painless extraction had been accomplished, thanks to 'a pain-killing liquid, specially prepared by the well-known dental surgeon, Dr. Morton'. Morton's practice was instantly besieged by sufferers from toothache, pleading for a painless extraction. Now Morton approached a surgeon at the Massachusetts General Hospital, Henry Bigelow, and begged him to arrange a demonstration. Bigelow agreed and talked his imperious chief, the same John Collins Warren, into allowing the ether to be given to a patient before an operation for a tumour. So on the appointed day Morton appeared in the operating theatre with his new device, more impressive than the ether-soaked cloth, for dispensing the vapour. He reassured the patient and introduced him to the beneficiary of his first successful tooth extraction, who offered further comfort. Warren and the audience of doctors and students watched as Morton worked on the patient with the breathing tube. After some minutes he straightened and addressed Warren: 'Sir, your patient is ready'. Warren made his incision, the patient made no sound, and after some 15 minutes the tumour had been extirpated from the jaw. When all was done Morton removed the tube and the patient came round. Morton asked whether he had felt anything, and received the reply, 'It was good'. Warren turned to his audience and spoke the words, often repeated, 'Gentlemen, this is no humbug'.

Henry Bigelow witnessed more successful operations under ether anaesthesia and wrote a report in the *Boston Medical and Surgical Journal*, which appeared in November of 1846, the month after Morton's original demonstration. He had some general ruminations on the effects of ether:

> ..... ether inhalation is well known to produce symptoms similar to those produced by the nitrous oxide. In my own former experience the exhileration has been quite as great, though perhaps less pleasurable, than that of this gas, or of the Egyptian haschish.

But, he went on to say, experiments with 'the oil of wine (ethereal oil)', which was 'well known to be an ingredient in the preparation known as Hoffman's [sic] anodyne' produced no such 'exhileration', but rather induced lassitude and a feeling of paralysis, the patient remaining conscious, but asking to be pinched or pricked to reveal to what extent perception of pain had been lost.

Bigelow was scrupulous in crediting Morton with the discovery of anaesthesia, which was no less than Morton noisily claimed, making no mention of Wells or of Jackson. He also wrote to Oliver Wendell Holmes, asking his advice on what the phenomenon should be called. The learned Holmes replied, 'The state, I think should be called *anæsthesia*. This signifies insensibility, more particularly (as used by Linnaeus and Cullen) to objects of touch. The words *anti-neuric, neuro-leptic, neuro-lepsia, neuro-stasis*, seem too anatomical; whereas the change is a physiological one. I throw this out for consideration'. (A leading gynaecologist and obstetrician later urged the use of *Eatokia* for anaesthesia applied in childbirth; it never caught on.)

Morton made an application for a patent on 'his' discovery, and demanded royalties from city and state for each use. He was challenged by Jackson who, ever the opportunist, now claimed that inhalation anaesthesia had been his idea all along, and denounced Morton as an ignoramus and a liar. Soon afterwards another contender entered the legal brawl: Crawford Williamson Long, a surgeon from Georgia had excised a tumour from the neck of a patient under ether anaesthesia in March of 1842, predating therefore even Wells's first efforts with nitrous oxide. He had gone on to use the procedure in amputations and childbirth, and had instructed colleagues, who had also then taken up his technique. But it was only in 1849 that he published an account of his work in the *Southern Medical and Surgical Journal*, and since publication represents the only valid claim to a discovery, his assertion of priority was rejected. Long later enlisted as a medical officer in the Confederate army in the Civil War, and at its conclusion was asked to supervise treatment of the wounded on both sides. Long died unrewarded in 1878. The unfortunate Wells, who did have a valid claim, was likewise squeezed out. He was mortified by the acclaim that the treacherous Morton and Jackson received, and tried to set the record straight in a bitter letter to the local newspaper, but to little avail. His contribution was at least recognised in Paris, where he was elected an honorary member of the Paris Medical Society, but the honour came too late. Deeply embittered, he had abandoned his profession, moved to New York, and had experimented with chloroform, to which he may have become addicted. At all events his increasingly erratic behaviour landed him in prison, accused, perhaps falsely, of an acid attack on two prostitutes. In 1848 he committed suicide at the age of thirty-three. The legal wrangles between the remaining contestants continued for two decades after his death. After ferocious lobbying of Congress, Morton, and to his disgust Jackson also, were awarded $100,000 apiece for the invention of inhalation anaesthesia, but this was revoked following a challenge by a lawyer acting for Horace Wells's widow. Yet neither man abandoned the quest for riches and fame. Morton's disreputable life ended in New York in 1868, when half deranged, he fell or leapt from his horse-drawn carriage and died a few hours later. He was 48. Jackson fared little better. He wrote a book on ether anaesthesia, reporting experiments on the patients in the lunatic asylum attached to the Massachusetts General Hospital, but eventually ended up as an inmate himself and died there in 1880, having reached the age of 75. As to the bones of contention, nitrous oxide fell out of use, except in dentistry, partly because the depth of anaesthesia that it engendered was inferior to that of ether, and partly because it caused often dangerous levels of oxygen-starvation. This was overcome twenty years later when nitrous oxide-oxygen mixtures were introduced. But it was ether that, starting in the late 1840s, became inseparable from the practice of surgery.

The word reached Britain in the form of a letter to a Boston-born doctor, Francis Boott, practising in Gower Street, the site of University College in London. It came from a family friend, Jacob Bigelow, a doctor, professor at Harvard, who was also a distinguished botanist, and the father of the surgeon, Henry Bigelow. 'I send you', he began, 'an account of a new anodyne lately introduced here, which promises to be one of the important discoveries of the present age'. He had taken his daughter to William Morton for an extraction under ether, and had been hugely impressed. Boott at once decided that he must acquaint the famous surgeon, Robert Liston at University College Hospital, just up the road, with this exciting news. But Liston was a famously sceptical and irascible man, and Boott was fearful enough to request a dentist from nearby Bedford Square to try it on a patient, so that he might satisfy himself the supposed discovery was no mirage. Emboldened by the outcome of this, the first test of ether anaesthesia in Britain, Boott sought an audience with Liston and told him the story. Liston, as it turned out, had also just heard about the miraculous effect of ether from none other than Bigelow's surgeon son, Henry, and resolved at once to try it out for himself.

On the agreed day doctors and students gathered in the operating theatre, and by way of a warm-up act, Liston's assistant, who had already experimented on himself, attempted to etherise a volunteer, a retired soldier. The man reacted by leaping to his feat with a roar and heading with aggressive mien towards the audience, fortunately collapsing as though pole-axed before he could inflict any damage. The audience, thus already rewarded, awaited the entry of Liston with his retinue and his patient. Liston was an imposing figure, six foot two (1.88 metres) tall in his green frock coat and boots. According to one account of his modus operandi, 'the first flash of his knife was followed so swiftly by the rasp of saw on bone that sight and sound seemed simultaneous. To free both hands he would clasp the bloody knife in his teeth'. Liston addressed his audience: 'We are going to try a Yankee dodge today, gentlemen' for making men insensible'. Ether was administered with a nebuliser and Liston, asking the students, as he always did, to time him, went to work. In two and a half minutes the diseased leg was amputated and by four and a half the wound had been stitched. The patient made not a sound until, as recollected by

Dr William Squire, the anaesthetist, he roused himself and moaned, 'Take me away; I can't have it done; I must die as I am'. Liston thereupon showed him the severed leg, and then 'stood motionless but tears were rolling down his cheeks'. Then he spoke: 'Well, gentlemen, this Yankee dodge sure beats mesmerism hollow' - for mesmerism, or hypnosis, had been in used in the search for ways of limiting pain, but the best succour until then had been the speed of the surgeon, which saved many patients from dying of shock.

Liston proselytised energetically for anaesthesia and he was fortunate in acquiring a partner in his endeavour. John Snow (1813-1858) casts a long shadow in the history of medicine. He was born into a poor family in Yorkshire, who could not afford to provide him with an education when his exceptional intelligence became clear. He developed an early interest in medicine, and at 15 was apprenticed to a doctor in Newcastle. Snow was and remained modest and retiring, pious, abstemious and a lifelong vegetarian. He saved money, qualified as a doctor and as an apothecary, and in 1836 made his way to London – on foot. He found lodgings amongst the poor in Soho and practised there until his early death. He was possessed of a restless curiosity, allied to exceptional intellectual rigour, and began in his spare time to conduct research in a variety of areas.** Snow's wide-ranging intellect had begun to focus on ether anaesthesia a year or two

---

* Snow is now mainly remembered for his famous study on cholera during the great epidemic of 1848. The story has been often told, but it is worth recalling that the disease, which in its most virulent form killed about half its victims, was most often treated by bloodletting, probably the fastest way to ensure a fatal outcome (p.). Opium was also commonly given, which may have eased the suffering, as also would gin and brandy. Snow suspected that the foul sewers had something to do with the spread of the disease, and he plotted on a map the geographical distribution of its victims. The epicentre in Soho was the pump in Broad Street, which served the local population as its main source of water. It is not now certain how accurate are the accounts of Snow's detective work, but the story goes that he investigated the death of an old lady in faraway Hampstead, and discovered that she had lived in Soho, believed the water there to be the purest of all and had bidden her sons to bring her bottles of it regularly. Snow caused the handle to be removed from the Broad Street pump, and the epidemic abated, although, in truth, it may already have passed its peak. Snow nevertheless was the first to conceive of the possibility of a water-borne disease, and his first publication (in 1849) on the subject, *Mode of Communication of Cholera*, stands as a monuments in the history of scientific analysis.

before the cholera outbreak forced itself on his attention. He devised an inhaler, and in 1847 he was already employing it at St. George's Hospital for tooth extractions, and soon after for more demanding operations. He made, as was his wont, a painstaking study of the problems associated with ether, and that year published a monograph, *On Ether*. His skills were quickly recognised by the more open-minded surgeons, among them Robert Liston, who evidently sought out Snow's services. The two men, so different in character, worked amicably together until Liston's premature death nine months later. Meanwhile surgeons and obstetricians and even veterinarians throughout Europe were taking up ether anaesthesia, and an enterprising Russian surgeon introduced rectal administration of the vapour, a procedure that had advantages and enjoyed a transient vogue. Ether, though, was not devoid of drawbacks: it could bring on vomiting and severe coughing, and it was of course highly inflammable and a major hazard in candle-lit operating rooms at night. Lively minds were intent on discovering other and better inhalation anaesthetics.

James Young Simpson (1811-1870) was the youngest of eight children of a village baker in rural Scotland. He was christened James Simpson and the origin of his adopted middle name has aroused much speculation: the most likely explanation is that he was always referred to in his turbulent youth as Young Simpson. Prodigiously bright, Simpson managed, despite his underprivileged beginnings, to enter the Medical School in Edinburgh, and at the age of 21 he was awarded the M.D. degree. He chose for a career the new and unfashionable speciality of obstetrics, and at the age of 29 was elected to the chair of midwifery, after a noisy campaign, and against the opposition of the professors on the committee. Simpson was a polymath, who made contributions to archaeology and other fields of scholarship, but it was as Scotland's premier physician and surgeon that he was venerated. His house became a meeting place for the intellectual elite, and every week he and two of his medical friends, George Keith and Matthews Duncan would gather for dinner and engage in discussion and experiments*.

Simpson had begun to offer ether to women in childbirth as soon as its value became known, but like Snow in London, he was not altogether satisfied, and the three friends began to try all the organic vapours they could find on themselves for anaesthetic effects. After dinner on a November day in 1847 the ladies, who had 'withdrawn' at the end of the dinner, returned to the dining room to find their menfolk either unconscious or in a state of high animation. Simpson, according to his own account, had brought out a bottle of chloroform, which he had forgotten was in his pocket, and tried its effects, and this was the result. Simpson decided at once that this was what he had been looking for. It acted rapidly, appeared to have no disagreeable side-effects and was not inflammable. (He did not of course know that it could cause liver damage.) He immediately tried it out on his patients – no question of course at the time of animal experiments or clinical trials. The first woman to profit from it gave tranquil birth to a daughter, she was persuaded to call Anaesthesia.

Chloroform is a simple substance with the formula $CHCl_3$ (composed therefore of a carbon atom linked to one hydrogen and three chlorine atoms), simultaneously discovered in the 1830s by chemists in three countries. None of them seem to have spotted its narcotic effects.

---

* A flavour of these evening activities can be gleaned from the diary of one of the guests at Simpson's table, the celebrated Danish writer, Hans Christian Andersen. He was travelling around Scotland with an English companion, Carl Joachim Hambro, founder of the merchant bank, who was apparently acquainted with Simpson. Andersen, a fervent admirer of Walter Scott, was fascinated with the strange country. On the Sabbath, he wrote to a friend at home, 'Everything is then at rest. Even the railway trains dare not run. All the houses are closed, and the people sit inside and read their Bibles or drink themselves blind drunk.' At the dinner a number of ladies were present, including Catherine Crowe, a novelist and poetess, whom Andersen much admired. The guests were treated to a demonstration of the effects of ether, and Andersen was shocked. 'I thought it distasteful', he later recorded in his memoirs, 'especially to see ladies in this dreamy intoxication; they laughed with open lifeless eyes; there was something unpleasant about it, and I said so, recognising at the same time that it was a wonderful and blessed invention to use in painful operations, but not to play with; it was wrong to do it; it was almost like tempting God.'

When Simpson publicised his observations chloroform quickly caught on, and very soon it had more or less supplanted ether for operations and in childbirth. In London John Snow had immediately carried out measurements of such factors as its solubility and persistence in the blood, the optimal concentration for different purposes and so on – studies reported in a mighty work of some 900 pages, *On Chloroform*, which appeared in 1858 after his death. Snow underscoreded its advantages, and the surgeons with whom he worked were soon persuaded. But in the wider world neither chloroform nor ether met with universal approbation, for surely to eliminate pain, which was so intimately linked to the human condition, was a presumptuous denial of the divine will. And had not God instructed Eve that 'in sorrow thou shalt bring forth children'? In Calvinist Scotland the opposition was particularly vehement, but Simpson was not easily intimidated, and hit back lustily. He conducted a correspondence with his opponents, among whom was a respected physician, Francis Henry Ramsbotham, ten years Simpson's senior. Ramsbotham was no religious bigot or obscurantist. He had genuine concerns, believing that anaesthetics were poisons and a danger to mother and baby, and that their effects had not been adequately tested - nor was he alone in this, for several other eminent figures, notably the great Magendie in Paris, took a similar view. Simpson responded that to deny women pain relief in childbirth was different in degree only from exposing them, as was still the practice in Vienna, to the risk of death from childbed (puerperal) fever. (The Viennese establishment has scorned the evidence adduced by Ignaz Semmelweis that the condition was contagious (p.) and continued to deliver the women in 'a bed still warm from a dead mother'.) The women, Simpson wrote, 'are doomed (and doomed unnecessarily and cruelly) to agony and torture'. They were 'sacrificed to suffer, as a fit-offering to the old medical prejudices regarding the propriety of pain'.

There were many other specious arguments. The professor of obstetrics in Philadelphia asserted in a letter to Simpson that if forceps were required during parturition pain was the best guide to their proper placement. Pain, moreover, was physiologically speaking 'the most desirable, salutary, and conservative manifestation of life force'. The woman was best sustained by 'cheering counsel', the learned professor went on, with more in similar vein.

Simpson replied to this nonsense that pain was no guide at all to placing the forceps, and that this was far better done when the anaesthetised patient could be properly examined. In Canada a medical journal invited the country's leading rabbi, who was also Lecturer in Hebrew Language and Literature at McGill University, to interpret the words of God as set down in the book of Genesis. Rabbi De Sola gave the desired answer: it was toil or labour that the woman had to endure, not pain, so anaesthesia was not contrary to God's will. Simpson, no mean scholar, had for his part already offered a translation of the Hebrew text. There were also some more rational worries, particularly about whether surgical skills could be compromised by the more leisurely pace at which operations would now be performed. There were jibes that the operating theatre clock might now be replaced by a calendar. Snow seems to have been one who preferred the surgeons of the old school, but no evidence came to light that speed of cutting saved lives, as it undoubtedly had done in the days before anaesthesia.

The breakthrough, in the end, came not from biblical exegesis but from a higher authority. In 1853 John Snow, who despite his retiring nature had become famous, was summoned to Buckingham Palace by Prince Albert. The Prince Consort, ever eager to learn about scientific advances and mindful of Queen Victoria's impending confinement, wanted to hear from the source about anaesthesia in childbirth. The conversation was evidently satisfactory for both sides, and when the moment came Snow was in attendance, together with the Queen's physician and her obstetrician. All went smoothly, and the delighted Queen was delivered of her seventh child, the future Prince Leopold. All religious and technical objections to the use of chloroform were instantly stilled, and soon after the daughter of the Archbishop of Canterbury was also treated to a painless delivery. James Simpson wrote to Ramsbotham with the unanswerable question: 'Will you be so disloyal as to abuse chloroform now that the Queen has taken it (and sent me too a kind message about it)?' In the event, it was to be another 14 years before Ramsbotham finally threw in the towel. The 5th edition of his textbook, *Principles and Practice of Obstetric Medicine and Surgery*, which appeared in 1867, 26 years after the first, was dedicated to 'Sir James Simpson, Bart, whose indefatigable exertions in the cause of science, and successful efforts to alleviate human suffering have rendered his name famous throughout the world'. His chapter on anaesthesia was unchanged however, but for the slightly grudging coda: 'Experience has fortunately proved that the gloomy anticipations, which I had formed respecting the dangers universally attending the administration of anaesthetics, have turned out to be, in some degree, fallacious; or at least it is not so great as I feared it would be; for the casualties that have resulted from its use during that period have been astonishingly few.' But in truth the battle had been won twenty years before.

Chloroform, so much in the news, penetrated the public consciousness and entered into art and literature. Here is the poet, W.E. Henley, who suffered miserably from bone tuberculosis, and had to submit to a series of operations:

> Behold me waiting – waiting for the knife.
> A little while, and at a leap I storm
> The thick, sweet mystery of chloroform,
> The drunken dark, the little death-in-life.

(His surgeon in Edinburgh was Lister.) Nor did its possibilities escape the peddlers of patent medicines. Quack preparations containing chloroform appeared on the market after about 1850, and much of the outrageous advertising was directed at the parents of babies suffering from teething colic or croup. Most of these concoctions contained opium, morphine or even heroin. Street's Infant Quieter, Atkinson's Baby Preservative, Dover's Powder, and in America, Godfrey's Cordial and Mrs Winslow's Soothing Syrup were typical of the hundreds of brand names on offer. In Britain the most successful and enduring was probably Dr J. Collis Browne's Chlorodyne. The name was an amalgamation of chloroform and anodyne, though it also contained morphine and other substances, and it was not originally conceived as quackery, for Dr Collis Browne was an Indian Army doctor who concocted it in 1848 as a treatment for cholera. By the time the doctor left the army and went into partnership with a London pharmacist, though, the claims for its powers had become truly extravagant: it would cure, the label assured the purchaser, everything from cholera, flu, bronchitis and flatulence to whooping cough and rheumatism. Seeing how profitable the nostrum had become, competitors stole the name and marketed their own chlorodynes. Lawsuits followed, and *The Lancet* and the *British Medical Journal* warned against the dangers of consuming these addictive potions, as many were now doing. Alarm also grew about the supposed use of chloroform by footpads and other criminals, who were reputed to ambush their victims with chloroform-soaked cloths.* It is doubtful whether chloroform was ever successfully used in this manner.

---

* Half a century later James Thurber was to write of his aunt, whose fear of being chloroformed by burglars was such that she would stack her possessions outside her door each night with a placard on which was written: 'This is all I have. Please take it and do not use your chloroform, as this is all I have'.

Chapter 6

THE NEW THERAPEUTICS AND THE RISE OF CHEMISTRY

Purity and wisdom

Chemistry, in the form in which we know it today, emerged in the latter half of the 18th century. Pierre Joseph Macquer (1718-1784), a prominent figure in the French Academy of Science, who trained as a doctor, but dedicated his career to the application of chemistry to commerce – to dyestuffs, ceramics and medicine – offered a definition of his calling that holds true today. It comes from his textbook, *Dictionnaire de chymie*, published in 1766, and later translated into several languages, including English:

The Object and chief End of Chymistry is to separate the different substances that enter into the composition of bodies; to examine each of them apart; to discover their properties and relations; to decompose those very substances, if possible; to compare them together and combine them with others; to reunite them again into one body so as to reproduce the original compound with all its properties; or even to produce new compounds that never existed among the works on Nature.

This is is a fair summary of what chemists strive for, and in particular organic chemists – those who concern themselves with carbon compounds, which include nearly all substances produced by living organisms, as well as drugs.

The notion that plant preparations, for example, are mixtures of different compounds, among which there might be one with useful physiological properties, really took hold at about this time, and chemists tried to find methods for separating the constituents and isolating whatever was of interest – the 'active principle', as it was termed. The new era arguably dawned in 1804 in a scientific backwater - the small Westphalian town of Paderborn. The protagonist in the story was the eldest son of the surveyor to the Prince Bishop of Paderborn and Hildesheim, and indeed the Prince's godson. He was destined to follow his father's calling, but when both father and godfather died the boy's mother could not raise the cost of the required training. And so, with little formal education, the young man enrolled in 1803 as apprentice in the court pharmacy. His name was Friedrich Wilhelm Adam Sertürner, and he was 21 when in 1804 he made his great discovery. Encouraged by his master, who (like many conscientious pharmacists and physicians) was troubled by the variations in potency of opium preparations, he had taught himself the methods of chemistry, and began experimenting with opium poppy juice. Sertürner's first paper, published in 1806, was masterly. In it he described the isolation of two new substances, one of them the narcotic active principle, morphine.

To achieve this Sertürner neutralised the acidic hot-water extract of crude opium with a base*, ammonia, and recovered a greyish precipitate. The residual liquid (the filtrate) from which he had collected the precipitate, gave rise to a second precipitate on addition of acetic acid (the mild acid of vinegar). Because this substance was insoluble in acidic, but soluble in a basic solution, he inferred that it was an acid, for salts were known to be generally water-soluble. He decided that the properties of anything he

---

* A base is the antithesis of an acid. Acids and bases neutralise each other with formation of water and a salt. So when, for example, sodium hydroxide, $NaOH$, is added to hydrochloric acid, HCl, the salt $NaCl$ (common salt) is formed. A strong base (like $NaOH$) is called an alkali.

isolated could be determined only by a test on a living creature, and so he tried it on a dog and on himself. The substance proved inert (and nor has any physiological activity been found since). He called it meconic acid, from the Greek for poppy. Sertürner now turned his attention to the first precipitate. He gave some to a dog and tasted it himself. It engendered an unpleasant feeling in him, and caused the dog after a while to become torpid, to stagger and then to vomit. Sertürner inferred that he was on the track of the active component, the true *principium somniferum*, the sleep-bringing principle. He next set about purifying it. He dissolved the material in acid, precipitated it again with ammonia, and repeated the operation. He now had sparkling crystals, soluble in acidulated water and in alcohol, which when redissolved and tested on the unfortunate dog, put it to sleep and all but killed it. Sertürner saved the animal with a dose of vinegar. To make absolutely sure he had obtained the full yield of active material and nothing else was left, he tried the filtrate from the final preparation of crystals on himself and another dog: this was what is now called a 'negative control', and indeed neither subject displayed any symptoms. Sertürner called his preparation morphium after Morphius, the Roman god of dreams. His paper revealed astonishing insight and prescience. He noted that his 'morphium' was a new type of substance with unprecedented potency; that replacing crude opium by a pure material would solve at a stroke the age-old bugbear of variable products and uncertain dosages; that testing the effects of newly discovered substances on living creatures was essential; that alkaline substances with powerful physiological properties were probably waiting to be discovered in other plants besides the opium poppy; and that useful, therapeutic compounds might even be lurking in the most poisonous of plants, and might act benignly when administered in sub-toxic amounts. The dismaying outcome was that so far as it was noticed at all, Sertürner's remarkable work was generally derided. This may have been because it emerged from the academic outback, and also probably because it drew attention to the basic character of the morphium, for it was an article of faith at the time that organic substances - acetic acid, lactic acid, tartaric acid and many more - were unarguably acidic. Bases, it was thought, simply did not occur in nature.

There followed a long gap in Sertürner's productivity. Scientific journals did not reach Paderborn, and he did not know, as he acknowledged in his later publication, of work in other countries, especially in France, which then led the world in chemistry and the study of drugs. Discoveries on opium products had been made in 1804, quite independently, by two Frenchmen. One was a Parisian pharmacist, Jean-François Derosne, the other Armand Séguin, assistant, or rather guinea-pig, over many years, to the late great Antoine Lavoisier, the father as is often said, of modern chemistry. Derosne had, like Sertürner, generated a precipitate by neutralising his mildly acidic opium extract, and published an account of this *sel de Derosne* in a French journal. It was however devoid of narcotic properties (but did later find some use as a cough suppressant). As for Séguin, he was a slippery character, and no great savant. He had served Lavoisier for five years, stoically enduring his role as a guinea-pig in metabolic experiments. He would be enclosed in a sealed rubber suit and have his intake of food and water, and his output of the products in urine, breath and sweat monitored for long hours. He avoided his master's fate on the scaffold, and attempted to continue the work, though with no useful outcome. Lavoisier's wife and collaborator, Marie Paulze had sought his assistance in preparing her husband's unpublished researches for publication, but she took umbrage when Séguin tried to claim more credit than was his due in the Preface. She also objected to his unwillingness to condemn those who had denounced Lavoisier and contrived his death.

Séguin continued to dabble in science, but his pronouncements on such matters as the efficacy of cinchona bark, which he insisted derived from glycerine, did nothing to advance human knowledge. Yet he did become rich, having acquired a position as scientist in charge of a tannery in Sèvres, charged with providing leather for army boots. (Although Séguin did effect some improvements in the tanning process the project in the end proved a fiasco.) Nevertheless, the persevering Séguin did read a paper on his opium extract to the *Institut de France* in 1804. The work had apparently been largely done by his able assistant at the *École Polytechnique*, Bertrand Courtois, whom we will encounter again. Séguin gave Courtois no credit, but in any case nothing was published until ten years later, because Séguin had other matters on his mind: he was a member of a consortium of businessmen, owners of a trading company, which dealt with the State. They were accused of profiteering and fraud, and Séguin - whose father had earlier been arraigned for corruption when treasurer to the Duke of Orléans, 'Philippe Égalité', famous supporter of the Revolution - may have felt himself particularly vulnerable. Faced with prison or worse, he managed to talk himself out of trouble and to get away with merely losing most of his fortune. By the time his paper on opium was published its revelations had been left far behind by Sertürner's continuing researches. Séguin, living in comfortable retirement after the fall of Napoleon, continued to instruct the world with pamphlets on a variety of topics, including the economy, gout and horse-racing, as well as scientific questions.

Sertürner, meanwhile, had moved in 1805 to a position as assistant in another pharmacy, this one in the small town of Einbeck near Göttingen, but had soon after opened a pharmacy of his own. But then in 1807 the town became part of the Napoleonic Kingdom of Westphalia, and to qualify as a pharmacist Sertürner had to complete a long course of study. He passed the examination, but in 1813, following the defeat of Napoleon at Leipzig and his banishment to Elba, Westphalia reverted to its previous status. Sertürner now found himself on the wrong side of the law, and a long period of legal wrangling ensued. It was only in 1816 that he found time to return to the study of opium. His plan was to improve the purification process, and scale up the production of his morphium. In addition to tests on dogs, he wanted to try the pure morphium on human subjects. And so it came about that he administered a weight of half a grain (30 milligrams – a considerable amount, and far beyond the dosages permitted today) dissolved in an alcohol-water mixture, to three boys, the oldest of whom was seventeen. He also swallowed an equal measure himself. The result was alarming and nearly fatal. At first little happened, so after 15 minutes they all took another half-grain. Immediately symptoms began to show themselves, first a severe headache, then weakness, twitching of the limbs and partial loss of consciousness. Sertürner, clearly terrified of what might be happening to his boys, managed to rouse himself sufficiently to drink a large amount of vinegar, which he also forced on his subjects. There was violent vomiting, which continued for hours, and then they all sank into a deep sleep. On waking they again started to vomit and other symptoms – pains in the head and body, constipation, narcosis and lack of appetite – persisted for some days.

In 1817 Sertürner published an account of the work and the consequences of his tests, and this time it did attract notice from a quarter that mattered. Joseph Louis Gay-Lussac (1778-1850) was one of the most important, and also one of the most attractive personalities in 19th-century science. At the time he was professor of physics at the University of Paris. (Later he moved to the Jardin des Plantes as professor of chemistry.) He already had a remarkable number of major discoveries to his name: he had established the relation between the volume and temperature of a gas; he had discovered that when gases combined they did so in fixed proportions, so that for instance two parts of hydrogen combined with one of oxygen to produce water; he had discovered an element (boron), and had shown that the recently discovered iodine (p.) was an element, the properties of which he defined in exacting detail; he had developed methods of determining the compositions of chemical compounds; and he had even invented a scale for the measurement of alcohol content in drinks. Most spectacular was his record balloon ascent, at no small risk, to 7 kilometres, from which he brought back samples of high-altitude air. Before that, he and the physicist, Jean-Baptiste Biot had ascended to 6.4 kilometres to determine whether the Earth's magnetic field changed with altitude, as had been suggested. (It didn't.) And as if this were not enough, he was a much admired teacher, and trained students, many of whom were to become famous. Now Gay-Lussac saw to it that Sertürner's talents and achievements were recognised. He arranged for Sertürner's paper of 1817, rendered into French, to be published in the leading French journal, the *Annales de Chimie et de Physique*, and it was almost certainly he who saw to it that this was followed by the award of the coveted Monthyon prize of the Academy of Sciences. It was Gay-Lussac who also proposed that Sertürner's name for his product, morphium should be replaced by *morphine.*

Sertürner's work, carried out in isolation in two pharmacies in small towns in north Germany, was a turning-point in the history of drug discovery. Above all there was his insistence on the prime importance of purity, for only a pure substance could be tested and administered in a reproducible manner. Morphine, it transpired, is one of a large class of drugs called alkaloids on the grounds that they were all basic (p.), or alkaline, and Sertürner's method of extracting and purifying morphine was equally applicable to the other compounds of this kind. Sertürner had made the point that morphine, and therefore probably all or many other such plant-derived substances, are poisons, and must be treated with the greatest circumspection. His paper bore in fact the title, 'On the most fearful poisons of the plant kingdom ....'.His surmise that many plants would yield such toxic, yet valuable compounds, which would enrich the therapeutic choices available to physicians, was soon proved correct.

Sertürner left Einbeck and established himself more grandly in Hamelin (Hameln), a somewhat larger town. For some years he occupied himself with improving and enlarging the preparation of plant alkaloids, and wrote several books. He was chagrined that, even though he had received a doctoral degree from the University of Jena in 1817, his work had had to wait for a French savant to be recognised, but he was soon showered with honours in his own country and abroad. The award of the Monthyon Prize by the Institut de France finally silenced the sniping of (among others) the insufferable Derosne, with his inflated opinion of his own contribution. In the last years of his life Sertürner became increasingly hypochodriacal and unstable, but he still pursued a number of interests, one of which was in firearms. He designed a breech-loading rifle, and experimented with the composition of bullets. There was also further chemical work: he showed that the strong alkalies, caustic soda and potash (sodium and potassium hydroxides), were compounds, not elements but this work was never published. Most remarkably, he wrote a paper on a cholera epidemic then ravaging the region, in which he concluded – well before Robert Koch discovered the existence of pathogenic bacteria – that a self-perpetuating agent was the cause of the disease, and that it was inactivated by high or low temperatures. For this acute insight he received no recognition. Sertürner died in 1841 at the age of 58.

The demand for morphine, and the products that followed soon exceeded anything that could be accomplished in high-street pharmacies, and in 1827 the first precursor of the modern pharmaceutical companies began to market a range of plant alkaloids: Heinrich Emanuel Merck (1794-1855) was the scion of a family which owned a pharmacy in Darmstadt, established by a forebear, in 1668. Heinrich Emanuel was a capable chemist, who turned his *Apotheke Engel* into a factory, producing compounds of high purity, which it supplied to doctors, pharmacies, hospitals and even to research chemists. The business passed to Merck's descendants, and later a subsidiary was opened in the United States.*" From little acorns mighty oaks do grow. The chemical formula of morphine was not definitively established until 1956.

In another scientifically obscure corner of Europe a young scholar entered on what was to be an illustrious career, a minor part of which would involve the testing of drug effects, mainly on himself. Jan Evangelista Purkinje** (the German version of his name, which wa properly written Purkině in

---

* Merck, Sharpe and Dohme is one of the world's major pharmaceutical companies. Merck and Company in the U.S. was transformed into an independent American concern when German commercial assets were impounded during the First World War.

** Purkinje was a remarkable figure, a polymath whose most famous work was in physiology and anatomy. His name is commemorated in a variety of anatomical structures and physiological effects that he discovered. Purkinje was born in a small town in Bohemia (then a part of the Austro-Hungarian empire) in 1787. At the age of 10 he was sent to a Piarist monastery in Moravia, close to the Austrian border, to be educated. The Piarists were a teaching order and the boy received a good education. He was moreover unusually bright, and quickly mastered German and Latin. He took holy orders, taught in Piarist schools, and prepared himself for university. At the venerable Charles University in Prague, where the teaching was conducted in German, he abandoned his religious studies and took up philosophy and science. In 1818 he wrote his doctoral dissertation on the physics of vision, an interest that remained with him throughout his career. Switching to biology, he progressed to the position of prosector, charged with the preparation of dissections for medical students, and acquired a profound knowledge of anatomy. Purkinje attracted the attention of a German professor in the university (whose daughter he married), and with his patronage was appointed in 1823 to a professorial chair at the University of Breslau, where he did most of his important work. In 1850 he returned to Prague and remained there until his death in 1869. Besides his extensive accomplishments in so many areas of biology, he took a leading part in the reform of scientific education and research in his country. As a Czech nationalist he took steps to introduce the use of the Czech language into education and into scientific publishing.

his native language) found the current materia medica archaic, and began in around 1825 a systematic examination of such drugs as he thought might be of value. He satisfied himself that the homeopathic doctrine was senseless, and for ten years categorised drugs by smell, taste and physiological effect. He tried out preparations of ipecac extracts in different forms; he studied the influence of digitalis on vision, and discovered that it caused dilation of the pupil; he observed the hallucinogenic effects of nutmeg, which was in wide clinical use at the time; he reported on the toxicity of turpentine, which was taken as an antihelminthic (to eliminate intestinal worms); and he experimented with camphor, still then in the mainstays of the remedies deployed by physicians. He reported that small doses caused a burning sensation in the stomach, while larger amounts led to severe stomach irritation a hot skin, general prickling, and heightened sensibility. Even greater doses gave rise to hallucinations, erratic behaviour and unconsciousness. These results were published and probably saved many patients from distress and worse due to reckless prescribing by many European doctors. After ten years of relentless self-experimentation Purkinje decided to discontinue this dangerous practice, probably out of consideration for his growing family, and dedicated himself to his most important work, which was yet to come.

Alkaloids abounding

It was in France that the predictions by Sertürner of a new age of chemically generated drugs were first realised. French chemistry was flourishing as never before. One of its elders declared that it was as if the immortal Lavoisier had risen from the grave. And chemistry concerned itself with pure compounds – exactly what the enlightened advocates of rational therapies now craved. A young pioneer in what came to be called natural-products chemistry was Pierre-Jean Robiquet, born in the city of Rennes in 1780. His father was a pharmacist, and the parents had high ambitions for their children. Pierre was to be an architect, but his education was brutally interrupted when both parents, suspected of attachment to the Girondins (the more moderate, therefore doomed, faction in the revolutionary Legislative Assembly), were arrested and their property impounded. The son, then aged 13, was sent to work first in a carpenter's workshop, then in a pharmacy in his home town, and finally in a factory making drugs for use by the navy. There he evidently developed an interest in pharmacy and chemistry. In time the family was reunited and Robiquet began his education in earnest, starting in Rennes and continuing in Paris, where he entered the laboratory of the noted chemist, Antoine Fourcroy, a former associate (and betrayer) of Lavoisier. There, with a fellow-aspirant, Louis Jacques Thénard, who was also to achieve eminence, Robiquet embarked on his first research project, the analysis of bladder stones. But after two years his progress was again interrupted, this time by military service in Napoleon's Italian campaign. Despite the privations he was forced to endure, the young Robiquet managed to attend some lectures at the Univeristy of Pavia in both anatomy and physics (the latter by the famous physicist, Alessandro Volta, who gave his name to the unit of electromotive force, the volt).

After Napoleon secured his foothold in Italy by victory at Marengo, Robiquet was sent home, to a military hospital in Rennes, and thence to the Val-de-Grâce military hospital in Paris. After six years as a hospital pharmacist, he entered the private laboratory of the celebrated chemist, Louis Nicolas Vauquelin to assist in the preparation of commercial products. He also qualified as a pharmacist, and opened his own small business. Robiquet made his first mark while in Vauquelin's employ: he isolated from the asparagus plant a simple substance, an amino acid, asparagine, which proved to be one of the 20 amino acids of which proteins are constructed. He later discovered several more amino acids, and also alizarin, the orange-red dye extracted from the root of the madder plant, which 50 years later formed the basis of the dyestuff industry. Robiquet began the ascent of the academic ladder when in 1811 he was appointed assistant professor at the École de Pharmacie, and apparently at much the same time *préparateur*, or assistant, in chemistry at the highly-rated École Polytechnique. In 1814 he was promoted to professor at the École de Pharmacie, where he remained until in 1824, in declining health, he resigned his professorial chair, which passed to his protégé, Joseph Pelletier. In 1826 Robiquet was elected President of the Société de Pharmacie, and many other honours had been heaped on him by the time he died in 1844.

Throughout Robiquet's active period the flow of important discoveries never ceased. In 1810 he had isolated cantharidin, the irritant, vesicant and supposed aphrodisiac, from Spanish fly. Much later Robiquet and one of his students isolated amygdalin from the seeds of the sweet almond tree. This is a glycoside, a compound made up partly of sugar residues. It is toxic, because a metabolic reaction in the body leads to the formation of hydrocyanic acid, but there were at one time high hopes for its value as a cancer treatment, and it was so used in some countries until the early 20th century. It was eventually recognised to be ineffective and dangerous, but it had a resurgence during the 1970s, when it reappeared as a notorious quack cancer remedy, laetrile (p.). But of all Robiquet's discoveries it was the alkaloids that most excited the interest of physiologists. First, in 1817, came noscapine (called narcotine by Robiquet) from opium, which still survives in some places as a cough suppressant, then caffeine in 1821, and finally, in1832, the crowning discovery, another opium alkaloid, codeine.

The priority for the discovery of caffeine has been disputed, for in 1819 a prodigiously gifted young chemist at the University of Jena, Friedlieb Ferdinand Runge (1795-1867) had also, unknown to Robiquet, purified an 'active principle' from a coffee bean extract. Runge was born in a village near Hamburg, where his father was the pastor. He began his working life as an apprentice in his uncle's pharmacy in nearby Lübeck. There he gave an early display of his talent and independence of mind by developing a research project on the side: he made a preparation containing atropine from the belladonna plant and discovered its mydriatic (pupil-dilating) effect, of which ophthalmologists made use for almost two centuries. After serving out his time in the pharmacy Runge entered the University of Berlin to read medicine, but completed his training at the University of Jena, with a thesis on atropine. In Jena he next turned to chemistry, intent on indulging his fascination with plant toxins, a subject on which he was already compiling a book. His research supervisor, a leading chemist of the period, recognised his pupil's talent, and introduced him to the Rector of the university – none other than Johann Wolfgang von Goethe. The great man had developed a deep interest in the progress of science, and was impressed by Runge. It was Goethe who suggested to him the problem he might take up next: it was to isolate an 'active principle' from the coffee bean, for coffee was regarded as a valuable psychotropic agent (as it would now be called), and thought by some doctors to have a fever-suppressing action. Runge succeeded, and dubbed his product *Kaffeebase*, or coffee base. Runge wrote up his work in 1819, and it was published the next year, three years ahead of Robiquet - the first but not the only time that Runge was deprived of recognition for a major discovery - under the striking title, 'Discoveries towards the Foundation of a scientific Phytochemistry [plant chemistry] – Coffee Base'. In 1822 he completed his second doctorate with a thesis on another natural product, indigo. After a short period teaching courses of technical chemistry and phytochemistry Runge embarked on the kind of scientific 'grand tour', in favour in Germany at the time, visiting research centres in France, Switzerland, England and Holland. In 1826, after his three *Wanderjahre*, he returned to Germany, and in in 1828 was appointed professor of chemistry at the University of Breslau. There he researched and taught for four years before taking up a post as scientific director at a state-owned chemical works in Oranienburg in Prussia. Runge's enlightened plans for the development of a chemical dyestuffs industry were thwarted by an ignorant commercial director, who eventually bought the organisation from the state and promptly sacked Runge. It was the end of Runge's career. He lived out his remaining years in poverty and died in obscurity in 1867.[*]

---

[*] Runge made a series of discoveries, which resonate through the history of organic chemistry. As related below, he anticipated the French researchers a second time in isolating quinine from cinchona bark, and again in the discovery of alizarin, which he prepared from the root of the madder plant. He could be said thereby to have sown the seed from which grew the German dyestuff industry. At the Oranienburg works he synthesised aniline and phenol (which he named carbolic acid), and showed that both could be recovered from coal tar residues. He synthesised Aniline Black, the first aniline dye, and was prevented by the obtuse commercial director from developing this line of research as he wished: it was left to W.H. Perkin in England more than twenty years later to prepare the first commercial aniline dye (Mauve), which changed the face of the industry. He made great strides in developing the production of coke and coal-gas. He wrote an enormously successful chemistry textbook, and a standard manual of plant chemistry among other works. Near the end of his life his achievements were to a modest extent acknowledged by a modest pension from King Frederick II of Prussia. But when in 1906 Perkin was invested with the highest award German Chemical Society had to offer (its Hoffmann medal) Runge's name was never mentioned.

Meanwhile in Paris, Robiquet too had been busy preparing his coffee extracts, and, probably at some time in 1820, he had crystals of pure caffeine. He knew nothing of Runge, and for some reason, having given an account of his own work at a session of the Society of Pharmacists, he neglected to publish his results. At much the same time, and in the same institute, the École de Pharmacie, another remarkable chemist, Pierre-Joseph Pelletier (1788-1842), was at work on the same problem. The son of a distinguished pharmacist, who had transformed the profession in his country (and in addition to his academic duties at the École Polytechnique, ran a pharmacy in the rue Jacob, which still bears the Pelletier name), Pelletier *fils* followed in his father's footsteps. An outstanding student at the École, where he qualified as pharmacist, he was awarded his doctorate in 1812, and three years later was appointed assistant professor in 'the natural history of drugs'. By this time the young man already had several major accomplishments to his name. In 1811 he reported a series of studies on plant resins – myrrh, opopanax, or sweet myrrh, bdellium, a more abundant myrrh substitute, galbanum, caranna gum and asafoetida, also called devil's dung. These all featured in ancient medicine, and some still found uses in medicine or in perfumery and in incense. Over the next four or so years Pelletier isolated and studied a series of other plant and animal products, among them amber and toad venom. His aim, like Robiquet's, was to find the active principle, or as they termed it, the *principe immédiat*, or *principe prochain*, in the crude natural material, with which the doctors and pharmacists of earlier generations had been content.

The work for which Pelletier became famous began in 1817. He had made the acquaintance of the formidable François Magendie (p.), with whom he undertook a search for the emetic substance in ipecac from the ipecacuanha root, and an investigation through animal tests of its physiological properties. Pelletier isolated the active principle, the *matière vomitive*, which turned out to be an alkaloid, as Magendie, who gave it the name, emetine, had predicted. (It is now also used to treat amoebic infections.) But perhaps the most important of Pelletier's discoveries was a brilliant, green-fingered student by the name of Joseph-Bienaimé Caventou. Like Pelletier, he had followed his father's calling and qualified as pharmacist in the service of the army. He had no sooner obtained a position in a hospital pharmacy in Paris than he threw it up to join Napoleon's army following the emperor's return from exile in Elba. After the defeat at Waterloo Caventou returned to Paris and resumed his career in a hospital pharmacy. In his spare time he wrote an introductory chemistry text to make a little money, and having become interested in the subject. In 1816 he published his first paper – on a chemical analysis of daffodils, followed by another on laburnum. But his profusely productive collaboration with Pelletier began in 1817, while he still occupied a lowly temporary position at the Hôpital Saint-Antoine, and continued for only about five years. It was enough, though, to secure Caventou a position at the École de Pharmacie, and later the chair of chemistry. But without Pelletier his creative fire was extinguished. Caventou sat on committees and taught at the École as Professor of Chemistry and later Toxicology until 1859, when he retired; he died at 82 in 1877.

Pelletier and Caventou's first collaborative success was again stimulated by Magendie - the preparation of strychnine from the *Nux vomica*, the fruit of the *Strychnos* tree. Pelletier had introduced the method of extraction with organic solvents, such as alcohol, benzene and ether, to obtain solutions of active materials from plant sources. It was in an ether extract of the seeds of the plant that strychnine crystals appeared. Magendie tested solutions of these crystals on dogs, and showed that the poison was carried in the bloodstream and not in the lymphatic glands, as the wisdom of the day had it. Magendie's interest in strychnine also stemmed from the use of preparations of *Nux vomica* and other members of the *Strychnos* family, such as the Saint Ignatius bean, in treating a variety of ailments, and also as a general stimulant. For many years it was prescribed for heart disease, muscle wastage, and a variety of other conditions, including incontinence. Strychnine is of course highly toxic, and incautiously ingested, causes rapid and painful convulsions, followed by death. A feature is the accompanying rictus, the *risus sardonicus*, and this macabre manifestation no doubt stimulated the prevalence of strychnine poisoning in early detective fiction. In England it titillated the public, which eagerly followed the more lurid murder trials; the notorious poisoners in the mid-19th century, both doctors, William Palmer and Neill Cream made abundant use of strychnine, then still a prescription drug. It was also used until even in the early 20th century as one of the earliest performance-enhancers for athletes. It is still used in alternative medicine in minute doses, as *Nux vomica* was in ancient times, to treat cancer, against which it has no demonstrable effects.

There is no known antidote against strychnine, but it is apparently inactivated when mixed with charcoal, which has the property of adsorbing (that is to say, tightly binding) many chemical substances. The efficacy of charcoal was demonstrated in 1813 by a French chemist, Michel Bertrand, who tested it first in animals, and then himself by swallowed 5 grams – a truly gigantic dose – of arsenic trioxide mixed with an excess of charcoal, and survived, but others tried and failed to repeat the experiment on animals. This was probably a question of the nature of the charcoal preparation, which has to be a very fine powder to provide the great surface area needed to adsorb a large amount of poison. (The material in this state is known as 'activated charcoal'.) In 1852 another Frenchman, Pierre-Fleurus Touéry, performed a like demonstration on a dog with strychnine, having first tied its oesophagus to prevent the animal from regurgitating the charge. The result did not convince his audience at the Academy of Medicine, who doubted whether the dog had been able to swallow through its constricted throat. Touéry thereupon mixed no less than one gram of strychnine with charcoal and swallowed it himself. This time there could be no doubt, for the foolhardy experiment indeed worked and Touéry displayed no ill-effects.

Pelletier and Caventou achieved another landmark when they purified the green-plant pigment, chlorophyll, a component in the machinery of photosynthesis. Then soon after Robiquet and Runge, they too isolated *caféine* – the name Pelletier gave it - and they went some way towards defining its properties, including its elemental composition. (Why the spelling was later changed - possibly to appease the Anglo-Saxons? – is unclear.) In his *Dictionnaire de Médecine* Pelletier recorded what it was that he and Caventou had really been after: the coffee plant was related to the cinchona tree, the source of quinine. So if, as some thought, coffee was indeed a weak febrifuge, then it might be a source of the only effective febrifuge known at the time, namely quinine. It was quinine, then, that they were hoping to find. If only Monsieur Robiquet had published his results, Pelletier grumbled, their task would have been considerably easier. But M. Robiquet, he added, should in any case receive the credit for discovering *caféine*. Poor Runge was long dead by the time 20th-century historians were able to set the record straight. Caffeine hardly qualifies now as a useful drug, although it has been widely employed by athletes to stave off fatigue and improve performance.

Runge was unfortunate a second time, for in preparing quinine he was again ahead of Pelletier and Caventou by perhaps a year, but his work seems not to have been noticed at the time. Attempts to obtain an active principle from cinchona bark began in the 18th century, and in 1745 a Portuguese naval surgeon by the name of Bernardino Gomes did recover some crystals after extracting a sample of the inferior grey bark with dilute acid and neutralising with alkali. He called the material cinchonine, but it seems to have done little good against malaria. Fifty year on, Antoine Fourcroy and his assistant, Armand Séguin (p.) both tried their hand, but their extracts were no more active than Gomes's. Then in 1817 Pelletier and Caventou made their first attempt, and produced yet another inactive powder from grey bark. Runge's 'Chinabase' was not crystalline, and was not tested against malaria, but he established that it was not cinchonine. Unaware of Runge's efforts in Jena the year before, Pelletier and Caventou in 1820 finally generated a sticky yellow substance from the highly valued yellow bark, which resisted all efforts at crystallisation but was highly active when tested in patients with malaria. They gave it the name quinine, from the *chinchina* or *quinquina*, the 'remedy of remedies' of the Peruvian Indians. Caventou insisted that they should make no pecuniary gain from their discovery, to which Pelletier, perhaps reluctantly, agreed. At all events the details of the preparation were published in full detail, and no patent application was made. It was Magendie who had most quickly grasped the implications of the discovery, and had tested the preparation, first on dogs and then on patients. Demand at once soared, and both Pelletier and Caventou began production on a larger scale in their own private pharmacies. In 1826 Pelletier procured 1500 kilograms of Peruvian bark, from which he extracted no less than about 50 kilograms of quinine. Later production passed into the hands of the nascent pharmaceutical companies, especially in Germany. Pelletier and Caventou duly received many honours, in addition to the lucrative Monthyon Prize from the Academy, and a fine statue (destroyed in World War II, but later replaced) was later erected in Paris to commemorate their discovery.

It was not the end of the partnership's achievements. They discovered two other alkaloids, brucine which existed along with strychnine in the *Strychnos* species, and veratrine from another toxic plant, but this turned out afterwards to be a mixture. Both were promoted by Magendie as specifics for several diseases, but before long they fell out of use, although brucine was reintroduced much later as a treatment for hypertension. The pair also isolated the red colouring matter, cochineal from the cochineal insect.

These discoveries set off a hunt, mainly in France and Germany, for more plant products, and medicinal alkaloids in particular. Many were found, for there was an abundance of toxic plants to explore. Several entered the pharmacopoeias, but few were of any great value. The most notable exception among those discoveries after the first great rush was Robiquet's codeine, said to be (at least after aspirin) the most widely used drug worldwide. Robiquet came upon it while trying more solvents in a search for more efficient ways to prepare morphine. It is the next most abundant of the alkaloids in opium after morphine, comprising upwards of 5% of the total, depending on the provenance of the poppy. It was shown much later to be chemically close to morphine (differing from it only by an added methyl group ($-CH_3$)), but very much weaker in its narcotic properties. It was initially a disappointment, although Robiquet and Magendie found that it retained the cough-suppressing activity of opium, and for a long time it was used only for that purpose, being free of the intoxicating effects of morphine. It was also sold as a treatment for diarrhoea. But in time its analgesic power, and lack of serious side effects were recognised. (Codeine is now usually sold in pills, compounded with aspirin or paracetamol.)

As for Pelletier, he continued his studies on plant alkaloids. He also isolated a number of previously unknown compounds, and also did valuable research on metal compounds, notably those of gold. He died at the age of 58, and Caventou, whose political views were the opposite of Pelletier's, paid his patron the compliment in his eulogy that he had been a 'partisan aussi sincère qu'éclairé de nos institutions monarchiques et constitutionelles' (a supporter, both sincere and enlightened, of our monarchical and constitutional institutions).

Organic chemists quarried the same rich vein for another century, searching for clinically useful plant alkaloids. Most were toxins, and quite a number came and went in the pharmacopoeias, as alarming side-effects made their appearance. One, which retained its interest, was ephedrine from plants of the *Ephedra* genus. This had in fact been known to the Chinese physicians from the start of the second millennium B.C., and was known to them and their modern followers as Ma Huang. It was used as a stimulant, a cough suppressant, and to treat more serious conditions, such as asthma and fevers. As a stimulant it was administered to minions of the ruling classes to encourage greater assiduity. The drug was first isolated from the plant by a Japanese chemist, Nagaioshi Nagai (1844-1929). He had studied medicine at the Dutch medical school in Nagasaki and pharmacy at the Imperial University in Tokyo. Like many aspiring Japanese scientists at the time, he continued his education in European universities, and did his first important work in the laboratory of the great German chemist, August von Hoffmann in Berlin, where he showed an aptitude for organic chemistry. His doctoral thesis concerned eugenol, which came into use as a local anaesthetic, and as a flavouring in the food industry. Returning to the Tokyo Imperial University, he began his work on ephedrine, which he purified in 1885. It was only in 1929, the year of his death, that his efforts were consummated by determination of the alkaloid's structure and its synthesis.

Stimulated by Nagai, Japanese physiologists investigated the properties of ephedrine, and discovered its mydriatic (pupil-dilating) action, and later its effect on the nervous system, resembling that of its close chemical relative, adrenaline (in American usage, epinephrine [p.]). Ephedrine has been used in our time as a general stimulant and enhancer of awareness and concentration, as a preventer of seasickness, as a decongestant, and most infamously as a slimming aid. In this it works in two ways: it suppresses appetite and disrupts carbohydrate metabolism, with a resultant diminution in body fat. Among other side-effects, it elevates blood pressure, and when it was used persistently for weight loss and by athletes seeking improved performance, it caused serious illness and several deaths. It now has some restricted clinical applications, and still occupies a place in traditional Chinese medicine.

Hail to the halogens

The halogens are a group of elements, of which by far the most abundant is ch;orine. It was discovered in 1774 by the Swedish chemist, Carl Wilhelm Scheele, but its identity as an element was established only in 1810 by Humphry Davy. Its name, from the Greek for green-yellow, was given to it by Gay-Lussac. The next, and in medical terms the most important of the halogens came to light in 1811. The history of iodine is rich in luck and serendipity. It could be said to have begun in China in the second millennium B.C. when ash of seaweed and sponges was discovered to cure goitre (p.). In Europe the history begins in medieval times or even earlier. The learned monk, Arnold of Villanova (p.) recorded in 1280 that burnt sponges were of value for treating goitre - the enlarged thyroid gland, which reveals itself as a gross swelling in the neck. Yet it was only in the first quarter of the 19th century that an understanding of the condition began to dawn.

Bernard Courtois (1777-1838) came from Dijon, where his father was a *salpêtrier*, a master of the important trade of saltpetre, that is potassium nitrate, manufacture. This salt, extracted from wood ash, was the indispensable constituent of gunpowder, for which the Republic during the Napoleonic wars had an insatiable demand. Courtois *père* had learned the trade at an institution, the Dijon Academy, in which Louis-Bernard Guyton de Morveau ruled. Guyton de Morveau was a respected chemist, and a man of influence. During the Revolution he discarded his patrician *participle*, and henceforth styled himself Guyton-Morveau, the name by which he rose to be a Deputy and then a member of the Committee of Public Safety. Courtois, having served for some years as his assistant, bought from him a small saltpetre plant. Courtois's sons joined their father in the business, but Bernard, the elder of the two, had wider ambitions, and chose to study chemistry and pharmacy in Paris under Fourcroy at the *École Polytechnique*. There followed two years of army service as pharmacist in a military hospital, after which Courtois returned to the *École Polytechnique*, this time in Thénard's laboratory. There he isolated morphine, only to have the credit stolen from him by the deplorable Séguin (p.). Whether from disappointment, want of a job or filial duty, he returned to his father's saltpetre factory in Dijon. It was there that by a combination of insight and luck, from which only others profited, he made a remarkable discovery.

The year was 1811, and business was bad, for the relentless demand for saltpetre had almost exhausted the supply of wood ash. The situation indeed was desperate because the British naval blockade was also impeding shipments of saltpetre from Chile and elsewhere from reaching the French ports (a situation that was to recur a century later in Germany during the First World War). Courtois, searching for alternative sources had the idea of trying the ash from seaweed, which was plentif Intentional ignorance: a hidtory of blind assessment and placebo ul on the beaches of northern France. Courtois's extraction procedures caused corrosion in the copper vats in which the process was conducted, and looking to other methods of breaking down the ash he tried adding sulphuric acid. Sulphuric acid mixed with water generates heat, which can even cause the water to boil, and as Courtois's brew heated up a purple vapour rose into the air. Where it condensed a deposit of shining black crystals appeared. Courtois suspected that he had found a new element, but he had a precarious business to run and a family to feed, so was unable to pursue his discovery further. Instead, he asked two chemist friends to take up the research and make his observations public. They did as he asked, investigated the properties of the new substance and some of its compounds, and told the story at a session of the *Institut de France* (which encompassed the Academy of Sciences). The report quickly came to the notice of Gay-Lussac, who began his own studies on iodine. Finally, in 1813 Humphry Davy, to whom Napoleon, who had a high regard for science and believed that it should transcend nationalities, had granted a *laisser-passer* despite the blockade, came to France with his wife to visit his French confrères. Gay-Lussac presented him with some of the black crystals, and back in London, Davy went to work and jumped the gun on Gay-Lussac by announcing that this was indeed a new element, with a resemblance to chlorine. This led to some acrimony. It was Gay-Lussac who suggested the name, *iode* (from the Greek for purple); in English it became iodine and in German *Jod*. As for Courtois, the true discoverer, he prepared and sold iodine to chemists, but the demand was evidently insufficient, the saltpetre business eventually collapsed, and he died in penury.

The therapeutic circle was not closed until 1820. That year inspiration struck in the mind of a Swiss physician and native of Geneva, Jean-François Coindet (1774-1834). The University of Geneva had at the time no medical school, so the young Coindet had headed for Edinburgh to pursue his ambition, where in 1797 he presented his doctoral thesis on the subject of smallpox. Two years later he was back in Geneva as physician-in-chief of the city hospital, where he wrought beneficial changes in treatment and in public health. In 1820, having heard that the new element, iodine, was abundant in seaweed, Coindet was struck by the thought that this was perhaps the active constituent which cured goitre. There has been some speculation that Coindet may also have had a nudge in the right direction from his son, who had been a medical student in Edinburgh. For during this time a chemistry lecturer, Andrew Fyfe, had presented a paper revealing that sponges, which had for so many centuries been used to treat goitre, were rich in iodine. At all events, Dr Coindet procured some iodine (which had been prepared by the young Jean-Baptiste Dumas, yet to emerge as the most famous French chemist of his time) on some patients with goitre. The results were dramatic: within a matter of a few weeks the swellings had softened and regressed. Coindet compared the efficacies of different preparation – the element in alcoholic solution (tincture), its compound, potassium iodide, KI, and a tincture made up of iodine and potassium iodide in dilute alcohol. He reported his success to the local learned society, the *Société Helvétique des Sciences Naturelles*, and after more trials, in two rather verbose papers in the foremost French journal, *Annales de chimie et de physique*.

But, alas, the wonderful remedy was, as so often, soon abused. First, whereas Coindet had specified the doses with caution, others gave it in huge excess, and indeed iodine in large amounts is a poison, so many sufferers fared badly. Coindet, suddenly caught up in a storm of abuse, countered with the assertion that iodine, when prescribed in whatever form in the right amount was harmless, and that the 150 patients whom he had treated were all in perfect health. But the continuing reports on the hazards of iodine sapped his confidence, and he began to wonder whether patients differed in their tolerance. He also sought other forms in which iodine might be given to attenuate any toxic effects: one was as potassium iodate, KIO_3, in animal fat. It was all to no avail: iodine in all its forms was proscribed and patients with goitre were made to suffer once more. Worst of all, iodine had been touted in many quarters as a panacea, offered in toxic doses to patients for all manner of ills, such as syphilis and scrofula. It was many years before iodine was rehabilitated as the only and sure treatment for goitre, but the notion that it might be some kind of cure-all persisted into the 20th century. The famous Hungarian biochemist, Albert Szent-Györgyi, who won a Nobel Prize for the discovery of vitamin C, the cure and preventative of scurvy, recalled a maxim that circulated when he was a medical student before the Great War:

> *Wenn du nicht weisst was, warum,*
> *Gebe dann Jodkalium,*

which can be loosely translated as
> If you don't know what or why,
> Give your patient some KI.

The beginnings of an understanding of the role that iodine plays in the body came in 1896 when its presence was discovered in the thyroid gland. Soon afterwards an iodine-containing compound, thyroxine was extracted. Goitre had been endemic in many parts of the world until a correlation was found with the composition of the drinking water: instead of the traces of iodine present elsewhere there was practically none in such localities. Addition of a little sodium iodide (cheaper than the potassium salt) eliminated the condition. 'Iodised' table salt, containing a trace of added sodium iodide, was also introduced, and before the 19th century was out not only goitre, but also the most distressing manifestation of iodine deficiency, cretinism (abnormal mental and physical development of children) had more or less disappeared, at least from Europe.

The antiseptic properties of tincture of iodine came to light in the late 1820s when it was found to kill many species of bacteria, and in 1829 a French doctor, Jean Lugol, concocted what became known as Lugol's solution, made up of iodine, potassium iodide, alcohol and water. It is to be found in pharmacies even now, more or less in that form. Another iodine compound, which enjoyed a wide vogue for a century or so, is iodoform, CHI_3, the analogue of chloroform. In the mid-19th century it was sometimes given for goitre, but its primary use was as an antiseptic. Its characteristic pungent bouquet was always associated with hospitals. It still finds occasional application as an antiseptic for wounds.

Discoveries of new elements proceeded apace in the first half of the 19th century, and not long after iodine it was the turn of another member of the halogen family, *bromine*. It is intermediate in weight between chlorine and iodine, but unlike those it plays no part in the chemistry of animals. Bromine salts are found in seawater, and there are organisms, such as algae, which incorporate it into compounds that play a part in their metabolism. A natural bromine compound with economic importance in ancient times was the famous Purple of Tyre, or Royal Purple (dibromoindigo), secreted by a marine snail. This reddish-purple dye was expensive and highly prized by the Romans. The element was discovered independently by a German in 1825 and a Frenchman the following year. Antoine-Jérôme Balard was a pharmacist, who taught himself and then others chemistry at the university in his home-town of Montpellier. He later became a professor at the *Collège de France* in Paris, where he did much excellent research and nurtured famous students, among them Louis Pasteur. When Balard discovered the new element he was 24 years old. He found it in seawater, while studying the seaweed from which iodine was extracted. He crystallised the sodium chloride (common salt) and directed his attention at the residual liquid (the 'bittern'). When he bubbled in chlorine a reddish-brown substance accumulated, which gave rise when warmed to a vapour with an unpleasant smell. Balard's further investigations led him to conclude that its properties were intermediate between those of chlorine and iodine, and he thought at first that it was a compound of the two – a compound that does indeed exist – but further study convinced him that he had found a new element. He called it muride.

Meanwhile across the Rhine another young chemist, Carl Jacob Löwig, was studying the properties of the same element, which he had extracted a few months earlier in 1825 from the spring water that bubbled up in the spa town of Bad Kreuznach, where he lived. Like Balard he had saturated the water with chlorine to release the bromine from its salts. When the water was shaken with ether the red-brown colour had entered the ether layer, and on evaporating the ether Löwig was left with the dark brown liquid, the pure bromine. He did not immediately publish his work, but took a sample of the new element to Heidelberg University, hoping to impress the famous chemist, Leopold Gmelin and secure an invitation to study at his feet. His overtures were successful, he was taken in as Gmelin's student and in time his successor. But in 1825 the appearance of Balard's paper must have been a nasty shock, for the discovery of an element meant instant fame, if not immortality, and in science priority is measured by publication date. Löwig's written account appeared in 1826, and so it is Balard who appears in the textbooks as the discoverer of bromine. The mandarins of the Academy of Sciences had applauded Balard's discovery, and so it was presented before the Academy and published in the *Annales de chimie et de physique*. It was probably Gay-Lussac once more who did not care for the name Balard had given the new element, the classical spirit prevailed, and it became *brôme* from the Greek for a stench.

It was clear that its parent compound in sea and fresh water was potassium (or sodium) bromide, and investigations by Balard, Löwig and other chemists soon brought to light more compounds, all analogous to those of chlorine and iodine. Pharmacists and doctors seized on the promise of new therapeutic riches. Because bromine is more abundant in nature than iodine, and was therefore cheaper it was at once tried for treating goitre, and all the other conditions for which iodine was widely prescribed as (ineffective) treatment; bromine and its compounds proved equally valueless. Somewhat later, in the mid-19th century, potassium (or sodium) bromide was found to act as a sedative. It was given in alarming daily doses (measured in grams) to agitated or hysterical patients to calm nerves and to quench sexual urges. Its deadening effect (known in France as *bromisme*) became legendary, and especially men confined together in prisons or barracks were, and perhaps still are often convinced that their drink was being laced with bromide, for how else to explain their depressed libido? Someone, it would always be said, had seen white powder being shovelled out of a sack into the tea. Out of this came the one valid medical application of bromides. An English doctor, Sir Charles Locock, starting from the commonly held premise that epilepsy is most often engendered by masturbation, conjectured that suppression of sexual arousal would in turn suppress epileptic seizures, and so, remarkably, it proved. Potassium bromide remained in use as an anticonvulsant, that is a treatment for epileptic or petit mal fits, until replaced by superior remedies with fewer side-effects.

In 1879 there appeared in Vienna a hefty and influential pamphlet with the title (in translation), *The more recent medicines: their application and action.* Its authors were Prokop von Rokitansky and Wilhelm Franz Loebisch. Rokitansky, or to give him his full name, Lothar Prokop Freiherr (that is Baron) von Rokitansky was the younger brother of the more famous Carl von Rokitansky, who gave his name to a series of diseases, was said to have carried out more than 30,000 autopsies in the course of a distinguished career and became the Rector of the University of Vienna. The brothers stemmed from the Bohemian aristocracy and played a prominent part in the intellectual life of the city. Prokop was a pathologist, as was his junior colleague, Loebisch, and together they compiled a formidable survey of the newest medicines of known or presumed effectiveness. This was to supersede the dubious collection of remedies, or supposed remedies, that the European doctors were rather randomly prescribing.

To conquer pain: local anaesthesia

'The last pain in our little finger', William Hazlitt averred, 'gives us more concern and uneasiness than the destruction of millions of our fellow-beings'. Allowing for overstatement, it is pain that was for all the millennia of human existence the greatest of all woes. At last, in the early part of the 19th century, following the discovery of laughing gas, nitrous oxide, came the means to render patients in the dentist's chair and on the operating table unconscious: anaesthesia with ether and chloroform dispelled much of the terrors of the surgeon's knife. At about the same time morphine preparations became available for the treatment of chronic pain, but what was still lacking was any effective local anaesthetic.

The best there was came from the South American Indians. The Incas had used an extract from the datura tree to relieve headaches. It contained a toxic alkaloid, which became known in the west as hyoscine or scopolamine (named after a botanist, Johann Scopoli). More widely used were the leaves of the coca bush, which the Indians chewed to combat fatigue and hunger, but their mild analgesic properties were also recognised. Knowledge of coca reached Europe in 1569 (p.), but another three centuries were to pass before any serious studies of its properties and possible uses were undertaken. Several European chemists tried to extract an active principle from coca leaves, but the potency of the material was weak and was further attenuated by the long sea journey. Finally in 1855 a German chemist, Friedrich Gaedcke managed to prepare a small amount of a pure material out of the mixture of several alkaloids and other compounds contained in the leaves. The quantity was too small to permit any detailed studies, but Gaedcke did describe its chemical properties and gave it the name, erythroxyline, from the name of the coca plant, *Erythroxylon coca*. By then reports of the interesting properties of coca were circulating, and so one of the moguls of German organic chemistry, Friedrich Wöhler, Professor at the University of Göttingen, resolved to examine Gaedcke's erythroxyline in more detail. For this, much greater quantities of coca leaves than could be procured from druggists would be needed, and Wöhler hit on a way to come by them. The Austrian Emperor, Franz Joseph had ordained an expedition by a frigate of the Imperial Navy, the *Novara*, which was to circumnavigate the globe. Wöhler asked the scientist attached to the mission, a geologist, to bring back a generous supply of the leaves. The *Novara* took three years over its mission, but on its return in 1859 Wöhler received the bulk of the 30 kilogram on board.

Wöhler entrusted his student, Albert Niemann with the task of preparing a useful quantity of the pure active substance. Niemann was clearly a highly able chemist. He had begun his career as a pharmacist's apprentice in his home town of Goslar, and while serving time in pharmacies elsewhere he enrolled in Göttingen University to qualify in his profession. He began research in Wöhler's laboratory, where he synthesised a new compound, which gained notoriety in the First World War under the name of mustard gas, bis(2-chloroethyl)sulphide. He described its malign effect on the skin, and recognised the hazard it presented. When presented with the consignment of coca leaves he succeeded in obtaining a good quantity of colourless crystals, and described the properties of their solutions in two papers published in 1862. The solution was weakly alkaline, like those of other plant alkaloids, was bitter to the taste, provoked salivation, and produced on the tongue a curious sensation of numbness, followed by a feeling of cold. This work formed the substance of Niemann's doctoral dissertation, in which the name, cocaine (*Kokain*) first appears. A year later, in 1861, Niemann was dead, of 'suppuration of the lungs', probably the world's first victim of mustard gas poisoning. The gas was first deployed on the battlefield by the Germans in Belgium in 1917. Niemann's preparative procedure for cocaine was later improved to give a higher yield by Wilhelm Lossen, another of Wöhler's students.

Niemann referred in his thesis to the possible applications that cocaine might find in medicine. There had indeed been stray reports in the medical literature of numbing effects of coca leaves on the mouth, and also of its euphoriant properties. In 1855 a German pharmacy was selling an extract of coca leaves for use against toothache. Then in 1859 an Italian doctor, Paolo Mantegazza described the symptoms of coca chewing, with which he had experimented in Peru; they included a furred tongue the next morning, flatulence and the more welcome sensation of general well-being. This, and no doubt other stories then circulating about the pleasures afforded by cocaine, inspired an Italian pharmacist, Antonio Mariani, working in Paris, to concoct a fortified wine, which he called *Vin Mariani*, described as *Vin Tonique à la Coca du Pérou*. It was first marketed in 1863 and its instant success drove Mariani to leave his pharmacy and set up a business to market the elixir. It was in fact one of many coca-wines, but much the most famous. Its rapturous reception is easily explained, for analyses of surviving samples have revealed a high concentration of alcohol and about a quarter of a gram of cocaine per litre, enough to subdue a horse. Doctors now widely prescribed *Vin Mariani* and other coca-wines as a stimulant and all-purpose tonic. It also found favour in high quarters.

Queen Victoria commended it, as did Pope Leo XIII, who even bestowed a Vatican gold medal on the manufacturer. *Vin Mariani*, though probably differently formulated, can still be bought in Italy.

A little later an American entrepreneur in Georgia, John Styth Pemberton, spotted the commercial possibilities of coca-wine, and in 1884 brought to the market a liquor labelled 'Pemberton's French Wine Coca'. It was prepared by steeping coca leaves in a sweet highly alcoholic brew, and was an instant success. But only a year later the local legislature passed a prohibition law, and Pemberton was compelled to omit the alcohol and convert his product, now carbonated, into a 'temperance drink', with at the same time extraordinary healthgiving nhancing and curative properties. In 1906 the Pure Food and Drugs Act forbade the incorporation of cocaine, and the drink underwent another transformation. It was henceforth made with residual coca leaves from which the cocaine, or at least the bulk of it, had been extracted for pharmaceutical use, and with the addition of the strongly flavoured kola nuts. These are the fruits of a tropical tree, and are rich in caffeine and theobromine, the caffeine-related stimulant in tea. For the new product Pemberton invented the catchy name of Coca-Cola.

Enter Dr Freud

The true importance of cocaine was as a local anaesthetic – the first of any consequence. There had been stray mentions, long before Niemann wrote his dissertation, of its numbing activity on the tongue and lips, and in 1855 a German pharmacist reported that toothache could be alleviated by chewing coca leaves. The first systematic investigation of the properties of cocaine was carried out by Vassily Konstantinovich von Anrep (1852-1927) at the University of Würzburg. Von Anrep was born into an aristocratic family originating in Estonia, or as it was then called, Livonia. He studied medicine in St. Petersburg, qualifying in 1876, and after serving for a spell as an army surgeon in the war between Russia and Turkey, he turned to research. The work for which he became, for a while at least, famous was done in a laboratory chiefly engaged in the study of plant alkaloids. Von Anrep tried the effects of cocaine on frogs and mammals and also on himself. He injected a cocaine solution under the skin of his arm and experienced a numbness which lasted for some 30 minutes, and he also tried it on his tongue. His most striking result emerged from an experiment on a frog: he immersed the animal's feet in two separate solutions, one containing cocaine, the other only salt. The first limb proved insensitive to both touch and heat, while the other (the control) responded normally. This work was done in 1879, and the report appeared in a German journal the following year. It took von Anrep another four years to compile a more complete account of his experiments, in which he also drew attention to the possible applications of cocaine in surgery. But he chose to publish the paper in a Russian journal, and consequently it was probably read by no-one at all in Western Europe or in America.*

Meanwhile in Vienna a drama of greater moment was unfolding. Cocaine in one or other form had become popular in much of Europe around the beginning of the 1880s for its pleasurable, more than any supposed medicinal effects. European travellers had also written popular accounts of the customs of the South-American Indians, including their practice of chewing coca leaves to ward off fatigue and boost energy. In 1883 a paper by Theodor Aschenbrandt, a German army doctor appeared in a medical journal. He had tried the effects of cocaine on a group of Bavarian soldiers engaged in manoeuvres, and found that their alertness,

---

* In 1904 von Anrep returned to St. Petersburg as chief medical inspector at the Ministry of Health. The next year he was elected to the state parliament, the Duma, and served in this capacity until the Revolution in 1917. As an aristocrat he evidently found it prudent to leave the country and seek refuge in London and Paris, where he remained until his death, without apparently entering a laboratory again.

endurance and military ardour were remarkably enhanced.* The paper was read by a a young neurologist in Vienna by the name of Sigmund Freud, who, it seems, was transfixed, and resolved at once to try it for himself. Freud became a proselytiser for cocaine, on which he published a series of papers, of which the most comprehensive. Über Coca (On cocaine – then called coca) appeared in 1884. He was also paid to recommend the cocaine preparations marketed both by Merck and by its competitor, the American pharmaceutical company, Parke Davis. He began to take 'small doses' regularly himself 'against depression, and against indigestion, and with the most brilliant success'. Writing to his fiancée, Martha in distant Hamburg he referred to cocaine as a *Zaubermittel* – a magic remedy – and in one love letter excitedly promised to come to her as 'a big wild man with cocaine in his body'.

Freud envisaged seven kinds of medical uses for cocaine: as a mental stimulant, a treatment for digestive complaints, an appetite enhancer for patients with wasting diseases, a treatment for morphine addiction, a drug against asthma, an aphrodisiac, and lastly as a local anaesthetic. Best of all, there was 'absolutely no craving for more cocaine after the first or even a frequently repeated dose of the drug'. It was only for the last of the seven proposed applications that cocaine established its immense value, while Freud's unshakable belief in the fourth (which had indeed been supported by two rather sketchy publications from America) was to

---

* The lesson was not lost on a later generation of German military leaders, for cocaine was even distributed to German recruits during the Second World War as a means of improving their performance in battle. It was infamously tried out in 1944 on prisoners in the Sachsenhausen concentration camp, when the victims were forced to march in circles, carrying heavy packs until they collapsed. The cocaine was administered in the form of pills compounded with 'Pervitin' (called amphetamine, and later 'speed', in the English-speaking countries [p.]), and morphine to limit pain. The results evidently satisfied the researchers, but the cocaine could not be produced in sufficient quantity for distribution to the army by the time the war ended. Pervitin or a close derivative, on the other hand, was given in bulk, so that over three months in 1940 more than 35 million pills were issued. Recent research has revealed that the abuse of Pervitin extended to the very top of the Nazi regime. Hitler's *Leibarzt* – his personal physician, the sinister quack, Dr Morell - had injecteded him daily with massive quantities of this and countless other dangerous substances, including crude steroid preparations, so that the Führer became a helpless addict.

lead to disaster. For Freud had a friend who was a morphine addict, and would serve as a guinea-pig. Ernst von Fleischl-Marxow was in sad case. He was a doctor who had been laid low by a terrible infection, caught apparently in the dissecting-room. His thumb had been amputated, he was afflicted by a neuroma, a nerve tumour, and was in constant pain. His illness had put paid to a highly promising career, for he was an admired neurologist and had made important contributions to the development of electroencephalography (EEG). He was now suicidal and hopelessly addicted to morphine. Freud, who had urged cocaine on several of his friends as a treatment for minor ailments, now started Fleischl-Marxow on a course of his favourite drug. At first the results appeared encouraging, but soon the patient's demand for the drug grew, until he was injecting huge amounts – as much as a gram per day – ruinous to his mental and physical state and to his bank account. Fleischl-Marxow experienced terrifying hallucinations, deteriorated quickly and died. Freud was denounced for professional dereliction and for laying a curse on the population, and he was forced to concede that he had been too sanguine in promoting the drug. It is thought that this distressing episode may have turned Freud against drug therapy of mental disorders generally, and thus set back the search for effective treatment of such states.

Freud's initial near-fanatical espousal of cocaine as a remedy for mental and physical conditions was offset by a missed opportunity to discern its true value. The glory accrued to one of Freud's colleagues at the University of Vienna, Carl Koller. Born in 1857 in Austro-Hungarian Bohemia, Koller was, like his friend, Freud, the offspring of a secular Jewish middle-class family, and also like Freud had studied medicine in Vienna. He was clearly an exceptionally able student, and while still an undergraduate had completed an acclaimed research project in developmental biology. He chose ophthalmology as his clinical speciality and was working in the eye clinic of the Vienna General Hospital when Freud approached him with a request for help. Wanting to discover how coca worked on the Indians of the Altiplano, his first thought had been to find out whether it increased muscle power. Would Koller then set up an experiment to test the proposition? Koller began by giving a friend a cocaine drink, and inspiration struck when the man remarked on the resulting numbness of the tongue. The phenomenon had been noted often enough before, but as the Hungarian biochemist, Albert Szent-Györgyi put it, discovery is seeing what everybody else has seen, but thinking what nobody else has thought. And the thought that now entered Koller's head was that cocaine might exert the same effect on the sensitive surface of the cornea. Many eye surgeons, including the professor of ophthalmology in Koller's hospital, had lamented the absence of a local anaesthetic, for eye operations were highly unpleasant ordeals for both patient and surgeon. General anaesthesia at the time was considered dangerous for eye surgery, and Koller had in fact tried a number of agents, such as potassium bromide, chloral hydrate and morphine, on the eyes of animals with no success.

Koller called on a young colleague in the university, Gustav Gärtner to assist with animal tests of cocaine, and together they dropped a cocaine solution into the eye of a frog. Within minutes the animal allowed the cornea to be touched without protest, while the other eye showed the normal avoidance response. After similar tests on a rabbit and a dog, Koller and Gärtner tried it on each other, and found that they could press their corneas with the head of a pin and feel nothing. Amidst much excitement, the first eye operation under local anaesthesia was performed on a patient with glaucoma. There was instant acclamation, and Koller prepared a report of his experimental results (though without at this stage mentioning the surgery), to be read at the meeting of the German Society of Ophthalmology in Heidelberg in September of the same year, 1884. Koller's minimal salary did not allow him to pay the train fare to Heidelberg, and a friend, Josef Brettauer was entrusted with the task of giving the talk. A paper on the successful eye operation was delivered by Koller himself a month later to the Vienna Medical Society, and published immediately after. Much excitement had been generated at the Heidelberg meeting, and an American doctor, Henry Noyes who was present, despatched a missive to the *New York Medical Record*, which appeared in print within days. The medical profession in Europe and America recognised the importance of Koller's discovery with unaccustomed alacrity, and the terrors of eye surgery were assuaged within weeks. Cocaine anaesthesia was also soon adopted for operations on the ear, nose, throat and rectum.

Sigmund Freud realised that, despite his consuming interest in cocaine, he had missed a major discovery, and with rather characteristic disingenuousness or perhaps self-deception, claimed to have alerted Koller to the possibilities of the drug as an anaesthetic. (He did, though, inscribe a reprint of one of his own papers 'to my dear friend, Coca Koller'.) Freud continued to take cocaine, and probably became at least mildly addicted. When, how and why he abandoned the habit was never clear. As for Koller, what should have been a triumphant career in Vienna, a world centre of medicine at the time, came to a melodramatic end, the indirect result of the pervasive Viennese antisemitism. Only a few months after his great discovery Koller was on duty in the hospital when a disagreement arose over treatment of a patient. A colleague, Fritz Zinner had applied a tourniquet to a wound, which Koller, believing that it might lead to the loss of a finger, removed. Zinner took it as an affront and called Koller an insolent Jew. Koller responded by slapping Zinner's face, and was challenged to a duel. Such 'affairs of honour', though still sometimes enacted, and especially by ardent young military reservists like Zinner and Koller, had been long prohibited in Austria. Koller inflicted two heavy gashes on Zinner's face. Both men were charged, and although Koller received a pardon later, it was clear that his future career was in doubt. Not long afterwards he took a position in Holland, but did not stay long, moving to New York in 1888. There he had a highly successful career, and died, laden with years and honours in 1944.

In 1884 Merck of Darmstadt began to produce cocaine on an ever-increasing scale, and other chemical concerns followed the lead. Later it was refined from a crude cake exported from Peru, and by the end of the 1880s it had become Merck's most profitable product. Eventually it was supplanted by atropine. The mydriatic (pupil-dilating) action of extracts from the deadly nightshade (*Atropa belladonna*), already mentioned, were known since ancient times. The alkaloid occurs not only in this, but also in other plants of the *Solanacea* family, and was first isolated in 1831 and subjected to a more detailed study by Friedlieb Runge (p.) twenty-five years later. It was a distinguished German doctor and pharmacologist, professor at the University of Breslau (now Wrocław in Poland), Wilhelm Filehne (1844-1927), who recognised the structural similarity between atropine and cocaine. If they were so closely related chemically and had a mydriatic activity in common, might their resemblance not also extend to anaesthetic characteristics? So it proved, but the activity of atropine was low. Filenhe, though, was not discouraged and proceeded to test a series of analogues, mainly prepared for him by chemists at the Hoechst company. Several were highly active as anaesthetics, but all had irritant side-effects. Attempts to find a satisfactory substitute for cocaine in eye surgery continued in several German laboratories, but none of the compounds were devoid of unpleasing side-effects. The closest was a fragment of the complex ring structure of cocaine, which was indeed a potent local anaesthetic but again failed on grounds of painful side-effects. Then in 1898 Richard Willstätter, a research student in Munich asserted that the structure for cocaine published six years earlier by a professor in the department, Albert Einhorn was wrong. This intelligence was not received kindly and the audacious young man was told to mind his own business. But Willstätter was not so easily deflected; he set about determining the formula of the closely similar, but functionally divergent atropine, and in 1898 deduced the correct structure and incidentally that of cocaine as well.*

---

* Willstätter (1872-1942) was one of the towering figures in the history of organic chemistry. His research supervisor was the most famous of them all, Adolf von Baeyer, who recognised his student's exceptional talent, and allowed him to write his doctoral thesis on the subject of cocaine. Willstätter was appointed to a professorial chair at the Swiss Technology Institute, the ETH, in Zurich in 1905, and he moved in 1912 to Berlin as professor at the university there and director of the state institute (Kaiser-Wilhelm-Institut) for natural products chemistry. Finally, in 1916, having been awarded the Nobel Prize for chemistry the previous year, he returned to Munich as successor to his patron, von Baeyer. In 1924, at the height of his fame and powers, Willstätter resigned his position. The debacle occurred in the course of a meeting of the university faculty when the appointment of a new professor of inorganic chemistry came up. Willstätter proposed the name of the obvious candidate, Richard Goldschmidt. This was met by loud muttering and a cry of 'again a Jew'. Willstätter, a secular Jew, gathered up his papers, wrote a letter of resignation, and never entered the university grounds again despite all attempts to coax him back, nor did he accept the many positions offered him in other countries. He did however continue to direct a laboratory in Munich, staffed by two people, one of whom was a faithful woman protégée, by telephone from his home. In 1934, after the Nazis came to power, Willstätter decamped to Switzerland, and died there eight years later.

Meanwhile however Einhorn had taken up the synthesis of cocaine fragments, based on his incorrect structure of the parent compound. The substances he prepared were quite simple compounds (benzene rings with commonplace substituents), but inevitably the compounds he had in mind eluded him. Nevertheless he sent his products to a pharmacologist in another university to test, and one, based on the erratic reasoning proved – undeservedly and unaccountably – effective. It was taken up by Hoechst, and quickly introduced into the market under the trade name of Orthoform, to be replaced later by a closely similar structure called benzocaine. The matter did not stop there, for local anaesthetics, many of which turned out also to have antiseptic properties, were highly profitable products, and there were many industrial organic chemists in Germany, France and elsewhere. Some compounds had greater potency, others some better solubility properties, and others again were easier and cheaper to prepare. Benzocaine was followed by novocaine, also called procaine, and procaine by dibucaine. Then in the 20th century local anaesthetics of quite different structural nature eventually displaced all of those inspired by cocaine. The most successful of the new generation was Xylocaine, generically called lidocaine in the U.S., and originally in Europe lignocaine. This proved to be a major advance in pain control.

The story of Xylocaine is a curious one. In 1935 a group of Russian chemists, driven by the observation that Central Asian camels, when grazing on reeds, would avoid one form, called *Arundo donax*, isolated from this species an alkaloid. They called it gramine (from the genus, graminaea, to which the plant belonged). It was characterised by a bitter taste. The previous year, a German organic chemist, who had taken root in Sweden, Hans Karl August Simon von Euler-Chelpin (1873-1964), who had by then redefined himself as plain Hans von Euler, had embarked on an examination of plant compounds, and particularly differences between those of normal and mutant strains. Von Euler was a very considerable organic chemist, who had done notable work on molecules of biological importance, and been awarded the Nobel Prize for Physiology or Medicine in 1929. He had found a strain of barley resistant to parasitic worms, which had been attacking crops. He isolated gramine, determined a probable structure, and thought it might be a suitable starting compound for the development of a pesticide. (The history of what followed has been unearthed by Professor J.A.W. Wildsmith.) In 1935, von Euler engaged the services of a young chemist, a recent graduate of the University of Stockholm, Holger Erdtman and asked him to attempt a synthesis of the alkaloid to confirm the structure von Euler had inferred. Erdtman discovered that his patron's structure had an error: a substituent group was in a different position in the (indole) ring system. His product, with the subtly divergent structure that von Euler had proposed, received the name, isogramine. As chemists did in those less restrictive days, Erdtman tasted his isogramine, and found that it anaesthetised his lips and tongue. This was interesting enough to induce von Euler to pursue the observation further. The isogramine was an irritant and unsuitable for clinical use, so derivatives were to be prepared as usual. Von Euler secured a small grant from the (then still embryonic) pharmaceutical company, Astra, and took on another young chemist, working towards his doctorate. Nils Löfgren and Erdtman synthesised a series of isogramine analogues in the hope of finding one that retained the desired but not the undesired property. The ten most promising products were given to von Euler's son, Ulf, a physiologist at the Karolinska Institute in Stockholm for testing on animals. (Ulf von Euler later discovered noradrenaline, and won the Nobel Prize like his father, in 1970, together with Julius Axelrod [p.].) But the test Ulf von Euler had chosen, on the corneas of rabbits, produced no very encouraging results: there was anaesthetic activity, but less powerful than that of the standard local anaesthetic then in use, procaine. Thereupon Astra and von Euler *père* lost interest. Erdtman, deprived of his income, left, while Löfgren headed for another department, and thence to a then-insignificant chemical and pharmaceutical company, Pharmacia.

But Löfgren had not lost interest, and by 1940 there was a new incentive: the war had begun in Europe and the supply of procaine, which came from Germany, ceased. Löfgren began again to synthesise prospective anaesthetics, and came up with a new compound, Lokastin, not as good as procaine, but it served the purpose. The following year Löfgren returned to the University of Stockholm as assistant lecturer in chemistry, assembled a group of enthusiastic undergraduates to help with the anaesthetic project, and was especially lucky to attract an enterprising medical student at the

Karolinska Institute, Bengt Lundkvist. Löfgren gave Lundkvist a newly designed compound, LL30 to try to evaluate. The student discussed the problem of assaying the activity with a friend, another medical student, Bengt Lagergréen. Lagergréen's research adviser was the only professional anaesthetist then practising in the country, Torsten Gordh, who lent him a book on the subject, duly passed to Lundkvist. With the help of the book Lundkvist performed a series of tests on himself with enormously encouraging results. Next, yet another medical student showed that LL30 had low toxicity. A patent application soon followed, but Pharmacia, though initially interested, decided against taking up the drug. The stalemate was resolved by another happy chance, when it turned out that the wife of an ophthalmologist, who had expressed interest in LL30 had a relative with a major commercial stake in Astra. The company was persuaded to fund a full clinical evaluation, conducted by Gordh, and after another three years, in 1949 Xylocaine, or Xylidone, as LL30 was dubbed by Astra, finally reached the market in Sweden and in Britain, and soon thereafter it received FDA approval in America. Lidocaine was an instant success. Löfgren and Lundkvist grew rich, the first became a professor, the second died young. Lidocaine found several other applications: it was the first of a family of drugs for the suppression of cardiac arrhythmias – irregular heart beat – and was used for this purpose in the 1950s, but may have occasioned as many deaths as it prevented (p.). It was found also to be an effective treatment for coughs, taken as an inhalant.

Chapter 7

THE RISE OF RATIONAL THERAPY

Clash of ideologies

If the emergence of a rational, experimentally based approach to the treatment of disease can be attributed to one man, that man was François Magendie. He has already made his appearance in the guise of a remorseless vivisectionist (p.), and of a tireless seeker after physiological truth. He sought in particular an understanding in physiological terms of how drugs acted, for disease was to him the physiology of the sick individual. If one did not understand the origin of the disease it was futile to grope in a state of ignorance for a cure; better indeed to do nothing and look to nature to heal the patient. Many contemporaries objected that this was a philosophy of despair - of therapeutic nihilism. Magendie was by temperament arrogant, disputatious and intolerant of dissenting opinions, and in the fractious atmosphere of the Parisian medical scene he paid a high price.

Magendie was born in 1783 in Bordeaux, the elder of two sons of a surgeon. The parents were freethinkers and ardent supporters of the Revolution, and when the sons were still young the father took the family to Paris to be closer to the centre of the action. Wanting his sons to learn to think for themselves, Magendie *père* would not allow them to attend school, until at the age of ten, young François rebelled. At sixteen he was

221

apprenticed to a surgeon at one of the great Paris hospitals, the Hôtel-Dieu, where he was allowed to perform dissections, and learned anatomy. Four years later he passed the entrance examination for the Paris medical school, and in 1808 emerged as Doctor of Medicine. During the brief period in the Faculty of Medicine that followed, Magendie contrived to quarrel with both the professor of anatomy and the professor of surgery. His first publication was a ferocious denunciation of the teachings of the much-admired Xavier Bichat (1771-1802), who had a large following in Parisian medical circles and beyond: the other French medical school of equal standing, the one in Montpellier, for instance, was wholly in thrall to his doctrines. (His name, like that of his follower, Broussais, appears in George Eliot's *Middlemarch*, in which Dr Lydgate, who has studied in Paris, plans a programme of experiments, inspired by Bichat's theories.) Bichat arrived in Paris in 1794 after service as a military doctor. His warm and outgoing personality and his inspiring teaching brought him ardent disciples at the Hôtel-Dieu, the largest and oldest of the Paris hospitals. Bichat was a vitalist: he held that the physiology of living organisms could not be explained by the laws of chemistry and physics, but was governed instead by 'vital properties'. He defined life as 'the sum of the functions by which death is resisted'. The Newtonian laws of physics impinged on the living organisms and were held at bay by the two attributes of living tissues, 'sensibility' and 'contractility', both of which were lost at the moment of death. He classified the types of tissue – twenty-two of them, as inferred from his anatomical labours – and their associated membranes in terms of the balance between the two influences. The differences between the various tissues ensured that they would be subject to different diseases. Bichat was thought to have performed six-hundred or so dissections of cadavers, many of them recovered from the guillotine and often putrescent. His early death probably resulted from a bacterial infection caught from one of them. His books - the 'Treatise on Membranes', the imposingly titled *Recherches physiologiques sur la vie et la mort*, and the immense four-volume 'General Anatomy, applied to Physiology and to Medicine', were regarded by his followers as sacred tablets.

Such was Bichat's reputation that Napoleon, hearing of his death, ordered that a commemorative statue be erected. Bichat's vitalist philosophy continued to be taught by the Paris faculty for another forty years. Claude Bernard (p.), writing long after the demise of vitalism, remarked that the modern medicine of his own time had its roots in the histological methods of Bichat. Little wonder therefore that Magendie's objurgations caused wide indignation when they were published. For whatever reason, Magendie resigned his post at the Faculty of Medicine, and switched his interests from anatomy to physiology. This was the moment when he embarked on a programme of animal experiments, examining the physiological effects of drugs. He devised a simple procedure, using a quill, of injecting solutions into a vein*, and made his first important discovery-that the drugs he tested were conveyed through the bloodstream, and not as was the current belief, through the lymphatic system. Magendie's insistence that the physiology of animals was akin to that of man also ran counter to received opinion, and led directly to the new science of pharmacology. As we have already seen, moreover, he used, wherever possible, the chemically pure 'active principles' that were then becoming available. This led to clinical regimes for administration of such substances as morphine and quinine. Magendie's talents must have been recognised by the more perceptive members of the Faculty, for in 1811 he was appointed to the position of demonstrator, charged with teaching anatomy, physiology and surgery. Then in 1813, having waited in vain for a position on the Faculty, he resigned once more, and set himself up as a private practitioner

---

* The needle syringe had not yet been invented. Primitive catheters had been used for experiments on blood transfusion, but the first injection of a drug directly into a vein probably took place in 1823, when Dr Enoch Hale in Boston experimented on himself with castor oil. This was in common use as a purgative (and remained so up to our own time), and Hale was motivated, at least in part, by the wish to find a means of administering it to patients who gad difficulty swallowing. He tried it on some rabbits with apparently little effect, and then injected some into his own arm vein. The apparatus was primitive and the whole process messy and slow. Some of the viscous liquid seeped under the skin, and after a short time unpleasant symptoms began to manifest themselves. The first was a disagreeable taste in the mouth, and was followed by headache, abdominal cramps, nausea and a stiffness in the muscles. Hale reported that it took some weeks for the effects to wear off completely. Castor oil, it was now clear, had toxic properties and needed to be used with care. A syringe with a fine enough needle to slide through the skin was developed only in 1853, independently by Alexander Wood of Edinburgh, and in France by by Charles Gabriel Pravaz.

and teacher. In 1822 he published a seminal work, the Formulary for the preparation and use of several new medicaments, in which he reasserted the importance of animal experimentation. 'Nothing is more false' he wrote 'than this belief [that drugs act differently in animals than in man]; twenty years of experiments of all kinds, be it in the laboratory or at the sick person's bedside, allows me to affirm that the manner of action of medicaments and of poisons is the same on man and on animals.'

Not until 1826 did Magendie achieve an appointment at the Salpêtrière Hospital, and four years later he was also placed in charge of the women's ward at the Hôtel-Dieu. Opinions differ about his skills as a doctor. He certainly made mistakes, notably in refusing to believe that cholera and yellow fever were contagious diseases and rejecting calls for quarantines, and also his scepticism over anaesthesia (p.). But despite his abrasiveness and hauteur towards his colleagues, Magendie treated his patients with kindness and understanding. His best service as a physician was his implacable opposition to bloodletting. His favourite student, Claude Bernard, now recognised as the greatest physiologist of the 19th century, and whose reputation eclipsed even that of his master, recalled fifty years later an account Magendie had given him of a hospital consultation. The question at issue was whether the patient should be bled from the right arm or the left leg. The debate 'could be compared to some of the best scenes on the comic stage, and [Magendie] predicted that a time would come when people would refuse to believe that in the most civilised city in the world in the first half of the 19th century, conscientious doctors could have contemplated such ideas'. Bernard testified that when he was a young doctor in the earlier part of the century, any doctor who did not bleed his patients, and bleed them severely, would be regarded as 'an ignoramus or a dangerous innovator'. Magendie was particularly vehement in his opposition to bleeding pneumonia patients, as was then the invariable practice. So radical were his views that that his housemen (interns) often felt duty-bound to disobey his injunction when he was not looking. Claude Bernard attested to this in one of his reminiscences. A young physician gave a presentation at a prize competition of the Académie des Sciences, the burden of which was that bleeding was the most effective treatment for pneumonia. Magendie, who was a member of the jury, objected. He did not bleed his pneumonia patients at the Hôtel-Dieu, and they recovered more quickly. One of his colleagues at the same hospital was also on the jury, and smiled at this. 'You don't bleed your patients, that is true', he said, 'but your housemen bleed them behind your back'. Magendie was appalled and complained the next morning to Bernard at this insubordination. 'I can assure you,' Bernard recalled, 'that from this time not a single patient was bled, and yet they recovered.'

Magendie's most important physiological researches were carried out at the Collège de France, where he had been appointed professor in 1831, and where he set up the first medical school laboratory. His single greatest discovery is enshrined in the Bell-Magendie Law. It was clouded by an ugly priority dispute with the English physiologist, Sir Charles Bell. Bell had tried cutting the roots of the spinal nerves of an animal and had found that severing one set (the anterior roots) impaired muscle contraction, on which cutting the others (the posterior roots) had a lesser effect. Magendie insisted that he had been unaware of Bell's work, which had been made public shortly before he began his own experiments, and there is no reason to doubt him, since he was always punctilious in giving credit to other researchers. Magendie's experiments were clearly more carefully done: he found that the anterior roots totally governed motility, whereas the posterior roots controlled sensory functions. Bell launched an intemperate attack on his rival, accusing him of outright plagiarism. Magendie replied in courteous and measured terms, giving Bell full credit for what he had done, and science historians now concur that Magendie was on the right side of the dispute. Magendie had many other accomplishments to his credit by 1845, when he resigned his appointments at the Hôtel-Dieu and the Collège de France (where he was succeeded by Claude Bernard), and retired to his estate. He died in 1855.*

Paris was for much of the 19th century the dominant centre of medicine in the western world. It attracted ambitious young physicians from all

---

* It is hard to imagine now the fascination and awe that the healing profession aroused among the public, most of all in France. The doctors of the day appeared in the thinnest of disguises in plays and novels, most famously in the novels and stories of Balzac, who was much interested in medicine, having even attended lectures in the Paris Medical School while a law student at the university. A literary scholar has counted up the number of doctors – 65 – who appear in the pages of the mighty sequence of novels, *La Comédie Humaine*. Dr Desplain, who features in many of Balzac's books, is the chief surgeon at the Hôpital-Dieu, the Baron Guillaume Dupuytren, son of a peasant, who gave his name to Dupuytren's contracture of the hand. Adored by his patients but detested by his colleagues for his rudeness and arrogance, he was one of the two professors who took offence at the young Magendie's presumption (p.). Another frequent part-player is Dr Horace Bianchon, drawn from Dupuytren's student, Jean-Baptiste Bouillaud, a noted cardiologist and Dean of the Paris Faculty. In *Le Peau de Chagrin* (in translation, *The Wild-Ass's Skin*), published in 1831, three medical luminaries are summoned to the bedside of the novel's unhappy protagonist, Raphaël de Valentin, and discuss the case across the prostrate patient, as though over a corpse. All are barely disguised representations of Parisian medical personages. Joseph Recamier, surgeon at the Hôtel-Dieu, Professor at the Collège de France, and a vitalist, appears as Dr Caméristus, François Broussais as Dr Brissat, and Magendie, most transparently, as Dr Maugredie. Balzac's perception of their personalities and professional creeds is exact. Caméristus is a follower of van Helmont (p.) and a believer in the 'vital principle' which 'evades all pharmaceutical remedies'; he advises a deep analysis of the patient's inner state, a search for 'the cause of the evil in the entrails of the soul and not in the entrails of the body'. He accuses Brisset of confusing cause with effect in asserting that the problem lies in irritation of the gastrointestinal tract, which can be treated only by drastic bleeding. '"Ever the absolutist, monarchic, religious medicine", Brisset muttered'. As for Maugredie, the man of 'distinguished intellect but sceptical and mocking disposition', who 'sees good in all theories but adopts none', and holds fast only to facts, he wears 'a sardonic smile' and merely urges his colleagues not to lose sight of the disease. In the end, after much debate and expounding of rival theories, the advice to the patient is to take the waters in Aix-les-Bains, and all ends badly. It is only the patient's faithful doctor and friend, the young Horace Bianchon (identified as Dr Bouillaud [p.]), who exhibits any compassion or concern (which appears less than fair to at least the real-life Magendie).

over Europe and, perhaps most of all from America, where the leading medical schools based their teachings on those of the Parisian oracles. Yet the Parisian medical community was riven by conflicting schools of thought and by fierce personal rivalries and animosities. Whose star was in the ascendant depended often on political posture. In the years after the Revolution those who had shown republican sympathies, and sometimes suffered for them, had the advantage. It also became possible for the first time for the sons of peasants and the proletariat to enter the professions, whereas after the restoration of the monarchy in 1830 a record of revolutionary leanings became a wasting asset. In the early years of the 19th century the acknowledged leader of the 'Paris school', which cleaved to the Hippocratic doctrine that the only guide to treatment was observation and experience (*'ars medica tota in observationibus'*), was Philippe Pinel (1745-1826), who had been a moderate revolutionary and opponent of the Jacobins. Though born into a family of physicians, he chose to study initially for the priesthood, but - oddly, considering his later views - developed an interest in drugs. From there he was drawn into the study of medicine, which he pursued in Toulouse and Montpellier. On his arrival in Paris in 1798, he met and impressed one of the leaders of the profession, Pierre-Georges Cabanis (1757-1808). Cabanis was opposed to blood-letting, and to the use of drugs, although he did on occasion prescribe antimony compounds, and iron for chlorosis. (The latter was a practice well ahead of its time, for chlorosis, an anaemia that imparts a greenish pallor to the skin and was then common in young women, is the result of iron deficiency.) Cabanis introduced his protégé to the celebrated *saloniére*, Madame Helvétius, hostess to a galaxy of intellectual and political luminaries, which included at different times the likes of Diderot, Condorcet, Thomas Jefferson, Benjamin Franklin, who proposed marriage to her, Talleyrand, and Napoleon himself). His future was now assured.

Pinel's greatest interest, which originated in the suicide of a friend, was in mental illness. Through his influential connections he was appointed physician to the infirmary at the Hospice Bicêtre, with responsibility for the care of some 4000 captives - felons, syphilitics and a few mental patients. His approach to their treatment was notably compassionate and enlightened. Like his patron, Cabanis, Pinel had little time for drugs, not even cinchona, and he especially condemned polypharmacy, the prescriptions of complicated drug mixtures. He was nevertheless an early supporter of vaccination and an opponent of heedless bloodletting. Most other members of the Parisian medical establishment, such as Jean-Nicolas Corvisart (1755-1821), personal physician to Napoleon, and his students, who included such great names as Laënnec, were also thoroughgoing sceptics. Corvisart, a heart specialist, took the principle to such outrageous lengths as rejecting the use of digitalis, the efficacy of which could scarcely have escaped a doxtor in his speciality. Laënnec, dying of tuberculosis, refused all purported remedies, and put his faith in the pure sea air of his native Brittany.

Pinel's famous disciple, Bichat shared, as we have seen, his mentor's scepticism concerning the use of drugs. Professors and their theories, they held, might come and go, but the materia medica remained practically unchanged, and was deployed in a mindless and indiscriminate manner. If, as Bichat believed, every disease struck at its own particular target, what use to administer a drug of which the site of action was unknown? Bichat did make an attempt to confront this question by way of some experiments on his patients at the Hôtel-Dieu to determine on which of the body's organs some of the common drugs exerted their effects. Nothing ever came of the plan, which was in any case terminated by Bichat's early death. A malign offshoot of the school of Pinel and Bichat was led by Bichat's most ardent admirer, Broussais. He unfortunately did not share his hero's scepticism, and diverged even further from his teachings in his uniquely bizarre and destructive conviction, discussed above.

There were fortunately also opponents of Bichat's views, of whom one of the most determined was Pierre-Charles-Alexandre Louis (1787-1872). He is often portrayed as the founder of what is now called evidence-based medicine. Louis was a working clinician, who had plied his trade in Russia for seven years before returning to Paris, where he had been trained. Mistrustful of clinical dogma, he set out to determine to what extent recovery from pneumonia was helped by bloodletting. He analysed data from case reports at the Charité hospital in Paris, and then he performed a controlled study, similar to that of James Lind on H.M.S. Salisbury nearly one-hundred years before (p.). He divided 77 pneumonia patients into two groups. All had been bled, but the first group only during the first four days after diagnosis, the second group later. The outcome of this, and much additional evidence, convinced Louis that it mattered not when and how much patients were bled, or even whether they were bled at all, except under certain defined circumstances. Louis's statistical methods were, by today's standards, less than rigorous, but they sufficed to prove that bloodletting was in general of only marginal benefit at best. Louis published several polemics, denouncing Broussais's methods. The Société d'Observation Médicale, which he founded, disseminated his principles, and made him especially popular with students from overseas, of whom Oliver Wendell Holmes was one. Louis's *méthode numérique* became, especially after the introduction of statistical refinements, the critical step in evaluation of therapeutic efficacy.*

The Parisian school was denounced from within France and outside as a nest of therapeutic nihilists. This was broadly true, although some doctors did still prescribe such dire remedies as antimony and calomel, as well as others that owed more to superstition than to science, such as viper's flesh, even after they had been expunged from the pharmacopoeia. The French, at all events, deplored the British enthusiasm for drugs, but, as the saw went, 'the British kill their patients, whereas the French let them die'. This was largely true, although the average patient was probably more likely to survive the attentions of a doctor in Paris than in London. Napoleon said of his personal physician, the highly esteemed Corvisart (p.), that 'In place of drugs he gives his patients a course in morality. Yet, does he do so badly? What is certain is that he consoles, and that is much'. The attitude of Corvisart and the rest of the Parisian establishment did not for the most part yield to the scientific transformation of drug therapy, led by Magendie and Claude Bernard. One of the last great figures of the Paris school was Armand Trousseau (1801-1867), who gave his name to 'Trousseau's sign' for malignancy, and was in many respects ahead of his

---

* Louis was also regarded as an authority on tuberculosis, on which he wrote a treatise, *Recherches sur la phthisis*. One of his patients was Chopin, whom he treated during his last illness.

time. He nevertheless asserted that science was all very well, but it induced clinical slackness: 'a little less of science', was his motto, 'and a little more of art'. The perceived antithesis continued to dog the practice of medicine for a long time.

An unusually clear-sighted view of the state of therapeutics in the mid-19th century appears in two books by a German physician, Carl August Wunderlich, born in 1815 to a father who was both a pharmacist and a doctor. Wunderlich was shocked by many aspects of medicine in Germany, and when he began to air his criticisms he incurred much hostility from his confrères. But in Stuttgart, where he eventually obtained a professorial position, he found listeners. In his book, *Behaviour of Body Temperature in Disease*, he introduced the measurement of temperature as a guide to the state and treatment of the patient, and his *Handbook of Pathology and Therapy* was equally innovative. But it was his youthful work, published in 1841, which established his reputation. It had the cumbrous title, *A Contribution to History and Evaluation of Present-Day Therapeutics in Germany and France*. The Parisians either offered their patients weak, and therefore useless remedies such as tisanes, or filled them with dangerous doses of dangerous substances. Broussais and his school were holding back progress. There was a lack of understanding of what purportedly therapeutic substances actually did, or of how individuals might differ in their needs. Nor was medical practice any more enlightened in Germany. Empiricism and the nonsense of Hufeland ruled, and the science of pharmacology had yet to be established. By the time Wunderlich died in 1877 the new move towards the rational application and development of drugs was well underway in France, and the rise of the synthetic dyestuff industry, especially in Germany, presaged the emergence of synthetic drugs.

Yet the credulity of many doctors and pharmacists even at the end of the 19th century can be gauged from such respectable journals as *Chemist and Druggist*, published in London. Opened at random these volumes offer startling advice, such as that below, proffered in 1889 on jaborandi. The jaborandi is a genus of tree, abundant in Brazil, the leaves of which found medicinal use among the Guarani Indians. The first report to reach Europe appears to have been written in 1570 by one Gabriel Soares de Souza, and tells that the Indians used it to treat diseases of the mouth. Later accounts credited it with the power to cure many ailments from the common cold to epilepsy. In 1874 a Brazilian doctor reported that it possessed exceptional diaphoretic (sweat-inducing) properties, and it also caused copious salivation. It therefore came into use as a treatment for dropsy because of the water that it caused the body to exude. The next year an alkaloid, pilocarpine was isolated from jaborandi leaf extract, and became a favoured treatment, not only for dropsy but also for dry mouth, and especially for Sjögren's disease, a condition marked by failure of the salivary and tear glands. Later still it was accidentally discovered to reduce the pressure of fluid in the eye, responsible for glaucoma, a common cause of progressive loss of sight. Here then is part of the entry in *Chemist and Druggist* on jaborandi:

The fact that the drug and its active principle do have a powerful effect on the hair is well known. Thus Professor G.H. Wheeler states that he saw a gentleman who became partly bald after an attack of small-pox, the remainder of his hair turning gray. By the use of a decoction of jaborandi and sage, not only did he recover his hair, but it was restored to its natural colour.

More, Dr E. Borel 'treated an old woman for hypertrophin of the left side of the heart' with jaborandi, 'and her hair, previously white as snow, commenced to be coloured'. The article then gives the formula for 'The Premier Hair Restorer', which comprises carefully specified proportions of 'sulphate of quinine', tincture of jaborandi, glycerine, eau de Cologne, bay rum and rose water. This is the level of reportage in volume upon volume of *Chemist and Druggist*, a kind of undertow beneath the advancing tide of rational therapy.

Chapter 8

IMMUNOLOGY: PREVENTION AND CURE

Invisible agents of death

Whether antibodies are to be regarded as drugs is a matter of semantic preference. What remains indisputable is they have saved more lives and suffering than all the synthetic and plant-derived remedies that ever were. The science of immunology grew out of the discovery and study of bacteria in the 19th century. Before that the great infectious scourges, which had tormented mankind ever from its emergence on the plane, were the subject of barely rational theories and superstitions. Why did diphtheria or cholera or the Black Death kill some people and spare others? Were the visitations punishments for unspecified transgressions? Could they be overcome by any means other than prayer, fasting and self-flagellation? From the time of Hippocrates such measures as breathing cold fresh air, submitting to the right diet and taking strenuous exercise were recommended by physicians. There was a widespread belief in diathesis, the theory that certain people were constitutionally prone to diseases, and could be recognised as such by their bodily features. An enduring theory was that disease was carried by a 'miasma' – bad air, fog from the sea and the like, and indeed when steam rose from a swamp in which mosquitoes were breeding, malaria ('bad air') would engulf the region (p.). The idea that tangible particles, too small to be seen, might be the bearers of contagion did appear from time to time, but drew little attention. Two Roman scholars, writing in the first century B.C. had articulated this belief. Lucretius, the poet and philosopher conjectured in his famous work, *De Rerum Naturae* that the dust motes dancing in a beam of sunlight were being bombarded by invisible particles (atoms) in the air, and that such invisible entities might also be the bringers of pestilence.* Some twenty years later in 36 B.C. another Roman, Varro (p.) warned against building too close to a swamp because tiny invisible airborne creatures could enter the body through the nose and mouth and cause disease. Such concepts were alien to the physicians of the two succeeding millennia, but a doctor and professor at the University of Padua, Girolamo Fracastoro (1483-1553), studying the spread of syphilis, 'the French malady', came to the view that it was transmitted by *seminaria*, or little seeds, too small to be seen, which could retain their virulence for years outside the body.

That tiny organisms, invisible to the naked eye, did indeed exist, were alive and moved was demonstrated in around 1670 by Antonie van Leeuwenhoek (1632-1723), the remarkable Delft draper who designed and constructed a superior microscope. With it he observed bacteria from his mouth, but he did not associate micro-organisms with disease; that came only two centuries later. Louis Pasteur (1822-1895) was born in the town of Dôle, the son of a tanner. At school he was bright though not remarkable, but he showed a particular aptitude for chemistry. He achieved a doctorate at the illustrious École Normale Supérieure with a thesis on crystals, and in 1849, at the age of twenty-seven, he was appointed professor of chemistry at the University of Strasbourg, having already the previous year performed one of the most famous and spectacular experiments in the history of science. This had emerged from his study of crystals and his early interest in the

---

* This showed astonishing prescience on all accounts. The effect on which Lucretius cogitated and its explanation is related to Brownian motion, the dancing of particles, such as pollen grains, suspended in water, and first reported by a botanist, Robert Brown in 1827, The effect was analysed in a famous paper by Einstein, which related the particles' excursions to the velocity of the bombarding water molecules, and became a cornerstone of modern thermodynamics. The interaction of the moving microscopic particles with light had by then also been explained by a leading Victorian physicist, John Tyndall.

phenomenon of fermentation*, for he had been drawn from the beginning to the chemistry of life.

It was now clear to Pasteur that fermentation must be encompassed by minute living organisms, For in a simple chemical synthesis there could be no way in which two compounds that were mirror images of each other

---

* In brief he had solved the riddle of optical activity, a property confined (in the absence of the organic chemist's art, and apart from certain crystalline minerals) to molecules produced by living organisms. An optically active substance will rotate the plane of polarisation of polarised in an either clockwise or anticlockwise direction. Polarisation occurs when a beam of light passes through a polarising prism, or these days through a sheet of Polaroid, or a film of a more modern material, such as is used in sun-glasses. The three-dimensional oscillation of the light wave is rendered planar (oscillating only in two dimensions, that is in a plane) and the orientation of the plane, whether up and down, for instance, or side to side, can be readily measured with a second polarising prism or sheet of Polaroid. A solution of an optically active substance will rotate the plane of polarised light passing through it in a clockwise or anticlockwise direction, according to whether it is 'left-handed' or 'right-handed'. Tartaric acid is a product of fermentation, and its solutions twist the plane of polarisation of polarised light passing through it to the right. But tartaric acid synthesised in the laboratory, with an identical formula to the natural product has no optical activity and does not affect the direction of polarisation. Pasteur decided that there must be an intrinsic asymmetry in the natural molecule, whereas the synthetic counterpart might be made up of a mixture of two forms of opposite symmetry, which would cancel each other out. He prepared crystals of a salt of tartaric acid, and with a lens he saw that the synthetic material consisted of equal proportions of crystals that were mirror images of each other, while the fermentation product contained only one of these forms. He separated the two crystal forms with magnifying glass and tweezers, dissolved them in water and showed that they rotated the plane of polarised light in opposite directions. This result was considered so startling and important that the Academy of Sciences demanded visual proof that Pasteur had not cheated. They delegated a distinguished elder of the scientific establishment, Jean-Baptiste Biot to watch the preparation of the crystals and perform the measurements of optical rotation himself. Biot was overcome by the beauty of the result. 'My child', he said to Pasteur, 'I have loved science so much during my life, that this makes my heart pound'.

could be discriminated. For this new type of life form Pasteur coined the name, micro-organism.* Back in Paris, first at the École

Normale and then at the Sorbonne, Pasteur plunged into what we would now call biochemistry, and in particular the study of fermentation. First he examined what happened when milk went sour and produced lactic acid: micro-organisms could be seen multiplying and when transferred to fresh milk would at once start the fermentation process. (He later extended his work on fermentation to the production of wine and beer, with important economic consequences.) His work showed that micro-organisms were everywhere and were carried in the air. Therefore when a culture medium, in which the organisms would be cultivated, was kept in sealed sterilised vessels it would indeed stay sterile, whereas exposed to the air, it would become host to the growth of what were to be called bacteria.** Pasteur next showed that the micro-organisms were specific in their action. Thus brewer's yeast would not turn milk sour, and was distinct from baker's yeast. In 1865 Pasteur, by now a respected public figure, was asked by the Minister of Agriculture to investigate a serious economic problem, the devastation of the silk industry in the south of the country, and even beyond, in Spain and in Italy, by a disease of the silkworms. Pasteur complained that he knew nothing of silkworms, but did as he was asked. It transpired that there were two separate diseases, and that both were caused by micro-organisms, revealed by Pasteur's microscope to be present in the chrysalis of the silk moth. The solution Pasteur devised was to examine a sample of a hundred or so moths and breed from the few that were free of the malign agent. To the objection that peasants did not possess the skills

---

* The word, bacterium, from the Greek, meaning a little staff, on account of the rod-like form of the first bacteria seen in the microscope, was initially introduced in Germany a few years later.

** This drew Pasteur into a fierce conflict with other biologists who clung to the doctrine of spontaneous generation of life, whereby life forms, such as maggots, were created, for example, through the putrefaction of meat. The issue was settled in a public demonstration. Pasteur's famous sealed 'swan-necked' flasks were designed to allow free access to air while excluding dust and other particulate matter. The flasks, containing sterile culture medium, can be seen to this day, the liquid within pure and transparent as it was a century-and-a-half ago. The unsealed flasks (the controls had been quickly contaminated with airborne germs.

to perform microscopic assays Pasteur replied that he had taught a little girl of eight to use the instrument without difficulty. That little girl was in fact Pasteur's daughter, Marie-Louise. Alternatively the moths could be sent, pickled in brandy, to a qualified person to examine. This did not altogether suppress the scoffing, but the industry was saved. The silkworm studies continued intermittently for some years

It was not until 1877 that Pasteur, convinced now that man's great scourges were caused by micro-organisms, at last turned his attention to human disease. First came anthrax, a disease at that time almost always fatal, and exacted a high price from sheep-farmers, who lost many animals to anthrax. A French scientist, Casimir Joseph Davaine, influenced by Pasteur's methods, showed that anthrax was transmissible between sheep, and microscopic rod-like bodies were found in the blood of infected animals. But the link to the disease was disputed, and the identification was made by Pasteur after long study and with the aid of a series of ingenious experiments. This can be said to have established once and for all the 'germ theory' of disease, and it led eventually to a vaccine. But the work carried out during the same period by Robert Koch in Germany had an equal claim to the discovery of the germ theory, and that led, as will appear, to an unseemly altercation between the two great men. Nor did it still the strident voices of the many sceptics who stolidly refused to believe in the existence of invisible animalculi. Among them were most of the French medical establishment, and such luminaries of the profession as Rudolf Virchow (1821-1902), the all-powerful doyen of German pathologists and anatomists. Virchow made many important contributions to the advance of medical science, but was also an opponent of evolution. Pasteur was particularly plagued by a maniacally obsessive Parisian doctor and professor, Charles-Félix-Michel Peter, whose mantra was 'disease is in us, of us, by us', in other words that it lies in the constitution of the victim, and does not enter the body from outside.

A revolutionary discovery, which was to have limitless implications for the prevention and treatment of infectious diseases, came fortuitously in 1879. It bore out spectacularly Pasteur's famous dictum that fortune favours only the prepared mind. Pasteur had chosen chicken cholera (a misnamed condition, unrelated to the human disease) as a model on which to conduct the search for possible treatments of this and other infections. He had established that an injection of blood serum from an infected chicken, or of a culture of the chicken cholera bacteria, into a healthy bird would induce the disease. In the summer of that year, when Pasteur returned from holiday, the first bacterial culture that he tested elicited a new and startling phenomenon. The chicken which received the injection did not die but showed only a mild and transient response. Pasteur did not simply discard the culture as others would have done, but inquired into its origin. It had been prepared, it turned out, by Pasteur's assistant, Charles Chamberland as usual, but had been overlooked when the laboratory closed for the vacation and left out on the bench. Pasteur had inadvertently used it instead of a fresh preparation. The serum from the injected chicken produced similarly innocuous effects in new recipients, but that was not all: those chickens now injected with a fresh, virulent bacterial culture did not die or become sick, whereas the controls – healthy unexposed birds similarly injected - all died. Pasteur had discovered an attenuated bacterial vaccine. Leaving cultures on the bench for months was not a convenient or reproducible process, so Pasteur treated fresh cultures by heating them. This killed the bacteria, but left an immunologically active residue behind. Pasteur surmised that this process might be quite generally applicable in infectious diseases.

Pasteur returned to the study of anthrax at intervals during the next decade, with the main aim of developing a vaccine. His succession of remarkable discoveries never stilled the vociferous carping by his opponents, but it was another sceptical gadfly who stung him into planning a dramatic demonstration. Hippolyte Rossignol was a farmer in Melun, south of Paris, · and also a vet and editor of the journal, *La Presse Vétérinaire*, which served him as the pulpit from which he could rant against Pasteur, germs and vaccination. Here, in January of 1881, is the start of one of his diatribes: 'Would you like some microbes? They have been introduced everywhere. Microbiaty is now altogether à la mode; it reigns as sovereign; it is a doctrine that may not be discussed, we have to concede without rejoinder, above all since its high-priest, the savant, Pasteur, pronounced the sacred word: "I have spoken. The microbe alone shall be the characteristic of a disease; it is henceforth understood and agreed, the theory of germs must bring it to the pure clinic; the microbe alone is eternally true and Pasteur is its prophet'. Rossignol conceived the idea of challenging Pasteur to a public trial of his fraudulent vaccine. Rossignol must have expected that the affair would lead to a hero's acclaim for him, a huge boost for his magazine, and ignominy for Pasteur. The president of the local branch of the Society of French Farmers, which was to sponsor the event, the baron de La Rochette called on Pasteur to negotiate the form of the trial – the numbers and kind (whether sheep or cows) of animals and so on. In the end it was agreed that twenty-five sheep were to be vaccinated before being infected with anthrax, while another twenty-five – the control group – were to be infected without prior vaccination. In the end there were also five cows and a goat in each group. The site of the experiment was the village of Pouilly-le-Fort near Melun.

There had been only partial success in laboratory experiments with existing vaccine preparations, but Pasteur's colleague, Émile Roux recollected later that Pasteur was sanguine about the prospects of a good outcome. Roux and Pasteur's assistant, Chamberland were both on holiday in April of 1881 when the arrangements for the trial were finalised, and Pasteur wrote to them both, begging them to return, because this would be 'a big and important event'. Roux felt that Pasteur had been foolhardy and that such a demonstration was premature, but the die was now cast. Roux knew, however, that an able veterinarian and follower of Pasteur, Henri Toussaint, who was pursuing similar lines of research in Lyon, had hit on a far better way than Pasteur's heating method of generating attenuated bacteria. He had experimented with chemical procedures of killing the bacteria, and the preparation he now gave Roux had been made with the antiseptic, carbolic acid (phenol). It was whispered that Pasteur deprived Toussaint of the credit for his discovery, but this was rejected by his supporters: for all his faults, which included arrogance and an often harsh

intolerance of contrary opinions, it seemed never to have been his practice
to steal credit from his confr` Conconfrères and subordinates.*

Pasteur arrived in Pouilly-le-Fort accompanied by Roux, Chamberland
and another young assistant, Louis Thuillier. The site was thronged
with peasants, farmers, vets and the merely curious, and Pasteur watched
as Roux vaccinated and marked the animals. Roux and Chamberland
would visit the animals daily, and Roux recorded that the conversations he
overheard revealed that there was little expectation of a positive outcome
of the trial. Some two weeks later a second vaccination was performed,
and another two weeks on, the inoculation with anthrax. According again
to Roux, as time passed Pasteur became increasingly agitated, wondering
whether he had after all over-reached himself**. But by the anext day his
self-assurance had returned, and indeed soon the word came that the
unprotected animals were dead or dying, while the vaccinated ones were in
perfect health. Pasteur and his three colleagues hastened back to Pouilly-
le-Fort and received the acclamation of the crowd. Pasteur insisted on
an autopsy of the dead animals to prove that they had died of anthrax,
and masses of anthrax bacilli were indeed found in their cells. It was a
sweeping success for Pasteur, and made his name famous throughout the
western world. The respected journal, *La Revue Scientifique* waxed lyrical:
'Pouilly-le-Fort is as famous as all the great battlefields, where M. Pasteur,
the new Apollo, no more feared to hurl oracles than might have the god
of poetry.' More trials were performed around France and elsewhere to

---

* Yet, as a meticulous comparison by the American historian, Gerald Geison, of
Pasteur's published papers with entries in his laboratory notebooks has revealed,
Pasteur claimed to have triumphed with his own dubious preparation, not Toussaint's
superior version, as he actually did. Geison found other such disparities between
Pasteur's claims and the reality. Clearly the great man was not above some sharp
practice when his *amour propre* was threatened.
** According to a later account by a scientist who had not been there, Pasteur was
informed that one vaccinated animal was sick. Pasteur thereupon panicked, accused
Roux of incompetence and demanded that it should be Roux, who as the guilty
individual should confront the critics, for he himself could not face the ridicule and
obloquy to which he would be exposed. We do not know which version is closer to
the truth. Certainly Roux was a devotee of Pasteur's (and his eventual successor), and
may not have been an unbiased reporter.

confirm Pasteur's result, including at an early stage one in which the blood of an animal suffering from anthrax was used as inoculums to prove once again that the disease was transmissible. Vaccines were soon prepared in sufficient quantity to immunise farm animals throughout France and elsewhere, and the economic problem that anthrax had posed to the agricultural industry all but vanished. One regrettable outcome, though, was that in Berlin Koch, as we shall wee, was filled with resentment: the adulation that Pasteur was attracting, at least from the scientists whose opinions mattered, was detracting from Koch's own brilliant achievements. Pasteur had encroached on his territory, against the dictates of professional etiquette, and worse yet, he was French.

The ultimate drama

The most dramatic demonstration of Pasteur's immunisation method occurred in 1885. He had been working for some years on eventso called hydrophobia. It is an agonising and at the time incurable disease resulting from the bite of a rabid dog and revealing itself only after an incubation period of a month. It engendered such fear that victims were often driven out of their villages and left to die alone, or were sometimes stoned to death. Rabies is a viral disease, affecting the nervous system. Viruses, which had not yet been discovered, are small enough to pass through any available filter and cannot be seen in the microscope, but they can induce formation of antibodies in the recipient in the same way as bacteria. Despite many attempts Pasteur had no success in culturing the infectious agent of rabies, and he decided that a new approach was needed. The way forward would be to cultivate the agent of a disease in the tissue that it normally affected. This was a bold move, but because the rabies virus grows in nervous tissue it is difficult to provoke its growth in an animal by injection of infected material under the skin, for then the disease will in this situation develop only after a long interval, often many months. The infectious material in this case was the saliva of a rapid dog, obtained at great risk to the operators, who had to restrain the animal while sucking up saliva specimens in a mouth pipette. The most direct access to the nerves is through the exposed brain, so Pasteur was advised to deliver the agent through a hole drilled in the skull of a dog. Pasteur, who had an abhorrence of vivisection and was appalled at the thought of the pain a trepanning operation would inflict on the dog, held back. The experiment was finally performed in his absence by his friend – later the second director of the new Pasteur Institute in Paris - Émile Roux. The dog, and others similarly treated later, developed rabies in two weeks.

The question now was how to obtain an attenuated preparation, and Pasteur found the solution with the help of an observation by Roux. Rabbits were susceptible to the rabies virus, and Roux had found that the spinal cord of an infected rabbit retained its virulence over long periods. Pasteur placed such an infected spinal cord in a vessel, exposed to air, but immersed in a sterile solution, allowed it to dry, and tested its virulence in dogs at intervals. After about fifteen days a pulverised sample no longer engendered rabies, and protected the animal against the disease. It remained only to determine whether the same remedy would work, as Pasteur fully expected, in a human. But a test involving injection of material derived from a rabid animal was a hair-raising proposition. Failure might have the direst consequences, as much for the person treating the victim as for the victim, who might conceivably not even have been infected by the bite. The dilemma presented itself to Pasteur on 6th July 1885, when a distraught mother sent her nine-year old son to Pasteur in hope of salvation. His name was Joseph Meister, and he had been badly savaged by a rapid dog. Pasteur, though a chemist and not a physician, resolved (or so it was related) to administer the injections himself. With great trepidation* he gave the boy a course of fourteen injections in the buttock and waited. Only after thirty days could Pasteur breathe freely, for the boy was in robust health and was returned to his family. Loyal to Pasteur, Joseph worked all his life, with an interruption for service in the Great War, as a caretaker in the Pasteur Institute and died by his own hand in 1940. It was put about that he had shot himself with his army

---

* Pasteur had good grounds for unease. Among them was another instance of his apparent way of trifling with the truth, uncovered by Gerald Geison (p. 141). Whereas Pasteur claimed to have tested his vaccine on hundreds of dogs, his laboratory notebook record tests on a mere handful, far too few for any firm conclusions about its efficacy.

revolver rather than allow the German occupiers access to Pasteur's tomb under the building, but this story is probably apocryphal. Not long after his success with Meister Pasteur treated a second victim of a rabid dog, a fifteen-year-old shepherd, Jean-Baptiste Jupille, who had been bitten while protecting a group of children from the dog's attentions. He too survived and is commemorated by a statue outside the Pasteur Institute.

Not surprisingly the entrenched medical profession was adamantly hostile to the rabies vaccine, and Pasteur was viciously attacked, accused of having caused deaths of patients who might not have contracted the disease (as not everyone bitten by a rabid dog necessarily did: the estimated proportion was 60%). His nemesis, the half-deranged Michel Peter vociferated: 'Pasteur does not cure rabies, he causes it'. Even within his own institute there were mutters of dissent, and the word 'assassin' was whispered, according to one of Pasteur's collaborators. In fact only a very few of the patients treated with the vaccine died, and would probably have succumbed to the disease in any event. A case which gave Pasteur much pain was that of a young girl whom he treated, even though she had been badly mauled and the interval between the attack and her arrival at Pasteur's door was already long. Implored by her parents to try all he could, Pasteur, knowing that the case was probably hopeless and that he would suffer if he failed, felt compelled to accede. The girl died, and her father wrote a moving letter, praising Pasteur for his selfless action, well knowing the damage it might do to his reputation. One of those who sided against Pasteur was the radical journalist, politician, and also physician, Georges Clemenceau (The Tiger, as he was later known), who was to become the Premier and leader of the country during the Great War. Over the course of the years thousands of people were treated with the Pasteur vaccine, and the death rate remained extremely low; thus history has vindicated Pasteur. It is remarkable that much of Pasteur's greatest work was done when he was already in fragile health, paralysed on one side from the effects of a stroke. He died in 1895 at the age of seventy-two, seven years after a second stroke had left him an invalid and incapable of continuing his work.

Robert Koch and the Four Precepts

The animosity between the two Colossi of 19th-century biology, Louis Pasteur and Robert Koch, by ten years his junior, reflected the hostile relations between their two countries. Heinrich Hermann Robert Koch was born in 1843 in Clausthal in Lower Saxony, the third of thirteen children of the manager of a mineral mine in the Harz mountains. The boy was something of a prodigy who excelled at school in mathematics and languages. He also came under the influence of a maternal uncle, who was a keen naturalist and imbued his nephew with a love of nature and science. With the intention of qualifying as a science teacher, Koch headed for the nearby University of Göttingen. There the lectures that fired his imagination were those of the anatomist, Jacob Henle, a leader in the emerging field of histology, the use of stains to observe and identify anatomical features in the microscope. Here was the seed from which grew Koch's transcendent career. But he was also captivated by the work of liuevaanother professor, Georg Meissner, who was noted for his research in animal physiology, and what came to be known as physiological chemistry. Koch, all ideas of becoming a school-teacher now forgotten, was studying medicine, and he undertook his first research project under Meissner's supervision. This involved analysis of the formation of a metabolic product, in which Koch was his own guinea pig. He had already received a prize for dissection, and now he was the author of a paper in a respected journal. More important was the conviction that his experience in the laboratory had inculcated of the indispensable need for animal experimentation when searching for the cause of disease.

Koch qualified in 1866, and planning to marry, was now in need of a job. What he found was scarcely glamorous – a post as physician in a home for disadvantaged children in a local village. But he also established a private practice, and still found time to pursue his interest in microscopy. A daughter was born the same year, but for Koch neither the marriage nor the work proved happy. In a prolonged effort to find a better position he settled, after several false starts, in the small country town of Rakwitz in Prussia. There, among the peasants, who sometimes paid him in kind, he set up a successful practice. He was a kind and conscientious doctor, well-liked and trusted by his patients. In 1870 the Franco-Prussian war began, and Koch, though excused from the draft by reason of his weak eyesight, volunteered, and spent the ensuing months tending the wounded and sick on the battlefield. Returning from the wars, he applied for the position of district medical officer, based in another small Prussian town, Wollstein (now in Poland). He again quickly acquired a reputation as a competent and caring doctor, and his practice thrived. At the same time he set out to do some serious research, generally by night, in a small laboratory separated by a curtain from his consulting-room. He had saved money to buy a microscope and a microtome, an instrument like a miniature bacon-slicer, used to cut sections of tissues so thin as to be effectively transparent, and capable of being penetrated by a dye and mounted on a microscope slide. Koch's industry was phenomenal: he kept all his activities in play, never refusing a call from a patient on a remote farm, and managing – for he was a convivial man – to take time to relax and drink with friends.

The research project on which Koch settled was animated by a local concern. Farm animals had been dying of anthrax, and occasionally the disease would also claim a human victim. Earlier work, especially by Davaine in France (p.), had suggested, but not proved, that the disease was transmitted by microscopic organisms. Remarkably, Koch's approach in this, his first study of an infectious disease, and the techniques he used, gave the impression of being finely honed from the outset. It was Athena, sprung fully formed from the head of Zeus. First Koch confirmed that the rod-shaped microscopic bodies were present in the cells in the hide of a cow that had died of anthrax. He then injected some of this matter into a rabbit, which sickened and died. Its fluids contained masses of the rods, and Koch could follow the growth of bacteria when a second rabbit was injected at different sites. Now to prove that the rods were the cause and not a consequence of the disease it was clear to Koch that he must culture the organism. What was needed was a sterile culture medium, and Koch's next inspiration was that the aqueous humour (the clear fluid under the cornea of the eye) would serve. He cultivated the bacteria in the sealed compartment between the microscope slide and coverslip, also realising that this must be done at something close to body temperature. This led him to a new discovery, for what he saw were threads along which motionless spherical bodies were disposed. Koch at once inferred that these were spores – a dormant form of the bacteria – and a search revealed that they were abundant in the soil where the local animals grazed. Koch wrestled with the problem of spore formation, and the reversion of spores to active bacteria. He inferred correctly that the spores must be able to persist for long periods in the soil. (This is why the small Scottish island of Gruinard remained out of bounds for so many years after 1942, when it was chosen as the site for experiments on anthrax as a biological weapon during the height of the Second World War.) Koch's would have been an astonishing feat under any circumstances, let alone for a provincial doctor working in isolation, in his spare time and with minimal equipment.

Koch could have been in no doubt that he had made an epic discovery, and the question now was how best for him, an unknown, to bring it to the attention of the community of scientists. Koch wrote a detailed report of what he had done and sent it to Professor Ferdinand Cohn, one of the grandees of German biological science and a leader in the field of bacteriology, director of the Plant Physiology Institute in Breslau, and editor of one of the most important journals. Cohn, it seems, groaned at the appearance of yet another claim to a scientific revelation from some amateur in an obscure corner of the country, but he looked at Koch's manuscript and instantly perceived its import. There was even a point of overlap with his own work, for he too had observed bacterial spores (though from another bacterium) in the microscope. In his letter to Cohn Koch had begged to be allowed to demonstrate his results and procedures, and Cohn acceded with alacrity. On the appointed day Koch collected his apparatus and preparations and took the overnight train, arriving in Breslau on a Sunday morning. By mid-day he was in Cohn's laboratory, assembling his demonstration. Over the next two days as his cultures matured he prepared slides, made drawings of the images, and inoculated animals. Cohn and his assistants inspected the results and were overcome with excitement. An account of what happened next can be found in the exhaustive (and exhausting) biography of Koch by Bernhardt Möllers.* 'Cohn sent a messenger to the Pathology Institute that someone should come at once, for Koch's thing was correct and highly interesting. As Weigert [see p.] had to perform a dissection Cohnheim [the distinguished director] went, and when he returned he said: "Now put everything down and go to Koch; this man has made a grand discovery, which in its simplicity and precision of methods deserves all the more admiration because Koch is shut away from all scientific contact and did all this work on his own, and indeed in absolutely complete state. There is nothing more to be done. I hold this to be the greatest discovery in the area of micro-organisms and I believe that Koch will astonish us again with future discoveries, and will put us all to shame'. Cohnheim's collaborators who hastened to inspect Koch's demonstration were of like mind.

During Koch's few days in Breslau both Cohn and Cohnheim worked with him, using their superior microscopes and taking photographs of the slides - then a quite new procedure, aimed at eliminating any subjectivity that might have gone into drawings of the images. Koch made a deep impression on all those present, both by his personality and his scientific acumen. Cohn and Cohnheim were henceforth his most fervent and influential champions. Kohn's next move was to send a trusted assistant to Wollstein to learn from the small-town doctor. A useful innovation apparently resulted from the visit, the introduction of white mice in place

---

* Möllers was Koch's last student, and the biography, *Robert Koch – Persönlichkeit und Lebenswerk* [Robert Koch – Personality and Life's Work], which runs to 756 pages, was clearly an act of homage and, according to the publisher's note, its author's life's work. The note further divulges that the book was in the course of production when the printing works in Hanover was destroyed in a Second World War bombing raid, and it appeared that all but a small part of the text had been lost. But some years later the remainder came to light after all. It was published in 1951, but in the interim its author had died.

of field mice as experimental animals.* Koch had also learned something of value during his visit to Breslau. Cohnheim's assistant, Carl Weigert had shown him his new technique of using the recently created aniline dyes for staining specimens for microscopy. Koch made abundant and highly profitable use of this procedure. Next, urged on by Cohn, Koch wrote up his work, which was published in a major journal and attracted immediate attention.

Cohn and Cohnheim conspired together to secure an appointment for Koch at Breslau University, but no positions were available. The best they were able to find for him was the post of community physician for the city, which Koch accepted in the expectation that he would be able to supplement the meagre salary by establishing a private practice. This proved more difficult than he had expected, and after a short and unhappy time he moved back with his family to Wollstein, where fortunately no successor had yet been appointed. Nevertheless Koch's name had become widely known, thanks to his paper on anthrax, and it was not long before a new opportunity came his way. With Germany now unified under Bismarck's chancellorship, national pride in intellectual and artistic achievements was leading to a proliferation of national institutions. Koch was offered a position at the newly founded Imperial Health Institution (*Gesundheitsamt*), and at last a full-time research career beckoned. He was supported by the Director of the institution, Heinrich Struck, a doctor, comprehensively ignorant apparently of contemporary science, and thought to have owed his position to long service as the Chancellor's

---

* Möllers records in his biography an anecdote related by Koch's daughter, later the wife of one of her father's colleagues. 'Eidam [the assistant delegated by Cohn to visit Koch] got Koch's permission to bring along his foster father, who was very interested in bacteriology, an old gentleman who loved children. The latter formed a friendship with the little daughter of the house [the teller of this tale], and he sent her after his return to Berlin some white mice, well accommodated in a cage in the form of a small carved house of several floors with little rooms, stairs and windows. The mice multiplied rapidly and formed a harmless diversion for the child, but because of their exceptionally high sensitivity to all manner of infections, they were especially appealing for Koch's experiments. So it happened that white mice were introduced into all bacteriology laboratories and became the most widely used experimental animal.'

personal physician. Koch, now 37 was given a laboratory, and he recruited two assistants, each of whom was to have an illustrious careers of his own. Their names were Gustav Gaffky and Friedrich Loeffler, both at that time army doctors.

Koch had formulated his famous *Four Postulates*, which guided his work, and by reason of his growing influence that of many others. His aim was throughout to discover the agent of a disease, and then a means of neutralising it. The 'four postulates' are rules for hunting down the micro-organism responsible for an infectious disease, and they are:

1. The micro-organism must be found in high abundance in the sick person or animal, but must be missing in healthy ones.
2. The micro-organism must then be grown in culture in the laboratory.
3. The cultured micro-organism must be shown to cause the disease when introduced into a healthy experimental animal.
4. The micro-organism must finally be isolated over again from the newly infected host animal, and seen to be identical with the original agent.

Koch knew that there would be certain cases in which the rules would break down, most commonly when the disease agent resisted culturing in the laboratory, but for the most part the postulates held up remarkably well through the years. Meticulous microscopy was an essential element in Koch's work. He kept abreast of improvements in optics, in photography and in histological stains, and his skills kept him always ahead of other bacteriologists. It was at his urging that the famous firm of optical instrument manufacturers, Carl Zeiss of Jena developed the oil-immersion objective. Koch also devised the plate technique for culturing bacteria, whereby a solution containing the organisms was applied to a glass dish containing a nutrient solution in which bacteria could thrive, set in a gel, originally of gelatine, later (and to this day) of agar from seaweed. The dish – today called a Petri plate or dish - would then be put into an incubator, and 'colonies' of bacteria would grow in patches in the transparent gel. Pure cultures, Koch said, were the very basis of bacteriology. Koch showed off his plate technique at the International Medical Congress in London in 1881, where he met Sir Joseph (later Lord) Lister, the pioneer of aseptic surgery, and no mean bacteriologist himself. Koch was enthusiastically received, and it was at that meeting that he also met Pasteur. It was their first and only (initially) amicable encounter: Pasteur reportedly congratulated Koch: *'Monsieur, c'est un grand progrès'*.

Koch, nonetheless, had certainly been irritated by Pasteur's talk at the congress, which had preceded his own, and might indeed have made greater mention of Koch's extraordinary work on anthrax five years before. Koch probably also shared the prevailing German detestation of all things French, for memories of the war, in which he had after all taken part, still festered.* At any rate, he kept his powder dry at the meeting and refrained from an open confrontation with Pasteur. Instead, he launched into an incontinent attack on his French rivel in print, in the first volume of the Reports of his Institute (*Mitteilungen aus dem Kaiserlichen Gesundheitsamt*), with additional arrows of contention from his disciples, Loeffler and Gaffky. Koch poured scorn on Pasteur's work on attenuated pathogens, especially anthrax, imputed to him incompetence in the use of impure sera. The paper Pasteur had given at the London meeting was devoid of new information, except that which was wrong. There was more in the same vein with separate contributions from Loeffler and Gaffky, offering evidence of Pasteur's experimental shortcomings. It was unprecedented and outrageous. Pasteur read a French translation of Koch's diatribe, and opted not to reply but to respond instead with a demonstration of his methods in Germany.

An opportunity had in fact presented itself, for a member of the Faculty of the veterinary school in Berlin had asked to try out Pasteur's anthrax

---

* The animosity was fully reciprocated, indeed Pasteur had, at the height of the war in 1871, returned to the University of Bonn the honorary degree with which he had been invested some years before. The scroll was accompanied by a letter averring that the sight of it was not hateful to him, and that he was disgusted by the sight of his name allied to that of the Emperor, *Rex Gulielmus*. This produced an equally florid and abusive response, ending with an 'expression of total contempt'. Attached also was Pasteur's 'libellous letter', returned to him so that it might not pollute the university archive.

vaccine. A strong committee, which included the redoubtable Rudolf Virchow, was set up to oversee the event, and Pasteur delegated his protégé, Louis Thuillier, to administer the serum. Koch was excluded, apparently on the technical grounds that the tests had been requested on behalf of the Prussian government, while Koch was employed by a body belonging to the German empire. Thuillier had called on Koch during his visit and had apparently been affably enough received. The master himself had shown him the culture methods and facilities of the laboratory, on which he reported approvingly to Pasteur after his return. Anthrax had tactfully not been mentioned. Thuillier also remarked that Koch was not popular with his colleagues, and implied that he was viewed as a bucolic boor, a judgement for which there is little other evidence. The result of the trials, performed on an estate in rural Prussia, was disappointing, but Pasteur asked for a second demonstration, which was a resounding success, and resulted in the adoption of Pasteur's method throughout the country. Pasteur was therefore riding high when he encountered Koch once more at the International Congress of Hygiene and Demography, held in Geneva later that year. Pasteur spoke on the subject of attenuation of pathogens, and when he sat down Koch was called upon to respond, but declined. His main reason was the linguistic clash: Koch's command of French was inadequate, and Pasteur had no German. Koch proposed therefore to save his response for a learned journal. Pasteur rejoined that he would await M. Koch's comments 'with confidence' and would reply when the time came. He wrote to Roux that Koch's behaviour had been ridiculous and he had made a fool of himself. He wrote to his son that the episode had been a victory for France, which was all he had desired. Koch did as foreshadowed and published a tract in which he again attacked Pasteur in intemperate terms, impugning his scientific competence and probity. Pasteur hit back in an article in the *Revue Scientifique*, after which both adversaries must have recognised that further public squabbles would do their reputations little good.

Koch's triumph: tuberculosis revealed

Koch's reputation in fact was at this time unassailable. He had suddenly become an international celebrity only a few months before. Fresh from his success in London, he had embarked on his most ambitious project. Tuberculosis was still probably the world's most feared disease. Statistics are sparse, but in most European and American cities it is known to have killed more people in Koch's time than any other illness. A mortality rate of around 5 per 1000 population per year was a common figure. Four forms had been recognised, although there was debate about whether they were indeed the same disease. Pulmonary tuberculosis, also known as consumption or phthisis, was almost invariably fatal; a second form was miliary tuberculosis, which was characterised by nodules that appeared in all parts of the body; another was scrofula, otherwise lymph gland tuberculosis or the King's evil (p.); and finally there was lupus, or tuberculosis of the skin. But it is the first that ravaged the population, most of all of the poor, living in overcrowded and insanitary conditions.

Pulmonary tuberculosis had been shown well before Koch took an interest to be an infectious disease by a French army doctor. Jean-Antoine Villemin (1827-1892) was born to peasants in the Vosges and orphaned at the age of thirteen. Though impecunious, he had ambitions to become a teacher, and an uncle helped him to an education, But in 1848, the year of revolutions, he was called up into the army and served as a medical orderly. His competence and intelligence propelled him into the School of Military Medicine in Strasbourg, where he qualified in 1853 as an army doctor. The following year he was posted to the Val de Grâce military hospital in Paris. There he set up a small laboratory in which he pursued his research in his spare time between tending his patients. He published his work on tuberculosis in 1865, and in 1866 was appointed a companion of the *Légion d'Honneur*, in recognition not of the excellence of is his science, but of his fearless and energetic activity during the cholera epidemic that had struck Paris. During the war with Prussia he was busy treating the many wounded, and probably again more for his clinical than for his scientific services, rose eventually to become Vice-President of the Academy of Medicine in the year before his death.

Villemin began his programme of research with four rabbits. Two he inoculated through cuts in the skin with pus from the lung of a patient who had died of consumption in the hospital shortly before. The other two animals, his controls, he injected with fluid from blisters elicited by burns. After a lapse of time he killed and autopsied the rabbits and found that the first two had developed tuberculous lesions, while the controls had remained healthy. Here was proof that tuberculosis was transmissible. After further series of experiments, spread over two years, Villemin presented his data to a session of the Academy of Medicine. There was little reaction from the audience, unaccustomed probably to investigations not conducted at the bedside. And what useful intelligence was to be learned from experiments on animals? But the opposition went deeper than that. 'Contagionism', as it was called, was regarded by its opponents as an arcane, almost medieval doctrine. It was, moreover, with its calls for quarantines and restrictions on trade, inimical to a flourishing economy and therefore carried a political burden. Thus it was that Villemin was ferociously attacked by intellectual ideologues. Even before he read his paper one of the most entrenched of these, Michel Peter, already known (p.) as Pasteur's most implacable and irrational adversary, went on the attack. 'The idea of the contagiousness of tuberculosis', he thundered, 'is almost universally, and almost without discussion, rejected by contemporary savants'. Everyone after all knew about the diathetic nature (p.) of the malady. All this was perhaps even true. After Villemin had delivered his paper two venerable figures rose to smother him in obloquy. One was a noted surgeon, Jules Guérin, who prefaced his remarks thus: 'Let us propose as a fact that tuberculosis is not contagious', and later he observed that even a consideration of the non-pulmonary forms of tuberculosis must lead to 'a general smile of incredulity' at the thought that the disease might be contagious. It was the putrid nature of the material taken from the patient in a late stage of consumption that was responsible for the state of Villemin's rabbits.*

And then a respected Academician, Hermann Pidoux launched into a long and impassioned tirade. He denounced the oversimplified notion that 'diseases are caused by diseases'. It would be, he said, as though diseases produced seeds, resembling those of a cabbage or the sperm of a rabbit. What more preposterous idea than that seeds of tuberculosis lurked within the tubercles, the small granular swellings within the lungs of the victims! The concept was animistic, medieval, superstitious. And at this level of cogency the debate continued.

The Academy declined to publish Villemin's paper, and he was compelled to publicise it privately. Spurned in France, Villemin's work did receive some attention across the Channel. Dr (later Sir) John Burdon Sanderson (1828-1905) was a man of many parts, a physician, eventually Regius Professor of Medicine at Oxford, a physiologist who did important work on the function of the heart, a bacteriologist, and a public servant who, when still quite young, was appointed Inspector to the Medical Committee of the Privy Council (the precursor of today's Medical Research Council).

---

* Guérin was also a persistent thorn in Pasteur's side, and was later at the centre of a scandalous episode at a session of the Academy of Medicine. According to his grandson, Louis-Pasteur Vallery-Radot, Pasteur had told his friends that he meant to crush this pest once and for all, and the opportunity came after a talk by Pasteur in October of 1880. Guérin directed a typically ill-informed diatribe at Pasteur, who responded with dismissive sarcasm. A vaccine was a vaccine, and Guérin's preposterous cavils nothing more than *logomachies* - word play. At this the infuriated octogenarian Guérin rose from his seat and attempted to launch himself at Pasteur. The president, Baron Larrey interposed himself between the adversaries, and Guérin was persuaded to leave. The next morning two men, announcing themselves as Guérin's seconds, called on Pasteur's with a challenge. Pasteur replied that, rather than fight, he would refer the matter to his own seconds (or witnesses, for the word, *témoins*, serves for both), namely the Permanent Secretary and the Annual Secretary of the Academy and editors of its publication, which included the reports of its sessions. Afterwards, tired of the interminable wrangling, Pasteur drew back and made a half-apology: it had not been his intention to wound the feelings of a colleague, only to defend the validity of his work, and there the matter was allowed to rest.

In that capacity and because he also had an interest in animal diseases, he was appointed to a Royal Commission set up to study the serious economic problem of rinderpest, or cattle plague, which was taking a heavy toll of cattle, especially in South Africa. Burdon Sanderson had studied Koch's work and communicated with Koch himself. He did as Koch would have done: he sought and found in the blood of infected cattle an agent capable of inducing the disease in a healthy cow, injected with blood of the infected animal. When Koch received the report of the Commission, he wrote an appreciative letter to Burdon Sanderson. It was therefore no surprise that Burdon Sanderson took note of Villemin's report, the more so because Villemin had also done notable work on a tuberculosis-like animal disease, glanders, which had been devastating the French cavalry horses. The Englishman went to Paris, met Villemin, discussed his results, and on his return set about repeating the experiments in his laboratory at University College in London. They succeeded in all important respects, but for a single mishap when one of the control animals turned out to be infected. The reason was never clear, but arose most probably through a mix-up in the laboratory. It was sufficient to prevent a full endorsement of Villemin's conclusions, and the report to the Privy Council left the outcome uncertain, and was accordingly seized on by the anti-contagionists. Villemin received scant recognition in his lifetime for his visionary work, but he did at least end up Professor of Medicine at the Val de Grâce Hospital and a General. But to Koch, as we shall see, the glory.

Koch set out on the same path that he had trodden in his work on anthrax, but tuberculosis was a tougher proposition. It resisted both detection under the microscope and cultivation in culture. Koch began by inoculating guinea pigs with tubercle tissue and induced lesions, but could see no micro-organisms. (The reason for the refractory nature of the tubercle bacilli was discovered much later: they have a fatty coating, which repelled the conventional stains.) Success came only when he tried staining with a dye that his assistant, Paul Ehrlich had been using, and at the 271st attempt came success. The blue colour gave poor contrast on the photographic film because of the low sensitivity of film then available to blue light, but Koch overcame the problem by applying a second stain (a so-called counter-stain) with a new dye, Bismarck Brown, also known as Vesuvin, a technique developed by Ehrlich. The tubercle bacilli, as they came to be called, stood out in pale blue against a strong yellow background. The result was another triumph of refined technique and preternatural patience. Koch would on these occasions shut himself away from all human contact in his small personal laboratory, and could not be disturbed. It is not surprising that the endless succession of such days and nights of intense absorption put his marriage under strain. Nor did he communicate with his colleagues, who saw only the remains of dead guinea pigs accumulating each day outside the door, but Koch was elated. In the course his labours Koch made another technical advance. He had found that a freshly prepared solution of the dye, Methylene Blue did not work, the colour appearing only if the dye solution had been allowed to stand for 24 hours on the bench before use. Koch deduced that the dye was being modified by something in the laboratory atmosphere. Ammonia was used in many preparations and was ever-present in the air in small amounts. Koch added a trace of ammonia to the dye and the problem was solved. He went on to show that all basic (the antithesis of acidic) compounds would do the same trick, and of the many he tried aniline (benzene with a basic amino group (-NH$_2$) attached) proved the best. (Soon afterwards Ehrlich introduced a new and better dye, the red fuchsin, which replaced Methylene Blue.)

Koch had next to overcome the culture problem. He had the advantage by now of access to material from tuberculosis patients in the nearby Charité hospital. One of the first observations he made was that the tubercle bacilli were at their peak just before the tubercles erupted, and their number then fell precipitately. Even with this information culturing remained difficult, and the bacilli began to reproduce only after a week or more in the culture medium. He had already shown that the bacteria were present in profusion in all bodily fluids of infected animals, and now he had cultured as many as were needed to infect guinea pigs. The animals developed tuberculous lesions, and so Koch had the necessary proof of transmissibility of the disease in accordance with his precepts. When he emerged from his room into the light and announced the results there was jubilation in the laboratory. It had been a prodigious labour. Koch had inoculated some 500 animals, had prepared and tested 134 cultures of the bacillus, and had examined specimens from close to one-hundred human victims of the disease and many more animals. It was a model of meticulous, indeed obsessive search after the truth.

Koch's problem now was to convince the many critics of the 'germ theory' that he had indeed made a momentous discovery, one that would be seen as a landmark in the history of biology and medicine. The obvious venue at which to break the news was the Physiological Institute of Berlin University, the world centre at the time for biological research. Over it however hung the formidable shadow of Rudolf Virchow, the ageing doyen of German biological science, the mean credited with establishing pathology as a respectable, rational discipline. And Virchow was implacably hostile to germ theory, and he had also opposed the creation of Koch's Imperial Health laboratory, which he saw as an intolerable slur on the primacy of his own Institute. There was thus a long-lasting *froideur* between the inhabitants of these two great research centres, and an intrusion by Koch with his despised theory into Virchow's realm appeared out of the question. Yet thanks to the relations that two of Koch's trusted assistants, Loeffler and Ferdinand Hueppe had struck up with the great physiologist, Emil du Bois-Reymond in Virchow's institute, the matter was arranged. It was a triumph for Koch, who had set up a demonstration of his results with a row of microscopes, so that all could see the slides for themselves. Paul Ehrlich, who was present, later avowed that the evening had proved to be the most important experience of his scientific life. Koch's paper, which appeared in print a few weeks later, caused a furore throughout the scientific world. It was reported in the leading newspapers, among them *The Times* in London, which printed a résumé provided by the physicist, John Tyndall, head of the Royal Institution, and famous for his work on light scattering, and for prov0ing the existence of airborne bacteria (p.).

Choler and cholera

In 1883 the progress of research in Berlin and Paris was simultaneously interrupted by a governmental imperative. Two years before, a cholera pandemic had erupted in Egypt. This feared disease had been identified by John Snow in London as a water-borne infection (p.). It killed at the time from one in five to one in three of those it infected (more in the prosperous countries when doctors might still bleed their patients). There had been in recent years a series of disastrous outbreaks in Germany (most famously in Hamburg in 1866, when Koch was still a district doctor), in France and in many other European countries. There were fears now that the highly virulent strain of the disease propagating in Egypt might find its way to Europe, and the governments of France and of Germany resolved to act. Commissions were set up, and members of Pasteur's laboratory and of Koch's were requested to travel to Egypt and discover the cause and prevention of the pestilence. Koch himself led the German expedition, which was better prepared and equipped than the French. Pasteur, too enfeebled by two strokes to take direct part, sent Émile Roux, Louis Thuillier and another young assistant, Edmond Nocard.

By the time they arrived the epidemic was declining, and Koch and his colleagues, first in Port Said and then in Alexandria, could not lay their hands on sufficient material to begin culturing. The French had better luck, at least to the extent that they came upon the corpses of a number of recently deceased victims of the disease. They dissected the tissues and identified, as they thought, micro-organisms, but these turned out to be nothing more than white blood cells. Much worse, Thuillier was one of the last martyrs of the epidemic. Roux and Nocard strove to save his life, but he died, with, according to the embroidered accounts that reached France, the words on his lips, 'Did we find it?' It was also said that Koch had been summoned to help save Thuillier's life, and assured the dying man that he had indeed found the agent of cholera, knowing full well that he had not. This too was apocryphal. The German team did however send a laurel wreath to lay on Thuillier's grave. No further fresh corpses were available, Roux felt they could do no more, and he and Nocard returned sadly to France.

As for Koch, he took his team to Calcutta, where an epidemic still raged and there were cadavers aplenty. Soon Koch's microscope revealed 'comma-shaped' organisms in the bodily fluids. Were these the cholera bacteria? A month later Koch had cultured them, but attempts to test their virulence failed, because no animals (including laboratory mice sent from Germany) would catch the disease. Koch did though find the same 'commas' in the local water, even drinking water. It was a reasonable supposition then, but no more, that these were the agents of cholera. Koch and his group returned home after an absence of eight months, during which time they had endured danger and hardship, as his letters to his wife and his beloved daughter testified. On his arrival in Berlin he was showered with praise and honours, and summoned for an audience with Kaiser Wilhelm I. That same year, 1884, there was a fresh outbreak of cholera in France, and Koch, eager to procure more samples from another source than India, hastened to Toulon. He quickly found the comma bacillus and showed it to Roux. Pasteur refused to believe that Koch had got it right and asked Roux to find the flaw, but Roux was convinced. The French press was indignant: why should a German intrude into a French affair, when France had the greatest scientist of all at its disposal. Koch of course had got it right.

A curious coda to the discovery of the cholera agent played out at the same time in Germany, where a cholera outbreak also occurred. Opponents of the germ theory of infectious disease were not yet mollified, and among the most prominent was Max von Pettenkofer, a man of varied accomplishments and high distinction. The son of Bavarian peasants, he had escaped from a life of toil, trained in chemistry, qualified as a doctor, and risen to the position of Professor of Medical Chemistry at the University of Munich. He had done important work in human nutrition and then in public health, for which he is best remembered. It remained his obstinately held belief that cholera lay in the soil, and that therefore Koch's cultures were little more than water, and could not possibly carry the agent of the disease. A man of conviction he decided to make a demonstration of this truth by drinking a culture, which he obtained from Koch's laboratory. He also made two of his assistants and three doctors share the ordeal. Pettenkofer suffered nothing more than a mild attack of diarrhoea, and the others seem also to have come to no lasting harm. Pettenkofer felt vindicated and Koch was discomfited. It was supposed that the assistant in Koch's laboratory who had supplied the culture had guessed Pettenkofer's intention, and not wishing to be an accessory to suicide and murder, had diluted it to the point of inactivity.

The phantom cure

With his cholera escapade behind him, Koch returned to face a host of problems awaiting him, both professional and personal. His health had deteriorated, and the ever more troubled relations with his wife could not have helped. His administrative duties and the burden of teaching and of speaking at conferences kept him away from the laboratory bench; the research was left to his assistants. Close to a breakdown, Koch left again, this time for an extended vacation in Switzerland, which seemed to restore his spirits. Then in 1885 he was appointed Professor of Hygiene at the University of Berlin, and director of the Hygiene Institute. Finally in 1890 Koch's hunger after discovery returned, and he addressed himself once more to the work he had left eight years before. His aim now was nothing less than to find a cure for tuberculosis. He struck out in a new direction, stimulated probably by the successes of his associates, Behring, Kitasato and Ehrlich, in breaking open the new discipline of immunology (pp.). Cloistered as of old in his personal laboratory Koch began to produce rapid results. He injected cultures of tubercle bacilli under the skin of guinea pigs that were either healthy or had been infected with the disease, and in the latter there appeared a remarkable phenomenon. A skin necrosis (death of tissue) set in around the site of the injection, a very high fever developed, accompanied by other severe symptoms associated with advanced tuberculosis. This state persisted for one or two days, and then recovery followed. To Koch it appeared that the bacilli which had infected the animal had been killed, and a cure had resulted, Koch tried his bacterial brew on himself. He ran a very high temperature with a violent headache, and was ill for some days.

Koch said nothing about his discovery to anyone, but dropped the bombshell – that a 'possible cure' for tuberculosis in at least 'some cases' could be effected by this new preparation, which he called *tuberculin* – at the 10th International Congress of Medicine in Berlin. It was an uncharacteristic and foolhardy move. Here was Koch, famous for his cautious, meticulous investigations, announcing a medical miracle, and failing even to consider the predictable brouhaha from press and public, which would ensure that his few words of caution were lost to view. Worse, he refused to divulge what his tuberculin actually was and how it had been prepared, even though secret medicines were forbidden in Germany. Koch's actions have never been properly explained, but there were suggestions that the Kaiser himself had been apprised of the supposed stroke of German genius, and wanted it broadcast to the world without delay. In Britain *The Lancet* was in no doubt: '.... all who are in any way acquainted with the circumstances under which Koch was practically compelled by his Government superiors and by his colleagues to make his premature statement at the International Medical Congress in Berlin will sympathise most deeply with him that he was compelled to break through his usual reticence'.

At all events, high drama ensued. Koch was engulfed in chauvinistic adulation. The Kaiser at once invested him with the Grand Cross of the Red Eagle, and the freedom of the city was conferred on him – a signal honour, previously bestowed on only three men.* Pasteur sent a telegram of congratulations, and medical journals and newspapers around the world hailed the greatest discovery in medicine ever made. Tuberculosis patients throughout the country flocked to Berlin in the hope of an instant cure, and in a vain attempt to meet the demand Koch got a pharmacist, a friend from his early days, to produce larger amounts of the drug. The chief chemist, August Laubenheimer of the Hoechst dye works approached Koch to negotiate manufacturing rights, but nothing seems to have come of this. A black market in tuberculin soon arose, and mountebanks selling spurious samples thrived. There were, to be sure, some sceptics. One was Arthur Conan Doyle, not yet the author of the Sherlock Holmes stories, but working as a doctor. He visited Koch's laboratory and reported with remarkable prescience that it was unclear whether tuberculin was indeed a cure, although it might prove in future to be useful for early diagnosis.

---

* They were Otto von Bismarck, The Prussian Chancellor who had united Germany, Helmuth von Moltke, military genius and the engineer of victory in the Franco-Prussian war, who was famously said to have smiled only twice in his life, first when his mother-in-law died, and secondly when he was told that the Swedes regarded Stockholm as a fortress, and the great archaeologist, Heinrich Schliemann, who had uncovered the treasures of Troy and Mycenae.

At the height of all the turmoil an upheaval was going on in Koch's private life: he had fallen in love with a seventeen-year-old art student (younger than his daughter who married one of her father's assistants shortly after, and more than thirty years Koch's junior), and was in the process of divorcing his wife. (The romance led surprisingly to a remarkably happy marriage, which endured up to Koch's death seventeen years later.) Koch tried to distance himself from the uproar over tuberculin. Some improvements were reported in patients, but the outcome overall was unhappy. A thousand or more doctors came to Berlin to acquaint themselves with the miraculous treatment, and patients in their thousands were inoculated with the ill-defined and highly variable tuberculin (also known as 'Koch's lymph'), and in the upshot it was adjudged generally useless, although there was little in the way of controlled trials. Some patients, it was thought, may have died of the cure. There were rumours that Koch had sold the secret to a pharmaceutical company for a vast sum, which perhaps he needed to regulate his family life. In the end he was forced to divulge the secret, though, the cynics said, only when it no longer had any pecuniary potential. It was indeed nothing more than an extract in glycerine of tubercle bacilli. At this stage Koch departed with his bride on a long voyage to Egypt, leaving the affairs of the laboratory in disarray. Koch never quite relinquished the hope that a real cure along the lines of tuberculin was still in prospect. He continued sporadically to work on the problem, and prepared a 'new tuberculin', which fared no better than the old.

Koch's reputation had assuredly taken a blow from the tuberculin fiasco, but he was still widely seen as an oracle on the subject of infectious diseases. And so in 1896 he responded to the call from the British Government to visit South Africa to find a way of eliminating the cattle plague, or rinderpest, which was killing off the local herds. Accompanied as always now by his young wife, he set about the task, but failed to identify or culture the pathogen. This was no fault of his, for it was a virus, which could not be seen or captured by Koch's bacteriological techniques. He then tried to develop a vaccine by Pasteur's method of attenuation, but this too failed. He would have continued had he not received the Imperial command to hasten to India, where the bubonic plague (the black death) had broken out, and was beginning to enter Europe by ship. The plague bacillus had already been identified in France by Alexandre Yersin (and is accordingly now called *Yersinia pestis*). The German commission, which had preceded Koch to Bombay, led by his former assistant, Gaffky, had shown that the disease was indeed the plague, but even with Koch's help it could make little headway. Next Koch was summoned back to Africa, this time to German East Africa where the plague had also surfaced. Koch established himself in Dar es Salam (in what is now Tanzania), cultured the bacilli but made little further impression, although he began to take an interest in other tropical diseases, especially malaria. He made a modest contribution to the problem of controlling the spread of that disease, but the science had been done by others (notably Ronald Ross and Charles Lavaran, who were both rewarded with the Nobel Prize). Koch was an indefatigable traveller, defying discomfort and danger in his pursuit of tropical diseases, but he made only one further significant contribution to the conquest of infectious diseases. This happened in Berlin, where he now directed a new Institute for Infectious Diseases, built specially for him. Georg Gaffky had isolated the bacterium responsible for typhoid fever, a serious problem in Germany and beyond, but it was Koch who conceived the the theory that healthy carriers of this and other diseases – people infected but not sick - must exist. This was an important insight, and later many such carriers were identified, a famous case being 'Typhoid Mary', the unfortunate cook, who infected 53 Americans, three of whom died, and passed the last twenty-three years of her life in quarantine.

In his retirement Koch travelled with his wife to America and Japan. He was fêted in both countries, but it was at a conference in the U.S. that he committed his second bêtise related to tuberculosis. The question at issue was whether human and bovine tuberculosis were unrelated or essentially the same, in which case the disease could be transmitted from cattle to people. That this was so had been perceived by Villemin, and Koch had initially agreed. Later though he had, by uncertain reasoning, changed his mind and vehemently asserted the opposite. It is all too reminiscent of the reply of an American Senator when asked his opinion by the journalist, Alistair Cooke, on a political issue of the day: 'Son, I've not made up my mind yet, but when I do I'll feel strongly'. Koch spoke at the International

Tuberculosis Congress in Washington in 1908, and loftily dismissed the belief, by then widely held by the American doctors, that bovine tuberculosis was a danger to man, and that the disease could be caught from the milk of infected cows. Koch's opinion carried weight, but the Americans for the most part stood firm. Final proof of animal-to-human transmission of tuberculosis came only later. Koch's pronouncement to the contrary inhibited research on the question, and failure to take the measures introduced in America almost certainly caused many deaths in Europe. Koch's lapse was eventually corrected by a process of sterilisation. It would have vexed him that this is known to the world as pasteurisation. Back in Berlin, Koch tried to resume work on tuberculosis, but the physical strength, which had made him such a fearless alpinist and sustained him through the hardships of work in Africa, had ebbed, and his heart was weak. He had received the Nobel Prize in 1905, not before time, for the award had gone to lesser men from its inception in 1901. It must have been a source of chagrin that the very first prize for medicine had been awarded to his one-time assistant, Emil von Behring. The ailing Koch departed to Baden-Baden to rest, and he died there in 1909, the year after his American and Japanese tour, at the age of 67.

Chapter 9

CHEMISTRY ASCENDANT

Heart's ease: amyl nitrite

The list of the medicines introduced during the first half of the 19th century included chloral hydrate, amyl nitrite, iodoform, salicylic acid, hyoscine and hyoscyamine, and pilocarpine. There were also a large number of others that were quickly discarded. The most important was undoubtedly amyl nitrite, which merits a section to itself. It is a simple chemical, first synthesised in 1844 by the French chemist, Antoine Balard, who achieved fame through the discovery of the element, bromine (p.). Fifteen years later Frederick Guthrie at Owens College in Manchester (which later became Manchester University) followed Balard's method, and reported in a paper in the *Journal of the Chemical Society* that the substance had a dramatic physiological action: having inhaled a little of the vapour, Guthrie found that his face had reddened, the artery in his neck was throbbing, and his heart was pounding alarmingly. More time passed before a doctor and physiologist, Arthur Gamgee, working in Edinburgh, took an interest in amyl nitrite and found that it strongly reduced the blood pressure. Gamgee demonstrated this effect to a friend, a doctor at the Royal Infirmary, Thomas Lauder Brunton.

Brunton (1844-1916) was something of a prodigy. He started research on the effects of drugs while still a medical student in Edinburgh, and broadened his education by time spent in leading European centres of medical learning. He developed a particular interest in the heart and its disorders, and by the time of the meeting with Gamgee he had achieved a high reputation as both a clinician and a researcher in physiology. (As a result he became a target of abuse by the anti-vivisectionists) Brunton at once had the happy thought that amyl nitrite might find a use in treating angina pectoris. His report on the matter, published in 1867, 13 with a description of the distressing nature of this condition – violent pain in the chest, often rising into the neck and extending into the arms, sudden in its onset, though transient. 'Brandy, ether, chloroform, ammonia, and other stimulants', he continues, had been the only treatments, which gave all too little relief. Brunton goes on to describe a particularly severe case of angina in one of his patients, which recurred each night and lasted for an hour or more. Various treatments were tried, but the only one that helped the patient was 'small bleedings of three or four ounces, whether by venesection or cupping'. Brunton inferred that relief resulted from a reduction in arterial blood pressure, and hence the possible usefulness of amyl nitrite struck him. Gamgee provided a sample, and Brunton applied a few drops of the liquid to a cloth over his patient's nose, whereupon the pain instantly abated. In time the blood pressure returned to its original level, but the angina attacks responded each time to the same treatment. Brunton, clearly elated, allowed himself some speculations about other conditions that might respond to amyl nitrite. These, it has to be said, proved unfounded, but Branton went on with some success to explore the effects of other related nitrites. Moving to London as professor at University College and St. Bartholomew's Hospital, he did further significant work in physiology and pharmacology and, anointed with many honours, crowned by the now extinct order of nobility, a baronetcy, he died in 1916. By then, and in fact soon after the discovery of its efficacy, amyl nitrite had gained wide currency as a treatment not only for the agonies of angina but for other forms of distress, even social. A few drops on a handkerchief, a pill under the tongue, or later some 'glass-pearls' – thin glass bubbles, which could be easily crushed in a piece of lace – were the usual means of achieving quick relief or a mild high.

We now know that angina is caused by fatty deposits (plaques), which constrict the arteries bringing blood to the heart and thereby impede the blood supply. The tension of the arterial walls is maintained by a layer of smooth muscle (which differs from the so-called striated muscle that allows us to walk and run). The action of amyl nitrite is to relax smooth muscle (and not only in the arteries), allowing the arteries to dilate and more blood to pass. Such insight was still in the womb of time in Brunton's day, but the hunt was on for physiologically active compounds amongst the many that chemists were now producing. Might there be, for instance, a compound bearing the nitro group ($-NO_2$) even better than amyl nitrite in combating angina, and free perhaps from its disadvantages – the transience of its effect and the headaches that it provoked? In 1878 such a compound came to light, and its properties were meticulously described in a paper published in four instalments in *The Lancet* by Dr William Murrell (1853-1912) of the Westminster Hospital in London. Its title was 'Nitro-glycerine as a Remedy for Angina Pectoris'.[*]

William Murrell studied medicine in London, and remained there throughout his working life, most of the time at the Westminster Hospital. In addition to his clinical duties, he pursued a busy programme of research into physiology, and into drugs and poisons. He published three widely used

---

[*] Nitroglycerine (more properly called nitroglycerol), which contains three nitro groups, was first prepared in·1846 by Ascanio Sobrero, Professor of Chemistry at the University of Turin. It soon transpired that the compound was a deadly explosive, and Professor Sobrero was the first to bear its marks on his face. It was, he decided, too hazardous to work with it, and he later remarked that he felt 'almost ashamed' to have been its discoverer. It nevertheless engaged the interest of mining engineers, and several containers of the liquid, known as 'blasting oil' were shipped to California. One of them blew up with disastrous results, and legislation was hastily introduced to prevent such accidents from happening again. A Swedish chemist and engineer, Alfred Nobel, took up the manufacture of nitroglycerine in the family armament factory. This proved a profitable undertaking, but when his younger brother, Emil and four other men were killed Nobel began to search for means of making the substance, if not wholly safe, then at least safer. (Even so the factory he later established in Germany was twice destroyed.) His solution was to absorb the liquid in kieselguhr clay, and the product was marketed as Dynamite. Nobel was troubled in later life by what he had wrought, and when afflicted with angina he apparently refused the nitroglycerine treatment.

books, one with the title *Aids to Materia Medica and to Forensic Medicine,* one on toxicology and one on how to deal with cases of poisoning. His work on the use of nitroglycerine was stimulated apparently by a discussion in a journal called *Medical Times and Gazette.* 'Mr. A.G. Field, then of Brighton', who was presumably a surgeon, since he experimented liberally on himself and on patients, reported on the effects of nitroglycerine, taken by mouth. In his famous paper in *The Lancet* Murrell quotes Mr Field's account of his experience: he had put two drops of a one-percent solution in alcohol on his tongue, and for three minutes nothing happened. Then 'he noticed a sensation of fullness in both sides of the neck, succeeded by nausea. For a moment or two there was a little mental confusion, accompanied by a loud rushing noise in the ears, like steam passing out of a tea-kettle'. There was a sensation of constriction about the lower neck, a pain in the stomach, and a feeling of lassitude; he sweated, he yawned compulsively, and his head ached. The symptoms passed, except for the headache, which persisted until the next day. Perhaps, thought Field, he was exceptionally sensitive to the substance, and so he tried it on some friends, who experienced similar sensations, and one of whom passed out. Two other doctors entered into the debate, and reported widely varying effects in themselves and their patients: perhaps the differences lay in the preparations, or perhaps indeed some individuals were more responsive to nitroglycerine than others. But another conjecture was that the effects had all been brought on by autosuggestion, perhaps through fear of the unknown. Murrell was dissatisfied by the conflicting reports and decided to try the substance on himself. He procured a 1% solution like Mr Field's and put the bottle in his coat pocket. He remembered it as he walked to his outpatients' clinic, opened the bottle and touched the cork to his tongue:

.... A moment after, a patient coming in, I had forgotten all about it. Not for long, however, for I had not asked my patient half a dozen questions before I experienced a violent pulsation in my head, and Mr. Field's observations rose considerably in my estimation. The pulsations rapidly increased, and soon became so severe that each beat of the heart seemed to shake my whole body. I regretted that I had not taken a more opportune moment to try my experiments, and was afraid the patient would notice my distress, and think that I was either ill or intoxicated. I was quite unable to continue my questions, and it was as much as I could do to tell him to go behind a screen and undress, so that his chest might be examined. Being temporarily free from observation, I took my pulse, and found that it was much fuller than normal, and considerably over 100. The pulsation was tremendous, and I could feel the beating to the very tips of my fingers. The pen I was holding was violently jerked with every beat of the heart.

The symptoms gradually subsided, and Dr Murrell felt able to continue with his work, although 'a splitting' headache persisted throughout the afternoon. Murrell was now convinced that the effects were not due to fear or anxiety. Clearly exhilarated by the exciting experience, he continued with his observations, trying the drug on himself in various forms 30 to 40 times. He then went on to try it on 35 people (presumably volunteers) to get a feel for individual variation. He made recordings of pulse-rate and blood pressure and the effects of varying the dose. Only then, and over a nine-month period, did he try the effects of nitroglycerine on three patients with severe angina. The results were remarkable: all three had been incapacitated by the condition, unable to work or to walk more than a short distance, and in constant fear of the next attack. Treatment gave almost instant relief from the attacks and forestalled further episodes, and after a course of treatment the patients were able to resume a normal life-style. Murrell was a quiet, modest man, who did not seek recognition, but in nitroglycerine he discovered a standard drug for angina pectoris, in use still after a century and a half.

Withering's legacy

It was almost exactly a century earlier that William Withering had hit upon the first effective drug for a different cardiac complaint, congestive heart failure (pp.). And yet it took long years for the value of foxglove for treating the disease to be universally accepted. Withering himself had not altogether understood the relation of dropsy (oedema, or in American English, edema, or swelling in either) to the heart.* In the 1830s French scientists set about isolating the active constituent of foxglove leaves, stimulated perhaps by the offer of a substantial prize by the Society of Pharmacy. A determined attempt was made by two Parisian pharmacists at the Charité hospital, Augustin Eugène Homolle and Théodore Quevenne. In 1841 they announced that they had obtained from an extract of the leaves of the common foxglove, *Digitalis purpurea* an amorphous, far from pure powder, though with good activity. They gave their material (which they incorrectly thought to be an alkaloid) the name, digitaline, and continued their attempts at further purification. Meanwhile another Parisian pharmacist was following a similar course and doing rather better. Claude-Adolphe Nativelle had extracted a similarly active amorphous material (though starting from another species, the woolly foxglove, *Digitalis lanata*), and succeeded in separating it into three chemical components. One of these contained the desired activity, and formed crystals. But these crystals, Nativelle found, were still impure. After further toil he finally collected crystals of the pure compound. He called it digitalin to distinguish it from digitaline, which carried the implication that it was an amine.

To Nativelle's chagrin it was Homolle and not he who was awarded the prize, Quevenne being debarred because he was a member of the Society. Nativelle angrily accused of Quevenne and the award commission of bias and corruption, and Quevenne responded to Nativelle's diatribe, as he called it, in a long and minutely detailed pamphlet published by the Society. The pharmacists and chemists took sides in this very public and intemperate altercation, and it seems that most supported Nativelle. The general tenor of professional opinion was reflected many years later, in 1869, when the Academy of Medicine bestowed on Nativelle one of its highest honours, the Ofila medal. Nativelle would no doubt have been pleased that a digitalis preparation is sold even now under the name of Digitalin Nativelle. By way of a further postscript, an incontestably pure

---

* It was not until the mid-19th century that the great English physician, Richard Bright (who made a speciality of diseases of the kidney, and gave his name to Bright's disease) discerned that dropsy could be a manifestation of a kidney *or* a heart disorder. He could distinguish between the two causes by the presence of albumin in the urine when it was the first. This would reveal itself by foaming when the urine was shaken.

preparation was made in 1879 by the great German pharmacologist (often called 'the father of pharmacology'), Oswald Schmiedeberg (p.). (This must have been particularly galling for the French, since Schmiedeberg occupied the chair of pharmacology at the University of Strassburg in the city (Strasbourg) that had been ceded to the Germans after the Franco-Prussian war only eight years before.)

The drug as eventually manufactured went under the name of digoxin (and later various other names), and is in use to this day, although its limitations gradually became apparent. One is that it is toxic in high concentrations (as was underlined when a male nurse who had worked in hospitals in New Jersey and Pennsylvania was convicted in 2003 of murdering 40 patients by this means). But in particular, it does good, does nothing, or does actual harm depends on the precise nature of the heart defect in each case and on associated conditions. It has found use for the treatment not only of heart failure but also of arrhythmias, such as tachycardia, characterised by erratic heartbeats. In the 19th century diuretics for treating congestive heart failure, came into use, as we shall see.

The heirs of Koch

Koch's part in the history of therapy can scarcely be exaggerated. His influence on those who sought inspiration by coming as assistants to his laboratory was all-encompassing. He had a dozen or so disciples and adherents who rose to great eminence in the late 19th and early 20th century. The most famous of them were two men of very different temperaments, whose lives and careers were for many years interwoven. They are Paul Ehrlich and Emil von Behring, or before his ennoblement plain Emil Behring. They were born one day apart in March of 1854, and died within two years of each other during the First World War. Ehrlich was a gentle and generous spirit, unassuming and admired and loved by his colleagues. Behring was very different personality: he was intelligent, well-read and had wide cultural interests with a particular leaning towards philosophy; but he was by nature solitary, secretive and mistrustful, prey to depression, yet too often pompous and overbearing. His relations with Ehrlich and with Koch were troubled, often acrimonious.

Like Robert Koch (and also his contemporary, Emil Behring), Paul Ehrlich was born into the lower middle (*Bürger*) class, but with a difference, for his parents were Jews. In consequence his name was expunged from the record during the Third Reich. The street in which Ehrlich lived during his years in Frankfurt, which had been changed to Paul-Ehrlich Strasse after his death, was given another name in 1938, and reverted only after the defeat of 1945. Antisemitism dogged Ehrlich's career. He was a sensitive man, and felt it deeply. Ehrlich was born in the Lower Silesian town of Strehlen (now Strzelin in Poland), where his father was an innkeeper and proprietor of a small liquor distillery. The son was an unremarkable student at the local school and later in the high-school (*Gymnasium*) in Breslau, but he was encouraged by his paternal grandfather, who had scholarly interests and a collection of books. But the formative influence on the direction that his life was to take resulted from his encounters with his cousin, older by a decade, Carl Weigert (1845-1904). Weigert, who was on course to become a prominent scientist, had studied in Vienna, Breslau and Berlin, had served as an army surgeon in the Franco-Prussian war, and had fallen under the spell of bacteriology. He was the first to discern the promise in staining bacteria for microscopy with the aniline dyes that Hoechst and other companies were producing, and in 1875 he wrote a manual on staining techniques. He was also one of the first microscopists to make use of the microtome to cut thin transparent sections of tissues (p.).

Ehrlich was profoundly impressed by what his cousin showed him, and began to experiment with histology while still a schoolboy. As an eighteen-year-old medical student at the local University of Breslau he was fortunate in one of his teachers, the celebrated anatomist Heinrich Wilhelm Waldeyer with whom he began research on the histology of different tissue types. Soon after, Waldeyer moved to Strassburg, as Strasbourg had become the previous year, with the first cohort of German academics, replacing the dispossessed French faculty. Ehrlich accompanied him, and within a short time had completed a study of lead poisoning, which presaged the great work to come on the action of drugs. Ehrlich's histological observations revealed that lead compounds were sequestered by the cells of solid tissues, a quite new concept. This insight, which came to Ehrlich so early in his career, gave an indication of the penetrating originality and clarity of thought that were to mark his scientific achievements.

From Strassburg Ehrlich returned to Breslau to conclude his medical studies. It was a stimulating environment, with Ferdinand Cohn and Julius Cohnheim (p.) at the apogee of their brilliant careers, and Ehrlich's cousin, Carl Weigert, then Cohnheim's assistant, also at hand. Taking advantage of the peripatetic tradition in the German universities at the time, Ehrlich also spent a term at each of the Universities of Freiburg and Leipzig. His work during this period led to his first publication based on the use of dyes: he discovered a type of white blood cell.* During his final term in Breslau Ehrlich was in the audience at a talk and demonstration on the life-cycle of the anthrax bacillus by an unknown country doctor, none other of course than Robert Koch. In 1878 Ehrlich presented his doctoral thesis, which had the title, 'Contributions to the theory and practice of histological staining'. It contained, among much else, the first description of the mast cell. For the next nine years Ehrlich earned his living as a doctor, eventually senior house doctor, at the famous Charité hospital in Berlin, continuing his research as time allowed, often by night. His situation improved when the Professor of Pathology, Theodor von Frerichs, discerning his exceptional talents, appointed him as his assistant, and allowed him time to pursue his own research.

Thanks to patience, relentless questioning of accepted wisdom, and a mastery of chemistry – a science to which he had been drawn since his schooldays - Ehrlich made great strides in the refinement of staining techniques. He applied these to the observation of bacteria in culture and especially in animal cells, but he also introduced a new and revolutionary concept, which he called 'vital staining'. He injected dyes into animals, generally mice, and dissected the animals to see what tissues might have

---

* This cell is characterised by internal granules, which are strongly stained with basic (as opposed to acidic) dyes, such as Ehrlich's Methylene Blue. He accordingly designated cell's of this type basophils (base-lovers). Ehrlich's basophil, now called a mast cell, plays an important part in the function of the immune system. Cells that are preferentially stained with acidic, rather than basic dyes, of which the dye, eosin was an archetype, are eosinophils.

taken up the colour. He quickly discovered that the highly water-soluble acidic dyes (which carried the negatively charged, water-seeking sulphonyl [-SO$_3$⁻] groups) scarcely revealed themselves in the tissues, whereas those containing basic (p.) groups stained both nerves and fatty tissue. Ehrlich conjectured that there might be a parallel with the alkaloids, which were basic, and were extracted from their alkaline solutions into such solvents as ether (as Pelletier and others (Chapter) had determined). The basic dyes in short were *lipophilic* – they sought fatty, rather than watery, media in which to mingle. This was a remarkable insight, far ahead of its time.

The strongest of these basic dyes was called Methylene Blue, synthesised by the great organic chemist, Adolf Baeyer some ten years previously. Ehrlich wondered whether, if this dye had such high affinity for nerve cells, it might not interfere with their action. Might it perhaps act as an analgesic? Ehrlich found a compliant clinician, who tried it on a few of his patients with painful conditions (an experiment which today would land the doctor in prison). It seemed indeed to lessen the pain, but this, the first synthetic 'magic bullet', did not enter clinical use, for it was found to cause kidney damage if given in the doses needed for effective pain relief. The dyestuff industry was generating new dyes of several chemical classes at a great rate. Ehrlich was drawn especially to the aniline dyes (first brought to his notice by his cousin, and he set out to test these and related compounds for activity against 'parasites', by which he meant bacteria, protozoa (such as the malaria parasite), or any other pathogenic micro-organisms. He enunciated a general rule to guide the strategy, which he expressed in Latin: *corpora non agunt nisi fixata*, that is to say, a substance acts only if it is. This prefigured the concept of receptors, elements in cells to which a poison or drug would specifically attach itself. (Nearly a century later (Chapter) this principle was extended to substances produced in the metabolism, such as hormones, which act on cells through their target receptors; thus many drugs act by attaching themselves tightly to such a receptors so as to deny access to the hormone or other metabolite.) A corollary followed from Ehrlich'srule : a therapeutic substance must have high affinity for a pathogen – it must, in his parlance, be 'parasitotropic' - but must not be 'organotropic', that is, must have minimal affinity for the cells of the infected organism. For such an agent Ehrlich coined the term, 'magic bullet' (*Zauberkugel*). The dyes which stained bacteria in the cell but not the natural cell contents possessed such selectivity, and might, by attaching themselves, smother and kill the bacterium. Ehrlich never found one that would be clinically applicable, but here nonetheless was the true conceptual origin of chemotherapy.

Ehrlich was still doing duty at the Charité when Koch, aware of the younger man's exceptional abilities, offered him a small room in his domain at the Health Institute in which he could pursue his research. 'Here', he told Ehrlich, 'you can do anything'. It was the beginning of a collaboration and a lasting friendship, for Ehrlich admired Koch enormously, and the intellectually charged environment that Koch had created was irresistible. Koch benefited equally from Ehrlich's presence. As a start, the new staining techniques effected a striking improvement in the images of Koch's tuberculosis bacilli in tissues. Ehrlich's restless questioning, agility of mind, and his outgoing personality also infected all within range. His friend and colleague, August Wassermann likened Ehrlich's temperament to champagne, but the torrent of words that flowed from him when his interest was aroused or a new idea sprouted in his mind could leave his colleagues bewildered. One of the assistants whom he acquired late in his career, the Englishman, Henry Dale (who was to achieve high distinction as a physiologist and Nobel Laureate) left this reminiscence: 'Everyone who visited Ehrlich at that time received a brief and cordial welcome before being immediately plunged into a turbulent stream of excited description of Ehrlich's latest scientific findings and theories, illustrated by diagrams in dye on any available surface, so that the visitor, even if his own interests and work lay in a related field of scientific research, soon felt he was losing the ground from under his feet, and there was nothing for it but to submit resignedly to the flood of words.'

It was Koch's famous lecture, which laid bare the nature of the tuberculosis agent, that had proved such an epiphany for Ehrlich, and led him eventually in new directions. In 1883 Ehrlich married, and soon there were two daughters. But in 1888 his life underwent an upheaval when it was discovered that he had contracted pulmonary tuberculosis, almost certainly in the laboratory. In the hope of a cure by a hot, dry atmosphere he resigned his appointment at the Charité and departed for Egypt, where he remained for two years. There was indeed a remission, and Ehrlich, who now had a position as one of Koch's assistants, entered into a turbulent association with another recently recruited assistant, Emil Behring. Inspired by Koch's work on vaccines, and temporarily discouraged by the lack of progress in his efforts at chemotherapy, Ehrlich was ready to turn his attentions to immunology, and when Koch suggested a joint undertaking with Behring - an assault on another much-feared disease, diphtheria – Ehrlich readily agreed. They began work in 1890, continuing in Koch's new Institute for Infectious Diseases.

Friends and foes: the Ehrlich-Behring axis

Emil Adolf Behring was one of thirteen children of an impecunious village schoolmaster in a remote village in West Prussia. Destined for a clerical career because the Church would pay the costs of his education, the young Behring found a better way: the Prussian army bred its doctors by recruiting bright young men to its military medical academy in Berlin. The stipulated commitment was a year's service for each term of medical education. Behring qualified and served in a series of garrisons, where his duties left him time for some research on the side. He developed a particular interest in wound infections, and his first scientific paper was a study of the efficacy of iodoform, widely used at the time as an antiseptic. His idea was that the suppuration of wounds was analogous to the rotting of meat. This could be prevented by such treatments as smoking which, Behring thought, must inactivate the agents of putrefaction. It was an enlightened idea, even if there was no outcome. His superiors must have gleaned that Behring was meant for something better than the routine of garrison clinics, for he was promoted and posted to a pharmacology institute in Bonn, where he was enabled to study chemistry, and also did some investigations on the blood of rats killed by anthrax, which, he recorded, contained an agent active against anthrax bacilli. After only a year in Bonn, Behring had his greatest stroke of luck: he was posted to Koch's Hygiene Institute in Berlin, where research on vaccines was in full swing. He arrived with a scientific question ready-made: what was it in the blood serum of the infected rats that protected other rats against the bacillus, and how might it be used to combat anthrax? It was on this problem that he began work, though without any immediate reward.

Behring was uncommunicative, and by no means popular with his colleagues, but he had high respect for Koch and for Ehrlich, and it was the genial and companionable Ehrlich with whom he struck up an improbable friendship. Behring also found common interests with an able Japanese visitor, Shibasakuro Kitasato (1852-1931), who had been working with the tetanus bacillus. Tetanus was the greatest threat to wounded soldiers on the battlefield, and would have been of acute interest to Behring, the army doctor. Koch's long-serving assistant, Friedrich Loeffler had made a major discovery: he had found that it was not the recently isolated diphtheria bacillus itself that caused the disease, but a soluble substance, a toxin, which it generated. The previous year Émile Roux and Alexandre Yersin in Pasteur's institute in Paris had made the same observation on bubonic plague, and had indeed isolated the secreted toxin, which they reported to be an enzyme. Now Kitasato found that the same mechanism also operated in tetanus, and he isolated the toxin from the blood of infected rabbits. Next, he together with Behring performed a celebrated experiment, which engendered what might now be called a paradigm shift (a much-abused term). They immunised a rabbit by injecting it with small, sublethal amounts of the tetanus toxin, thus rendering the animal immune to infection by tetanus. What, they wanted to know, was the basis of the immunity? What they found was that the filtered serum from the animal's blood contained something that neutralised the toxin. When therefore some of this serum was injected into mice or rabbits the animals were unaffected by an injection of toxin, in an amount that would have killed an untreated animal many times over. The activity survived for months outside the animal. The immunity could even be passed from animal to animal. Behring and Kitasato called the mysterious substance an 'antitoxin' (*Gegengift*), and noted in the classic paper in which they reported their work, that not only did the antitoxin confer immunity, but it could also be employed therapeutically. Thus an animal already infected and sickening with tetanus could be cured by an injection of an antitoxin preparation. Here was the start of serology. How the credit was to be divided is difficult now to judge, but it does appear that Behring exerted himself to minimise Kitasato's contribution, and switched the order of names on the famous paper against the wishes of Koch, the director of the laboratory. This was probably the reason why Kitasato did not share the Nobel Prize that eventually accrued to Behring. Indeed, Roux too had isolated the toxin in Paris at the same time, and developed an effective serum, so the Nobel Prize should by rights have been shared three ways.

Behring now set his sights on an even higher target. Diphtheria was the greatest scourge of children in the 19th century. It was sometimes called 'the strangling angel' because of the distressing constriction of the airways that all too frequently ended in death. At first all went well, but unfortunately for Behring, Kitasato returned to Japan in 1891, and he now had only one loyal collaborator, the only man who could tolerate his erratic moods, Erich Wernicke to help him. (Both Kitasato and Wernicke later complained, though only after Behring's death, that their contributions to the discoveries associated with Behring's name had never been properly acknowledged.) The urgent problem was to produce the antitoxin, or antibody, as we would now call it, in sufficient amount for clinical use. For this purpose large animals were needed, and in some numbers, and these would have to be housed and fed. A sheep and a few lambs were available, and Behring found accommodation for them in stalls erected in the arches under the elevated railway line nearby. But the small grant, which was all that the ministry was willing to offer, and what funds Behring and Wernicke could find from their own limited resources were clearly insufficient to run what amounted to an industrial-scale operation. A benefactor was at hand however. Friedrich Althoff reigned over the Prussian Ministry of Spiritual Education and Medicine. An erudite, adroit and enlightened mandarin, he had been responsible for the reform and expansion of first the Prussian, and after unification, the German university system. He saw it as his mission to support the best scholars and researchers, and he knew how to hew through the thickets of the university bureaucracy and get his way. He was a man of liberal disposition with no time for antisemitism or the rampant anti-Catholicism that also permeated Prussian institutions. Late in his life Ehrlich expressed his gratitude to Althoff in a moving letter. He owed Althoff his career, he wrote, which but for Althoff's constant exertions to rescue him from antisemitic prejudice, would have lain fallow.

It was Althoff who had been behind the foundation of Koch's institute, and he now came to Behring's rescue also. The state had neither the means nor the desire to involve itself in a commercial manufacturing enterprise, but August Laubenheimer, chief chemist and chairman at the Hoechst Dye Works (founded in 1863 as the Teerfarbwerke [Tar dye works] Lucius, Meister und Brüning at Höchst-am-Main near Frankfurt) approached Behring with a view to a collaboration. This would require the consent of both the ministries of education and of war (since Behring was still on the payroll of the Prussian army). Althoff saw to the one and the Surgeon-General of the army agreed to the other, but with the proviso that Behring was to make no pecuniary profit from the arrangement. Althoff mediated, and a five-year agreement was signed with the option that it could be abrogated after one year if Hoechst so chose. Hoechst drove a hard bargain: the company was to receive 50% of the profits when sales finally ensued. Meanwhile the company would provide generous funds for research, material for immunisation would be prepared in Koch's institute, and Hoechst would produce the serum. Laubenheimer, a former professor of chemistry had been mostly concerned with dyes, but had dipped a toe into biologicals with the manufacture of the successful analgesic, antipyrine. Interested as he now was in pathogenic bacteria, he balked at the idea of research requiring animals. His reservations were apparently overcome by the company chairman, and stalls for large animals were constructed.

If all went well commercial serum production would start within the year. But all did not go well. Serum samples from sheep and a dog prepared in Koch's institute were tried on eleven children suffering from diphtheria in the Charité Hospital and appeared to have worked well enough, for nine of them recovered. Yet these numbers were still too low to represent proof of efficacy. Tests at Hoechst had revealed alarming variability of the inoculum samples received from Berlin, most of which were too weak. Behring sank into a sulky state of despondency. Koch, who said Behring must be treated like a child, urged him to seek help from Ehrlich, and it was Ehrlich's good cheer that eventually lightened the atmosphere. Ehrlich had been dividing his time between the Institute and a small laboratory of his own that he had set up, and he had become interested in antitoxins and their possible uses. Within a short time he had achieved remarkable results.

Working with goats, he had made a discovery of the first importance - that antibodies in the blood of the mother could pass to her offspring in the milk. This changed the thinking in the nascent field for two reasons: it brought into the open what became known as 'passive immunity', meaning that immunity against something (a pathogen or vaccine for instance) could pre-exist in the blood of an animal that had never been exposed to that agent; and secondly it meant that immunity could be transmitted from one animal (or human) to another.

Ehrlich went further: he formulated his 'side-chain' theory of the toxin-antitoxin reaction. He was in no doubt that this was chemical in nature, and he conjectured that it resembled two pieces of a jigsaw fitting together. An antitoxin (the antibody) that had been produced by the animal (or person) in response to an intruder such as a bacterium, would afterwards recognise and neutralise another such bacterium. It would do this by engaging with projections ('side-chains*') on the surface of this new but identical bacterium. A bacterial toxin on first entering the body acts in the same way as the parent bacterium, by engaging with side-chains on the surface of a cell (which we would now call receptors), and thereby disrupting the normal biological processes in that cell. The animal reacts by producing more new receptors in an attempt to recover its previous function, and these structures also lie in wait for a later invasion (assuming the organism recovers from the initial assault). This scheme prefigures to a remarkable degree the 20th-century research, which led to an understanding of what is now called humoral immunology. The antitoxin, which could be produced in an animal, was the first functional example, as Ehrlich saw it, of the 'magic bullet' – the missile that would destroy its target (the 'non-self') without injuring the host organism (the 'self').

This was still not all. Ehrlich immunised mice against the deadly plant poisons, abrin and ricin (notorious in our time as a means of assassination favoured by the operatives of certain totalitarian regimes). He developed a method of immunisation with gradually increasing amounts of the toxin to

---

* Ehrlich's side-chains are not to be confused with side-chains in their modern meaning. There are the parts of the 20 kinds of amino acids of which proteins are made up that differ one from another.

generate sera of high potency. He placed the general method of evaluating the potency (antibody titre in today's terminology) of the resulting serum on a quantitative basis, most importantly by measuring the lethal dose of toxin that the immunised mice could tolerate. Ehrlich, then, was no novice in immunology, and as Koch had perceived, no-one was better equipped to help Behring out of his difficulties. Ehrlich went to work to improve Behring's preparations and establish assays for measuring and controlling their strengths. It was in the event he rather than Behring who was responsible for making the vision of a clinically effective and reliable product a reality after barely a year of intensive work.

This set Hoechst on the path to a mighty commercial coup. In 1894, after only a few months of development, the company sold some 75,000 vials of anti-diphtheria serum, and before long diphtheria mortality had fallen by half. It was soon decided that a product of such importance must be regulated by the state, and Koch was charged with overseeing the arrangements. Behring had fallen out with Ehrlich, who felt he was being treated as a subordinate and denied credit for his indispensable contribution. A dismayed Althoff tried with partial success to heal the breach. The two men sealed an agreement to divide the profits from the sale of the Hoechst serum equally, and Behring at least became rich. But Ehrlich was later persuaded by Hoechst to forego his share when the contract was renewed. Behring finally fulfilled another longstanding ambition: he had wanted a professorial chair and his own research institute. He had importuned Althoff endlessly with threats to resign from Prussian employ and defect to Russia if he did not get his wish. The issue was the more pressing for him because he had by then taxed Koch's patience too far, and relations were at a nadir; Koch wanted him out. This was at least in part because Behring had refused to submit to Koch's rule that researchers must not lay claim to commercial profits arising from discoveries made in his institute. Once again Althoff indulged his turbulent protégé. He could not create new university positions, but in 1894 a professorial chair became vacant at the University of Halle, and Behring was appointed. Then after only a year a better prospect came in view at the University of Marburg, close to Frankfurt and the Hoechst works. The election of a new professor had to be approved by the ministry, but the wishes of the Faculty were seldom overridden. The Marburg faculty had chosen its own candidate, but Althoff succeeded with threats and blandishments to get his man appointed. And so Behring left Halle for Marburg where he remained for the rest of his life, living in some splendour in the Villa Behring with his new young wife and burgeoning family, fêted by the local intelligentsia and entertaining regally. When Behring's wife contracted diphtheria vials of the best serum were sent from Hoechst, and her life was saved.

Among his university colleagues Behring had few friends. As a teacher he was not a success; his lectures were largely about his own work, and ill-informed about other areas, and caused resentment among the students. Nevertheless Behring was now famous, adulated as 'saviour of the children' and rich. He was showered with honours, which included elevation to the nobility – he was now Emil von Behring, and his honorary appointment as a state counsellor meant that he was henceforth to be addressed as Excellency. (Ehrlich did the decent thing and sent a message of congratulations.) Orders of chivalry were conferred on him at home and abroad, and even the French made him a Chevalier of the Légion d'Honneur. His desire, though, to attend Pasteur's seventieth birthday celebrations were thwarted because he fell ill and also because Pasteur, whom he had always revered, was still an implacable Germanophobe, and did not want to receive him. Pasteur's portrait nevertheless remained on the wall of Behring's study until his death, next to those of Bismarck and of Frederick the Great. In 1901 Behring was awarded the first Nobel Prize for Medicine. (Wilhelm Conrad Röntgen was the first Nobel Laureate in Physics for the discovery of X-rays.) The award to Behring was arguably deserved, but it must have seemed to others absurd that he should have been recognised before Koch especially. It is striking that of the many nominations by scientists from around the world, not one came from Germany.

Ehrlich by this time had achieved some independence as head of a vestigial serum testing institute in a Berlin suburb, and was later to enter into a far better arrangement in Frankfurt. Behring asked to have the evaluation of his sera done in Ehrlich's institute, but Ehrlich had had enough, and wanted nothing further to do with his one-time friend. Behring occupied himself with the problems of side-effects of serum treatment that had revealed themselves, and with improving tetanus treatment. (The prophylactic use of the tetanus serum was to save many lives among the soldiers in the trenches of the Western Front in the Great War.) Behring and his assistants also developed a new procedure of immunisation against diphtheria, and finally also a vaccine for protecting calves against bovine tuberculosis. Yet there were no notable breakthroughs. Ehrlich, still simmering with resentment in November of 1899, vented his feelings in a letter to a friend, quoted in her romanticised memoir of Ehrlich by his secretary, Martha Marquardt. Behring, he wrote, 'was only reaping what he had sown .... That he imagined I would, for a ridiculous wage, work for [his institute] I can well believe, so that new discoveries and millions would accrue to him. He has only me to thank for the diphtheria success'. He goes on to detail the poor potencies Behring was achieving in his serum preparations, compared to Ehrlich's; and when, with the utmost difficulty he finally got Ehrlich's methods to work, 'he tried to discredit me, saying that I knew nothing about immunology, that he had advanced much further than me, etc. ..... I always get quite angry when I think about this dark time, and on the dexterity with which B. at that time masked my scientific participation'. 'Retribution has not been lacking', Ehrlich continues with evident satisfaction, for 'he could see how far he got *without me* after our parting. All is aborted, his work on plague, cholera, glanders, streptococcal infection, no advances in the diphtheria area, only hypotheses and pseudo-precise number games - and all this with an abundance of means and a horde of workers ...... Naturally, you can see with what rage he is filled. He wanted to be the sole ruler, who after the crushing of Koch prescribed the rules for the whole world, and at the same time earned great sums - a superman, but fortunately without a super brain'. Such a discharge of spleen was highly uncharacteristic of the good-natured Ehrlich, but the provocation was clearly great. He concluded his letter, 'Down with the mammonisation of science'. (A century on, we can see, of course, that it was Behring's philosophy which eventually prevailed.)

There was, however, a development of no small importance in Behring's career. It followed a terminal quarrel with Hoechst, which even Althoff could do nothing to mitigate. Behring severed his association with Hoechst, and used his Nobel Prize money to set up his own company dedicated to the production of serums at Marbach near Marburg. Behringwerke, founded in 1904 eventually grew into a mighty concern, which survived the Second World War, but in 1952 was absorbed by its old rival, Hoechst. The plant remained a major supplier of vaccines until, many years later, it was broken up and most of the parts were sold off. All that now remains is a modest biotechnology company. As for Behring, depression had increasingly taken its toll, his health had failed, and he died in 1917 at the age of 63.

Ehrlich combats sleeping sickness

While running his small serum evaluation operation Ehrlich was still tied to Koch's institute. Depressed by his relations with Behring and the animosity that also festered between Behring and Koch, he had grown eager to escape. There was no longer anything, he wrote to his cousin Carl Weigert, to keep him in Berlin. Antisemitism had held him back in Prussia, as it had Weigert, and he set his sights on Frankfurt, where Weigert had found a position in a hospital. Frankfurt had been an autonomous free city before German unification, and a long liberal tradition still prevailed. It had, however, no university, a source of chagrin to the city fathers and the intelligentsia. The Prussian regime evidently took the view that the single institution of higher learning – the Philipps University of Marburg – should suffice for the state of Hesse. The citizens of Frankfurt had other ideas, one of which was to force the Imperial hand by founding a succession of high-calibre institutes. Frankfurt was also less corrupted by the antisemitism which had so impeded Ehrlich's career, and it was Ehrlich who, in 1899, was invited to head the new Royal Institute for Experimental Therapy, incorporating also the Berlin serum institute. The arrangement owed much yet again to the benign manipulator in the shadows, Friedrich Althoff. It was he also who ensured that the Johann Wolfgang Goethe University sprang up in the city soon afterwards.

Settled with his family in Frankfurt, Ehrlich soon became a part of city's intellectual society, and in an article in the district newspaper he elaborated his current thinking about the therapy of diseases. The local prominence that he attained resulted in due time to a great stroke of good fortune. The widow of the leading Jewish banker in Hamburg, Georg Speyer, was living in Frankfurt, and was looking out for a scientific institution to establish to commemorate her husband's name. She consulted her brother-in-law, a chemist and industrialist, who suggested Ehrlich as the man who could best bring the plan to fruition. The sum on offer was generous, and the Georg-Speyer-Haus came into being in 1906, next door to the Institute of Experimental Therapy, with Ehrlich in the saddle. Althoff tried yet again to heal the rift between Ehrlich and Behring, and urged renewed collaboration. Ehrlich would have none of it, and explained why he could never again work with Behring in a very long letter to his old patron.

In any case, by the time of his arrival in Frankfurt Ehrlich had decided that serum therapy held no further answers to the challenges presented by the great majority of serious diseases, such as cancer and syphilis. It was time to return to chemotherapy and the quest for the 'magic bullet', cast in the laboratory, and not in an animal. Organic chemistry held the key, he decided. Ehrlich began work on cancer, and while he found no magic bullet he lit the path that his successors would take. With a clinical colleague, Hugo Apolant, he developed the method of transplanting human tumours into experimental animals; he showed that cancer cells grew much faster than the cells of healthy tissue; and, most importantly, he and Apolant discovered how normal cells in connective tissue (the matrix surrounding nerves, blood vessels and the like) could be transformed into malignant (sarcoma) cells. In his search for substances that would target a malignant cell, or again an invader, such as a bacterial pathogen, Ehrlich returned to his first love, dyes. He proceeded to test as many dyes as he could find, as well as other compounds, for activity against trypanosomes. These are protozoa (micro-organisms, much larger than bacteria, some even than cells) responsible for a number of tropical diseases, notably sleeping sickness, carried by the tsetse fly. Ehrlich had previously had mildly promising results with another protozoan, the malaria parasite, with his familiar dye, Methylene Blue. His choice of trypanosomes was dictated by the discovery by French researchers that mice could be infected with two species of the organism, and that the infection could be transferred from one animal to another through the blood. When, moreover, the sick mice were injected with an arsenic compound, arsenious acid, the trypanosomes disappeared from the blood, though only to return and kill the animals two days later.

Ehrlich was fortunate in acquiring the services of an able Japanese assistant, recommended to him by his friend from Berlin days, Kitasato. Kiyoshi Shiga had isolated the bacterium responsible for dysentery while in Kitasato's laboratory in Tokyo. (It was named *Shigella dysenteriae* in his honour). The French group generously supplied Ehrlich with trypanosome cultures. The first candidate compound that Ehrlich and Shiga tried was another arsenical in the hope that it might prove more effective than arsenious acid. Atoxyl was a commercial product, supplied by a chemical company in Berlin, and was to prove a starting point for the programme that led to Ehrlich's most famous achievement. It had little effect on the trypanosomes and was put aside. Ehrlich and Shiga then went on to test more than one-hundred compounds, mainly dyes, on mice infected with trypanosomes. The best, which Ehrlich named Nagana Red, did little more than arsenious acid, but he thought its limitations might have been a consequence of its low solubility. He therefore asked a chemist at another dye works to synthesise a more tractable derivative (bearing an additional water-seeking sulphonyl group). This product, named Trypan Red, worked: the infected mice were cured, but the efficacy of the dye was confined to only one of the species of trypanosome. This was not good enough, and Ehrlich struck out in another direction. All the same, since sleeping sickness was a serious problem in parts of Africa, the published report on Trypan Red by Ehrlich and Shiga generated interest, and it was tried out on people suffering from the disease. The results were discouraging, for distressing side-effects quickly made themselves felt: Trypan Red affected the optic nerve, and was apt to cause blindness, possibly even death, and its use was quickly abandoned.* A modified form of Trypan Red was also tried out by Koch on gravely ill patients during one of his expeditions to Africa, but again with unsatisfactory results. The effort had not been waster, however, for Trypan Red came into its own as a specific for the treatment of the parasitic animal disease, babesiosis.

Ehrlich furibundus: syphilis cure and the syphilis war

The development to which Ehrlich's name was to be for ever linked was now on the horizon. He had been surprised to hear of the observation reported by a parastologist at the Liverpool School of Hygiene and Tropical Medicine that the commercial arsenical preparation, Atoxyl cured mice of trypanosomiasis. This was the opposite of what he and Shiga had concluded in their grand survey of compounds, but then, they had tested the compound on trypanosomes in culture and not in mice. They therefore repeated what the Liverpool workers had done and reproduced their result. This suggested to Ehrlich that the Atoxyl had undergone a

---

* This was not the end of the quest for a trypanocidal drug. A research group at the Pasteur Institute in Paris, led by Maurice Nicolle (1862–1932), one of three brilliant brothers – Charles, director of the Pasteur Institute of Tunisia received the Nobel Prize for his work on typhus, and Marcel was a distinguished art critic – had procured a huge number of drugs from the Bayer company in Germany and tested their activity against trypanomiases. They eventually found one with high potency, and called it Trypan Blue. Side-effects precluded its use in humans, but it found wide application in farm animals. Meanwhile an assistant of Ehrlich's had joined Bayer, and stimulated the company's chemists to prepare more dyes and their derivatives, and test them for trypanocidal activity. Their efforts finally bore fruit only in 1917, two years after Ehrlich's death, with the synthesis of Bayer 205. Not wanting companies in other countries to manufacture the hard-won compound, Bayer did not disclose its structure, but they had filed patents on earlier and less effective products. From these Ernest Fourneau, the chief chemist at the Pasteur Institute, divined a number of possible formulae for Bayer 205, synthesised several of them and found one, Fourneau 309, that was equally active and was in fact the very same molecule. Because Bayer had kept the formula of Bayer 205 to themselves, they were unable to file a patent, and so could not prevent Germanin, as they called it, from being produced and brought to market by other companies. Germanin, also called Suramin, is still a standard remedy for trypanosomal diseases.

metabolic transformation in the mouse, which converted the essentially inert compound into a trypanosome killer.* The structural modification would probably, Ehrlich thought, have been a simple one – a type of commonplace reaction known to chemists as a hydrolysis or a reduction). The obvious course therefore would be to prepare a series of modified Atoxyls to test for anti-trypanosome activity in cultures. But when Ehrlich contemplated the formula of the compound it seemed to him that it must be altogether inert and not susceptible to simple modifications, for it bore no reactive groups that could easily be chemically altered. But then Ehrlich found that Atoxyl would react with a reagent that would normally target an amino group (-NH$_2$), not evident in the formula. Surely then the formula assigned to the compound by the man who had synthesised it, the French chemist, Antoine Béchamp was incorrect. The chemical company in Berlin, which supplied the Atoxyl would not hear of it, but Ehrlich asked a colleague, an organic chemist, to help, and toget, her they arrived at the correct formula. (The compound was phenylarsenamide)

Next came another development: a German veterinarian had been trying Atoxyl with some success on chickens infected by a parasitic disease, then called spirillosis. There had also been reports of a weak effect against syphilis, but the benefit to patients was offset by the drug's toxicity, and it was never widely used. Then in 1905 Ehrlich heard from his friend from student days, Albert Neisser in Breslau - the man who had discovered the causative agent of gonorrhoea, the gonococcus – that Atoxyl combatted that disease a great deal more effectively than syphilis. This got Ehrlich interested, for he had been thinking about the horrors of syphilis, and how it might be tackled. The research group at the Pasteur Institute had found that monkeys could be infected with syphilis, and Neisser thtereupon began to try possible therapies on infected monkeys in Java. At Ehrlich's suggestion he tested two arsenic compounds, which, toxicity aside, indeed proved effective. Ehrlich was now fired up, the more so because the syphilis parasite had been seen under the microscope two years earlier by a young German doctor, Fritz Schaudinn, working with

---

* This was another remarkable insight on Ehrlich's part: substances that are metabolically converted into a pharmacologically active agent are now known to be numerous, and are referred to as 'prodrugs' (Chapter ...).

a professor of dermatology, Erich Hoffmann. Earlier workers had missed it because, like the trypanosome, it was thin and thread-like, and almost transparent. In appearance it was in fact rather similar to the trypanosome, to which Schaudinn and Hoffmann supposed (wrongly) that it must be related. Schaudinn's discovery was met with general scepticism, for there had previously been a succession of false sightings of the parasite, and it cost him great effort to convince the world. He gave it the name, *Spirochaeta pallida*, reflecting its pallor (but it was later renamed *Treponema pallidum*). What finally closed the circle was the discovery that chicken spirillosis was very similar to the syphilis spirochaete, and that both shared a physical resemblance to the trypanosome. Ehrlich had received a visit from Hoffmann, and was clearly convinced by the specious similarity between the syphilis and trypanosomiasis agents, a misapprehension that did no harm at all. With the target, as he thought, clear in view, Ehrlich could begin the serious hunt for a magic bullet. Atoxyl was to be the starting point – the 'lead compound'.

For all the progress in diagnosis and identification of the causative agent, there was still no sign of any in the treatment of syphilis. Mercury, with all its dire side-effects, so often worse even than the disease (p.), was still the only effective treatment. Ilya Metchnikoff (1845 – 1916) at the Pasteur Institute in Paris, with whom Ehrlich was to share the Nobel Prize, did show that a calomel salve, applied before exposure to the spirochaetes would prevent infection, and in the German military it was dispensed as a prophylactic. But of course once the parasites had entered through the skin it was too late. Arsenic compounds seemed the most promising recourse, if only one could be found with an acceptable level of toxicity. Ehrlich wanted a drug which would be highly effective in killing the spirochaetes, so that one definitive dose would cure the patient, who would not then need to be exposed to a long course of poison. More especially, there would be less time for resistant strains of the parasite to emerge. (This had been observed in cultured trypanosomes, and is familiar today in infectious diseases and even cancer [p.], for all of which Ehrlich's principle holds.) Ehrlich's plan of attack was to synthesise and test as many arsenic compounds, starting with derivatives of Atoxyl, as would be needed before the right one was found, all to be tested against both trypanosomes and the spirochaetes of syphilis.

This would be a meticulously planned, exhausting, immensely laborious campaign, demanding willing and capable collaborators. Here Ehrlich was fortunate: he had an excellent organic chemist, Alfred Bertheim, the man who had found the correct structure for Atoxyl, and in 1909, two years into the project, Sahachiro Hata joined the laboratory. He was another alumnus of Kitasato's institute in Tokyo, and he had learned to infect rabbits with the syphilis spirochaete by procedures just developed by a pair of Italian workers. This means of assaying the flood of new compounds that Bertheim was producing greatly expedited the process of selection. By then compounds 306 and 418 had already been found to show some promise when tested by Albert Neisser in Breslau, and compound 306 had also done well in killing trypanosomes. All of them were now also examined by Hata. The number of compounds rose into the six-hundreds, but Ehrlich apparently was not dismayed, and with compound 606 his persistence was at last rewarded. Hata recorded an unprecedented level of potency, and low toxicity.

Ehrlich was cautious, and did not immediately announce the development, but he did enter into an agreement with Hoechst to manufacture and market compound 606, should clinical trials prove successful. Two doctors in remote hospitals were invited to test samples on a small number of syphilitic patients. Encouraged by the outcome, Ehrlich now initiated what was probably the most extensive clinical trial that had ever been undertaken. He sent 65,000 vials of the compound to several carefully chosen treatment centres. The compound was dissolved in dilute alkali, but other media, such as alcohol-water mixtures were also tried. The solution was administered by injection into the muscles of the back, a somewhat painful process, which caused quite severe local inflammation. The doctors reported miraculous results: even many patients with advanced disease were reported cured. Considering that today something of the order of 10,000 compounds (often produced, to be sure, by combinatorial chemistry [p.]), and at least a decade of clinical trials are typically needed to bring a new drug to market, Ehrlich's achievement seems truly remarkable. Hoechst gave compound 606 the name, *Salvarsan* (from *salvare*, to save, and arsenic). Ehrlich gave his account of the discovery and performance of compound 606 at the Congress of Scientists and Doctors, held that year

(1910) in Königsberg. Several doctors, including Neisser, also spoke with enthusiasm about the impending revolution in treatment of syphilis. Word at once spread and the press and the regime exulted: the great scourge was about to be consigned to history. Hoechst sent Salvarsan samples to all the doctors in the country as a loss leader, and at first there were only plaudits and gratitude.

But it was not long before there were less welcome reports. A single injection was commonly insufficient to stop the progress of the disease, so a course of several treatments was recommended. There were also mild side-effects, but these were seldom troublesome. Those with neurosyphilis, whose central nervous system had been penetrated by the spirochaetes - about one in twenty – did not improve. This was because Salvarsan could not cross the barrier shielding the nerves. Ehrlich was well aware of this and had warned against it. Yet when such patients deteriorated or died it was sometimes attributed to poisoning - for it was after all an arsenical - by Salvarsan. There were also instances of infections caused by the use of impure, instead of distilled water in preparing the injections. Soon a vociferous anti-Salvarsan party arose. In the overwhelming proportion of cases Salvarsan worked with remarkable reliability. Ehrlich countered hostile criticisms by pointing out that there had never yet been a totally harmless remedy against a serious disease, and he asked his critics to consider the failure rate in surgery. Was this an argument for letting patients die? Many doctors also complained, with some justice, about the price Hoechst was charging for the drug, which was later reduced. Moreover, research did not end with Salvarsan, and Ehrlich and the Hoechst chemists effected an important improvement, which went far to eliminate unpleasant side-effects. They were able to design a Salvarsan derivative with far better solubility properties, which could therefore be injected in a much smaller volume. This, compound 914, called Neosalvarsan, came on the market only a year later.

All along doctors had been besieged by desperate syphilitics demanding the miracle drug. Quacks peddled fraudulent preparations. Rumours of deaths circulated. The worst miscreant was a dermatologist in Berlin, who was also doctor to the Moral Squad of the police. This man, Richard

Dreuw denounced Salvarsan at a meeting of the Dermatology Society of Berlin, asserting that it had been released prematurely without proper testing, that it was toxic and deleterious to the unfortunate patients. The Chairman intervened, and the report of Dreuw's lecture was rejected by the Society's journal. Dreuw thereupon put it about that the truth was being suppressed by the 'Salvarsan Syndicate'. The director of a Berlin hospital, who was also a cousin of Ehrlich's approached the city magistrates with a complaint against Dreuw's calumnies, and they instructed the police to terminate the malefactor's contract. Yet Dreuw's obsession did not abate. He persuaded some members of the Prussian parliament, the Reichstag, to take his side, and one notoriously antisemitic newspaper in Switzerland, *Der Samstag* (Saturday) printed a venomous article, attacking Ehrlich. A Frankfurt paper, by contrast, likened the Jewish Ehrlich to Christ. This drew a riposte from the *Samstag* accusing him of profiteering through Hoechst, and several German papers joined in with antisemitic diatribes, one even declaring that 275 people had died from Salvarsan treatment, and an incalculable number had gone blind or suffered terrible neurological damage. Ehrlich responded in a newspaper article that more than a million people had already been treated with Salvarsan, and so 275 deaths was a remarkably small number, considering also that simple incompetence would have been responsible for some of them. And what would have been the cost in lives had the patients not been treated?

The vocal minority made little impact on the homage heaped on Ehrlich as saviour of the syphilitics. He was received by the Kaiser, made a privy counsellor of the highest grade, which entitled him, like Behring, to the title of Excellency, and many honours came his way from his own country and abroad. The one which must have meant most to him made good an injustice of seven years earlier, for in 1908, not before time, he was awarded the Nobel Prize, shared with Ilya Metchnikoff of the Pasteur Institute. The citation made particular mention of Ehrlich's work on the evaluation of serum potency, an achievement for which he should have at least shared the Nobel Prize with Behring.* Yet the sniping did not end, and one particularly annoying episode close to home upset Ehrlich greatly. A Frankfurt scandal sheet with the grandiose title of *Der Freigeist, moderne Zeitung für alle kulturellen Interessen* (The Free Spirit, modern Periodical for all cultural Interests) printed an allegation that Karl Herxheimer, a distinguished professor and head of the dermatology clinic in the city hospital had forced prostitutes to submit to injections of the 'untested drug, Salvarsan'. Some, the article asserted, had gone blind, become paralysed, and suffered other dreadful consequences. Herxheimer, it went on, had been driven by greed to indulge in financial machinations, involving the sale of Salvarsan, and was no better than a murderer. Ehrlich, who was badly affected by the furore surrounding Salvarsan, wanted Herxheimer to ignore the noxious gadfly, who published his paper from a one-room flat. But Herxheimer – a Jew, who was to die in 1942, at the age of eighty, in the Theresienstadt (Terezin) ghetto in Czechoslovakia - wanted blood and insisted, to Ehrlich's dismay, on clearing his reputation and exacting retribution. Ehrlich was to be his star witness in the ensuing libel case. (The two men would probably have known each other, for during his formative years Herxheimer had been an assistant in the Frankfurt Pathology Institute to Ehrlich's cousin, Carl Weigert.) Before the affair came to court a mass meeting took place in the great hall of the Frankfurt Stock Exchange, addressed by, among others, the perpetrator of the article, the half-deranged Dreuw from Berlin, and the editor of the *Samstag* from Basel. Frenzied accusations flew: Ehrlich had not only poisoned the sick with Salvarsan, or alternatively, according to others, hadn't even invented it - that honour belonged to Hata, or should it be 00?

---

* That he had not received the prize earlier, and in particular had not shared it with Behring, was due to the adamant opposition of a member of the Nobel Committee of the Swedish Academy. This dissident was the Swedish physical chemist, Svante Arrhenius – himself a Nobel Laureate - who refused to accept that for every molecule of toxin that entered an organism thousands of anti-toxin molecules could be generated. The idea seemed to him to run counter to the principles of thermodynamics. The nature of such phenomena as enzymic catalysis had not at that time been unravelled, but Arrhenius's posture still appears blinkered to an extraordinary degree. He relented in later years. It was equally unjust that Koch was not awarded the prize until 1904, four years after Behring.

When the case came to court panic seized the defendant. He was barely coherent, and expostulated that a State conspiracy was behind everything. Dreuw too had thought the better of what he had evidently promised to say, and he now tamely conceded that he personally had had no experience of Salvarsan beyond once witnessing an injection. Herxheimer in evidence stated that he had been using Salvarsan for four years in the municipal hospital without encountering any cases of blindness or paralysis, except from quite other causes, nor had any patient died of it. The defending advocate requested a psychiatric examination of his client on grounds of a manic disposition. The court found the defendant responsible for his actions and guilty of libel, and sentenced him to a year in prison, when the prosecution had asked for only six months. Ehrlich had also given evidence, and his equilibrium had been severely tested by the ordeal. He wrote to the editor of the leading German medical periodical (the *Deutsche medizinische Wochenschrift*), fulminating against the rabble that the trial had exposed to view – nature curists, opponents of vaccination, quacks, anti-vivisectionists and antisemites, all united in showering him with filth. In another, later letter to the same organ Ehrlich compared his experience with that of Koch during the tuberculin debacle; but by comparison with the deluge of ordure he had been forced to endure, the resilient Koch had been sprinkled with rose-water, and was able to turn his back on his adversaries. Nor did the attacks on Ehrlich cease, although the press throughout the country mostly supported him. Dreuw's vituperation did not let up, and continued for years after Ehrlich's death. Ehrlich tried to set matters straight in an extended article in the respected paper, the *Frankfurter Zeitung*, in which he gave an account of the cost of Salvarsan, and explained that a generous slice of the profits was going towards the advancement of medical research.

Despite the many irritations, Ehrlich was famous, and inundated with world-wide acclaim; he was invested with orders of chivalry from Germany and abroad, he was a State Counsellor entitled to the honorific of Excellency, and he was elected to the membership of some eighty academies and other learned bodies, and he had also become rich. The Salvarsan wars had left their mark, but the quarrels were superseded by other concerns when, in August of 1914, the First World War broke out. The grim event had at least, Ehrlich remarked, brought him 'Salvarsan peace'. Yet, deeply depressed as he was, he nevertheless signed, along with Koch and Behring, the infamous Fulda Declaration, headed 'Appeal to the Culture-World'. It rejected as a foul calumny the perfectly valid Allied accusations against the German army, which had been perpetrating atrocities in Belgium. (Nearly all German intellectuals, called upon to sign did so; Einstein was the most famous and publicly noisy exception.) Ehrlich's health was precarious, and his addiction to strong cigars – he smoked 25 a day – must not have helped. At the beginning of 1915 he suffered a mild stroke, from which he recovered. He still visited his laboratories daily, and made plans for a fresh chemotherapeutic assault on cancer, but over the winter he grew weaker, and his wife took him to a sanatorium in Bad Homburg to regain some strength. He died there of a heart attack in August, 'cheerful, conversational and intellectually alert', his wife wrote to a friend, up to the end. It was presumed that, had he lived, he would have received a second Nobel Prize, this one in chemistry, and shared with Hata.

Ehrlich was laid to rest in the Jewish cemetery in Frankfurt. Behring came to pay his respects. According to Martha Marquardt, the 'old, sick man [he was 61] dragged himself with difficulty, leaning heavily on his stick, in the funeral procession to the last resting place of Paul Ehrlich. He had composed a fine obituary and later published it. But here in the face of death, by the open grave, he could only stammer a few words: "Now you too are at rest, you dear friend. Yours was ever a sensitive soul. And if we hurt you ... forgive!"'.

Chapter 10

MIRACLE DRUGS

Pain and the willow

Halfway into the 19th century physiologists and physicians began to take a new interest in body heat. Credit for the invention of the clinical thermometer is generally ascribed to the 16th-century scientists and doctor, Sanctorius Sanctorius of Padua, but it was another 250 years or so before the small, calibrated clinical thermometer was developed. In 1868 Carl Wunderlich (p.) published an influential book on the relation of body temperature to disease and the measurement of temperature as an aid to diagnosis and treatment. Whereas it had been generally supposed until then that a high temperature in fevers was nature's way of combating the condition, the paradigm now shifted in the opposite direction. A high temperature signified that the disease had the upper hand, and conversely, if the temperature could be brought down the disease would abate. So now many doctors would plunge patients into a cold bath to reduce a fever. There were certainly a few antipyretics (temperature-reducing substances), or febrifuges, such as quinine, which was effective against 'intermittent fever', that is to say malaria. Quinine was therefore classed as an 'antiperiodic', but it was also used, ineffectively, against fevers of all other kinds. Febrifuges were conflated with analgesics, or painkillers, since fevers were associated with such symptoms as headaches and joint aches.

Analgesics at the time were few. Opium was the indispensable stand-by, either by itself or in the form of laudanum (p.), and there was of course alcohol, while` many essentially inert plant products could be found in the old herbals. The most popular patent fever remedy from the mid-19th century until the early 20th was *Warburg's tincture*, also marketed as Dr Warburg's Fever Drops, Warburg's vegetable Fever Drops, Tinctura antifebrilis Warburgii and other variants. Carl Warburg was born in Mainz around 1805. Whether he was related to the illustrious Jewish Warburg clan, which produced so many scientists, bankers, publishers and other notables, is unclear. He studied medicine in Heidelberg, travelled in Latin America and is thought to have first concocted his nostrum while in British Guiana (now Guiana) in 1834, as an antipyretic for use against tropical fevers. It came to Europe in 1839, and in two later trials it was adjudged a success. The problem was that the composition of Warburg's tincture was a secret, the mark of a quack medicine, and it therefore attracted the opprobrium of many members of the medical profession. Nevertheless, it sold in huge quantity, and was endorsed by Queen Victoria and by the explorers, Sir Richard Burton and Dr David Livingstone (a doctor), among many other famous people, and Warburg became a celebrity in England and other countries. He set up a plant in Surrey to meet the rising demand for his product. Warburg was no charlatan, in the sense that he evidently had total faith in the efficacy of his medicine, and he claimed to have given away large amounts of the potion gratis to the needy. It was, he maintained, better than quinine, which merely relieved the fever, while his tincture cured. Despite the disapproval of much of the medical establishment Warburg's nostrum received many commendations from doctors who thought it better than quinine. They included the Physician in Ordinary to Queen Victoria and the personal physician to King William of the Netherlands.

Among Warburg's most fervent supporters was Surgeon-General W.C. Maclean, Professor of Military Medicine at the Army Medical School, and physician at the Royal Victoria Military Hospital at Netley on the English south coast. In an article in *The Lancet* in 1875, in which the composition was finally disclosed, he proclaimed it the best of the known remedies against malaria. He forgave Warburg for so long concealing the formula of his tincture for reasons of '*res augusta domi*', meaning straitened domestic circumstances, in other words that the man needed the income from the sales to feed his family. "Would any man in his senses, or who has any regard for the welfare of his patients", Maclean rhetorically demands, "refuse to administer James's Powder [highly toxic – see p.], Battley's Sedative Liquor, or Ruspini's Styptic, because their inventors refuse to make known the composition of these remedies?" The short answer to this might have been 'yes'. But the General is not yet done. On a current of purple prose he takes his readers on a stirring tour of the Empire: "Many will say, "After all, this vaunted remedy is only quinine concealed in a farrago of inert substances [as indeed it was] for purposes of 'mystification'". To this objection my answer is, I have treated remittent fevers in every degree of severity contracted in the jungles of the Decan and Mysore, at the base of mountain ranges in India, on the Coromandel Coast, in the pestilential highlands of the northern division of the Madras Presidency, in the malarial rivers of China, and in men brought to this hospital from the swamps of the Gold Coast, and I affirm that I have never seen quinine, when given alone, act in the manner characteristic of this tincture, and although I yield to no one in my high opinion of the inestimable value of quinine, I have never seen a single dose of it given alone .... arrest an exacerbation of remittent fever, much less prevent its recurrence, while nothing is more common than to see the same quantity of the alkaloid in Warburg's tincture bring about both results". Maclean does add, however, that "In the terrible remittent fevers described by Livingstone and his followers, the form of purgative prescribed by the great traveller, and known to his people as "Livingstone's Rousers", may be promised. By no authors is the necessity for careful nutrition and due stimulation so much insisted on as by the companions of the immortal explorer ...."

At the foot of the article the composition and mode of preparation of Warburg's tincture are set out. Quinine was the active ingredient, but there were no less than fourteen other constituents, all of them seeds, roots or extracts of plants; one, called Confectio Damocratis, 'which', says *The Lancet* in a footnote, 'consists of an immense variety of aromatic substances, was once officinal [in common medical use], and is to be found in the Ph. Lond; [the London Pharmacopoeia] 1746'. A few years later the remedy also appeared in the form of tablets. It was not sold merely as a febrifuge, but also as a treatment for scurvy, dysentery, consumption, scrofula, delirium tremens and more. The British Government, which had been supplying the tincture to soldiers in colonies around the world, awarded Warburg the rather niggardly sum of £200. He is said to have died poor in London in 1892, aged 87. His medicine at least did no harm.

This was still a time of untested remedies based on rumour and local lore. Typical is a comment published in 1902 in the *The Lancet* under the title, 'Old beliefs concerning tobacco'. 'The belief that tobacco-smoke is a disinfectant has long been popularly held', it begins, 'and *The Lancet* has been lately invited by the *Daily Chronicle* to "spare a moment from the pursuit of germs" to speak upon the point.' The tone of the article is cautiously sceptical. It relays reports from France and elsewhere of the killing of pathogenic bacteria in culture by high concentrations of tobacco smoke, and of the supposed immunity of tobacco workers to the plague, but it concludes: 'As yet, at any rate, there is nothing authoritative to be said'. But a decade later, in 1913, the editorial tone is very different. The title this time is 'The germicidal properties of tobacco smoke', and it begins, 'It is not surprising to learn that tobacco smoke is inimical to the activity of micro-organisms, since it contains, amongst many other things, pyridine, which has been shown to be a powerful germicide'. (Pyridine has a strong and disagreeable smell, which the nose, at least, does not detect in tobacco smoke, so one would guess that its concentration must be minute, and its practical effect imperceptible; nor is it in reality 'a powerful germicide'.) 'Definite experiments have recently been made', the article informs its readers, 'which show that tobacco smoke rapidly destroys in particular the comma bacillus of cholera'. Then follow accounts from the medical officer in the Greenwich workhouse in London that the tobacco-smoking inmates show resistance to epidemics. In Hamburg during a cholera epidemic 'it was reported that not a single workman engaged in the cigar factory in that city was attacked by the disease'. And then 'amongst a body of 5000 cigar makers only 8 cases and 4 deaths from the cholera occurred'. (*The Lancet* does not disclose whether they all smoked or whether merely handling the tobacco sufficed.) Experiments had shown moreover that tobacco smoke killed both cholera and pneumonia bacilli, and perhaps prevented 'some forms of nasal catarrh'. The article enlarges on the use of pyridine in medicine in France, and concludes with the warning that excessive smoking may be counter-productive, and lower resistance to the incursion of dangerous bacteria. *The Lancet*'s unaccustomed credulity in 1913 stands in bizarre contrast to the tone of the earlier article, but is by no means unrepresentative of the medical literature of the period.

Almost at the same time the first fully synthetic and highly effective bactericidal compound was discovered and became a tragic cause of an iatrogenic disease. Julius Morgenroth (1871-1924) was a doctor and bacteriologist, whose choice of career had been inspired by the cousins, Weigert, with whom he had worked after qualifying in medicine, and Ehrlich, who had engaged him as his assistant at the serum institute in Berlin. Morgenroth rose to the position of director at the bacteriology division of the Institute of Pathology at the Charité Hospital, where he set out on a search for antimalarial compounds. It had not proved possible to infect mice with malaria - species of the malaria parasite that infect mice were discovered only later – but Morgenroth found that mice infected with trypanosomes recovered when treated with what was still the only effective agent against malaria, quinine. Deciding to make do, he proceeded to test the effects of related molecules against trypanosome infections, some of which gave mildly encouraging results. Then a chance and unrelated observation intervened: Morgenroth found a freakish similarity of behaviour between trypanosomes and pneumococci, the bacteria responsible for the most lethal form of pneumonia, both of which could, in the test-tube, be dispersed by a particular solvent system. On the remote chance that this reflected a deeper similarity between these very different organisms, Morgenroth tried some of the quinine analogues on pneumococcus-infected mice. One (ethylhydrocupreine) was astonishingly effective against an infection that had long resisted every compound doctors and scientists had thrown at it. Morgenroth's compound was equally effective against infections in other species of animals, but pathological examination revealed frequent damage to the optic nerve. There appears to have been little attempt to conduct proper human trials before a small pharmaceutical company put the compound on the market under the trade name, *Optochin*. The result was that some hundreds of patients were blinded. The compound found an application during the Great War in the treatment of wounds, since it worked on other bacteria also, and more lastingly in an assay for discriminating between different species of streptococci species, for which it is still used.

Willow, willow

Aspirin appears in the Oxford English dictionary in lower case. In the early part of the 20th century it had already entered the language. When the railwayman, Jimmy Thomas, who was elected a Member of Parliament in 1910 and held several ministerial offices, complained of 'an 'orrible 'eadache', and the great lawyer and politician F.E. Smith recommended he try 'a couple of aspirates', the quip would have been lost on no one. Considering the chemical simplicity of acetylsalicylic acid, it seems surprising now that its path to the clinic and pharmacy was so strewn with rocks. The bark of the willow is mentioned in the earliest medical and herbal texts, but then so are most parts of most of the common plants. It is listed as an analgesic in the Ebers papyrus and by Hippocrates. The bark and leaves are commended by Dioscorides for eye and ear complaints (and the finely ground leaves taken in wine with a little pepper as a contraceptive). The more restrained Hildegard of Bingen in the 12th century regarded willow extracts as a remedy for fevers and aches, while the ever-optimistic Culpeper imputes to them the usual plenitude of curative properties. But for its discovery, or rediscovery in modern times we have to thank a member of the remarkable tradition of English savant-divines, the Rev. Edward Stone (1702–1764).

The son of a Buckinghamshire farmer, Stone graduated from Wadham College, Oxford, where he later returned as a fellow and sub-Warden, having served in the interim as vicar in a village near Oxford. Oxford Fellows, all at the time in holy orders, were not permitted to marry and retain their fellowship. The way out, which Stone evidently took, was to acquire one of the keenly sought-after college-owned livings, and become a country parson. Thus Stone settled in the Oxfordshire town of Chipping Norton. He wrote books of theology and one about the transit of Venus across the face of the sun, a perpetual preoccupation of astronomers. It was in Chipping Norton that Stone, at the age of fifty-six, paused during a stroll along the local stream to take his ease by a willow tree, and was inspired to break off a piece of bark and apply it to his tongue. The taste was extremely bitter, and Stone was reminded of another bitter bark, one known to have powerful curative properties, cinchona. Might the willow not then have a similar quality, and replace the very expensive Peruvian bark for the treatment of agues? Agues, or recurrent fevers, were common in England and would most often have referred to the cyclical flare-up of malaria. Stone, ignorant presumably of medieval writings on the subject, made another connection. Agues were associated with water and marshes (p.), and the willow was 'a tree that delights in a moist or wet soil'. The ancient tradition that God had provided a cure close to where any sickness would breed was never far from pious minds. 'That this might be the intention of Providence here', Stone recorded, 'I must own, had some little weight with me'. He followed up his conjecture: he cut a sizeable amount of bark, dried it out in an oven owned by the local miller and then ground it to powder. It was not long before he found an opportunity to test its effect on a man in the grip of a fever. He cautiously fed the man a little of the powder, and perceiving no ill-effect, increased the dose. After the first treatment the fever paroxysms abated, and after the second dose the fever was gone. A single success, Stone clearly realised, was no kind of evidence, and he proceeded to treat sufferers from fevers over a period of five years. He worked out a dosage regime, and found that there were only rare cases of what must have been malaria in advanced stages, in which his treatment was not fully effective. In those cases he supplemented the willow powder with a little Peruvian bark with gratifying results.

It is now clear, of course, that the willow bark was no cure for malaria, against which only the Peruvian bark was then a specific. Yet it mitigated the symptoms by relieving, at least temporarily, the fever and attendant headaches. Either then Stone was deceived in seeing a permanent cure, or the agues were in many cases not really intermittent fevers. For Stone, though, the time had now come to make the discovery public, and he wrote a letter to the Earl of Macclesfield, President of the Royal Society. 'Among the many useful discoveries which this age has made', he began, 'there are very few which better deserve the attention of the public than what I am going to lay before your Lordship.' The letter was read before a session of the Royal Society, and in June of 1763 it was published in the Society's journal, the *Philosophical Transactions*. And there it lay, waiting for a man of science a century on to discover it. The word must somehow have spread however, because in scattered doctors' surgeries and pharmacies willow bark was used as a valued treatment for the symptoms of the ague. As for Stone, he returned to the study of astronomy, and died suddenly a year later in 1764.

That was how matters rested for the greater part of a century, although there were sporadic reports of preparations of willow bark extracts, the first in 1826 from two Italian chemists, and then in 1828 Joseph Buchner, a pharmacist in Munich boiled up some of the bark and recovered a yellow, partly crystalline mass, to which he gave the name, *salicin* from *Salix*, the generic name for willow species. The following year a French chemist, Henri Leroux did it better, and obtained a good yield of colourless crystals, but did little to investigate their properties. Another decade passed before in 1838 an Italian chemist, Raffaele Piria, working in Paris, improved the method further and recovered what was probably a single pure compound. He recognised its acidic character, and called it *salicylic acid*, and went on to prepare a new derivative, salicyl alcohol.* Meanwhile, in 1831, there had been an interesting development. A Swiss pharmacist, Johann Pagenstecher, with an interest in folk remedies of a kind by then largely out of fashion, had been exploring plants with supposed analgesic properties. One such was the Alpine meadowsweet, which was well-known as a remedy for toothache. He collected the flowers, distilled them, as chemists and alchemists used to do, and recovered a clear fragrant liquid. This, Pagenstecher found, indeed had the desired analgesic properties, and

---

* Simplifying the chemistry grossly - oxidation of an alcohol produces an aldehyde, which in turn can be oxidised to an acid. Thus an alcohol is characterised by the group – C-OH, where C is carbon, O oxygen and H hydrogen; drinking alcohol, ethyl alcohol, has the formula C_2H_5OH. The group, -CHO identifies an aldehyde, while the acid derived from it by oxidation contains the group –COOH. An ester, which results from the combination of an acid of this kind with an alcohol, contains the group –COOR, where R can be, for example a methyl (-CH_3) or an ethyl (-C_2H_5) group, or something more complex.

he reported as much in a brief paper in a Swiss journal, *Pharmacie*. There it caught the eye of a German chemist with an interest in plant alkaloids, Karl Jacob Löwig, who repeated Pagenstecher's extraction and obtained from the mixture of substances an aldehyde (see footnote above), which he oxidised to the corresponding acid. This product he called *Spirsäure*, from *Spirea ulmaria*, the meadowsweet. (*Säure* is the German for acid, reflecting the sour taste.) Löwig published his report in 1834, not knowing that his *Spirsäure* was nothing else than salicylic acid, described and named six years previously by Raffaele Piria.

The next related discovery was made in 1843 by a French chemist, Auguste Cahours, who examined the leaves of the wintergreen plant, from which oil of wintergreen was obtained. This was (and is) favoured as a treatment for coughs, as an embrocation for muscle aches, and sometimes as a flavouring. It proved to contain a generous proportion of methyl salicylate (an ester [see footnote above] of salicylic acid), so here was another compound of the same chemical family with analgesic activity. Progress continued at the same leisurely pace. Another ten years elapsed before, in 1853, an eminent French chemist from Alsace, though then a professor in Montpellier, Charles Frédéric Gerhardt pulled off the synthesis of salicylic acid. It was a laborious process, the yield was low and the product remained obstinately contaminated with reaction by-products, but Gerhardt went a step further: he chose to block the hydroxyl (-OH) group by a type of reaction called acetylation, which converted it into $-OCOCH_3$. Why he did this is not clear, but the resulting compound was *acetylsalicylic acid*, known to us as *aspirin*. It was still impure, and Gerhardt, having apparently little interest in commercial applications, he published an account of his work and let the subject drop. It was to be another half century before the wonder drug arrived to spread its benison. Meanwhile the acetylation procedure was repeated in 1859 by a chemist in Innsbruck, by the name of von Gilm, who apparently obtained a pure product. Another ten years on, in 1869, a report appeared of yet another synthesis of acetylsalicylic acid, this time from a German chemist, Karl Johann Kraut. Unlike his predecessors, Kraut passed on his method to a small company, the Chemische Fabrik von Heyden, where for the time being it languished.

A few years later, a prominent German chemist, Hermann Kolbe (1818–1884) tried his hand at synthesising salicylic acid with little success.* (He had originally refused to believe that it even existed, holding instead to the view that all reported preparations had been nothing more than the familiar compound, benzoic acid.) Fourteen years later, in 1874, having by then succeeded the great Justus von Liebig, the country's most renowned chemist, as professor in Leipzig, he fared much better. His motives at the time were far removed from any desire to bring succour to ailing mankind, for he had another vendetta on his hands. August Kekulé von Stradonitz, a francophile German, who had worked with Charles Gerhardt and had also spent years in Paris and in London, and was one of the founders of structural chemistry, had formulated a theory of the structure of benzene. This was the then-mysterious but centrally important molecule, C_6H_6, which lies at the root of organic chemistry, of most drugs and of the great majority of the molecules of life. Its ring structure came to Kekulé, as he recalled it, while in a reverie one night on the upper deck of a London bus carrying him from his lab to his digs. He saw in his mind's eye molecules dancing around one another, until one, like a snake eating its tail, turned into a closed ring. It was one of the critical insights in the history of chemistry, but Kolbe would have none of it. He had a theory of his own and he was proposing to prove it by isolating isomers (compounds with the same atomic composition but different structures) of certain benzene derivatives, of which salicylic acid was one. In this he failed, but he did find a simple and cheap way of synthesising the compound, a great deal better than Gerhardt's.

---

* Kolbe, then a professor at Marburg University, was a belligerent and disputatious man, coarse, assertive, intolerant and dogmatic. He was antisemitic, resented the power of the Prussians, and nurtured above all an obsessive hatred of all things French. He may thus have been motivated by the desire to assert his superiority over Gerhardt. Kolbe whipped himself into a chauvinistic frenzy during the Franco-Prussian war of 1870-1. He was especially infuriated that the French Academy of Sciences would not remove the universities of the lost Alsatian cities of Strasbourg, Mulhouse and Metz from the title page of its journal. Following the attempt at a rapprochement between the learned societies of the two countries some time after the end of the war, Kolbe resigned from the German Chemical Society in a rage.

In the world of clinical practice the promise of willow bark, and of salicin had not been altogether forgotten. Some doctors still prescribed it for fevers and rheumatism. Some, with an interest in chemistry, had remarked on the chemical similarity between salicylic acid and phenol (carbolic acid), the first disinfectant adopted by Joseph Lister in his surgical ward, and now in wide use throughout Europe and America. It was, however, corrosive and poisonous, as soon became clear to operating theatre staff. The notion of using it internally to kill the bacteria responsible for serious diseases, such as typhoid, arose but was soon abandoned.*

What of salicylic acid then? Carl Buss, a doctor on St Gallen in Switzerland was one who thought the risk was worth taking. The condition of his typhoid fever patients improved; their temperature fell and their fever diminished. Yet the typhoid infection remained, so the acetylsalicylic acid was no disinfectant, but it was a very effective antipyretic. Buss wrote up his findings in 1875, and his publication did much to encourage its wider use.

The following year there appeared in *The Lancet* a long paper by Dr Thomas Maclagan, medical superintendent of the Dundee Royal Infirmary. It had the title, The Treatment of acute Rheumatism by Salicin, and begins with a survey of all the methods recommended for the treatment of this painful condition – everything from purgatives and diaphoretics to aconite, quinine, lemon juice, sulphur, mercury and 'tincture of muriate of iron' [ferric chloride in alcohol]. But he, for his part, was a 'miasmatic' he believed that diseases entered the body from the environment (p.).

---

* It had its adherents; in Britain it was used by a few doctors in association with iodine. A trenchant letter to *The Lancet* in 1889 declared it useless, and reveals the exasperation of practitioners at the flood of pharmaceutical products entering the chemists' shops. Dr F.M. Pope inveighed against its use against enteric fever (typhoid). 'At the present time, when every week, almost every day, brings its new drug, each in turn praised as being the greatest discovery of modern therapeutics, it is of importance that any fact which contradicts already published opinions on the action of any drug should be as widely circulated as the original statements.' Dr Pope tabulates the results of a controlled trial of the phenol-iodine treatment on his typhoid patients, showing the same proportion of deaths in the treated patients as in the (admittedly ten times larger) control group. Enough said, he suggests.

He held, moreover, like the Rev Edward Stone, that 'nature seem[s] to produce the remedy under climatic conditions similar to those which give rise to the disease'. Therefore, if, as was taken for granted, rheumatic fever (which Maclagan uses interchangeably with 'acute rheumatism') arises predominantly in cold and damp places, this is also where one should look for the curative organisms, most obviously the various species of Salicacea – the willows. 'Salicin', Maclagan instructs his readers, 'has long enjoyed a reputation for tonic and febrifuge properties, and was at one time a good deal used as a substitute for quinine. It has of late years, however, gone very much out of use, and it does not now even find a place in the British Pharmacopoeia.' He tried salicin on himself and then on his rheumatic patients. 'The results', he declares, 'exceeded even my most sanguine expectations' – body temperature fell, pain receded. Maclagan then recounts in minute detail the progress of six of his patients on salicin. He concedes that the small number precludes any definitive conclusions, but all of them benefited mightily from the treatment. The salicin acted as both febrifuge and analgesic, but should not altogether replace earlier methods of treatment. Maclagan also alludes to three favourable reports, which had appeared only weeks earlier from German doctors. One of Maclagan's readers contributed a heartening anecdote in a letter to the journal. Dr Frederick Ensor relates an experience of his own during his service as District Medical Officer in a town by the Orange River in the Orange Free State. He was called to treat a Dutch woman in the throes of a fever and close to death. He had done what he could, dosed her with calomel and 'Dover's powder', 'and rode away'. Two months later he was pleased to find her fully recovered, but, she informed him, it was no thanks to his ministrations; an old Hottentot shepherd had given her a decoction of willow shoots, and in a trice she was restored to health.

Maclagan's article had clearly found wide resonance. Salicin or salicylic acid (which he had found less satisfactory than the crude extract, presumably because of impurities) were taken up in major hospitals in Britain and in Europe, and were used to treat other conditions than just rheumatism and rheumatic fever, such as gout. Maclagan, feeling perhaps that he had done enough, left Dundee and settled in London, where he set up a highly successful practice and became physician to royalty and the *haut monde*. In

Leipzig meanwhile, Kolbe was busy. Carl Thiersch, a surgeon in the local hospital, who befriended Kolbe and became his family doctor, had wanted to replace the corrosive and poisonous phenol as a disinfectant in surgery, and was not alone in speculating that salicylic acid might be the answer. Thiersch seems to have stimulated Kolbe's interest in salicylic acid, beyond his preoccupation with Kekulé's benzene theory. Soon Kolbe's visions of pecuniary gain were also piqued by an approach from another direction. No sooner had he announced his successful synthesis than he received a visit from Friedrich von Heyden, a former student of one of Kolbe's colleagues. Von Heyden had established a chemical manufacturing concern – the very one to which Kraut had passed his method of synthesis - and was proposing to market the compound. Kolbe, sniffing lucre, entered into an agreement. The business thrived, but legal problems about patents and marketing rights soon arose. Kolbe, though, had convinced himself that salicylic acid had quite remarkably curative and rejuvenating properties. He seems to have been something of a hypochondriac, for he treated himself with salicylic acid for stomach upsets, blisters in his mouth, kidney stones and bad breath, amongst other nuisances, and found that it cured them all. More, it acted as a tonic, and from 1874 he took to drinking huge volumes of watery salicylic acid suspensions daily, which so improved his general sense of wellbeing and vigour as to create the expectation of great longevity (prefiguring perhaps the low-dose aspirin pills which are now meant to reduce the risk of strokes and heart attacks). His faith in salicylic acid as a cure-all was enhanced by a domestic episode, when he gave it to his daughter, who had contracted diphtheria. When Dr Thiersch arrived some days later on the scene he allowed the treatment to be continued, and the girl recovered. Whether it played some part in the cure is uncertain, although reduction of the fever could have done some good, but when tested against cholera and typhus it proved ineffective.

Persuaded that the wondrous chemical must, in addition to all else, be a peerless antiseptic, Kolbe first persuaded the captain of a ship bound for the tropics to add salicylic acid to the water butts to prevent bacterial growths. When this failed Kolbe had a ready explanation: the salicylic acid was absorbed by the walls of the wooden containers. He was not discouraged, and successfully promoted the methyl ester (see above), the active ingredient, which he had synthesised, of oil of wintergreen, as well as a tooth-powder based on salicylic acid. His greatest effort went into the marketing of salicylic acid as a food additive to prevent or retard spoilage. This was successful up to a point, but after brief storage meat and other solid food was said to acquire an unpleasant taste. Salicylic acid did better when added in small quantities to beer and wine, and it was used in the German drinks industry for some time, until proscribed by new food additive regulations. Curiously, there is a much later account (in 1903) in *The Lancet* of the excellence of salicylic acid as a food preservative. The two authors could find nothing against it; they thought it would serve well those impoverished people who could not afford gastronomic luxuries, and best of all, it would keep them away from 'intoxicating drinks'. Kolbe's high expectations of revolutionising the food industry were dashed nonetheless, nor did he ever disprove Kekulé's theory of benzene structure, which was after all correct, but his disappointment would have been assuaged by the wealth that salicylic acid brought him.

Pharma ascendant

The genesis of Big Pharma, as it has now come to be known, followed closely on the emergence of the dyestuffs industry in Germany. If that industry had a single begetter, this man was the son of a London builder. William Henry Perkin was born in 1838. His father was determined that he should become an architect, but the City of London school which he attended was one of the few that taught science, and the boy was captivated by chemistry. His teacher, who had studied at the Royal College of Chemistry under the famous chemist, August Wilhelm Hofmann, interceded successfully with the father: the young Perkin enrolled under Hofmann at the age of fifteen. The benign Hofmann (a German, whom the Prince Consort, both a German, and keenly interested in science, had lured to London), gave the young Perkin impossibly difficult projects, including the synthesis of quinine – something not accomplished until 1944. From such stiff challenges Perkin learned his craft. He became Hofmann's assistant at seventeen, and to make time for research of his own he also set up a laboratory at home. There over the Easter holiday on 1856 he made his first great, though accidental, discovery. It had been recognised that coal tar, the sticky black residue remaining after carbonisation of coal to make coke, or its gassification to make coal gas, was rich in a variety of aromatic and other carbon compounds. (Aromatic to a chemist means a compound containing a ring with double bonds, as in the archetype, benzene. The designation is historical not literal. The aromatic compounds are the most versatile in all of chemistry.) Perkin wanted to make quinine starting from a coal tar product that sufficiently resembled it in structure to serve, he thought as a starting point. The attempt failed, and Perkin tried again, setting out this time from aniline (aminobenzene), one of the simplest and most abundant constituents of coal tar. This time he was rewarded with a black mass of the kind that chemists would normally throw away in disgust, but Perkin tried dissolving it in alcohol, and a rich purplish blue solution resulted. It seemed to him like a dye, and when he immersed a piece of silk in the solution it acquired a colourfast and light-resistant brilliance. Perkin sent a sample to the famous Pullar dye works in Scotland, and the management were enchanted. After further work Perkin left Hofmann's laboratory and set up a factory to manufacture his dye.

After many vicissitudes the business broke into profit. The dye was marketed first as Aniline Purple, then Tyrian Purple - after the famous Roman dye, derived from a marine mollusc and used to colour the imperial togas – and finally *mauve*. Under this name it took the fashion salons of Europe by storm, and the French word entered the English language. In time Perkin's business diversified, and he began to produce the coal-tar-derived starting material for a plethora of synthetic dyestuffs. The most eager purchasers were the German dyeworks, of which some half dozen were dominant. The most important were Hoechst, the Bayerische Anilin und Soda Fabrik (Bavarian aniline and soda works, better known as BASF), and Farbenfabriken vormals Bayer (Colour works, formerly Bayer). German organic chemistry led the world and the country's dyestuff industry was now able to establish its pre-eminence It was the ever-widening choice of dyes that so effectively helped Ehrlich (Chapter) to his discoveries. With so many first-rate chemists, a dynamic management and the support of a science-friendly government, a move into pharmaceutical products became an obvious departure for these commercial juggernauts. As for Perkin, his fortune secured at the age of thirty-five, he sold the factory and devoted the rest of his life until his death in 1907 to pure science. The mantle fell on his elder son, William Henry Perkin, Jr, who became a virtuoso of organic synthesis and professor of organic chemistry in Oxford.

Kolbe's salicylic acid synthesis lent itself well to the industrial scale, and the demand for the substance, not only as an antipyretic, but also as an intermediate in the synthesis of dyes and other commercial products, was growing, And yet it was far from a satisfactory medicine: it was unpleasant to take, it irritated the throat and especially the stomach, and often caused internal bleeding and sometimes tinnitus (ringing in the ears). Some patients preferred to put up with the pain rather than take the stuff. What was needed then was a derivative with the antipyretic and analgesic properties of salicylic acid, which was no longer an irritant. One attempt to modify salicylic acid by turning the acidic (-COOH) group into an ester (p.), thereby blocking it, was made by a Polish biochemist working in Basel. Marceli Nencki (who gave his name to a leading biochemistry institute in Warsaw), made such a product, which he called *Salol*, in 1883, although with a view to intestinal antisepsis. It was quite insoluble, but was metabolised to salicylic acid and phenol in the small intestine, and therefore exercised some benign effect. It enjoyed a brief vogue despite its modest efficacy.

Fevers, though, were a fashionable preoccupation in the medicine of the day, and the competition to invent an effective febrifuge was intense. Most products on the market were largely or wholly worthless. Organic chemists were groping in semi-darkness for antipyretic compounds and analgesics. Two successful products came about by purest accident. The scope of the activity of quinine was still unclear, and its formula still unknown. Methods of synthesising a class of compounds called quinolines had been developed in Germany, and in 1882 a chemist at Munich University, Otto Fischer synthesised a number of quinoline derivatives in the hope of discovering an antipyretic, guided only by an incorrect structure that had been proposed for quinine. One of his compounds indeed proved, when tested on animals and people by a prominent pharmacologist at the University of Erlangen, Wilhelm Filehne, to work tolerably well. It was offered to Hoechst, who proceeded to manufacture and sell it in 1883 under the name of Kairin. It did not last long, for it was not only antipyretic but also toxic. Other derivatives were prepared and duly marketed by Hoechst, but all had drawbacks, mainly of toxicity or cost.

Next, an assistant of Fischer's, Ludwig Knorr made a variant of one of the quinoline compounds with advice from Filehne on the basis of another incorrect formula. It was a much better antipyretic than what had gone before. Its true formula was not established until later, but Hoechst, to whom it was once more offered, called it Antipyrin and, even though it was expensive and its action was of short duration, launched it on the market with great éclat. It was rapturously received, and the New York Times, for instance asserted that '[a]mong the many remedies that have been discovered to alleviate the ills of suffering humanity none is more important than Antipyrine'. Next came Antifebrin. In 1886 two doctors, Arnold Cahn and Paul Hepp in what, since 1871 had been the German city of Strassburg, placed an order for naphthalene from a pharmaceutical supply house. Naphthalene was a coal-tar product (later familiar as moth-balls), and had found limited use for killing parasites. Cahn and Hepp meant to give it to a patient with an infestation of intestinal worms. What they were sent in error was a quite different compound (though also derived from coal tar), acetanilide. The two physicians clearly did not notice the absence of the moth-ball smell, and dosed a patient with the supposed naphthalene. It did not kill the worms, but did bring down his fever. Hepp communicated the curious discovery to his brother in the chemical industry, and in short order acetanilide was on the market as an antipyretic, produced by the Kalle Company in Frankfurt. Antifebrin was moderately effective, much cheaper than Antipyrin, but anaemia was a side-effect. Hoechst reacted to the impudent competition from this relative midget of a company by acquiring it and selling their Antifebrin as a Hoechst product. The third highly profitable analgesic appeared only a year later from a different source. Carl Duisberg (1861–1935) was engaged as a promising young chemist in 1883 by Carl Rumpff. the chairman of what was then the modest drug company, Farbwerke Friedrich Bayer. He married the chairman's niece and by dint of exceptional organisational abilities, persuasive powers and commercial acumen rose rapidly through the hierarchy. At a young age he was head of research, and from 1900 headed the company throughout its evolution into one of the world's greatest industrial concerns. It was he who in 1887 perceived possibilities in the antipyretic but dangerous acetanilide, and asked another able young chemist at Bayer, Oscar Hinsberg to synthesise analogues of the compound in the hope of finding one that retained the analgesic virtues without the toxicity. The result was *Phenacetin*, still as later emerged, toxic, but far less so than the parent compound. Phenacetin was the first of a series of acetanilide derivatives with progressively better antipyretic and analgesic properties and lower toxicity, of which the most durable, also originally from Bayer, is *paracetamol*. Hinsberg conjectured that paracetamol might be a metabolic product of phenacetin, which does the analgesic work in the body, and many years later this was shown to be the case. Such was the instant demand for phenacetin that Bayer were driven to produce it in recycled beer bottles. It was the most widely sold and profitable pharmaceutical product that had then ever been seen.

Aspirin!

Duisberg, presiding over Bayer's irresistible rise, was still on the look-out for even better antipyretics, encouraged perhaps by the increasing demands created by Europe-wide influenza epidemics. The drug-development operation comprised a research section, synthesising new compounds, and a pharmacology section, charged with testing them for medicinal properties and side-effects. The first was headed by a chemist, Arthur Eichengrün, the second by a pharmacologist, Heinrich Dreser. Both men were confident and assertive, but their personalities were very different, to the extent that friction was almost inevitable. Eichengrün (1867–1949) was born in Aachen, the son of a fabric-merchant. An outstanding student at Berlin University, he had done the research for his doctoral thesis at the University of Erlangen, a stronghold of organic, and especially medicinal chemistry, and in 1896 he had joined Bayer and quickly proved his worth. He was quick-witted, imaginative, and by nature ebullient, gregarious, and reputedly something of a womaniser. Dreser (1862–1924) had come to Bayer in 1897 from the University of Göttingen, where he had been an

Ausserordentlicher (that it Assistant) *Professor* in pharmacology. He was, by contrast, stiff, formal and unyielding. There seems to have been antipathy from the outset, and the clash was not long in coming.

Eichengrün was given a free hand by Duisberg, and resolved at an early stage to look into salicylic acid analogues, starting with the acetyl derivative, acetylsalicylic acid. He entrusted the syntheses to one of his subordinates, Felix Hoffman. Hoffman went to work and within a short time he had a satisfactory preparation. This was later hailed as a great achievement, but in truth it was, in chemical terms, a rather modest step, for we may assume that Hoffman, and for that matter Eichengrün, must have been aware of the published accounts of syntheses of the same compound by Gerhardt (which was even to be found in a prominent German journal and in German), by von Gilm and by Kraut. All the same, Hofmann's preparation was evidently pure, for when Dreser's pharmacologists tested it on animals no ill-effects were recorded, and the results were highly gratifying. The next step should have been more extensive trials, especially on patients in hospitals, but Dreser would have none of it. He spoke of (spurious) evidence that the parent compound, salicylic acid had caused heart damage, and declared the derivative valueless. Eichengrün, fully aware of its potential, was appalled, but Dreser was adamant. Thereupon Eichengrün took the initiative. Having first tried the acetylsalicylic acid on himself, he sent samples to a doctor with whom he was acquainted, and who was also the Bayer representative in Berlin. This man distributed samples to several other doctors and to a dentist for evaluation. In short order highly enthusiastic accounts came back – patients' rheumatic pains had receded without adverse effects, and a martyr to toothache had found instant relief – all of which Eichengrün relayed at a managerial meeting. Dreser, predictably incensed by Eichengrün's temerity in going over his head, denounced the reports as typical examples of 'Berlin bombast'; the drug, he insisted, was worthless. A year's delay ensued before Dreser took up acetylsalicylic acid again. One may surmise that Duisberg had intervened, probably at Eichengrün's urging, and prompted also by an especially insistent report on the drug from a doctor in Halle. The reasons behind the tergiversation was never fully explained, but one conjecture has been that Dreser's prolonged opposition may have been due to his

313

overriding concern with another new product, diacetylmorphine (heroin), of which he had high hopes.

Now that he had no choice in the matter Dreser embraced acetylsalicylic acid with the fervour of a convert, and it was he who published the first paper on its superior qualities. The added irony was that of the three men involved it was only Dreser who profited financially. According to his contract with Bayer he would receive royalties on any compound that his division brought to market. Eichengrün and Hoffman, on the other hand, would profit only from patented discoveries, and acetylsalicylic acid was not new, and could not be patented. It could, however, be given a new and catchy name. Various ideas were aired, such as Spirea and Euspirin. Eichengrün voted for Aspirin, even though others thought the overtone of aspiration might mislead doctors and patients, but he finally had his way. Thereafter there remained only the problems of large-scale production, advertising, and fending off rivals.

Eichengrün was associated with several more important innovations for Bayer, and left in 1908 to start his own chemical company, the Cellon Werke in Berlin, where he invented a number of lucrative products, most famously the fire-resistant material, acetylcellulose. But Eichengrün was a Jew, and so in 1938 his company was 'Aryanised' and taken from him. He survived because protected by his Aryan wife, but in 1943 he was arrested for failing to add Israel to his name on a document, as the Nazi racial laws demanded. He was released after four months but deported in 1944 to the ghetto at Theresienstadt (Terezin), and was one of the few inmates not sent to their deaths in Auschwitz before the arrival of the Soviet Army. Liberated, he settled with his wife in Bad Wiessee, a spa town in Bavaria, where he died, though not before asserting his claim to the development of aspirin, which he had even done in a letter despatched by an unknown route from Theresienstadt to IG Farben in 1944. As for the other *dramatis personae* in the aspirin story, Duisberg died, still in harness, in 1953; Hoffman left the laboratory, ended his career in the Bayer sales division and died in 1946; and the egregious Dreser grew immensely rich from his share of the sales of the most lucrative drug in commercial history, and retired early from the company. Bayer merged in 1925 with BASF and several smaller companies to form the giant IG Farben conglomerate. (The name in full is IG Farbenindustrie - IG from *Interessengemeinschaft*, literally, associates with common interests, and Farben, colours or dyes.) At its zenith it employed some 120,000 people, including 1,000 chemists. After the Second World War, IG Farben was again split into its three major component parts, Bayer, which continued to produce pharmaceuticals, including of course the eternally profitable aspirin, BASF and Hoechst.

This was by no means the end of the aspirin story. In the first place IG Farben, which enthusiastically supported the Nazi regime from the moment in 1933 that Hitler became Reich Chancellor (manufacturing amongst other useful items the Zyklon B supplied to the extermination camps), proceeded to reinvent the past. Aspirin was given a prominent place as a great German (that is Aryan) discovery in the Hall of Honour in the German Museum in Berlin. Eichengrün's name had of course been expunged (as it also was from the creation of acetylcellulose), and his contribution to pharmaceutical history was supplanted by a new myth. Hoffman and Dreser were now the sole inventors of aspirin. Hoffman's father, the story ran, suffered from severe arthritis, and salicylic acid had eased his pain, but at the cost of intolerable side-effects. The son resolved to eliminate these by creating a benign derivative, retaining however the full analgesic power, whence aspirin. In 1949 the now aged Eichengrün tried once more to reassert his claim to the discovery. He chronicled for the second time, and published in a journal, *Pharmazie,* his recollection of the events that led to the discovery of aspirin. A few weeks later he was dead.

Pharmazie was an obscure organ and few pharmacists, much less scientists, would have read it. Then in 2000 Professor Walter Sneader of Glasgow University unearthed the article and searched the Bayer archives in a determined effort to uncover the reality. He found nothing in the chronology or in the surviving notes by the participants to contradict Eichengrün's account, and in particular his insistence that Hoffman had not known why he had been asked to synthesise the salicylic acid derivative. Eichengrün had presumably felt it prudent to keep his peace after he had been so traduced because it was no time for a Jew in Germany to speak up in his own defence, and his position was undoubtedly precarious. His

80th birthday, in any event, was celebrated with many tributes in learned journals, and thanks to Sneader, his reputation as the begetter of aspirin has been posthumously vindicated.

Eichengrün and aspirin made Bayer great, but the company managers did not always get their own way in the world of commerce. They tried to secure a patent in Germany but were denied on the grounds that the compound had been known for half a century and there was nothing novel about the manner of synthesis. Yet in Britain and the United States the patent application was, perversely, approved. The judgement was soon put to the test when challenged by Friedrich von Heyden. His company was producing aspirin and started to sell it in Britain, inviting Bayer to sue. In 1905 Bayer, as expected, took the Chemische Fabrik von Heyden to court for infringement of patent rights. Both sides lined up distinguished British and German chemists to give evidence on their behalf. Von Heyden's case was simple: his company had indeed infringed Bayer's patent, but in their submission the patent was invalid for the most obvious reasons. The judge heard the evidence, denounced the Bayer patent as preposterous, and their case deliberately misleading, and found for von Heyden. In Britain there was henceforth a free-for-all in the aspirin market. In the United States Bayer acted more discreetly: they set up a subsidiary with its own factory, and Bayer aspirin flooded the market. The promotion of aspirin worldwide was the first such undertaking by a commercial concern, and the shape of things to come.

It was inevitable of course that aspirin, like any other drugs, would eventually display some side-effects. Occasionally allergy developed, and blood clotting disorders could be aggravated, but more frequently reports appeared of stomach ulcers and other digestive problems. To mitigate these last effects the 'soluble' or 'dispersible' aspirins were developed. The salts of acetylsalicylic acid, such as the sodium salt, still had poor solubility, and the answer was to compound salicylic acid with sodium bicarbonate, so that the effervescence (evolution of carbon dioxide) on contact with water generated a much more finely divided suspension with no large particles that could irritate the throat and settle on the stomach linings. Especially in America many mixed preparations, containing caffeine or additional antipyretics, became popular. By the end of the 19th century the preoccupation with fevers had waned - they had been gradually recognised as symptoms not causes of diseases – and marketing of aspirin and other antipyretic products was henceforth based on their analgesic properties. In time aspirin had to compete once more with acetanilide-derived and similar compounds, and although it remains to this day the most widely bought of all medicaments, such competitors as Tylenol, Neurofen and Ibuprofen have at least in some measure replaced it.

Yet there was still more to be learned about aspirin, for in 1950 Dr Lawrence L. Craven, a GP in the town of Glendale in California published a paper in the *Annals of Western Medicine and Surgery* – not a journal that most doctors and researchers in the academic mainstream would probably have seen – and another in the same year in the *Journal of Insurance Medicine*, on how aspirin could prevent heart attacks. Craven (1883-1957), born in Iowa, qualified in medicine at the University of Minnesota, and spent the remainder of his life in Glendale. He was clearly a thoughtful and perceptive man, as the story he told in his publications testified. Like most GPs at the time his duties included performing minor surgery, mainly the removal of tonsils (a prevalent practice at that period) and of adenoids. For 36 years, he wrote, he had carried out these procedures with no instances of postoperative haemorrhages, and then, six years before his publication, all this had suddenly changed: haemorrhages started to occur with alarming frequency. Craven was in no doubt as to the cause: the onset of the problems had coincided with the introduction of analgaesic chewing-gum. This contained aspirin and was given to the patients after their operation to alleviate the pain. Craven did a simple experiment: he measured the time for clot formation in blood to which a small amount of aspirin had been added, and found that it was very considerably retarded. He had discovered an unsuspected property of aspirin, and it led him to a wild conjecture. If aspirin inhibited the blood clotting process, might it not, he wondered, prevent the formation of a thrombus in a damaged coronary artery, the common cause of heart attacks?

Craven had a second argument. Heart attacks were more frequent in men than in women, and it was well-known that women were much more prone than men to swallow aspirins to soothe trivial aches and pains. In 1948 he had begun giving aspirin to 400 of his patients, and by the time he wrote his paper in 1950 none had suffered heart attacks. Of course there had been no control group, which would have been difficult to arrange in a busy general practice, and no screening of the patients in the study, as Craven was well aware, but the results, he believed, spoke for themselves, and he thought that men might be well advised to take a small prophylactic dose of aspirin each day to reduce the chance of a heart attack or a minor stroke. Craven wrote only two further papers, one in 1953, the other in 1956, shortly before his death. In 1953 he moderated his position, suggesting that it was men between the ages of 45 and 65, who were overweight and sedentary, and therefore more predisposed to coronary thromboses or strokes, who should take prophylactic aspirin. Craven also reported that he had done an experiment on himself, which consisted in dosing himself with a dozen aspirin pills a day for five days, at which point he had been afflicted with a violent nose-bleed. This did not recur until he performed the experiment a second time. In his final paper he summed up his observations of no less than 8000 patients in Glendale. Only nine had died of what were thought to be heart attacks, but proved on autopsy to have been aortic aneurysms (weak regions of the artery, which become distended, and can spontaneously burst). This seems improbable, and in any case, time intervals and details of the patients and their states of health were undefined. And then, in 1957, a few months after the publication of his last paper, Craven must have compounded the scepticism that already existed by dropping dead at the age of 74 with a heart attack. Nevertheless, he had received communications from a number of doctors elsewhere in the country to the effect that they too had had good results by prescribing aspirin to their patients. But so far as the medical establishment was concerned his papers had all the effect of a pingpong ball dropping into a vat of treacle. Craven's evidence was 'anecdotal', not properly controlled or analysed, and besides he was an obscure GP in an obscure town. Or perhaps the papers had simply not come their way. Had someone listened however, many lives might have been saved over the next decade and more.

It was only ten years after Craven's death that he was fully vindicated. American researchers confirmed his results and what he inferred from them, and did much more: they discovered the manner of action of aspirin on the clotting system. Minute concentrations of aspirin act on the blood platelets, highly specialised cells which play a central role in what is known as the clotting cascade. Together with a blood protein, fibrin they form a plug to seal a wound. This requires the platelets to form aggregates, or clumps, and aspirin interferes with this process by preventing release of an essential molecule from the platelet's interior. It is now generally agreed that a low dose of aspirin every day reduces the likelihood that a thrombus – a blood clot – will form in a coronary artery and provoke a heart attack. In the late 1960s there was a further development, when the action of a class of compounds found in most cells was uncovered. These compounds are the prostaglandins (a misnomer, because they were first identified by the Swedish biochemist, Ulf von Euler [p.] thirty years earlier in sperm, and wrongly supposed by him to originate in the prostate gland). The prostaglandins have a number of functions in the body, one of them in blood clotting, and another in eliciting the inflammatory response to a physiological insult. Aspirin impedes this prostaglandin action also, and functions therefore as an anti-inflammatory agent. This attribute of aspirin was clear almost from its inception, but what emerged only later was that the effect on inflammation was quite separate from its analgesic action. Salicylic acid, which is merely aspirin (acetylsalicylic acid) without its acetyl ($-COCH_3$) group, is (side-effects notwithstanding) an analgesic, but it does not combat inflammation. Aspirin, then, is the archetypal miracle drug, with its three disparate beneficent effects – against pain, fever and heart damage. There are now other, and more powerful drugs, given to people at risk of strokes, and thromboses (such as the deep-vein thrombosis we are warned to beware of on long flights) generally. Clopidogrel is an anti-platelet agent, devised by Sanofi in France, and under the trade name of Plavix is one of the best-selling drugs in the U.S., and to a lesser extent in European countries, where an older (and cheaper) compound, first synthesised in the 19th century, dipyridamole (Persantine) is often preferred. (Both are given together with aspirin.)

IG: search and find

Bayer (and later IG Farben of which it became a part) enjoyed tolerable success after aspirin, but nothing on the same scale for another three decades. Chemistry was still the company's strength, and it was on synthetic compounds to counter bacterial infections that the directors had set his sights. Under Duisberg's guidance Bayer had in the early 20th century achieved high eminence as a centre for drug research with facilities unmatched in the world. Chemists, pharmacologists, pathologists and others in the universities, no longer turned up their noses at a position in commerce, for the advantages were many. For the first time talented young scientists were looking to Bayer, Hoechst and other companies for the prospect of a productive (and lucrative) career. One of them was Gerhard Domagk, born in 1895 in the small town of Lagow in the Mark Brandenburg, in what is now Poland, and where his father was a teacher. The son had begun his university studies in Kiel when the Great War began, and he at once joined the élite Leibgrenadier (Emperor's bodyguard) regiment. After three months in Flanders he received a serious head-wound. He recovered and was next sent to the eastern front as a medic, and there had his first experience of battle wounds and of the infections, especially the feared gas gangrene, which killed more soldiers than bullet or shell alone. His experiences made a deep impression on the young man, and probably directed his career into research. He returned to his medical studies in Kiel, specialising in pathology and bacteriology.

Gas gangrene was caused by anaerobic bacteria of some species of *Streptococcus*. It was usually fatal, and the only treatment was amputation of the affected limb (if a limb was the site of the infection) before the bacteria progressed further. It took some years for doctors to recognise that, since the streptococci are anaerobic they do not thrive in the presence of oxygen, and so the best hope of preventing or interrupting the course of an infection was to leave wounds open to the air. Graduating in 1921, Domagk began his research career in the university hospital in Kiel. He found a congenial patron, moved with him to the University of Greifswald, and thence, two years later, to the University of Münster, where he was appointed *Privatdozent*, in effect an untenured (and meagrely paid) lecturer.

Domagk's research in Münster focussed on phagocytosis, an important function of the immune system, executed by specialised cells (phagocytes), which engulf and destroy intruders, such as bacteria. His publications on the subject caught the eye of Heinrich Hörlein, the director of research at Bayer. Hörlein evidently thought phagocytosis, and probably immunology generally, an area with medicinal potential, and offered Domagk a position with good laboratory facilities and scope for assistants. Domagk, who now had a family to support with slender prospects of promotion, seized the opportunity. Access to the huge resources that Bayer had to offer, the promise of supporting staff, and no doubt a much enhanced salary, would all have been hard to resist. Many years later, when he had become famous, Domagk was asked why he had left the academic world for industry. His reply was that he had felt he would be able to help more people that way. Domagk joined Bayer in 1927, and so began an association that endured for the rest of his life and led eventually to a Nobel Prize.

Hörlein was a chemist, who had joined Bayer in 1909, having mastered his craft under Ludwig Knorr (p.) at the University of Jena. At Bayer he had made his mark by the synthesis of dyes, and then of the barbitone hypnotic drugs (sleeping draughts, also called soporific). Hörlein espoused Ehrlich's chemotherapeutic principle, and especially the power of dyes and their derivatives to kill bacteria. There was still wide scepticism in the medical profession about the future of laboratory-made, rather than plant-derived drugs, but Bayer had had some success with synthetics. Before Domagk's arrival the work had been led by a former assistant of Ehrlich's, Wilhelm Roehl, who had resuscitated his patron's line of investigation into sleeping sickness (trypanosomiasis), based on azo dyes*, which had been extensively studied by German chemists.) From Roehl's work, after a long and arduous search, had emerged Bayer 205, otherwise suramin or Germanin (p.), which had had such dramatic success in Germany's African colonies. He had then moved on to a search for an antimalarial drug to compete with quinine, then in short supply, and had found one, marketed under the name of Plasmochin in Germany and Plasmoquin elsewhere, though later its name was changed to pamaquin. Roehl's career was cut short at the

---

* Azo compounds have at their centre two nitrogen atoms, linked by a double-bond, -N=N-.

age of forty-eight by septicaemia, which struck him down on a field trip in Egypt in 1929. Domagk, who stepped into Roehl's shoes, was already deeply immersed in a programme to discover synthetic antibacterial agents. He never returned to immunology, his first love. Atebrin (initially and confusingly called Plasmochin E) appeared after Mietzsch and others at IG Farben had supposedly synthesised no less than 12,000 compounds, and became famous under still another name, mepacrine.*

Hörlein's philosophy of drug discovery was to go after his quarry by a systematic attack on a broad front. It was Ehrlich's way, vastly magnified. One started from a compound, generally a dye, which had shown some faint promise, often in quite another context, and would modify it chemically, by adding or subtracting or moving around elements of the structure. Each new compound was to be tested in animals, generally mice, which were consumed in their thousands. It was taken for granted that the path to success might be long – years, even decades - and certainly labour-intensive. It required skill, stamina and endurance, and the resources that only a large concern like Bayer could support. There was no parallel outside Germany. Domagk's targets were streptococci, of which there were many species, and within each species many strains, but there was also the hope that a chemical agent might appear which could kill all, or at least many species of bacteria. Streptococci were responsible not only for gas gangrere but also for other wound infections, common forms of septicaemia (blood poisoning), which had killed Roehl, puerperal (childbed) fever, and many other dire conditions, and there was no effective treatment.

---

* When war came again in 1939, and Britain could no longer procure antimalarials (or other drugs) from Germany, the synthesis of pamaquin and mepacrine was entrusted to the chemists of ICI (Imperial Chemical Industries). In 1942, to meet the demands of the troops in India and Burma, ICI supplied 32 million tablets of pamaquin and 50 million of mepacrine. Later the company's chemists developed two better chemically related antimalarials of their own, Paludrine and chloroquine, although the last had been prepared some years earlier, but not apparently further studied, by IG Farben. Chloroquine is still a standard treatment and prophylactic, although much restricted in efficacy because of the emergence of resistant strains of the parasite.

Domagk's plan was to test the many compounds that the Bayer chemists had produced over the years, and synthesise as many more as were needed until Ehrlich's magic bullet turned up. His first task was to settle on a strain of the most dangerous species, *Streptococcus pyogenes*, which would be lethal in both humans and his test animal, the mouse. He isolated such a strain from the cadaver of a victim of the disease in a local hospital. Next, he needed to develop a culture medium in which the strain could be propagated. This too was quickly accomplished. He now began his assays with gold compounds, some of which showed mild activity, but were uniformly toxic. Next he tried a series of compounds of arsenic, again too toxic to be of use. Then Domagk started on one of Ehrlich's favourite azo dyes as the 'lead compound' or point of departure. Two first-rate organic chemists had been allocated to him, Josef Klarer (1898-1953) and Fritz Mietzsch (1896-1958). Klarer had learned his trade at the Technische Hochschule (the Technical University) in Munich under Hans Fischer (celebrated for his work on a class of compounds, the porphyrins, which occur in such important biological molecules as chlorophyll and the red oxygen-carrying protein of the blood, haemoglobin). Klarer had been badly wounded in the Great War, and had a manic and unstable streak, and at the same time a preternatural talent for organic synthesis and capacity for intensive work. Mietzsch had obtained his doctorate at the Technical University of Dresden in dye chemistry, and it was a class of dyes that he had been engaged to synthesise at Bayer's Leverkusen works when he joined the company. While contemplating the structures of the so-called triphenylmethyl dyes he was struck by a superficial resemblance to that of quinine. Might they then have therapeutic potential? Hörlein, hearing of Mietzsch's idea, arranged for his transfer to the Ebersfeld laboratories and entry the world of drugs. In collaboration with Roehl he played a major part in the development of Plasmoquin, and then of the more effective Atebrin. Mietzsch was more phlegmatic than the volatile Klarer, and, many years after the events here related, he succeeded Hörlein as head of research. Besides the highly talented Mietzsch and Klarer, Domagk had at his disposal a group of six technicians to help with the animal assays.

Domagk and his assistants tested some 4,000 compounds. He had put his faith in azo dye derivatives, and Klarer and Mietzsch provided him with more than 500 compounds in the first two years. Few had given any encouragement In 1930 Klarer's Compound 487 (designated Kl-487), which contained a chlorine atom, showed the best, though still weak, activity. Some showed signs of working against different strains, or in the test-tube but not in animals. Another gave faint hope and a patent was taken out. More than three years had passed, and gloom must have hung heavy over Domagk's department, yet the work continued and the mice died, as well as many rabbits and guinea pigs. Then in 1932, Hörlein made a suggestion. It was not based on any logical inference, only something he had done when still working as a dye chemist to improve the strength of binding of a dye to wool: he had introduced a negatively charged sulphonyl group (-SO_3). Try a sulphur substituent, he suggested. With nothing to lose, Klarer did so - but not quite, for what he inserted into the dye was not a sulphonyl group but mo, from a readily available compound, easily derivatised to allow coupling to the dye. It was October 1932. The first attempt yielded Kl-695, and the result was breathtaking. Domagk was away, and it was one of his assistants who tested the compound, and informed him on his return that he would soon be famous: all the mice that had received an injection of Kl-695 were alive and well, and all the controls were dead. There were no detectable side-effects, but the puzzle was that the compound had no effect on the streptococci in culture, nor did it rescue animals infected with other bacteria. Klarer continued, and another thirty-five compounds on, with Kl-730, the results were even better: much smaller doses protected the mice against the lethal streptococcus strain, though again with the same puzzling features. A minor drawback was that the deep red dye turned the mice red, but the colour faded in a day or two. There was another strange aspect, which might have put Domagk and his chemists on their guard, namely that the sulphanilamide substituent could be placed in any position in the large parent dye molecule with little effect on the activity. There was at all events rejoicing at Bayer after more than three years of unremitting failure, and Kl-720 was given the name, *Streptozon*. More compounds were made and tested on other bacteria, and intensive studies of mouse pathology revealed that the drug caused kidney damage, though only at very high doses. It also appeared that the dye survived in the bloodstream and in the acid conditions of the stomach, and was excreted in the mouse's urine.

There was silence now from Bayer. No patent application was made, for if an effective cure for stretptococcal infection could result from taking a sulphanilamide conjugate in any position on the dye skeleton, a whole series of such drugs could be made, and Bayer could scarcely apply for a patent on each of the many opetions. No human trials were initiated, but some samples of the substance were sent to a few physicians, and the word leaked out that Bayer had a cure for streptococcal infections. A flood of inquiries ensued from doctors with sick patients, sometimes members of their families. It was a curious situation, for here was one of the most startling coups in the history of drug discovery, and no report had been published, no statement made, and there had been no announcement at any scientific meeting. And meanwhile the research was continuing apace. Could the sulphanilamide group perhaps also exert a curative activity when attached to something other than the Bayer dye? The possibility was explored, and indeed Klarer soon had another compound, Kl-821, in which sulphanilamide was linked to a quite different backbone and which was also effective. This only made the patent problem still worse. On the other hand, it now appeared that Streptozon had appreciable killing activity against some other bacteria, notably staphylococci. These are responsible for suppurating wound infections, abscesses and especially meningitis, of which there had been serious epidemics. The name of the drug therefore had to be changed: it was henceforth *Prontosil*, in which guise it added abundantly to the fortunes of Bayer and those therefore of IG Farben. There was only one further innovation – the introduction of hydrophilic (water-seeking) substituents into the molecule to render it more water-soluble, and therefore suitable for injection. This successful product was *Prontosil solubile*.

The first report by Domagk on Prontosil appeared in a German medical journal in 1935, mentioning only the first results, obtained nearly three years before, and giving scant details. The 100 percent cure rate in mice, so cursorily stated, seemed to many doctors and pharmacologists much too good to be true. Then Domagk's own young daughter pricked herself with a needle. The wound became infected and soon she had a raging streptococcal infection. Her father brought some Prontosil from the laboratory, and after several heavy doses she began to respond. The fever subsided, and after a day she returned to health and vigour. Another victim, who was brought back from the brink, was Ronald Hare, a bacteriologist at St. Mary's Hospital in London. Hare had been infected by a bacterial culture from a patient with puerperal fever when a sliver of broken glass penetrated his finger. By good fortune a colleague, the distinguished doctor and bacteriologist, Leonard Colebrook had begun an investigation of the efficacy of Prontosil and was able to treat him. Hare recovered. Hörlein had visited London a short time before this episode and had spoken about the new drug at a meeting of the Royal Society of Medicine. In the audience had been Henry Dale (p.), who asked Bayer for samples to be evaluated in England. It was the cautious and conservative Colebrook who ultimately satisfied himself of Prontosil's power by a controlled trial on patients in the 'septic wards'. Publications in *The Lancet* in 1936 did much to spread the good news about Prontosil around the medical world.

Debacle: the Gallic riposte

While Bayer and Hörlein and his myrmidons had been congratulating themselves and wrestling with problems of names and patents, in distant Paris a small group of researchers at the Pasteur Institute were slipping the lead into the boxing glove. Ernest Fourneau (1872-1949) was the head of chemistry at the Institute and Bayer's nemesis, for he had already cracked the puzzle of the undisclosed sleeping sickness cure, Bayer 205 (p.). He now wanted to discover the secret of the mysterious Prontosil. Fourneau was an accomplished operator, both inside the laboratory and beyond. Ernest François Auguste Fourneau was born in Biarritz into a family of hoteliers: his father was a chef at one of the resort's grand hotels. Like many of the leading French chemists before him, Fourneau passed through the rigorous training offered by the School of Pharmacy in Paris and qualified as a pharmacist. At the same time he developed a keen interest in organic chemistry, and he attended courses in the subject and showed exceptional talents. This was to be his career, and he wisely decided to study with some of the great masters in the craft of organic synthesis in Germany. He worked for three years, first under Gattermann in Heidelberg, then Emil Fischer in Berlin and lastly in Munich with Richard Willstätter, all names that echo down the history of chemistry. Fourneau made the most of his opportunity: in addition to very considerable accomplishments in the laboratory, he became fluent in German, made many friends, and remained throughout his life an ardent Germanophile, a foible for which he would later pay the price.

Returning to France in 1902, Fourneau renewed an earlier contact with the three Poulenc brothers, small-time chemical suppliers, and persuaded them to form a research-based company, which he would direct. This was the genesis of the Établissements Poulenc Frères, which later merged with the Société chimique des Usines de Rhône to form the largest pharmaceutical concern in France, Rhône-Poulenc. Success was not long in coming: Fourneau synthesised a new anaesthetic, which swept the market. Until then a number of products with names such as Nirvanin, developed in Germany, and inspired by cocaine (on which Fourneau had worked in Willstätter's laboratory in Munich not long before) had held sway. ut Fourneau's new compound, though, was better on all counts. It was less toxic and had no irritating after-effects. It was given the name amylocaine, but was marketed as Stovaine – a play on Fourneau's name, for a *fourneau* is a cooking stove, and its inventor was fluent in English. Stovaine made the company (and Fourneau) rich. Fourneau retained his connection with Poulenc Frères after his move to the Pasteur Institute, and it was there that he synthesised another profitable drug, manufactured and sold by Poulenc. This was an improvement on Ehrlich's Atoxyl, which had cured sleeping sickness, but with the risk of serious neurological side-effects, including blindness (p.). The new compound, acetarsol, was sold under the name of *Stovarsol*.

By the time Fourneau decided to investigate Prontosil his name was already familiar to pharmacologists. He had indeed been offered, and had rejected, a position by Duisberg in Bayer's operation in France. His collaborator at the Pasteur Institute, Daniel Bovet has left an impression of the man's personality. Fourneau was a *bon vivant*, courtly, immaculately suited, groomed and perfumed, his white goatee beard trimmed. A laboratory explosion had deprived him of the sight of his right eye and left him with a limp. He was well-connected and cultured, and sought after in the Parisian salons. In the laboratory Fourneau was affable but distant. Bovet tells us that the heads of the divisions. Bovet tells us that the heads of divisions in the Pasteur Institute, the *chefs de service*, were generally addressed by their staff as *Père*, but never Fourneau, who was always Monsieur to his colleagues. Fourneau had assembled a highly able and close-knit team of young researchers. Daniel Bovet (1907-1992) was an Italian, born in Switzerland and educated at the University of Geneva, whose later achievements in developing the first effective anti-histamine, and then a mucle relaxant, used in surgery brought him a Nobel Prize in 1957. Bovet was married to the sister of the group's bacteriologist, another Italian, Federico Nitti (son of a famous politician and prime-minister after the end of the Great War). The other two members of Fourneau's team were Jacques Tréfouël (Fourneau's assistant, and later head of the Pasteur Institute), and his wife Thérèse Tréfouël.

When the news of Prontosil seeped out of Germany Fourneau scanned the details of the patent and divined what the formula, more or less, must be. He and his team proceeded to synthesise some candidate compounds and had them tested in animals by two experienced bacteriologists, Constantin Levaditi and Albert Vaisman at the Institut Alfred Fournier, the laboratory of the 'French League against Venereal Hazard'. The best compound was similar to Prontosil in its efficacy, and almost immediately it also proved itself in patients with deadly streptococcal infections. Levaditi and Vaisman quickly had a report in print, to the great displeasure of Hörlein, who denounced it as plagiarism. Fourneau wasted even less time. Only three months after Domagk's sketchy publication the French had their *Rubizol* on the market. The Germans were infuriated and cried foul, but worse was to come. Further related compounds were prepared and tested, and then one day, as Bovet relates, when a number of mice were being divided into groups of four to be injected with the latest products, he found that he had four left over. On an impulse he injected them with the virulent streptococci, followed by sulphanilamide, the colourless substituent in the Prontosil (and Rubizol) structures, which was inseparable from the activity. He was startled to find that the four mice were alive and well. If this result was real it followed that the large and complex molecule that Domagk's chemists had so laboriously synthesised was unnecessary. As Bovet later put it, the large, complicated red car had a simple white engine. Further assays confirmed the result. The sulphanilamide proved to be more effective even than Prontosil, did not colour mice or patients pink, and had no discernible side-effects. It was moreover cheap and easy to prepare. A report was forthwith published under the names of Tréfouël, Bovet and Nitti in the organ of the Society of Biology, the *Comptes rendus de la Société de Biologie*. Fourneau selflessly, but tactfully removed his name from the author list.

When the French publication reached Ebersfeld it struck like a bombshell. The most authentic description came from a German physiologist who was in the Bayer laboratory at the time and gave an account to Bovet many years later. Initially there was disbelief, then doubt, followed by experiments hastily executed, which upheld the French results, and finally there were recriminations. Why had the chemists been made to labour more than three years to no purpose? Why had so much money been so heedlessly spent? Why had so obvious a possibility not been considered by anyone? German science would be held up to ridicule. It would be the end of Bayer's patent, or so it must have seemed. Hörlein rallied his forces. Sulphanilamide was a commonplace compound, known to chemistry since 1908*; it had long been produced at the Leverkusen plant for use as an intermediate in various syntheses, and could clearly not be patented. The French answer was the obvious one: synthesise some close analogues with the same, or with luck perhaps a little better therapeutic potency, and it was not long before a new patentable drug, *Septazine* was put on the market by Rhône-Poulenc. Hörlein saw it differently. The Bayer name, he thought, would ensure that doctors and patients would prefer to put their faith in Prontosil, and so for a time it proved. There was, however, another theory, voiced by Fourneau and firmly espoused by many European researchers: they thought it scarcely credible that such meticulous and experienced

---

* The synthesis had been reported in that year by an Austrian chemist, Paul Gelmo, who had then been lost to view. He had, it transpired made his career as a chemist in the Royal and Imperial Printing Works - until, in 1949, a compatriot discovered that he was still alive and in Vienna. He was sought out and questioned about his work of four decades earlier. An account published in the *New York Times* the same year revealed that he had not made the connection between the compound he had synthesised so long ago and the substance that was which was now such a priceless remedy.

workers as the Germans could have omitted to try sulphanilamide for possible anti-bacterial characteristics, given that its presence in Prontosil and its relatives was indispensable for activity and worked wherever in the complex skeleton it was placed. An accusatory letter from Hörlein to Fourneau even hinted at it. Hörlein evidently found it hard to stomach the smugness of the French; the Bayer group, he told Fourneau were far ahead of the Pasteur, they were merely more fastidious in examining all aspects of their compounds' properties.

It seems this bluster can almost certainly be put down to understandable pique. The best evidence against hidden motives on Hörlein's part comes in fact from Daniel Bovet, who relates in his memoirs the story of a colloquy in 1981 with a surviving member of Hörlein's laboratory in Eberfeld. Ernst Auerhagen had been engaged by Hörlein as a physiologist in 1933 and had had regular contacts with Domagk's group. He had found Hörlein formidably intelligent, more feared than liked by his colleagues, and, like Domagk, autocratic by nature. He testified to the devastating impact of the article in the *Compt. rend. Soc. Biol.*, and he reacted with astonishment and indignation to the suggestion that Hörlein would have concealed so important a discovery as the therapeutic activity of sulphanilamide. This, he told Bovet, would have been wholly contrary to what was known of the man's character, for Hörlein had always opposed as a point of principle any secrecy in matters concerning drugs. Auerhagen had a ready explanation for the gaffe: the Germans, he said, were in thrall to the cult of dyes, from which a mighty dyestuff and pharmaceutical industry had arisen. Also, the shade of Paul Ehrlich, 'the man with the blue fingers', hovered over the country's bacteriologists and pharmacologists, and indeed his favourite Methylene Blue had made a great impact on therapeutics. Yet the history of science is replete with examples of failures to take note of what appeared obvious in retrospect and to break out of a set pattern of thought. It is worth recalling also that the highly accomplished French group found their way to sulphanilamide only by accident. Auerhagen offered an explanation for the long period of silence which followed the discovery of Prontosil: it was the relentless and meticulous testing on more animals of more species, a practice which continued unabated, and without which the drug would never have come to light in the first place.

The upshot

Domagk, looking for a way to save face, insisted without evidence that Prontosil was more specific in its action than sulphanilamide, which had a disseminated effect. The assertion became even less plausible when Jacques Tréfouël's deduction that Prontosil was broken down metabolically to release the active portion, sulphanilamide was proved correct. Bayer, though, had more pragmatic interests. Not only did the company advertise relentlessly the virtues of Prontosil, but it also embraced sulphanilamide, which it produced and sold under the name of *Prontosil album* (white Prontosil!) or elsewhere *Prontalbin* and *Prontylin*. The original Prontosil was now *Prontosil rubrum*, or 'red Prontosil'. Hörlein also took immediate measures, like the French, to repair the omission and look for modified sulphanilamides, preferably with improved properties, which could be patented. An able young chemist, Robert Behnisch was taken on and set to work with the help of Klarer and Mietzsch. The outcome was a pair of new drugs with modest and transient success, called Diseptal A and Diseptal B, later renamed *Uliran* and *Neo-Uliran*. Taken orally, they proved an unexpectedly useful treatment for gonorrhoea. More importantly, the success of sulphanilamide set off a frenzy of activity in pharmaceutical companies around the world, all intent on producing a patentable version of the original. Domagk ceased to concern himself with Prontosil and its offspring, and took refuge in cancer research.

In 1939 the Royal Swedish Academy announced the award of the Nobel Prize for Physiology or Medicine to Gerhard Domagk for 'recognising the antibacterial activity of Prontosil'. This curious citation betrays a certain unease among the grandees in Stockholm. Domagk had not invented or created Prontosil, nor did Prontosil long endure as the antibacterial of choice. Hörlein, in his lecture at the Royal Society of Medicine three years earlier, had expressed himself in the same cautious manner: the 'discovery' of Prontosil was due to Mietzsch and Klarer, while the 'observations' were made by Domagk. The two chemists who had toiled so heroically for over three years to produce new compounds by the hundreds, were bitterly resentful at seeing their work reduced to a footnote. Klarer, in particular, distanced himself from Domagk and struck out in another direction.

There was an echo of the conflict on the tenth anniversary in 1943 of the first therapeutic application of Prontosil, when Domagk published his reflections in a German journal. The text, under the title, 'Ten years of sulphamidotherapy', contains the tortuously worded sentence, 'In December 1932 the German chemists, Mietzsch and Klarer submitted on the basis of our experimental results a patent on the preparation of sulphamide compounds, which without that would have had no especial interest'. In the very next issue of the same journal there appeared a second article under the names of Domagk, Klarer and Miezsch, with the challenging title, 'Once more: ten years of sulphamidotherapy'. The authors note pointedly that their names appear in alphabetical order, and thet 'they contributed in equal measure to the solution of the problem'. The likelihood is that Mietzsch, who, after all, conceived the project in the first place, was the main guiding force. Bovet sagely observed of Domagk, 'the scientist makes the discovery, but the discovery makes the scientist'.

The award of the Nobel Prize seems perverse in another way: it was Fourneau and his group who had come up with the important discovery, and had opened a new avenue of drug research. The Prize therefore might arguably have gone to Fourneau, perhaps with Bovet, or at least might have been shared by Domagk and Fourneau. The French maintained a dignified silence. An added irony was that, by reason of a ruling of the

Nazi regime,* Domagk was prevented from accepting his prize. It was not until 1947 that he was able to shake hands with the King of Sweden, but under the terms of the Prize the money that went with it reverted to the Nobel Foundation. Klarer and Mietzsch were at least rewarded for their efforts by their cut of the patent rights on Prontosil and its satellite drugs.

Domagk returned to his laboratory in Eberfeld. Unlike Hörlein, he had not joined the Nazi party, and did his best to stay out of trouble. The Second World War began and research was now concentrated on materials for the treatment of wounds, and also on the growing problem of tuberculosis. Homosulphanilamide, called *Marfanil*, proved effective against forms of gas gangrene and tetanus, and even better was *Sulphathiazole*, a complex sulphanilamide derivative, synthesised by Behnisch, and used to treat a wide range of bacterial diseases, including pneumococcal pneumonia meningitis and staphylococcal infections. The prolific Behnisch also produced a related compound (benzaldehyde thiosemicarbazone, given the trade name, Conteben), with activity against tuberculosis. When properly tested later it proved to be too toxic to the liver to be useful, but it was the basis for somewhat more successful attempts. This progress was all the

---

* Three years earlier the Nobel Peace Prize had been awarded to a heroic journalist and pacifist, Carl von Ossietzky, who had spoken out against the depredations of the Nazi regime from the outset. He was imprisoned in a concentration camp when the award – an overtly political gesture by the Scandinavians – was announced, and Hitler forbade any German citizen henceforth to accept a Nobel Prize. Ossietzky was already dead, a victim of tuberculosis and maltreatment. Two German scientists were awarded the Nobel Prize for Chemistry at the same time as Domagk's in medicine. They were Richard Kuhn (an Austrian before the *Anschluss*, the absorption of Austria into Germany) and Adolf Butenandt, both of whom supported, or at the very least tolerated and profited from the regime, but they too were made to sign letters of refusal composed by party officials. An appeal to the Reichsmarschall, Hermann Göring elicited only the reply that the Nobel Prize was unwelcome to Germans. Domagk, who had written an apologetic letter to the Swedish Academy on receiving news of the award, was arrested and spent a week in a Gestapo prison. (He later related that when a warder asked him what crime he had committed he replied that he had won the Nobel Prize for Medicine. He then heard the warder tell a colleague in the corridor that he had a madman in his cell.) Domagk's house was searched, and after his release from prison he was prevented from attending a scientific conference at which he was to speak, on the pretext that he was ill.

more remarkable because of the impediments with which Domagk and Behnisch had to contend. There were destructive bombing raids and many privations, and the recurring problem imposed by the Nazi regime of an interdiction on the use of animals in research.* With the end of the war Domagk not only had his Nobel

Prize (minus the money) reinstated, but became an object of adulation as the inventor of the Sulfa drugs, as they were now called, and many honours were conferred on him from around the world. As for his employers, IG Farben there were questions to be answered. An Allied military court was set up to investigate the company's activities in the foregoing years. Twenty-three of the senior figures in the company were arraigned on charges of plundering property in occupied countries, of complicity in crimes against peace, membership of the SS, supplying material (Zyklon B) for the murder of victims in concentration camps, and, worst of all, enslavement of forced labourers in the company's own camp-within-a-camp in Auschwitz-Monowitz, which housed the Buna factory. Twelve of the accused were sentenced to periods in prison (from which they

---

* The original legislation, promulgated for the state of Prussia by Hermann Göring in his capacity as Prime Minister, condemned transgressors to confinement in a concentration camp until such time as sentence was pronounced. The ban was soon extended to Bavaria and other regions and caused consternation in the pharmaceutical laboratories. Hitler and many of those who surrounded him were devotees of what is now called 'alternative medicine', of homeopathy, herbal healing and the like. Their tender concern for animals contrasted bizarrely with their attitudes to people. Hörlein was compelled, at some risk to himself, to intercede and had trying encounters with representatives of the regime. When the consequences of a ban on animal testing for the supply of medicines to the military was made clear, the legislation was modified to allow some loopholes, but laboratories like Bayer's were forced to prepare applications for all projects involving the use of animals and to submit to regular inspections. As time went on it became easier to violate the regulations, and often the authorities would turn a blind eye. This was not the only problem Hörlein had to contend with, for IG Farben and Hörlein himself had become a target for hostility from the Nazi-controlled press for their international interests. The fruits of its research, it was said, were assisting foreign powers. Patents merely made new discoveries available for foreign exploitation, and a patent embargo was accordingly imposed on grounds of military necessity. To give away military secrets was an offence punishable by death. Pharmaceutical profits were instantly compromised.

First Do No Harm

were quite soon released), and the remainder were acquitted. Among this group was Hörlein, who emerges from the turmoil as an essentially honourable man. He had, it appeared, put a stop to consignments of drugs to Auschwitz on learning that they were destined for experiments on captives (for which the leading SS doctor was executed). Hörlein, despite his membership of the Nazi party, which had allowed him some room to negotiate with the regime, seemed to have had little sympathy with the Nazi movement. In Paris, on the other hand, Ernest Fourneau was less fortunate. He had continued to enjoy life among the *beau monde* throughout the occupation, and it did not escape notice that he had found the company of the occupying Germans congenial, had indeed attended functions at their Embassy. He was denounced as a collaborator but was not persecuted beyond dismissal from his position as a *chef de service* at the Pasteur Institute. He remained in the laboratory however, and busied himself once more at the bench, but no discoveries of note had emerged by the time he died in 1949.

The march of the Sulfa drugs

The end of the war saw also an end to the dominance of the German pharmaceutical industry. Large research-based companies had sprung up in Britain, and especially in the United States, boosted in no small measure by the possibilities that the so-called Sulpha (or Sulfa) drugs had opened up. In the late 1930s this had begun to turn into a free-for-all. In the ensuing decade, before the appearance of the antibiotics, thousands of new compounds were offered to doctors or sold over the counter. Most of the Sulpha drugs had low toxicity, but taken, as they often were, in excessive doses, they could engender serious side-effects. An infamous episode with a different cause unfolded in the United States in 1937. Sulphanilamide had acquired a sudden cachet when it saved the son of the President, Franklin Roosevelt, from impending death by septicaemia, and it became widely prescribed. A doctor in a small town in Mississippi had administered a preparation marketed as Elixir Sulfanilamide by a small pharmaceutical operation in Tennessee, S.E. Massengill and Co. Within a day all thirteen of the doctor's patients who had received the drug were desperately ill or dying. Soon after, a doctor in Tulsa, Oklahoma saw several of his patients, mainly children, die, apparently of kidney failure, after taking Elixir Sulfanilamide, and contacted the American Medical Association. The Food and Drug Administration, the FDA, was alerted and an investigation was immediately begun at the University of Chicago. It turned out that the Massengill Company had distributed 700 bottles of their medicine to doctors and sales representatives, and another 600 to pharmacies to sell over the counter. The new drug, of foreign provenance and uncertain purity, was the immediate suspect, but the true explanation quickly came to light: Harold Watkins, Massengill's chief chemist, seeking a way to bring the insoluble sulphanilamide into solution and make it palatable, especially to children, had found a solvent. It was diethylene glycol, and he had for good measure also added some red dye and a raspberry flavour. Diethylene glycol is toxic.* Massengill sent recall notices, but without any urgent warning. The company claimed through its lawyer that the Elixir had been fully tested, but an FDA investigation revealed that no tests had been done. The Elixir caused 107 deaths and probably many more cases of kidney damage. Soon after, the famous 1938 Food, Drugs and Cosmetic Act was passed into law by Congress. One consequence was that less than twenty years later, the FDA averted the thalidomide catastrophe in America (p.). Harold Watkins shot himself, whether by accident or intent was not established. It could be said that his culpable negligence in the end saved incalculable later misery.

The way of discovery: fortune and the prepared mind

One problem associated with the use of heavy doses of sulphanilamide resulted from its low solubility. This could lead to the formation of crystals in the kidney, which might then pass into the urethra with painful consequences. More soluble derivatives were developed, the first of which, sulphacetamide (trade name, *Albucid*), was prepared by German chemists

---

* It was then, and still is used as an antifreeze, and has been at the centre of other scandals, most recently when it was discovered in wine, added to enhance body and sweetness. Consumers of the wine were injured, and considerable economic damage to innocent growers also resulted.

at the Schering laboratories in Berlin, and was used for some years, especially for urinary tract infections. There were many more variants, but much the most important sprang in 1938 from the laboratories of a modest English pharmaceutical company, May & Baker in Dagenham, not far from London. The head of research, Arthur James Ewins (1882-1957), the son of a railway worker, had started his career as a seventeen-year-old laboratory assistant at the Wellcome Physiological Research Laboratories, where he worked with several distinguished scientists, including Henry Dale (p.). Ewins acquired a London University chemistry degree through evening classes, and at the age of twenty-four was made head of the chemistry division at the Wellcome. In this capacity he became more closely associated with Dale, who thought him an able chemist with an unusual talent for developing a research project, if somewhat lacking in imagination. Then in 1914 Dale left to become the first director of the new National Institute for Medical Research in London, and Ewins accompanied him.

Almost immediately the Institute was turned over to the demands of the war. Much of the effort went into the development of medicines to replace those no longer available from Germany, and the work brought Dale and Ewins into contact with British pharmaceutical manufacturers, including May & Baker. This led in 1917 to Ewins's departure from Dale's institute for the May & Baker laboratories, then in south London, as director of research. Came the end of the war, and Ewins was able to develop new interests. The company did well in an unspectacular way until, in late1935, the news of sulphanilamide broke, and the decision was taken to follow where Fourneau and later Bayer so profitably led. Whether this was due solely to Ewins, as director of research is unclear, for there may also have been some discussion with the management of Rhône-Poulenc, which had acquired a controlling share in May & Baker. Ewins's plan, at all events, was to explore the effects of introducing substituents on one of the two nitrogen atoms in the molecule. Ewins had a small group of capable chemists at his command, one of whom, George Newbery had already pulled off the synthesis of Prontosil, based on the information in the German patent, though just after it had been accomplished in Foutneau's laboratory in Paris. Newbery and another of Ewins's chemists, Montague

Phillips set about producing new derivatives, which were then sent for testing to one of the country's leading pathologists, Lionel Whitby at the Middlesex Hospital in London.* Whitby assayed dozens of compounds from May & Baker for their antibacterial activity in mice, and for a long time there was no sign of any improvement on the parent compound. Then one day in October of 1937 Dame Fortune smiled in Dagenham.

The sequence of events has been reconstructed by the historian of science, John E. Lesch (*The First Miracle Drug – How the Sulfa Drugs Transformed Medicine*) from a transcript of a conference on the history of the discovery, held in 1961. A May & Baker researcher, perhaps Newbery, came upon a dusty bottle on a laboratory shelf. L.E. Hart, one of the chemists, recalled that it had reposed, to be precise, on the front of the third shelf to the left of a cupboard. It contained 2-aminopyridine, a simple enough compounds, which had been prepared in 1930 by another May & Baker chemist, Eric Baines for use by a colleague, who had long since left. The compound had thus never been put to the forgotten use for which it had been intended. What then prompted the decision seven years later to take this bottle, rather than any other, off the shelf and use it for an unrelated synthesis? Merely, it seems, the accidental circumstance that it sat in a visible position at the front of the shelf. Baines thought, though, that anyone asking him to synthesise some 2-aminopyridine could have wanted it only for the purposes of the sulphanilamide project. As he explained to a curious colleague, 'You would set out to try and make something, and you would find something on the shelf, and you would try it'.

It was Newbery who performed the coupling reaction, or at any rate instructed a laboratory assistant identified only as 'Alexander', to do so. Montague Phillips had played a part in defining the final step after coupling (deacetylation) to yield the desired product. The sulphapyridine, as it was termed for short, was entered in the laboratory log as T693.

---

* Whitby was an imposing figure. Heroic service in the Great War had deprived him of a leg, despite which he re-enlisted as a colonel in the Royal Army Medical Corps at the start of the Second World War. He ended his career as a knight of the realm, Regius Professor of Physic (that is to say Medicine) at Cambridge University, and finally its vice-chancellor.

This was later designated *M&B 693*, under which name it became famous. (A canard appeared in the press that 692 such compounds had previously been prepared and tested, but such numbers referred in reality to compounds synthesised for a wide range of projects.) Whitby was away when the sample of T693 reached the Middlesex Hospital, and there were no streptococcal culture on hand, so Whitby's assistant injected doses into mice infected with the deadly pneuococci. The results were startling: all the mice survived. On Whitby's return further assays were performed on mice infected with streptococci, staphylococci, meningiococci and gonococci. T693 gave protection against all of them. This was unprecedented. Ewins, on receiving the news, sent a sample of the compound to a pharmacologist for toxicity tests. It proved harmless in therapeutic doses. Several members of the laboratory at May & Baker thereupon swallowed doses of T693 with no ill-effects, and soon thereafter it was tried on a dangerously ill human subject, a farm worker, who quickly recovered.

The next step was to adapt the laboratory preparation to the industrial scale. This proved to be no trivial matter. Amongst other problems, one of the intermediates in the synthesis of 2-aminopyridine was highly explosive, and the problem was only overcome with the help of chemists or chemical engineers from Rhône-Poulenc, and not before there had been one serious accident. A report by Whitby on the prodigious new drug in *The Lancet* and clinical trials on patients in a hospital in Birmingham followed, and it seemed clear that M&B 693 was indeed the magic bullet which everyone from the time of Ehrlich had sought. Later of course a more rigorous search revealed that, like every other drug, M&B 693, pushed to the limit, had side-effects, in particular the formation of crystals in the urethra, which could cause distressing blockages. Nevertheless, the drug almost instantly rendered obsolete the erratic serum therapy, which had previously given the only hope of a cure for lethal infections, and the many wholly ineffective treatments commonly used. In the United States M&B 693 was made under licence by the Merck company and sold as Sulphapyridine Merck. In the years that followed well over a thousand sulphanilamide-based drugs were produced, some with advantages over Sulphapyridine, such as slower elimination from the body through the kidneys, most merely patentable variants. One of the most useful, sulphathiazole, M&B 760, is still prescribed, mainly to treat gonorrhoea. By far the greatest number of new products emerged from the rapidly expanding pharmaceutical industry in the United States.

The Sulpha (in America Sulfa) drugs undoubtedly saved thousands of lives on the battlefields of the Second World War. They were even used prophylactically in the U.S. Army, and reportedly caused a large reduction in the incidence of infections. The crowning moment for the Sulpha drugs came in December of 1943 when Winston Churchill, returning from the Tehran conference with Roosevelt and Stalin, which was meant to establish the new world order after the war, was smitten with pneumonia. Landing in Cairo in a perilous state, he was seen by army doctors, who wanted to treat him with the latest 'miracle drug' penicillin, which had just come on stream. His personal doctor, the egregious Charles Wilson, Lord Moran, refused to consider (in which the second accompanying physician, Dr Bedford apparently concurred), and insisted on a sulphanilamide, probably M&B 693, which happily worked. Later Moran (known in the profession as 'Corkscrew Charlie' by reason of his well-known deviousness), put it about that it was penicillin which had worked the wonderful cure. He was Dean of St. Mary's Hospital Medical School in London, where Fleming (p.) observed the effect of the *Penicillium* mould on a bacterial culture, and Moran wanted to advertise the lustre of his School. As for Churchill, he made a joke of the episode, deliberately conflating his doctors, M and B, with May & Baker.

There was no Nobel Prize for M&B 693, even though it undoubtedly saved many more lives than Prontosil and its immediate successors ever did. Who in any case would have merited the crown? Would it have been Ewins, who initiated the project? Or perhaps his distant superiors at Rhône-Poulenc who may have wished it on him? Perhaps Newbery, who took the dusty bottle off the shelf, or Baines who put it there? Phillips perhaps, who thought up the deacetylation reaction, or Alexander the laboratory assistant, who actually performed the synthesis? The history of science is rich in such accidental discoveries to which no single person can lay claim, and which are often dignified by the word, serendipity. There were at least competent people to exploit their luck. It was only Phillips who loudly complained that his contribution had received no commendation or reward; he thought this was a consequence of his proletarian origins (not unlike that of Ewins). Ewins was rewarded by election to the Fellowship of the Royal Society, but none of the others seem to have profited.

A final twist to the sulphonamide story arose out of the observation that the effect of the drugs on infected wounds was attenuated by abundant pus (white blood cells), and also when there was much dead tissue. Whitby remarked also on the time lapse before the bactericidal effect set in. He conjectured that it impeded the assimilation of essential metabolites on which the growth and multiplication of the bacteria depended. In 1940 two researchers in Oxford, Paul Fildes and a young research fellow in his laboratory, Donald Woods tackled the problem. They found that tissue extracts, and even an extract from yeast cultures, inhibited the action of the drug. These, and the white cells all had in common, then, a constituent which destroyed or sequestered either the drug or something in the bacteria on which it acted. It was this second possibility that was a major insight. Suppose, they argued, that the sulphanilamide compound resembled something the bacteria required to grow and derived from the environment – the wound for instance - in which they thrived. If this was so the drug might act by competing with the vital metabolite at the point at which it acted. Thus, when the surrounding tissue supplied more of the metabolite it could overcome the action of the drug. Woods set out to search for such a molecule in tissue extracts, guided by what was then known of bacterial metabolism. One of the compounds known to be implicated in bacterial growth, which at the same time looked rather like a sulphanilamide, was para-aminobenzoic acid (PABA for short). PABA was available from the major chemical supply house, and Woods bought some. He later described the moment when he examined the bacterial culture to which the drug and PABA had been added and saw that the bacteria were alive and doing well, as the most exciting event in his life. The drug was competing with the metabolite. The discovery had implications far beyond the mechanism of action of Sulpha drugs. It was what the philosopher of science, Thomas Kuhn termed 'a paradigm shift', for it redirected much of the thinking in physiological and biochemical research. First it implied that the bacteria had, in effect, receptors for metabolic compounds or drugs – the concept prefigured a half century earlier by Ehrlich (p.). Secondly it introduced the principle of competitive inhibition – of two substances competing for a site at which one of them normally exerts its action. Obvious as this may seem to us now, it was certainly not so then, and it became a guiding precept in much of the drug research that came after. As for the Sulfa drugs, their pre-eminence waned as resistant strains of bacteria emerged, and more especially when penicillin and other antibiotics were discovered and almost entirely supplanted them.

Chapter 11

ANTIBIOTICS: THE NEW AGE DAWNS

Prehistory

The term is an old one, but 'antibiotic' gained its modern meaning with the discovery of penicillin. Indeed, the Oxford English Dictionary defines **antibiotic *n.*** as 'A medicine (such as penicillin or its derivatives) that inhibits the growth of or destroys micro-organisms'. Earlier definitions restricted antibiotics to compounds produced (like penicillin) by micro-organisms. But today the spread of resistance of pathogens to the available natural antibiotics makes the need for new, often purely synthetic compounds ever more pressing. The term, antibiosis, or *antibiose*, was coined in fact in the late 19th century by a French microbiologist, professor at the Medical School of Nancy University, Paul Vuillemin, but did not enter the vocabulary of scientists, much less the public, until a century later, and then it was suddenly on everyone's lips. So much for the semantics then, but the substance has lain more deeply buried under a layer of obfuscation, legend and hyperbole. It had been put about and was universally believed that the discovery of the first antibiotic, penicillin sprang from a flash of inspired insight by a bacteriologist at St. Mary's Hospital in London, Alexander Fleming in September of 1928. This distorted version of the events had its origins in the relentless publicity generated by Fleming's obstreperous Greek wife, Amalia, by the accounts offered by Fleming himself, and by the then Dean of St. Mary's Hospital Medical School, the aforementioned Lord Moran, and amplified by early biographers, and a chauvinistic press.

The belief that moulds and other fungi possessed curative virtues originated in ancient times. There are allusions in Hippocrates and Pliny, and in the folk medicine of European and Asian countries to the application of mouldy bread to wounds to prevent or eliminate infections. Over the years many physicians, biologists and others studied the effects of moulds on infections and on cultures of micro-organisms, and some made attempts to extract the substances responsible. Thus, in 1870 John Scott Burdon Sanderson (whose work on animal parasites we have already encountered [p.]), a doctor and physiologist, then at St. Mary's Hospital in London, two generations before Fleming, noted in 1870 that a bacterial culture medium contaminated with mould would not support the growth of the bacteria. He imparted the information to his friend, Joseph Lister, whose interest in antisepsis was already well-known (p.). Lister investigated further, and even treated a nurse with infected wounds with a *Penicillium* mould. (The name derives from the dog Latin, *penicillum*, a paintbrush, alluding to the mould's appearance, and given to it by Alexander Fleming.) Next came William Roberts, a doctor, later professor of medicine in Manchester, who wrote in 1874 that he had found the growth of bacteria to be incompatible with that of 'fungi' in the same culture. The next year John Tyndall (p.) at the Royal Institution in London took an interest in the phenomenon and gave a demonstration of the killing of bacteria by *Penicillium* moulds. Tyndall's were much the most thoroughly designed experiments that had yet been done. He tested culture media in the form of broths prepared from a wide range of animal and plant tissues, set up numerous replicates and watched for the arrival of bacteria and mould spores from the air, for like Pasteur, he had established that bacteria and other micro-organisms were carried on the breeze. Sometimes, he found, the cultures contained growing bacteria, sometimes moulds, but never both. Where a mould had established itself the bacteria, if there were any, had turned into a dead sludge, and where there were thriving bacteria, no mould grew. It was, he wrote, 'the struggle for existence between the bacteria and the *Penicillium*. 'In some tubes the former were triumphant, and in others tubes of the same infusion the latter was triumphant!' Vuillemin, for his part, saw antibiosis as part of a general phenomenon, the inverse of symbiosis (the interdependence of two life forms). On this interpretation antibiosis could be taken, rather profitlessly, to include the relation of predator to prey, and the killing of animals or plants by parasites. Pasteur had summed up the principle very simply in 1877: 'La vie empêche la vie' – life impedes life. He was concerned of course only with microbes, and described quite explicitly the failure of a micro-organism to thrive in a favourable medium if that medium was also host to a different organism. He even foresaw therapeutic promise in such systems.

In the last two decades of the 19th century there were a number of publications along these lines, describing an antagonism between two bacterial species, and even some reports of cures through the expulsion of a pathogenic by a benign bacterium. This was later termed 'replacement therapy'. A probably impure bactericidal substance from a cultured bacterium – a true antibiotic – was prepared during the 1890s by two German bacteriologists, Rudolf Emmerich and Oscar Löw. Its origin was a species of bacteria found in green wounds, then called *Bacillus pyocyaneus*, but now known as *Pseudomonas aeruginosa*. He bactericidal substance was exuded by the bacteria when the culture aged, and it killed a range of pathogens *in vitro*. This *pyocyanase* as its discoverers called it in the mistaken belief that it was an enzyme (thus a protein), raised high hopes. It came into quite wide clinical use, and was indeed the first antibiotic ever deployed in hospitals, but it was erratic in its activity and quite toxic, and after a brief vogue was abandoned.

In 1896 and 1897 came the first properly scientific studies of antibiosis by *Penicillium* moulds. Bartolomeo Gosio (1863-1944) was a highly accomplished Italian microbiologist and doctor, head of the research department at the State Health Service in Rome. At the time he was studying the causes of pellagra, a disease which afflicted the poor, whose diet often comprised little but maize. It was not then known that the pellagra was the result of a vitamin B deficiency, and Gosio had the idea that it might be linked to an infestation of the maize by a mould, as ergotism is to a mould in grain (p.). He did indeed find a mould – a *Penicillium* – in his sample of stored maize, and out of it he prepared a water extract, and from that extract crystals of an antibiotic. The substance inhibited the growth of anthrax bacilli. This, as Howard Florey wrote forty years later, was the first preparation of a crystalline antibiotic. It was not penicillin, for the mould was not *Penicillium notatum*, but another species, *Penicillium brevicompactum*, and the antibiotic was later given the name, mycophenolic acid. It was never used to treat infections, for it proved to be a powerful immunosuppressant – a substance which suppresses the function of the immune system – but many years later it found its application in transplant surgery to prevent rejection of the donor organ.

The second discovery, more remarkable in that it was made by a young army officer, Ernest Dufresne (1874-1912) studying at the military medical service hospital in Lyon. Dufresne had noticed that the colonial Arabic stable boys would store their horses' saddles in a warm, damp room to encourage the growth of mould. When questioned they told him that the mould would prevent or reduce the development of saddle-sores. This piqued Dufresne's interest, and he decided to study the properties of moulds for his doctoral thesis. In a careful series of experiments he first treated guinea pigs, infected with typhoid, with mould from the leather, and found that they did not die. Then he prepared extracts from the common *Penicillium glaucum* mould and injected it into guinea pigs which he also dosed with typhoid bacilli. Unlike the controls, these animals again survived. Dufresne failed to interest the grandees of the Pasteur Institute in his discovery, and they may not in fact have troubled to read his communication, so all that remained was his thesis. Nor in fact did his military duties allow him the opportunity to continue his work. Dufresne died of tuberculosis at the age of thirty-seven.

So it continued. In 1908 a Swiss, Adriano Sturli (1873-1964) published a paper on a 'toxin' contained in *Penicillium glaucum*. This had the effect of preventing the growth of anthrax bacilli added to a culture. Over the next few years a doctor working at the Pasteur Institute in Paris, Albert Vaudremer (1866-1943) published a series of studies on a mould of a different kind. *Aspergillus fumigans* is one of hundreds of species of *Aspergillus*, widespread in nature, familiar in the kitchen as contaminants of starchy and sugary foods, and for the most part harmless. Vaudremer found that an extract killed tubercle bacilli in culture, and encouraged by this result and by the lack of toxicity, he and his clinical colleagues tried it on patients in hospitals and sanatoria. In 1913 Vaudremer told that over the preceding three years the extract had been given to more than 200 patients. None had suffered any ill-effects, but, as to the outcome, he was cautious and unwilling to assert that such improvements as there had been might not have reflected merely instances of spontaneous remission of the disease. The extract has a place in history as the first antibiotic used in the clinic, but its efficacy remained uncertain. Nevertheless, *Aspergillus fumigans* later yielded four different antibiotics, and more were derived from other *Aspergillus* species. During the period from 1923 up to the Second World War the pace of discovery accelerated. The first substantial advance came from the laboratory of André Gratia (1893-1950), working at the Institut Pasteur de Brabant in Brussels and the Free University in the same city. Gratia and his colleague, Sara Dath described in 1925 the effect of *Penicillium glaucum* on a culture of anthrax bacilli: the turbid culture became clear, signalling the lysis (that is to say bursting) of the bacteria, which become almost transparent on shedding their contents. They inferred that the mould secreted a substance that destroyed the bacteria. But Gratia's main interest at the time was actinomycetes, also known as 'ray fungi', a curious group of filamentous bacteria with attributes of fungi. They live mainly in soil and derive their nutrients from decaying plant or animal matter. Actinomycetes were to acquire huge importance in the hunt for better antibiotics, prefigured in Gratia's researches. He and his team found that their species of actinomycetes had the capacity to destroy a wide range of pathogenic bacteria. The filtered preparation from the cultures were injected into rabbits and guinea pigs, which were not incommoded, notwithstanding the deadly character of the bacteria from which the solution had been derived. These were sensational results, and their impact deepened when Gratia was able to report in 1930 that many human subjects with serious infections had been successfully treated, apparently without appreciable side effects. Gratia went on to do much distinguished work but never pursued his discovery of antibiotics any further. This was said to have been the result of a long bout of illness which kept him away from the laboratory. His strains of moulds died, and he had other interests, to which he was evidently eager to return. Why Gratia's therapeutic preparation fell out of use is equally unclear, but doubt about the importance of his contribution is beyond doubt.

The rise and rise of Alexander Fleming

In a letter to *The Lancet* by in 1999, many years after the events here related, three scientists from the Free University of Brussels, where Gratia is plainly not forgotten, remind the journal's readers of the man and his work. The great bacteriologist, Jules Bordet, under whom Gratia learned his trade, might have said, they suggest: 'My boy, the trouble with you is that you do not baptize your children'. For Fleming, when he gave it the name, penicillin, was no closer to identifying the active constituent in the *Penicillium* extract than Gratia had been. In truth, the real handicap under which Gratia, and indeed Gosio, Duchesne and the others laboured was that they had no Howard Florey to seize the problem and run with it.

Alexander (Alec to his friends) Fleming was born in 1881 in Ayrshire in Scotland, the seventh of eight children of a farmer. The family's circumstances were difficult, and at the age of fourteen Alexander moved to London to find work. He received his education through evening classes at the Regent Street Polytechnic (which seventy years later metamorphosed into the University of Westminster), while working first as an office-boy and then as a clerk in a shipping agency. But he had higher ambitions and great determination, and in 1902 he won a scholarship to St. Mary's Hospital Medical School, which, after graduating in 1908, he never left. At St. Mary's he caught the eye of the imperious Professor Colonel Sir Almroth Wrighoringt, a man of strong opinions and much influence.* Wright, who was something of a pioneer in the application of vaccines, had founded (and directed until he retired at the age of eighty-five) the Inoculation Department at St. Mary's, and he was notoriously intolerant

---

* George Bernard Shaw had come to know Wright, a habitué of London literary circles, and had been allowed to visit the laboratory. There he supposedly overheard a conversation about which of two patients should be treated with a serum of which too little was available for both. Shaw tapped his nose and said, 'I smell drama'. This encounter gave rise apparently to Shaw's great play, *The Doctor's Dilemma*, in which Wright appears as the physician-immunologist, Sir Colenso Ridgeon.

of drugs. When the Great War came Wright, who had served in the Royal Army Medical Corps in the Boer War, returned to the colours with the rank of Colonel. He persuaded the military authorities to set up a hospital in Boulogne, dedicated to the treatment of infected wounds, and there Fleming joined him, and acquired his enduring interest in bacteriology and the treatment of infections. He never deviated from this objective to the end of his working life. In time he was to succeed Wright as head of what is now the Wright-Fleming Institute at St. Mary's Hospital.

Fleming was a skilful and methodical laboratory worker. His first, and as he rightly believed best discovery came in 1922, sparked characteristically by an accident. He took advantage of the cold from which he was suffering to see what kinds of bacteria might be reproducing in his nasal secretions. He plated out a sample on the agar gel in a Petri dish (p.) and by the next day colonies of various kinds of bacteria were growing. On closer examination the dish disclosed to Fleming that a few of the colonies appeared to be dissolving. Fleming scraped such a colony from the agar and again cultured (sub-cultured in the jargon) the surviving bacteria in a liquid medium. Into this he dropped a little of his nasal mucus and was delighted to see the bacterial suspension clearing. The inference was that the dissolving colonies on the Petri dish belonged to a previously unrecognised bacterial species which was susceptible to a component of nasal mucus. Fleming guessed that this would turn out to be an enzyme, and so indeed it transpired when it was isolated many years later. Fleming called it lysozyme, and the susceptible bacterium (with the benefit of Almroth Wright's classical education), *Micrococcus lysodeikticus*. Lysozymes (differing in detail from Fleming's enzyme) are ubiquitous. They turned up in many bodily fluids from tears to saliva, and also in egg white. They give protection against a select number of infections by dismantling the cell wall that encases the bacteria. But lysozyme has no effect on the major pathogens, such as streptococci and staphylococci, and although Fleming invested much time in studying it further, it never found any practical application, nor did it excite much interest.

The vastly more important discovery – perhaps more properly rediscovery – came about seven years later by an outrageously improbable chance. Doubts have always surrounded the sequence of events, mainly obfuscated apparently by Fleming himself. In 1928 he was working on staphylococci, especially the dangerous yellow *Staphylococcus aureus*. That summer he broke off his work for a five-week holiday, and because of the restricted bench space in his cramped laboratory he pushed the many Petri dishes containing experimental cultures into a corner to allow one of his colleagues access to the bench during his absence. On his return in September he inspected the plates, recorded what they revealed, and and dropped them into a tray of disinfectant. (The glass Petri dishes would be cleaned, sterilised and re-used, whereas the plastic ones in use today are thrown away.) It was at this time that Merlin Pryce, an assistant of Fleming's who had recently left, appeared in the laboratory to ask how the work had been progressing. To illustrate a point he was making Fleming grabbed a handful of the Petri dishes from the top of the pile in the disinfectant vessel and therefore not immersed. While showing one of these to Pryce something caught Fleming's attention. 'Here's a funny thing', he said. The agar in the dishes, which had lain on the bench the last five weeks, had become mouldy, but in this dish a clear ring could be seen around one spot of mould. (The plate is now a historical relic in the care of the Science Museum in London.)

Fleming decided to follow up his observation. He consulted a mycologist (an expert on fungi, including moulds), C.L. LaTouche, who had a laboratory on the floor below. LaTouche opined, wrongly, that the mould was *Penicillium rubrum*, when it was in actuality *Penicillium notatum*. (Both are relatively rare species.) Fleming scraped away some of the mould from the agar plate, cultured it and tried its effect of a filtered extract on different species of pathogenic bacteria. The results were most interesting: the extract stopped the growth of the bacteria, even at high dilution. Fleming injected it into a mouse and a rabbit and observed no ill-effects. A young assistant of Fleming's volunteered to test it on himself for any toxic effects. He cultured a sample in milk, and reported that the solid mould tasted not disagreeable – rather like Stilton cheese. Again there were no consequences. Then Fleming dropped some extract into the eyes of a laboratory technician, who was suffering from the eye infection, pneumococcal conjunctivitis, and was instantly cured. (This gave the greatest satisfaction to Fleming, a keen and highly competitive sportsman and captain of the St. Mary's Hospital shooting team of which, with a match in prospect, the technician was a member.) Thereafter, although there were no proper clinical trials, or even tests on infected animals, the antiseptic, as Fleming called it and to which he gave the name, penicillin, was used to treat a few cases of skin infections. It was also used sporadically, so Fleming later said, to soak bandages on infected wounds. He had clearly lost all interest in any wider applications that might flow from his discovery, and now saw only one purpose that it might serve. He had been struck that the mould did not kill all bacteria, and there was one, on which his interest happened just then to be focussed, that was totally resistant. *Haemophilus influenzae*, a pathogen originally thought to cause influenza (which is actually a viral disease), is the agent of a variety of unpleasant infections. It was also notoriously difficult to culture and isolate. Fleming's idea was to use penicillin to eliminate contaminating bacteria from *Haemophilus influenzae* cultures.

Fleming seemed to be fixated on this modest aim, and in so far as there was further progress at St. Mary's towards isolating the active constituent from the mould, it was not due to him, but to two young doctors, both in their twenties, who were doing stints in the laboratory at the time. Stuart Craddock (the man who had eaten the mould) and Frederick Ridley (later a distinguished ophthalmic surgeon), made a brave attempt to isolate the active principle from the mould extract – the true penicillin. They proceeded as chemists did (and do): they tried extraction from the watery solution with solvents, and then drying their extracts under vacuum to prevent oxidation. They also examined a range of storage conditions in an effort to find those in which the product would be most stable. In this they had only limited success, for the penicillin always lost its potency in a matter of days. They did however establish that it was a small molecule, not a protein, and they managed to obtain preparations of much increased potency in impeding the growth of bacteria. Fleming, whose ignorance of chemistry seems to have been rather comprehensive, took no interest in this work, but did not oppose it. He made no further contributions to the evolution of antibiotics, and for close on a decade penicillin lay dormant.

The most remarkable aspect of the story up to this point is the confluence of improbabilities that led to Fleming's observation, which was much more a product of luck than those of his predecessors, Gosio, Duchesne, Vaudremer and Gratia. First Fleming had picked a Petri dish at random out of the disinfectant bath, only because Merlin Pryce had happened to call on that day, before the plates had been washed; secondly it chanced to be one of the few that had not sunk into the disinfectant fluid; then a *Penicillium* spore had entered the room five or six weeks before and settled on this one plate; that spore had belonged to the uncommon *Penicillium notatum*, which happened to be the species that produces much the largest amount of penicillin (otherwise any clear zone on the plate would almost certainly have been too insignificant to catch the eye). Ronald Hare, a doctor and microbiologist who was at St. Mary's at the time and made a study of the circumstances surrounding Fleming's discovery, noted that when American pharmaceutical laboratories began to explore the properties of *Penicillium* moulds in the 1940s they found only three species out of some hundreds that produced high concentrations of penicillin. One of those three was the *Penicillium notatum*, which La Touche in his mycology laboratory on the floor below Fleming had been culturing. Not only was this an uncommon species, but Hare also tells us that the windows of Fleming's laboratory were never opened for fear of allowing cultures of pathogens, kept on the window-ledge, from falling on passers-by in the street below. But there was more: Fleming had assumed, as did others, that penicillin functions, like lysozyme, by dissolving the bacterial cell wall, but this is not so. An Oxford microbiologist, A.D. Gardner showed that it exerts its killing effect during cell division, and therefore acts only on growing bacteria, and not at all on mature, established colonies. So, says Hare, the *Penicillium* spore must have been on Fleming's famous plate before he seeded the bacterial colonies. Yet Fleming would surely not have wanted to perform an experiment on a dish contaminated with a ripe growth of mould. Bacteria grow much faster than moulds, so the patch of *Penicillium* must have appeared during the days or weeks that the plate was left on the bench. How then could the established bacterial colonies around the mould have been lysed? Ronald Hare's suggestion was that Fleming, a habitually forgetful and disorganised worker, had omitted to put his seeded plate in the incubator, as was the standard practice, to bring about bacterial growth overnight. From the weather records for the period in question Hare learned that early August that year, when Fleming had left for his family holiday, was unseasonally cold. Under these conditions mould grows well, but the bacteria lie more or less dormant. There followed a period when the temperature rose from 16°C (60°F) to 27°C (80°F), at which the growing bacteria would have encountered penicillin and promptly burst. Hare even did experiments to support his inference. At any rate, no better explanation of the mystery has ever been offered.

There is no doubt that Fleming was an astute, if messy, laboratory worker with an eye for the odd and unexpected – some of those who worked with him testified to that – and he loved, as he would put it, playing with bacteria. He even cultivated a hobby of making pictures, much admired, from bacteria of different colours, plated out in artistic patterns. He was a kindly and affable man, well liked by his colleagues, but at best a middle-rank scientist, as he himself recognised. Certainly he seems to have been a poor judge of what was interesting and important. As a shrewd self-publicist, though, Fleming was masterly. There is no reference in his publications to Gosio, Gratia or any of those who preceded him in the discovery of the antibacterial properties of *Penicillium*, even though, as a punctilious reader of the literature he would certainly have known of their work. He was careful to leave it to others to inflame the press with proclamations of an epic discovery by the modest, publicity-shy Scottish genius, toiling devotedly in his dingy little lab by Paddington railway station for the benefit of humankind. This was certainly the impression he made on the horde of newspapermen who made a track to Praed Street (where a blue plaque now marks the spot). Fleming certainly made no attempt to minimise his contribution, and was abundantly rewarded. Even in America his picture found its way onto the cover of *Time*. The lists of his medals, honorary degrees, freedoms of cities and other marks of esteem, occupy several pages in his various biographies. He died of a heart attack in 1955. It was left to a far greater scientist than Fleming to turn penicillin into a milestone in the march of medicine.

The taciturn Australian

That great scientist was Howard Walter Florey (1898-1968). He was the antithesis of Fleming, the intellectual magpie, flitting from one transiently alluring object to another. Florey's way was to seize on an interesting problem and pursue it with remorseless thoroughness to its conclusion. Born in Adelaide, Florey qualified as a doctor at the local university. Soon after, he took ship for England, and went first to Oxford to gain experience in neurophysiology under one of the commanding figures in the field, Sir Charles Sherrington. After two years he moved to London for a year of research at the London Hospital, and thence to Cambridge, where he branched out into new areas of physiology, especially the mechanism and control of mucus secretion and its supposed relation to inflammation. His talents were recognised, and in 1931 he was appointed Professor of Pathology at the University of Sheffield. By then he was married to another Australian doctor, who later joined him in the laboratory, but the union was turbulent and his wife was eventually displaced in his affections by an Oxford colleague, Margaret Jennings. Florey's was indeed a somewhat abrasive personality; he could be brusque with his colleagues and had little respect for authority, but he was loyal to his associates and unyielding in his principles. In Sheffield he built up a strong research group, continued his work on mucus and made more useful contacts, most importantly Edward Mellanby, who left Sheffield to become the head (the Secretary) of the Medical Research Council, and remained his steadfast patron throughout the ensuing years. In 1935 the opportunity for which Florey had been waiting presented itself: he became head of the newly established Dunn School of Pathology in Oxford.

Florey had seen Fleming's paper on lysozyme, and discerned a possible link to the physiological function of mucus, for he had found evidence that mucus interfered with bacterial growth, and moreover lysozyme, which breaks down the long, stringy molecules, made up of sugars, in the cell walls of certain bacteria, occurs in mucus. It was something of a blind alley because Florey soon determined that it was nothing more than the viscosity of the mucus which impeded the proliferation of bacteria. He continued nevertheless to study lysozyme, and to expedite the work he engaged a biochemist, an ebullient young emigré from Berlin, Ernst Boris Chain (1906-1979). As a Jew he had had the foresight to leave Germany when Hitler became Chancellor in 1933. He had worked briefly in London and then in Cambridge under the great doyen of British biochemists, Frederick Gowland Hopkins, who commended him to Florey. For some time at least, he and Florey got along very well. Florey seems to have admired Chain for his varied talents, especially his near-professional skill as a pianist. Chain was put to work on lysozyme, to find out what it really was and to discover its substrate, the molecule on which it acted. It was so widely distributed in animal tissues that what it was actually doing there was an obvious question to ask. All that was known was that it attacked one known species of bacterium. With help from other members of the laboratory Chain proved that it was an enzyme, and that the substrate was one of the sugar-like constituents of the bacterial cell wall. Florey felt at this point that there was little more to be gained from further work on lysozyme, and he and Chain began to think in terms of searching for other interesting natural compounds – Chain thought enzymes – with bacteriolytic (bacterium-disrupting) activity of a more useful kind. A search of the existing literature on the subject threw up many papers about preparations with activity against some of the major pathogens. Among them was Fleming's publication of 1929, and Chain, assuming that the 'penicillin' would prove to be another kind of lysozyme, thought it would be a good starting point. Florey agreed, and settled on a three-pronged attack on bacteriolysins. Penicillin was to be pursued in parallel with two other promising substances, one secreted by a soil bacterium, *Bacillus subtilis* (which much later found its way into biological washing powders), the other from *Bacillus pyocyaneus*, which we have already encountered (p.).

In throwing himself into the study of penicillin, Chain had at least one lead. None of the work that the two junior members of Fleming's laboratory had done on penicillin had been published, or was ever mentioned by Fleming, who clearly had seen no interest in it. But an attempt to purify penicillin had been made by an excellent chemist, Harold Raistrick at the London School of Hygiene and Tropical Medicine. Raistrick had a particular interest in the chemistry of moulds, and he and an assistant had got as far as extracting some of the penicillin activity into weakly acidic watery solution, and thence into ether. But here they reached a dead end, because when the ether solvent was evaporated away, the solid residue remaining had no activity. The active principle was obviously unstable, and to proceed further would have demanded arduous exploration of stability limitations and effects of solvents. Since Fleming himself had indicated that the penicillin held little therapeutic promise – a view in which Raistrick's clinical colleagues, with the unerring judgement of their calling, concurred - Raistrick, who had other interests to occupy him, abandoned the project. His paper, published in 1932, on the elusive properties of the antibacterial component of the mould 'juice' must nonetheless have indicated to Chain that it was no enzyme, for enzymes are proteins, and proteins are not soluble in ether. While still fixated on lysozyme Chain had asked Florey to provide help in setting up the demanding techniques required for the purification of an enzyme from animal material. He had already identified the man for the task - Norman Heatley (1911-2004), whom he had met in the laboratory in Cambridge.

When Florey approached Heatley with the offer of an appointment in Oxford, and Heatley agreed to come, with the proviso that he did not wish to be answerable to Chain, whose temperament he evidently found hard to endure. Heatley was a quiet man ....with a self-deprecatory sense of humour, given to the kind of understatement that was alien to Chain's nature. In one of his reminiscences Heatley recalled Chain's insistence that they were looking for a yellow compound. 'How do you know it is yellow?' Heatley demanded. 'But I'm telling you', was the heated reply. (Penicillin is colourless.) Heatley was a virtuoso of laboratory technique, with an exceptional ability to design and build apparatus. Chain and his assistants were baffled by the problem that had previously defeated Craddock and Ridley at St. Mary's and then the much more experienced Raistrick at the London School of Hygiene and Tropical Medicine – how to recover the active material from the mould extract. It was Heatley who succeeded where Chain had stalled, and solved the problem, expressing only embarrassment that he had not thought of the answer sooner. That answer was back-extraction: the compound (whatever it might be) was soluble in water, and if the water was weakly acidified it could be transferred into ether or a similar water-immiscible solvent when this was shaken up with the water extract. But how to retrieve it from the ether without inactivating it? Heatley merely shook the ether solution with alkaline water and the 'active principle' returned to the water layer, leaving behind the myriad of unwanted mould components in the original water extract. (Chain, who persisted in his belief that penicillin was an enzyme, had scoffed at Heatley's insight.) The activity, measured by how much the solution could be diluted and still inhibit the growth of bacteria, was greatly increased, although it later turned out that the proportion of antibiotic still amounted to less than 1% of the total material in the mould. It was Heatley who devised the apparatus for accurate and economical assay of the precious material and another device for culturing the *Penicillium notatum* mould, a sample of which had survived in London at St. Mary's. Remarkably the back-extraction method had been anticipated ten years earlier in Fleming's laboratory, where Lewis Holt, a chemist, was trying his luck on penicillin. Fleming took no interest, and Holt gave up after a week or two because of the instability of the product. Holt's effort was discovered by Ronald Hare in a notebook at St. Mary's long after Fleming's death.

In 1938 with war threatening, Florey's paymasters, the Medical Research Council realised that antibacterial agents would become increasingly important and urged that all the laboratory's efforts should be dedicated to developing methods for the large-scale production of penicillin. Florey had never concerned himself with any practical uses that might flow from his researches. He was 'not interested', he wrote, 'in suffering humanity – I don't know that it ever crossed our minds about suffering humanity; this [the preparation of penicillin] was an interesting scientific exercise'. (As history has shown, but governments seldom recognise, nearly all the most important and most beneficial discoveries have been stimulated by such undiluted curiosity.) Matters now moved swiftly in Florey's institute. His friend from Cambridge days, Paul Fildes suggested adding yeast to the culture medium, which increased the growth rate threefold. *Penicillium* moulds require oxygen, and therefore were seen to grow best in shallow dishes with a large surface area. Here again Heatley found the solution. First he procured bedpans from the local Radcliffe Hospital, and when this proved successful he designed large dishes with the desired properties. By a happy coincidence Florey had an Australian friend, a general practitioner, working in the Staffordshire pottery town of Stoke. Dr Stock replied to Florey's inquiry by telegram, recommending the only manufacturer he thought might be equal to the task. Heatley sent a sketch to James Macintyre & Co. Ltd., and three days later travelled to the factory in Burslem, where was astonished to find that three prototype vessels, not yet fired, were waiting for him. After several days in the kiln they were sent to Oxford and were found satisfactory. Another 174 vessels were ordered and production began. Florey procured funds from the Medical Research Council to employ six women, the 'penicillin girls', who for a meagre wage tended the production line. A further innovation, lyophilisation, also called freeze-drying, proved immensely important. This allows labile substances like penicillin to be concentrated from dilute solutions without anything as destructive as boiling off the water.* Heatley set this up, and after a few months there were 100 milligrams of a brownish solid product, sufficient for animal trials, which were conducted by Florey.

Heatley related how he and Florey took turns to observe the first batch of inoculated mice through the night. By 3.45 a.m. the last of the control animals, which had been infected with streptococcus was dead, while those which had also been given penicillin were in vigorous health. It was a moment of exaltation. Exhaustive tests on mice and other animals followed until Florey was at last satisfied that the material was safe and effective, and the amounts and duration of treatment required for a cure of a mouse or man had been worked out. By then it was 1940 and the war had started in earnest. Florey feared that if there were an invasion and the German army reached Oxford the enemy might take possession of the laboratory

---

* Lyophilization was the invention of Tadeusz Reichstein, the Polish-born organic chemist at the University of Basel. He did it to satisfy his constant craving for coffee while he worked. He had tried preparing concentrates which he could dilute with hot water for instant satisfaction, but all of them were tasteless if not offensive until he hit on lyophilisation, which became the basis of Nestlé's instant coffee preparation. The principle is simple enough: the watery solution is 'shell frozen', that is frozen in a rotating vessel to form a thin film of ice. A high vacuum is then applied to the vessel, which can be gently warmed to hasten the process, and the frozen water gradually evaporates, leaving the solute in the vessel. Reichstein shared the Nobel Prize in 1950 for his work on the isolation of corticosterone and other important steroids (p.) from adrenal glands (p.).

and especially of the mould, and make their own penicillin. He therefore made plans for the destruction of all samples should the dread event occur, and to preserve the vital strain he and Heatly smeared cultures inside their clothes.* That August a paper with the title, 'Penicillin

as a chemotherapeutic agent' and with seven authors, their names arranged in alphabetical order, appeared in *The Lancet*. It caused surprisingly little stir, except in the mind of Fleming, who turned up in Oxford to see what had been achieved 'with my old penicillin'. It must have seemed a deliberate provocation to Florey and his colleagues. But the challenge now was to try penicillin on a human subject.

Further purification was achieved by another technique which had come into use in recent years, column chromatography.** There were still vicissitudes that had to be overcome. At one stage the activity of the product dropped alarmingly, and it was another member of the group, E.P. Abraham, who discovered that traces of an enzyme which destroyed penicillin was

---

* Florey remained anxious to keep penicillin out of German hands. The microbiologist, Miltom Wainwright has discovered in Florey's archive correspondence from 1944 relating to this question. German chemists had evidently made inadequate attempts to prepare penicillin, having come by samples of material, possibly from American prisoners-of-war. Wainwright conjectures that penicillin may even have saved Hitler's life after he had been wounded in the assassination attempt of the 20th July of the same year. The German pharmaceutical industry was hardly in a state to embark on a programme of antibiotic production, and it appears that an application was made to the Ciba (later Ciba-Geigy, and eventually Novartis) company in Switzerland for help. Florey, at all events, received a letter from Ciba requesting a sample of the *Penicillium notatum* mould. Florey communicated this to Mellanby, giving his opinion that the request should be denied. 'It seems highly undesirable', he wrote, 'that the Swiss should have it as this would mean that the Germans get it'. Better therefore that wounded German soldiers should be allowed to die. Florey also warned Fleming that he should not accede to any request from the Swiss.
** There are today many variants of this technique, but they all work on the same principle. The solution is applied to the top of a long column, a glass tube, containing a material that binds weakly but to different degrees the constituents of the mixture of compounds in the solution. When a solution of appropriate salts in water is allowed to flow through the column the various components accompany it at different rates, depending on the extent to which they are bound to the column material, and are collected one after another in the outflow.

present, but could be removed by chromatography. With each successive step to eliminate the impurities which made up the bulk of the original crude 'mould juice', the activity rose, and at the beginning of 1941 Florey judged that there was sufficient active material for a human trial. It was resolved after consultation with doctors that healthy volunteers should not be subjected to this new compound of uncertain toxicity, and that instead it would be best to search for a patient suffering from a fatal condition and judged to be beyond recovery. Mrs Elva Akers was such a patient, adjudged by her doctors to have no more than a few weeks to live, and she agreed to be the guinea-pig. There were no serious consequences, but the patient's temperature rose distressingly. This effect was transient, and was found to be the result of a small amount of a pyrogenic (temperature-inducing) impurity. Florey returned to his animal experiments, and further column chromatography eliminated the pyrogen from the preparation. Florey and his clinical advisers now decided that it was safe to invite healthy volunteers for further trials. The results were satisfactory: there were no ill-effects, and the penicillin was eliminated quickly in the urine. Charles Fletcher, the hospital doctor who had been collaborating in the undertaking now came up with a real patient. Albert Alexander, an Oxford policeman was dying from rapidly spreading streptococcal and staphylococcal infections. Massive doses of sulphapyridine had failed to arrest the spread, and the doctors had run out of options. Dr Fletcher brought the entire supply of purified penicillin to the bedside and administered at intervals four intravenous shots of the precious preparation. By the next day the patient had undergone a remarkable transformation: his temperature had fallen to normal, and the discharge from his many abscesses had ceased. The supply of penicillin was now exhausted, but enough was recovered from the patient's urine for a few more injections. For ten days all went well, but then the staphylococci reasserted themselves, and Albert Alexander died.

The production of penicillin in Florey's institute continued apace, and several new patients, all of them in extremis, were treated. The outcome in each case was dramatic, but a half-dozen successful cures did not amount to a clinical trial. The production line at the Dunn School was already fully stretched and quite incapable of generating the amounts of material that would be needed. Florey and his patrons at the Medical Research

Council tried hard to stimulate commercial interest, but with little success. Eventually a small company in London agreed to culture the mould and supply the crude filtrate for purification in Oxford. But - especially with the war gathering pace and bringing with it a flood of battle casualties – the need for production on an altogether larger scale was becoming increasingly urgent. The prospects in Britain were poor, and Florey and Henry Dale and Mellanby at the Medical Research Council turned their gaze across the Atlantic. The help was enlisted of the Rockefeller Foundation, which had given generous support to several laboratories in Britain over many years. At this point Chain raised a new question: should the process of penicillin production be patented? (Penicillin itself, as a natural product, could not qualify for a patent.) Chain later insisted that he had not envisaged the purpose of such a move in terms of personal gain, but rather to ensure that commercial profits would go towards the funding of future fundamental research. Florey was doubtful, but pressed by Chain, he put the question to Henry Dale and Edward Mellanby, who presided over the primal source of support for the penicillin project, the Medical Research Council. Bot were scandalised by the suggestion, for to place any commercial constraints on the production and sale of drugs discovered under the Council's aegis would be wholly unethical. The consequences of their dictat were soon to become apparent.

In June of 1941 Florey and Heatley made the long, circuitous journey by air to New York, and began a protracted round of discussions with experts on moulds and fermentation in Government and commercial institutions. Heatley spent some months at the laboratories of the Merck pharmaceutical company, working with Andrew Jackson Moyer, an authority on the cultivation of micro-organisms. Together they developed new procedures for the growth of *Penicillium notatum*, and the preparation of penicillin, but when, after a suspiciously long interval, a description was published it bore only the name of Moyer. The reason behind the surreptitious elimination of Heatley soon became clear, for it was Moyer who took out the patent. Chain had been vindicated. In the meantime the facilities at the Dunn School had been much improved with the introduction of clever innovations by a protégé of Heatley's, Gordon Sanders, and it remained the main source of penicillin in Britain until I.C.I. (Imperial Chemical

Industries) began production. By 1942 the value of penicillin was clear to all, and it had substantially supplanted the Sulpha drugs for the treatment of infectious diseases*.

A myth and its genesis

In August of 1942 Alexander Fleming had surfaced once more. He appealed to Florey for a sample of penicillin to treat a patient at St. Mary's. This was a personal friend with a streptococcal infection. Florey sent what material he had, and Fleming's friend was saved. Some days later a leading article appeared in *The Times* under the title 'Penicillium', announcing the discovery of a miraculous new drug with a passing allusion to Oxford. This was followed the very next day by a letter from Sir Almroth Wright, which included the following passage:

I would, with your permission, supplement your article by pointing out that on the principle *palmam qui meruit ferat* [the palm to him who merits it] it should be decreed to Professor Alexander Fleming of this laboratory.

---

* Penicillin, as we shall see, did not act against all pathogens, and in exploring the limits of its efficacy, some appalling acts of barbarity were committed. Perhaps the most shameful occurred over the three years from 1946 to 1948, when a joint U.S. and Guatemalan team, led by John Cutler, a U.S. Health Service doctor, carried out experiments on captive Guatemalans - prisoners in a gaol, patients in an insane asylum and soldiers. The aim was to determine whether penicillin, already known to be reasonably effective against syphilis, could also prevent the emergence of the disease after infection. In all 696 people were infected with syphilis, some by infected prostitutes sent into the gaol, the rest by inoculation in the penis, the arm or the face, or by injection into the spinal fluid. Another 772 subjects were infected with gonorrhoea, and 142 with chancroid (a painful sexually transmitted bacterial disease. The project was supported by several U.S. Government bodies and by the Guatemalan regime. Cutler evidently specialised in such experiments, for he had also been engaged in the infamous Tuskegee episode – the U.S. Public Health Service syphilis experiment – in which, starting from 1932, some 600 poor, rural black men in Alabama were infected with syphilis and left untreated so that the progress of the disease could be observed. In 2011 the U.S. Secretary of State and the Secretary for Health made a formal apology on behalf of the country at large when the Guatemalan experiment was brought to light by the researches of a historian at Wellesley College in Massachusetts.

For he is the discoverer of penicillin and was the author also of the original suggestion that this substance might prove to have important applications in medicine.

This untruth bore immediate fruit, for the same day journalists converged on St Mary's and were treated to interviews with Fleming, who evidently made no attempt to minimise his claim to the brilliant achievement. In *The Times* next day there was a counterblast from the Professor of Organic Chemistry in Oxford, Sir Robert Robinson*, affirming declared that 'a, bouquet at least, and a handsome one, should be presented to Professor H.W. Florey'. But the damage had been done, and it was not in Florey's nature to engage in a public contest. He refused to speak to journalists, and made no public statements, to the evident chagrin of his dedicated co-workers, who hoped that he would do something to set the record straight. He did, though, write an aggrieved letter to Sir Henry Dale, asking whether an account of the actual events might be published, for, he told Dale, Fleming's assurances of restraint amounted to nothing. There was evidence on all sides of Fleming's duplicity, of his insinuations that the discovery and development of penicillin had been his own, with only

---

* Robinson, a distinguished chemist, who was awarded the Nobel Prize for Chemistry in 1947, had taken an interest in both lysozyme and penicillin, and had deduced – but wrongly -its structure. He had been contradicted by Chain, something to which the imperious Robinson was not accustomed, and a row had developed. In the end the correct structure was determined by X-ray crystallography in 1949 by Dorothy Crowfoot Hodgkin, another (later) recipient of the chemistry Nobel Prize. A further respect in which Robinson was wrong and held up progress in the production of useful amounts of the antibiotic was in opposing the proposed investment in fermenters; he held the unshakable belief that the future lay in his own trade of chemical synthesis, in which he was indeed a master. A total synthesis lay in the future, eventually achieved not by Robinson but by John Sheehan in America (see below), but it proved to be too laborious to be scaled up for commercial production. Robinson's main contribution to penicillin had been to prepare the first crystals, although this was also done at about the same time at the Squibb pharmaceutical company in New Jersey by Oscar Wintersteiner. It was a surprise to both chemists that their penicillins were not identical, but differed in one substituent group in the core of the structure. The samples were evidently extracted from different strains of mould, and were termed penicillin F and penicillin G; they differed in small ways in their properties.

'a few final flourishes' from the Oxford group. Dale in response offered no comfort but only reasons why Florey should swallow his resentment and maintain a dignified silence. A later appeal to Sir Edward Mellanby, the Secretary of the Medical Research Council, brought the same answer. What mattered, said Mellanby, was not the delusions of the public and the press, but the opinions of Florey's peers – the scientists – who fully understood the situation. The public perception would in any case prove ephemeral, and the truth would surely emerge.

In this Mellanby was wrong, for he had not reckoned with Lord Moran or with Lady Fleming (p.) and the hagiography which she commissioned from the writer, her husband's first biographer, André Maurois. Nor does Mellanby seem to have given any thought to the inevitable Nobel Prize that the Royal Swedish Academy would award for penicillin. And so the myth became firmly and enduringly entrenched in the public consciousness. In 1954 the Nobel Prize for Physiology or Medicine was bestowed jointly on Fleming, Florey and Chain, and it must have seemed to many of the participants in the work that Norman Heatley was the most conspicuous loser. But the Prize can be awarded to no more than three people, and this was by no means the only occasion on which the distribution of credit for a major advance might have appeared unjust. Fleming's contribution to the new age of therapeutics was trifling compared to that of Florey, and owed much to pure luck. Had earlier workers been fortunate enough to stumble on a growth of a *Penicillium notatum* strain, they too would have discovered penicillin. And yet it was Fleming's brief report that set the direction of Florey's research. (An Oxford Professor of Medicine fifty years later put it like this: 'without Fleming, no Chain or Florey, without Florey, no Heatley, without Heatley, no penicillin'.) Fleming himself seemed to have recognised his limitations, and at least in the company of scientists, he gave full credit to the Oxford group. In his authoritative biography of Fleming Gwyn Macfarlane cites a letter which he received from a distinguished microbiologist and chemist, W.E. van Heyningen, who knew Fleming well and liked the man. Fleming, he found, was 'easy-going, modest, uncritical and gregarious', and popular with his colleagues. Fleming 'told me often that he didn't deserve the Nobel Prize, and I had to bite my teeth not to agree with him. ... I don't know whether he took a different line with laymen, but if he'd have liked to pretend to be a great scientist with me and others of his scientific colleagues, he had the sense to know that none of us were any more impressed with him than he was himself.'

Fleming was honoured with a knighthood and innumerable honorary degrees, medals, memberships of scientific academies, and the freedom of the boroughs of Chelsea and Paddington, in addition of course to his share of the Nobel Prize. His portrait appeared on the cover of *Time* in the U.S., and the then-popular British magazine, *Picture Post* elected him Man of the Year. His remains now repose in Westminster Abbey, in the company of Newton, Nelson, Wellington and other national heroes. Florey in the end did even better: he was made a knight, Provost of Queen's College, Oxford, President of the Royal Society, a member of Order of Merit, and ended up Baron Florey of Adelaide and Marston. Chain also became Sir Ernst, and lesser honours were bestowed on other members of the Oxford team. A half-century after the event, someone finally remembered Normal Heatley, and Oxford University bestowed on him an honorary degree of Doctor of Medicine. The story of penicillin is, it could be said, an affirmation of Paul Ehrlich's maxim of the three G's: what the scientist needs is *Geduld, Geschick, Geld* – patience, skill and money. Florey and his team had the first two in great measure, and as much of the last as could be spared, given the conditions of the time.

A world of antibiotics

The stupendous success of penicillin set off a search for more antibiotics, and it was not long before a profusion of active natural antibacterial substances came to light. Some destroyed (lysed) the bacteria, others stopped them from reproducing. The problem was that the majority were toxic at the doses needed to eliminate infections. Nor was penicillin even the first antibiotic to be isolated. In 1939 René Jules Dubos (1901-1982), a French microbiologist, who in later life became famous as a thinker, an environmentalist and a writer. Dubos graduated from the Institut National Agronomique in Paris, became captivated by antibacterial compounds, and in 1924 made the decision to pursue his career in America. On the ship he encountered one of the leaders in this very field, Selman Waksman (of whom more later), and enrolled as a Ph.D. student under Waksman at Rutgers University in New Jersey. His next stop was the Rockefeller Institute for Medical Research (now Rockefeller University) in New York, and there he remained for most of his life. At the Rockefeller he had the good fortune to alight in Oswald Avery's laboratory. Avery, one of the outstanding scientists of his time, was the man who identified the carrier of genetic information as DNA, and Dubos was put to work on the system which led Avery to this momentous discovery. Dubos's task was to find a bacterium that would attack the lethal pneumococcus on which Avery was working. The expectation was that such a bacterium would have to secrete an enzyme capable of breaking down the polysaccharide (sugar-based) protective capsule encasing the pneumococcus. After a long search, a soil bacterium with this property, *Bacillus brevis* was found in the New Jersey cranberry bogs, but the active substance that it secreted was not an enzyme. From the *Bacillus brevis* cultures Dubos, with the help of a biochemist, Rollin Hotchkiss, extracted and purified not one but two compounds. These they called *gramicidin* and *tyrocidin*, and both turned out to be peptides (short chains of linked amino acids, such as make up the much longer chains that constitute proteins). Both were active against common pathogens, but proved too toxic for internal use. Gramicidin is still used to treat infected wounds. There were in retrospect two important outcomes of Dubos's work, transcending by far its direct practical value. In the first place it directed attention to the riches lurking in the myriad soil bacteria. The second was the effect on Florey of the four papers that appeared in 1939, which as he later owned persuaded him that penicillin was a practical proposition.

Dubos had another shrewd insight: he knew about the frequency of mutations in micro-organisms, and warned against the dangers that the development of resistance would present. It was not long after penicillin came into use that his forebodings proved justified, and the euphoria of the post-war decades began to evaporate. Yet even in 1969 the Surgeon General of the United States could tell Congress that 'it is time to close the book on infectious diseases and to declare the war against this pestilence over'. And in 1968 Professor Lawrence Garrod of St. Batholomew's Hospital in

London, had spoken of the ravages of bacterial infection, which 'no-one recently qualified, even with the liveliest imagination, can picture', and similarly opined that such times were gone forever. Penicillin, and before that the Sulpha drugs, had indeed wrought a remarkable change in clinical practice from the time when hospitals all had 'septic wards', harbouring dying people, many of them young. Sadly, it was not long before that the limitations of penicillin (like the Sulpha drugs) were beginning to reveal themselves. The hunt for new antibiotics had in fact begun much earlier, initially with the dual aims of discovering a product with a broader spectrum, effective that is to say against a wider range of pathogens,* and of generating something that could be patented.

Chain, who had fallen out with Florey over the patenting issue, had moved quickly in this direction. He had left Oxford for a position at the Istituto Superiore di Sanità, the state institute of health research, in Rome, but he had also approached the Beecham pharmaceutical company outside London, offering his services as a consultant. At his urging Beecham agreed to try modifying the primal penicillin in the hope of hitting on some derivatives with new and interesting properties. The Beecham chemists knew their business, but they also had a slice of luck: they discovered what was essentially the core of the penicillin structure, a molecule called 6-aminopenicillanic acid, 6-APA for short, in the 'mould juice'. This, a minor by-product of the fermentation process, was the perfect starting material for the synthesis of penicillin derivatives. Soon a series of substances with resistance to the destructive penicillinase enzyme secreted by some bacterial strains, and a broader spectrum of activity, or both, went into production. Methicillin, cloxacillin, dicloxacillin, flucloxacillin, ampicillin and a few others largely displaced penicillin. Similar objectives were being pursued by the Bristol Company in America, aided by one of the leading

---

* In particular, penicillin was effective only against Gram-positive bacteria, and by no means all of those. Gram-positive bacteria are those that take up the purplish Gram stain devised by the Swedish bacteriologist from whom it takes its name. The majority of the most virulent pathogens, including the streptococci and staphylococci, are Gram-positive, but there are many others, such as the agents of typhus, dysentery and gonorrhoea, which remain colourless when exposed to Gram stain, and are thus termed Gram-negative.

organic chemists at the Massachusetts Institute of Technology, John Sheehan, who had pulled off a *tour de force* in synthesising both penicillin and 6-APA, but the process could not be scaled up to a commercial level. A prolonged patent wrangle nevertheless resulted. Many of these products remain in use still, for particular purposes.

Nemesis, in the form of widespread antibiotic resistance, followed close on the hubris of over-confidence, uninformed use, and the avarice of the agricultural industry. Doctors took to prescribing penicillin prophylactically, and it and, later other antibiotics, could be bought over the counter. They were widely taken to treat the common cold and flu, which like all other viral infections, are untroubled by antibiotics, and penicillin was also added to cough-drops, moth-washes and even hand-soaps. Worse yet, poultry breeders made the catastrophic discovery that birds fed antibiotics reached maturity on less of their usual feed. This was because the antibiotics eliminated most of the gut bacteria to which chickens, like all vertebrate animals (ourselves of course included), and that normally absorb their share of nutrients. Their absence also causes anatomical changes in the animals, which make an additional contribution to faster growth. Growth promoters, as they are called, came into universal use in the agricultural industry around the world, and both governments and the pharmaceutical companies, which produced the antibiotics, disregarded all warnings. Antibiotics from the effluvia of factory-farms turned up in rivers and drinking water, and resistant strains of pathogens started to appear. Neither did the introduction of antibiotics designed to be fed only to animals solve the problem, for they were too similar in their chemistry to some of those in human use, so that resistance developed against these also. As the magnitude of the disaster revealed itself, some governments took action. Sweden and Denmark were the first to proscribe the use of antibiotics as growth promoters and in veterinary practice. Others, and also the main producer, objected noisily: farmers would go bankrupt and the agricultural economy would collapse if restrictive proposals were implemented. The British and the Belgians held out longest, but after prolonged opposition they too gave way. No farmers went bankrupt, nor did the economy suffer perceptibly. But the damage had been done.

From the sewer to the clinic

The disastrous consequences of antibiotic misuse lent urgency to the search for new antibiotics, but the pharmaceutical companies showed little interest. The fact is that a drug that cures a disease and is then no longer needed is far less profitable than one used to treat a chronic, or at least long-lasting, condition. Some important discoveries did follow close on the heels of penicillin, though almost entirely in academic or state institutions. So, in 1945 Giuseppe Brotzu, Professor of Hygiene, and Rector of the University of Cagliari in Sardinia (and later mayor of the city) was struck that, at a time when typhoid fever was rife on the island, young people were bathing in the sea around the main outlet of the city's untreated sewage, and gorging on the raw shellfish thriving in its vicinity. Why were they not all coming down with typhoid? Brotzu, who read the medical journals, knew about the work going on in Oxford, fell to wondering whether micro-organisms in the sewage might not be giving rise to an antibiotic. He sampled the effluvium from the sewage pipe, tested it on by agar-plate assays against cultures of typhoid bacilli, and found that it indeed killed them. Despite his very limited laboratory resources and his many duties, which included supervision of the local public health service, he managed to make considerable further progress. He identified the organism responsible for the antibacterial activity as a mould, *Cephalosporium acrimonium*. He next prepared an extract, which contained the active substance, though still in very impure form. Brotzu felt that he was onto something important because in further tests his preparation killed the agents of typhoid, cholera and brucellosis (variously also known as undulant fever, Mediterraneam fever and Malta fever) – all Gram-negative bacteria against which penicillin was ineffective.

But Brotzu had now reached the limits of his resources, and he could do no more than publish a brief report in Italian, and in a Sardinian medical journal. This appeared in 1948, and made all the impact of a raindrop falling into the ocean. Brotzu did however send a copy of his paper to a friend in London, who brought it to the attention of the Medical Resaerch Council. The MRC told him to try Howard Florey in Oxford, and this drew an immediate response. Brotzu provided a sample of his extract and Floret's colleague, E.P. (later Sir Edward) Abraham went to work on it. Abraham and his collaborator, Guy Newton established that Brotzu's preparation contained not one but five compounds with antibiotic activity. Abraham called them cephalosporins, but found them in most respects disappointing. Their activities were low, and tested on a wider range of bacteria than Brotzu had had to hand, they worked primarily on Gram-positive species. They were also chemically very similar to the penicillins. One of the compounds seemed nevertheless to have some promise, for it had no detectable toxicity, was resistant to the penicillinase enzyme, and had a moderately broad spectrum of activity. This was cephalosporin C, and attempts to interest industrial concerns in preparing it on a large scale drew a response, though mainly in America. The chemists of the Eli Lilley company set about the task, and also began to explore semi-synthetic derivatives. The structural core of the compound was isolated, like that of penicillin (6-APA) from cultures of the mould, and spawned a series of derivatives. In 1964 the Eli Lilley researchers found one with all the desired characteristics – stability, a broad range of activity against both Gram-positive and negative pathogens, and minimal toxicity. This was marketed as Cephalosporin *tout court*, and remains the most widely prescribed of all antibiotics. Brotzu at least received an honorary degree from the University of Oxford.

The campaign against resistant pathogens continued, and in the view of most bacteriologists is unlikely ever to end. It has never been more than two or three years before the first reports of resistance against a new antibiotic. Methicillin, long the first line of defence against *Staphylococcus aureus* infections, met its match in the methicillin-resistant strains of the bacterium, the notorious MRSA. A large proportion of humanity is host to staphylococci and other potentially pathogenic bacteria: they live on our skin, in our noses, our ears and other orifices. The trouble begins when they migrate to a location where they should not be, such as the lung or the colon. In the United States and Britain some 60% of the *S. aureus* cultured from patients in hospitals are MRSA, and it is the sick and those with wounds, whether from surgery or accidents, who are most susceptible to a lethal spread of the organism. The pattern has been repeated for other antibiotics and other pathogens. The dearth of treatments for Gram-negative species is of especial concern. One of the leading American researchers in this area has come up with an acronym for the pathogens considered most dangerous: ESCAPE, standing for *Enterococcus, Staphylococcus, Klebsiella, Acinetobacter, Pseudomonas, Enterobacter* species. Fewer and fewer of the major pharmaceutical companies are now engage in antibiotic research. It has become harder, and antidepressants and statins, which reduce cholesterol levels, are vastly more profitable. The future is clouded.

Antibiotics and the White Plague

For all the impact of the penicillins and cephalosporin in the clinics, they were almost no help in combating the most feared of all infections, tuberculosis. From its peak in the early 19th century when it accounted in England for one in every four deaths, pulmonary tuberculosis (consumption) had declined, but a hundred years on it was still essentially incurable. There was no evidence that the fresh-air-and-rest regime actually worked, and the sanatoriums that spread like a rash around Europe and America in the later 19th century did little more than offer some comfort to those who could pay. Neither the toxic gold compounds, nor the many other speculative cures in vogue in the early 20th century and before (pp.), had any proven therapeutic value. The agent of the disease, *Mycobacterium tuberculosis*, or Koch's bacillus (p.) is a small bacterium with a coat, unique to this and other members of the *Mycobacterium* genus (such as the organism responsible for leprosy). It is made up in large part of fatty, waxy compounds, highly resistant to chemical attack. The exceptionally slow rate of multiplication of the bacterium added to the obstacles it put in the path of the researcher. A turning point came in 1943. Selman (*né* Zolman) Abraham Waksman was born in Russian Ukraine in 1888. Denied entrance to university by the ubiquitous antisemitic prejudice, Waksman emigrated in 1910 to the United States. The young man made a favourable impression on another Russiam emigré, a professor in the agricultural faculty of Rutgers University in New Jersey, and he was awarded a scholarship to study at Rutgers, where he remained for the rest of his working life. His aspirations were high, and he moved smoothly through a Ph.D. to a junior position on the faculty. For his speciality he chose the micro-organisms in the soil,

371

and within a short time he had established himself as an authority in the field, and had built up a thriving research group.

It was probably his brilliant student, René Dubos (p.) who induced him to turn his attention to the prospects of discovering new antibiotics – the word was coined by Waksman (but see p.). In 1940 he and a colleague proceeded to study the properties of actinomycetes, an unusual class of soil bacteria with certain of the characteristics of a fungus. From cultures they obtained an extract with powerful activity against a range of pathogens. They named the active constituent actinomycin, but it proved a disappointment for its high toxicity against animals ruled out its clinical use. (Later research in other laboratories revealed that Waksman's preparations, renamed actinomycin A, contained several closely related compounds, and in 1951 actinomycin D was isolated in Waksman's laboratory, and under the name of dactinomycin, came into use against a number of infections, and most of all in cancer therapy). Waxman and his acolytes had at any rate acquired experience in the growth of bacteria on a relatively large scale and on the fractionation – that is separation of components – of extracts. It was against that background that Albert Schatz (1920 – 2005), whom Waksman described as his best student, entered the laboratory.

Schatz sprang, like Waksman, from a Russian Jewish family. He was born in Connecticut, where his parents derived a modest living from a Christmas-tree farm, but the son was bright and personable enough to secure a modest scholarship at Rutgers University. His agriculture studies were interrupted by the war: he was called up in 1941 and sent to work in a military hospital in Miami. Discharged two years later on grounds of health, he returned to Rutgers and joined Waksman's busy laboratory. Schatz was as eager as his patron to discover new antibiotics, and especially one that worked against tuberculosis. Perhaps because of a common belief that the soil harboured whatever it was that caused the scourge, soil micro-organisms may have seemed a propitious point of departure, but of course Waksman's laboratory led the world in this rather recondite field. There had also been some indications from earlier work of Waksman's that some soil samples were indeed hostile to the mycobacteria. Schatz began his quest using a harmless species of *Mycobacterium* to assay his culture extracts, but soon decided to switch to the real thing – *Mycobacterium tuberculosis*. This was a dangerous move, for several dedicated researchers had become infected by their own cultures, had developed pulmonary tuberculosis, and some had died. Schatz was consequently treated as a leper, a carrier perhaps of the feared disease.

Schatz went to work with ferocious determination, often spending nights as well as days in the laboratory. It was only two months of prodigious labour, culturing and assaying innumerable strains of actinomycetes against an array of pathogens, before he found two strains which prevented the *Mycobacteria* from dividing. One came from a soil sample, rich in manure, the other from a chicken with a supposed throat ailment, brought by a local farmer to the poultry pathology department of the university. The professor who examined the bird knew that Schatz was searching for new bacterial strains, told his assistant to take a throat swab and bring it to Schatz. He cultured both his new specimens, and shown the grey-green colonies on the culture plates, Waksman became seriously interested. He dubbed the bacteria *Actinomyces griseus* from their unusual hue, and diverted the work of the laboratory into studying their properties and those of their extracts. Schatz now varied the composition of the culture medium to find conditions for optimal growth, prepared extracts and tested them for antibiotic activity. This, he was thrilled to discover, was prodigious, and extended over a wide range of pathogens, including Gram-negative species, and most excitingly the tuberculosis bacilli. Even better, the product, now called *streptomycin* to distinguish it from the largely useless actinomycin, proved to possess very low toxicity in animal tests, initially on chick embryos. The bacterium from which the streptomycin came was renamed *Streptomyces griseus*. (Waksman later claimed that he had discovered the bacterium and first cultured it, but he probably knew that this was untrue for a second reason as well, namely that it had been reported by a Russian bacteriologist in 1914.)

The first paper on the discovery was published in 1944, with Albert Schatz as the lead author. The paper elicited a visit to the laboratory by a veterinary surgeon, William Hugh Feldman from the Mayo Clinic in Rochester, Minnesota, one of the foremost centres of medical practice and clinical research in the country. Feldman and his colleague, an eminent physician, Corwin Hinshaw wanted to carry out more exhaustive animal tests, and finally try the effect of the new substance on consumptive patients at the Mayo. Could Waksman – that is to say, Schatz – provide sufficient material for the purpose? Waksman agreed, and Schatz went to work at his usual frenetic pace to meet the needs. The animal results with Schatz's material fulfilled all expectations, and so the time had come to approach a pharmaceutical company, Merck of New Jersey was known for its capacity to produce pure preparations on a clinically useful scale. Merck agreed, apparently with some misgivings, to go ahead, and towards the end of the following year, 1945, Hinshaw and Feldman began treating patients. The results were electrifying: dying patients were pulled back from the brink, and as the news spread, demands for streptomycin came from all quarters.

Waksman and Schatz had some months earlier taken out a joint patent on the discovery, but settled informally that neither would derive any profit from the sales. Waksman, though, had broken this accord before it was made, for he had entered into an agreement with the Rutgers University Foundation that would give him 20% of all monies the Foundation should receive from royalties. (These, it was true, went largely, but by no means entirely, into supplying the needs of the laboratory, and they eventually made Waksman extremely rich.) Schatz knew none of this, but when Waksman presented him with the patent application to countersign, he demurred. Waksman, according to Schatz's account, became enraged and threatened to use his connections to ensure that his protégé's career in science would be over. Schatz signed. Complaints to the university fell on deaf ears. Waksman had form: he had been involved in a similarly acrimonious affair some years earlier, when a member of his laboratory let it be known that he had been deprived of proper credit for a discovery. But the university authorities sensed that streptomycin would bring in a great harvest of wealth and renown, and they wanted no scandal. Public acclaim followed the reports of the new 'miracle drug', but it was Waksman on whom it fell, and not Schatz. The adulation clearly went to Waksman's head, and his benign persona began to show cracks. He was suddenly in huge demand. In the U.S. he received the ultimate accolade of an appearance on the cover of *Time*. In Europe he embarked on a triumphal tour of the leading scientific institutions, and was hailed as 'the Einstein of biology'. In none of the accounts of the great discovery was Schatz's name ever mentioned. Schatz, who had liked and admired his patron, seemed now to have been expunged from the record. Bitter and helpless, he turned his back on Rutgers, and took a position in a Marine Biology laboratory in California. There was also the question of the royalties, and Schatz was hard up. He wrote to Waksman with a series of questions, to which he received a curt and dismissive reply. Schatz's contribution, Waksman now informed him, had been a very minor one to the heroic struggle that led to the discovery and production of streptomycin. He had repaid the unstinting help he had received from his professor in helping him to his Ph.D. with shameful ingratitude.

This was too much for Schatz, who initiated a court action, which limped on for a year before an out-of-court settlement was agreed. The judge found for Schatz, on the grounds that the patent had named him and Waksman as co-discoverers of streptomycin – that both had signed the document stating, 'They verily believe themselves to be the original, first and joint inventors of an improvement in the same' (that is, streptomycin). He ruled that Waksman's royalties should be reduced by half to 10%, that Schatz should receive 3%, and that the remainder should be divided between the other members of the laboratory (including the glass-washer) who had participated in the work. But the Rutgers faculty and the scientific establishment at large were outraged. The lawsuit was an assault on the reputation of the profession. And who, in any case, was this upstart, a mere graduate student, who had the temerity to pit himself against a faculty grandee, one to whom he owed his career? At this rate every professor would live in fear of calumny by one of his students. And so Schatz was cast into outer darkness, with little chance of finding a position in any institution that counted. Worse was to come, for in 1952 Waksman was awarded the Nobel Prize for Physiology or Medicine. Schatz again sought justice: he wrote to the King of Sweden and to several distinguished scientists in the field, none of whom replied, except Dr Feldman who wrote a sympathetic letter.* Schatz could not make his voice heard above the mutter of disapproval. Waksman must nonetheless have felt insecure, for he now began to rewrite history. Schatz's contribution, he reiterated, had been trivial; he, Waksman, had searched for and found the critical strain by taking throat swabs from a sick chicken brought by a farmer, and it was he alone who had isolated the antibiotic for testing. These were lies, although their perpetrator may well have come to believe his own fabrications, just as the ageing King George IV firmly believed that he had led a decisive cavalry charge at the Battle of Waterloo. It was more difficult, however, to explain away the patent, which bore the name of Schatz as co-discoverer of streptomycin, or the recollections of students who were present when Schatz first saw the effect of the two actinomycetes strains on the tubercle bacilli, nor yet the striking fact that of all the hundreds of publications that bore Waksman's name it was only on his first and critical paper with Schatz that the student's name had been placed first.

Neither Waksman's autobiography, *My Life with the Microbes*, published in 1958, nor his later book, *The Conquest of Tuberculosis*, makes any mention of Schatz. "In the antibiotic programme", he writes in the first of them, "I was assisted by nearly fifty graduate students and visiting investigators. Without them I could never have accomplished what I did. They were the fingers of my hand, which, as a unit, accomplished a great task. This teamwork might be compared to that of an orchestra, with the conductor leading and assigning the task to each member, none of which would have produced any symphony afterwards." This was as close as Waksman ever came to tipping his hat in the direction of Schatz and his other hirelings. He was at pains to distance himself from any such gift of fortune as threw penicillin into Fleming's lap. He described the hard road to the discovery like this: "We went about it the hard way. We isolated freshly some tens of thousands of cultures of different microbes. [Much use here of the regal 'we'.] Theses were tested for their activity against bacteria. Ten percent of

---

* Hinshaw also felt that he and Feldman might have shared the Prize. His story was that a delegate from the Nobel committee had come to investigate their merits, but had been warned off by a member of the Mayo Clinic directorate, who had doubts about the correctness of their work. Yet another disappointed man was Jørgen Erik Lehmann, whom we shall meet shortly.

them were found to possess such potentiality ...." Further sifting, he tells his readers, brought the number down to "ten new compounds .... Only one of these proved to be a successful agent, streptomycin."

Now this is clearly a brazen perversion of history, but we should pause to consider whether there is anything to be said in Waksman's defence. The affair is far from unique in the annals of science. There have been many resentful graduate students and other junior researchers who believed, often with justice, that their part in an important scientific advance had been discounted. Nor was Schatz *vs* Waksman the only legal action arising out of such a cause. Yet the question must be asked whether the aggrieved party could have made the great discovery working in isolation. Schatz had the advantage of an environment, built up by Waksman over many years, dedicated to the study of soil bacteria. Waksman had developed the techniques of culture and assay that had become routine, and it was in this same laboratory that the first usable antibiotics were discovered, even if by another outstandingly able student, René Dubos. Moreover, Waksman had turned over much of the effort of his research group to the pursuit of antibiotics, so streptomycin did not come out of the blue. In a reminiscence written long after Waksman's death his younger colleague, H. Boyd Woodruff related the following episode: 'Dr. Waksman appeared in the laboratory one day. He was highly agitated. "Woodruff", he said, "drop everything! See what these Englishmen have discovered a mold can do. I know the actinomycetes can do better!" Thus was initiated the first search in Waksman's laboratory for antibiotics from actinomycetes.'

Even Schatz did not demur at the naming of Waksman as co-discovered on the streptomycin patent. A study of the contretemps between the professor and his student, published in 2004 by William Kingston, even produces legal reasons why Schatz needed to be named as co-discoverer in the patent application. Kingston also suggests that Schatz's account of what happened is a distortion, that Waksman had set a veritable army of students and assistants to work, screening bacteria – a routine assembly-line occupation, demanding care, but little in the way of skill or perspicuity - and that any of the others thus engaged could equally well have struck lucky. This may be wholly or partially true, but none of it excuses Waksman's behaviour in traducing Schatz, disparaging his contribution in such venomous terms, and misrepresenting history in so many respects, nor indeed the uncompromising hostility of the panjandrums of the scientific establishment towards Schatz. Rutgers University made partial amends in an obituary of Schatz, published in its magazine, *Rutgers Focus*, and there have been several historical attempts, notably that of Milton Wainwright in a persuasively argued article, to vindicate Schatz posthumously; and there is also a book (*Experiment Eleven*) by Peter Pringle. As between their conclusions and those of William Kingston, readers of these accounts can make up their own minds. Schatz also had his say, first in a Pakistani dentistry journal, of which he happened to be an editor, and later in a book, published shortly before his death. His co-author was Inge Auerbach, a survivor of the Terezin ghetto, where she caught pulmonary tuberculosis, and only much later was treated with streptomycin and cured. After Rutgers, Schatz, the outcast, nevertheless had a successful, though rather erratic career in science. He worked in several universities and Government laboratories in the United States, and was a professor for some years at the University of Chile. He participated in the discovery of another antibiotic, nystatin (active against infections by yeasts and fungi), was politically active, published many papers and three books, received marks of recognition in the form of honorary degrees and awards, and died in 2005, aged 82. Waksman remained active for some years after fame enveloped him, and died in 1973 at the age of 85.

After streptomycin

Streptomycin was seized on by clinicians and patients. Its power to cure tuberculosis appeared magical, and it undoubtedly saved many lives and assuaged much misery. But it was not very long before the euphoria began to fade. Not all patients responded, and resistant strains of the mycobacteria appeared. Chemotherapy research had meanwhile been continuing. At the Bayer laboratories in Germany Gerhardt Domagk was back in action after the rigours of the war, when research had all but come to a halt. The collapse of sanitation and medical services in the bombed cities, malnutrition in the population, and prisoners-of-war returning from overcrowded and insanitary camps brought about a tuberculosis epidemic. The Sulpha drugs were practically useless against mycobacteria, but Fritz Mietzsch and his highly able young colleague, Robert Behnisch synthesised a series of new compounds, the sulphathiazoles, which had shown some promise in animal tests carried out in 1939. Thus encouraged, Behnisch had broadened his search for new organic structures, and in 1941 had produced a series of the related thiosemicarbazides. Some of these compounds were already familiar, having been used as intermediates in the synthesis of sulphanilamides. Several showed further promise, and as soon as the work resumed at the war's end, Behnisch set about making hundreds of variants on the structural theme. Three of them were startling in their potency against tuberculosis. Domagk found that they could all cure infected guinea pigs at remarkably low concentrations, with no apparent side-effects. One was chosen for human trials, and Domagk persuaded sceptical physicians in a tuberculosis hospital to treat a few patients. Elated by the results, Domagk prepared a report, couched in overheated terms, and indeed the number of subjects was too small, and the procedures too sketchy to permit any firm conclusions. The drug was called tibione (TB-one), and was patented by Bayer under its later trade name of Conteben. But under the legislation imposed by the occupying powers in Germany the patent carried no legitimacy. Two American doctors, one of them Corwin Hinshaw from the Mayo clinic, visited Bayer and bore away a supply of Conteben. Clinical trials in America produced an altogether less dazzling outcome, for the drug proved ineffective against the most deadly forms of tuberculosis. Still, it was judged useful in treating lesser infections, and remained in use for some years until better therapies emerged.

In the same year, 1944, that saw the discovery of streptomycin, a Swedish doctor, schooled in Denmark, with a thorough knowledge of chemistry, and a record of successful research, Jørgen Erik Lehmann (1898-1989) found, by clever inference, a new molecule with activity against tuberculosis. He had been set on his course by a publication from an American chemist, turned pharmacologist, Frederick Bernheim at Duke University in North Carolina. Bernheim had been studying the metabolism of mycobacteria. He had added a variety of substances to cultures to see which might affect the metabolic rate, and therefore also the rate of growth. In particular, he had focussed his attention on benzoic and the related salicylic acid, on the grounds that these compounds bore a close similarity to a known metabolite of streptococci. The strategy worked: Bernheim found that when either compound was added to his culture of mycobacteria the oxygen consumption, reflecting the growth rate of the bacteria was enormously increased. Bernheim published a brief report, and then began to search for an analogue of benzoic or salicylic acid that would act on the mycobacteria in the opposite sense to the parent compound. Here he was applying the principle of competitive inhibition formulated at about this time by Donald Woods (p.), according to which an inactive analogue of a metabolite might swamp the action of that metabolite and bring the metabolic cycle to a halt.

Bernheim and his colleagues synthesised 49 such derivatives, mainly containing chlorine or iodine atoms in the benzene ring at the centre of the benzoic and salicylic acid structures. A few worked in stopping the spread of tuberculosis in infected guinea pigs, but there was only one that did not kill the animals as well as cure them. This one compound was tried on a few patients, but nothing more was heard of it. At the Sahlgrenska Hospital in Gothenburg, where he ran the chemical pathology laboratory, Jørgen Lehmann read Bernheim's paper, and decided to follow the same route. His first step was to repeat Bernheim's observation with salicylic acid, and to his surprise, he failed: there was no accelerated oxygen consumption or faster growth. Lehmann did not give up, and looked for possible reasons. The only difference he could discern between Bernheim's experiment and his own was that unlike Bernheim his mycobacteria were of a harmless strain (which of course was much safer for the experimenter). He procured a virulent strain, and now the experiment worked. Pondering the possible modifications that he might make to the salicylic acid structure, he decided to try introducing an amino ($-NH_2$) group into the ring, probably on the basis that this was a feature of the Sulpha drug structures. There were four positions on the benzene ring of salicylic acid at which a new substituent could be inserted.* Lehmann thus had a choice of three positions

relative to the pre-existing substituents, at which to introduce the amino group. Two of the aminosalicylic acids had been synthesised in the remote past in Germany, but Lehmann especially wanted one of the others, probably by reason of an analogy with the sulphonamides. The synthesis of this *para*-aminosalicylic acid (*p*-aminosalicylic acid, or PAS, as it became known, although 4-aminosalicylic acid is the proper chemical usage) turned out to present difficulties. Lehmann had already approached Ferrosan, a pharmaceutical company in Malmø, with an invitation to collaborate, and it was their chief chemist, Karl-Gustav Rosdahl, who overcame the problem, and at the end of 1943 delivered the compound to Lehmann. How many products Ferrosan prepared for Lehmann is not clear, but PAS was a triumph, albeit a delayed one. After successful animal assays, a limited clinical trial also proved encouraging, if not yet dramatic.

Yet Lehmann's published report met by apathy. He did not have the resources for a full-scale clinical trial, and there was in any case wide scepticism about the prospects of a chemical remedy for tuberculosis, a subject with a sorry historical record. There had been a number of specious claims over the years, one of which, especially, was too recent and too embarrassing to have entirely faded from doctors' memories. A professor of physiology in Copenhagen, Holger Møllgaard had, for no discernible reasons, tried curing tuberculosis-infected guinea pigs with a compound of gold. It had produced alarming results of organ damage and shock, which Møllgaard chose to interpret

---

* The benzene ring is hexagonal, and in benzoic acid is carries one substutuent group, a carboxyl (-COOH) in the ring. This group makes the compound an acid. Salicylic acid is defined by two substituents, each projecting from the ring at different (actually adjacent) corners, a carboxyl group and a hydroxyl group, -OH. There are thus in salicylic acid four corners at which an additional substituent could be introduced. Its position is traditionally designated *ortho* (if it is adjacent to the carboxyl group), *meta* (if it is at the next-but-one corner), or *para* (if it is three corners away, and thus at the opposite vertex of the hexagon). These are casual descriptions, inadequate, especially for defining more complex structures, and the rigorous nomenclature employed by organic chemists uses numbers. Thus *para*-aminobenzoic acid, for example, ir properly designated, 4-aminobenzoic acid.

as the release of toxins from disintegrating mycobacteria, resulting, as he claimed in many cases of recovery. He applied for a patent on the compound gold thiosulphate, under the name, Sanocrysin, and published a book on his discovery in 1924. The news it brought was received with enthusiasm in some places, and caution in others. The *Journal of the American Medical Association* pointed out with some acerbity that Møllgaard had not discovered a new compound, for gold thiosulphate had been prepared for the first time in 1845, he had merely given it a new name, and, the editorial warned, more work needed to be done before the claims for its usefulness could be taken seriously. Sanocrysin (which was also touted as a treatment for arthritis) was fiasco, and probably harmed many patients.

The consequence of the tepid reception accorded to Lehmann's work was that it took more than two years before PAS came into wide clinical use. Even then, it was upstaged by the much more flamboyantly promoted streptomycin. PAS was to reveal its real value only later, after the limitations of streptomycin had become apparent. It was neurotoxic, could cause deafness and other afflictions. Worse, striking initial cures were often reversed as resistant strains of the tubercle bacilli emerged. PAS had advantages over streptomycin: the starting materials were cheap, and there was no toxicity. Then it became known that William Hugh Feldman, of the Mayo Clinic had contracted streptomycin-resistant pulmonary tuberculosis, and that his life had been saved by PAS, administered by his colleague, Corwin Hinshaw. With the rapid spread of drug resistance generally came the realisation that no single drug was likely to retain total efficacy for long. While the drug kills the bacteria against which it was found effective at the outset, the few mutant individuals resistant to the drug – which could be one in a million or far fewer - would survive and multiply. If instead the patient is treated with two drugs with different modes of action on the bacterium, then the chances of strains resistant to both would be vastly reduced. This is now a general principle of drug treatment for infections and also for cancer, which presents, as will be seen later, a similar problem of drug-resistance. It was thus an obvious strategy to treat tuberculosis patients with two drugs, streptomycin and PAS together. This indeed vastly improved the chances of a cure, and became, after too long a delay, the standard way to treat patients.

In retrospect it is clear that the development of PAS was no less important than that of streptomycin, and Lehmann apparently felt justifiably aggrieved that his contribution was not recognised by the Nobel committee. A share of the prize with Waksman (and arguably Schatz) would have appeared just. Lehmann explored several more derivatives of salicylic acid, but none were better than the first. The search for more and better chemotherapeutic agents continued elsewhere, and in 1951 there was a breakthrough. The light dawned more or less by chance and at the same moment in three laboratories, a remarkable example of simultaneous discovery. E.R. Squibb & Sons in New Jersey was one of several pharmaceutical companies on the hunt for anti-tuberculosis drugs. By the beginning of 1951 its chemists had synthesised some 5000 new compounds for testing in mice. The emphasis was on thiosemicarbazide derivatives ('thio' implying the presence of sulphur atoms), which had been the basis of antibacterial substances prepared in the Bayer laboratories. In one of the best of these compounds a pyridine ring* was linked to the thiosemicarbazide. The preparation showed some activity, but history repeated itself once more when the intermediates in the complicated multi-step synthesis were also tested as a matter of routine. One was found to possess remarkably high activity, more than ten times greater than streptomycin. The compound was isonicotinyl hydrazide, or *isoniazid* for short (which was to find a quite different use a few years later [p.]). Meanwhile, not far away in Nutley, New Jersey, a group of researchers under Robert Schnitzer at Squibb's competitors, Hoffmann-La Roche had also been on the wrong track. Schnitzer, who had worked in the Hoechst laboratories, had arrived in America in 1939, a refugee from Nazi Germany, and lucky to escape, having served time in a concentration camp. A pharmacologist, he was struck by the weak antitubercular activity of nicotinamide, a member of the class of B3 vitamins. This stray fact had been noted by a French doctor by the name of Vital Chorine, whose interest was in leprosy. In 1945 Chorine had been trying the effects of the available vitamins on rats infected with the leprosy bacillus, *Mycobacteria leprae*, closely related, as its name implies, to *Mycobacterium tuberculosis*, and it was nicotinamide,

---

* Pyridine is a hexagonal ring like benzene, but with one of the carbon atoms replaced by a nitrogen. Pyridine compounds are numerous in nature; the bases designated C and T in DNA are familiar examples

albeit in very large doses, that had suppressed the development of the disease. It was then an obvious step to try it on guinea pigs injected with a tuberculosis culture, and indeed a large dose of nicotinamide prevented, or at least delayed, the onset of the disease. That same year there was another straw in the wind: another French practitioner, Ernest Huant, a cancer specialist, sought to alleviate the unpleasant effects of radiation treatment, especially on the skin, by giving his patients nicotinamide. His reasoning was that this was the vitamin which kept the deficiency disease, pellagra (literally, 'the angry skin') at bay. Perhaps therefore it might also heal the skin lesions caused by the X-rays. This would have been a futile hope, but Huard noticed something else: the patches on the lungs, visible in the radiograms of patients who happened also to have tuberculosis, seemed to regress under this treatment. Huard wrote a cautious note in a minor clinical journal, suggesting that tuberculosis specialists might want to look into this unexpected phenomenon.

Tuberculosis researchers were willing to try anything, and they did indeed confirm both Huard's and Chorine's observations. Fumbling in the dark, they conjectured that a metabolic property of the vitamin might be responsible for its effect on the tubercle bacillus, but research in an industrial organisation, the Lederle Laboratories in New York State, showed that this was not so, for closely related compounds which had no vitamin B3 function in animals still possessed anti-tubercular activity. This set off a wider search for pyridine-containing compounds with greater activity. Schnitzer and his colleagues at Hoffman-La Roche synthesised several such compounds, and found, like their compeers at Squibb, that an intermediate used in a series of demanding multi-step syntheses - isonicotinic acid hydrazide – had remarkable antitubercular activity. Far away in Germany, Domagk and his chemists had entered the same maze as the Americans and emerged at the same exit. Domagk, as it happened, travelled shortly afterwards to the United States and did a tour of conferences and laboratories, without divulging what he had discovered, for trials of the efficacy of isoniazid were still in progress. Neither did the Americans reveal that they were in possession of the same knowledge.

A leading specialist in the treatment of tuberculosis at the Cornell Medical School in New York had been invited by Squibb and had agreed to evaluate the new drug in patients, when a few months later, he was approached by the clinical director of Hoffmann-La Roche with the proposition to participate in clinical trials on a highly promising tuberculosis drug of their own. This of course turned out to be the very same isoniazid under another provisional trade name. The Hoffmann-La Roche product was already in the hands of two doctors at another site in New York, the Sea View Hospital. They reported astonishing results: forty-four seriously affected patients with little hope of recovery responded dramatically with a rapid alleviation of all their symptoms. In Germany meanwhile Domagk's friend, Phillip Klee was also getting results in his hospital in Wuppertal, close to the Bayer plant. But it was in New York that the storm broke. An announcement was made, and the press besieged the Sea View Hospital. Pictures were even shown of patients before and after – in bed in a state of seeming decomposition, and then dancing in the wards. Almost immediately public hysteria erupted, and soon after, a black market in the meagre supplies of the drug then to hand. Isoniazid was represented as (yet again, but justifiably) a 'miracle', and was moreover cheap and easily prepared. It manifested its worth most spectacularly when it was given in conjunction with streptomycin and PAS as a threefold 'combination therapy'. Tuberculosis could now be almost infallibly cured, but inevitably, though time only after some decades, new strains appeared with resistance even to this treatment.

When the circumstances of the isoniazid discovery were revealed, a wrangle ensued about priorities, patents and trade names. It was terminated by a rude shock for all parties when someone read the literature and found that isonicotinic acid hydrazide had been synthesied in 1912 at the Karl-Ferdinands University (the German university in Prague, in which Einstein once held a professorial chair, now amalgamated with the Czech sister-institution as the Charles University) by two research students as part of their research project for the Ph.D. degree. No medical relevance had been foreseen, or indeed considered, and the publication had excited no interest. It lay undiscovered like a time-bomb, for the earlier synthesis meant that isoniazid could not be patented. Had the publication by the two students come to light sooner, no pharmaceutical company would have considered embarking on a research programme based on the compound, and suffering humanity might have been deprived for ever of a life-saving medicine. Isoniazid remains a cornerstone of tuberculosis therapy even today. All the pharmaceutical companies could do was to synthesise new pyridine derivatives in the hope that one or other would prove better, or at least not inferior to isoniazid, and could be patented.

At the same time, the hunt for new and better antibiotics from the soil never let up. In 1943 the chairman of Lederle Laboratories asked a recently retired Professor of Plant Pathology at Cornell University whether streptomycin was the last word in such antibiotics, or whether a continued search might prove worthwhile. The professor, Benjamin Duggar, an expert on soil bacteria told him that there were better fish in the sea than had yet been caught. Duggar was forthwith invited to prove it, and he took up the challenge. He asked his friends around the country to send him soil samples, and within weeks, working with two assistants, he had a culture of a streptomycetes species, which was secreting a bright yellow material with a remarkably broad range of antibiotic activity. The bacterium was christened *Streptomyces aureofaciens*, and the antibiotic – unusual in that it contained a chlorine atom – *chlortetracycline*, was later given the commercial name, *Aureomycin*. Lederle supposedly sold 20 million dollars'-worth of the drug in the first year. This was the first of the tetracycline antibiotics (so-called because the core structure consists of four fused carbon rings). This set off a search by competitors for more such finds, and soon oxytetracycline, tetracycline *tout court*, and others soon came to light.

New antibiotics by the dozen, and later by the hundred, appeared in the ensuing years, few of them without their drawbacks, but one that deserves mention, though not entirely for happy reasons, is *chloramphenicol*, also known by its trade name, *Chloromycetin*. It was Parke Davis who, in 1943, engaged the services of a botanist at Yale University to set up a screening operation to find promising bacteria from soil samples from around the world. Chloramphenicol came from a bacterium found in a soil from Venezuela, and given the name, *Streptomyces venezuelae*. It had a broad spectrum of activity. It worked on Gram-positive and Gram-negative bacteria, and appeared to afford the best defence against infectious diseases yet discovered. The structure was determined by a Parke Davis team, led by a remarkable chemist, Mildred Rebstock, who followed up by synthesising the molecule. It was licensed only in 1949, but hit the market with a sensational impact, which propelled Parke, Davis to the top of the roll of the world's most profitable pharmaceutical companies. Chloromycetin had seemed devoid of significant side-effects, but after a few giddily successful years tragedy supervened. Reports came in of deaths from aplastic anaemia – the destruction of the bone marrow, which produces the blood cells. The victims were few, but the effect deadly, and there were also instances of lesser damage to the bone marrow. Sales abruptly fell, and there were lawsuits. Chloramphenicol nevertheless retained its place in the pharmacopoeias, and continued to be used, though in much more cautious amounts than before, for certain conditions, including typhoid and meningitis, and most safely in eye-drops.

So far as the treatment of tuberculosis was concerned, streptomycin was supplanted by other antibiotics, and PAS by various more expensive products. By-products of the search for anti-tubercular drugs were compounds active against leprosy. Before effective synthetic remedies became available the only known treatment was the foul-tasting, practically unassimilable chaulmoogra oil, and later its active principle, chaulmoogric acid, both of limited efficacy. From the pursuit of sulphanilamide drugs emerged a relatively simple, easily prepared molecule with powerful bactericidal properties. It was synthesised simultaneously, though not for the first time, in Domagk's laboratory and by Fourneau in Paris. (It had in fact been first reported in 1908 by Germans chemists.) It was rejected for clinical use by reason of its toxicity, but tested against *Mycobacterium leprae*, it proved active enough to be rehabilitated. This drug, *Dapsone* became a standard treatment, and gave rise to a series of improved derivatives, synthesised and marketed by American pharmaceutical companies. Another notable advance was the discovery of a new group of antibiotics, structurally unrelated to streptomycin, though found in a related species, *Strepromyces mediterranei* from soil of a Provençal pine forest. These were isolated by workers at the Milan chemical concern, Leppetit, and named rifamycins after their favourite gangster film, Rififi. The best member of the group was rifampicin, which became the preferred treatment for both tuberculosis (together with isoniazid) and leprosy, for which it was (and is) administered in combination with dapsone or its derivatives. Later the infamous teratogenic (birth defect-inducing) drug, thalidomide was rehabilitated as an effective treatment for a number of diseases, among them leprosy (p.).

The emergence of isoniazid-resistant strains of the *Mycobacterum tuberculosi* was an incentive to the search for other similar compounds, and of the many that were synthesised, it was pyrazinamide that has best stood the test of time. The compound was simultaneously made in the laboratories of the Merck and Lederle companies. The quest for more effective and less toxic anti-tuberculosis drugs, continued in the Lederle Laboratories, and eventually bore fruit in 1961. This was a quite unrelated structure, found apparently by a more or less random search. Ethambutol (Myambutol) is still used today, most often as part of a cocktail with any of pyrazinamide, isoniazid and rifampicin. With the rise of 'multi-drug resistance', and most devastatingly, the so-called 'extensively drug-resistant' strains of tuberculosis, the therapeutic options have been largely exhausted, and the need for new drugs has become desperate.

This then is far from the end of the antibiotic story, for the battle against resistance can never be won. The best hope is to contain the menace as long as some at least of the available antibiotics remain effective, while searching for new ones that the pathogens will not yet have seen. In 1953 the Eli Lilly company came up with vancomycin, isolated from a bacterium discovered in a soil sample sent from Borneo by a missionary. It proved active against penicillin-resistant staphylococcal infections. But unfortunately it had many toxic effects, and appeared to have no future. Yet some four decades later, when distraught clinicians were searching for anything that would neutralise a resistant infection – especially by the much-feared methicillin-resistant *Staphylococcus aureus*, MRSA - it was brought out once more. It became at once 'the antibiotic of last resort', that is to say must not be used except in extremis. This directive was intended to delay as long as possible the emergence of pathogen strains resistant to its action. Such strains have been relentlessly appearing, and at a much faster rate than new antibiotics. There have been attempts to develop semi-synthetic derivatives of vancomycin - a complicated structure of amino acids linked together in a ring, and coupled to sugars – and one of the derivatives, teicoplanin (Tagocid), with a different range of side-effects is in use as an alternative to vancomycin. There are now a variety of other unpleasant species of bacteria that have become resistant to all the antibiotics that doctors can throw at them. Their names – *Klebsiella pneumoniae*, *Enterococcus faecium* (of which vancomycin-resistant strains (VRE) turn up especially in hospitals), and others - are unfamiliar to the public, with perhaps two exceptions. One is *Escherichia coli* (*E. coli*), the common bacterium that thrives by the trillions in our guts, but gives rise to pathogenic, even deadly strains; the other is the famous *Clostridium difficile*, which can cause serious intestinal distress, and is more apt to erupt when antibiotic treatment has killed off the benign *E. coli* and other species in the gut, thus allowing the alien species, now devoid of competition, to take root. The last estimate put the annual world death toll from antibiotic-reistant *C. difficile* at about 14, 000, and rising fast.

There is one more important family of antibiotics, the carbapenems, which, like the penicillins and vancomycin, intervene in the process by which Gram-positive bacteria build their cell walls (though at a different point in the metabolic reaction sequence). The carbapenemes derive from yet another species of soli bacteria, *Streptomyces cattleya*. In 1976 Japanese researchers isolated from it a highly effective antibiotic, but thienamycin, as it was named, proved too unstable for clinical use, as well as too reluctant to enter a human cell. Yet such was its potency in the test-tube against the most dangerous pathogens, and so comprehensive its reach, that attempts began almost at once to make derivatives free of the drawbacks of the parent compound. In 1985 one such reached the market: imipenem is given to the patient together with another compound, cilastatin, which blocked the action of an enzyme in the kidney that would otherwise destroy the drug. The combination is sold as Primaxin or Cilasafe. Then in 2005 the Sinogu Company of Japan gave the world doripenem, called Doribax or Finibax, administered by injection, and highly effective. These carbapenems are reserved for the treatment of life-threatening infections, and are considered, like vancomycin, 'antibiotics of last resort''. But even so, resistant strains of pathogens have already made an appearance. One other natural product in which high hopes have reposed surfaced in a 'high-throughput' screening programme (p.), run by what was then Merck. The compound was one of the no less than 250,000 natural substances that the screen encompassed. It occurs again in one of the multitude of known species of *Streptomyces, S. plaensis,* and is called platensimycin. Like the foregoing antibiotics, it thwarts cell wall assembly, but seems still to be in an experimental stage of development.

There is also however another means of treating some resistant infections, which, repugnant as it appears, is nevertheless very effective. There were occasional reports over some decades, followed in 1958 by a scientific paper in a respectable medical journal, of 'faecal microbiota transplant therapy', or less obliquely, faecal transfer. The plan was, and is, to infuse into the patient by enema (or more recently also by a nasal tube through the duodenum) faeces from a healthy donor, who has been rigorously screened for infections by pathogenic bacteria or parasites. The principle is that normal gut bacteria, which abound in the faeces, can drive out the *C. difficile,* just as the infection by *C. difficile* drives out the normal and beneficial micro-organisms. Successful treatments were reported at intervals through the following years, but the first full clinical trial was begun only in 2012 in the Medical Centre of Amsterdam University in Holland. The control group of patients were treated in the conventional manner with vancomycin. The trial was stopped after a short time because it was quickly obvious that the faecal therapy was vastly superior, generally clearing up a recurring infection after the first delivery. The conquest of 'hypervirulent' *C. difficile,* which first announced itself in hospitals in 2000, seems now to be almost complete. Faecal therapy has been urged

---

* A difficulty for the doctor is to make the right choice of antibiotic, which is contingent on a correct identification of the pathogen. This is a time-consuming process because the bacterium has first to be cultured, and in serious cases speed of diagnosis and treatment is critical. A solution to the problem is now in view, for if its DNA can be at least partially sequenced (p.) then reference to a database will at once disclose the species and strain of the bacterium. DNA sequence determination with modern technology is quick, and the falling cost promises to make it widely accessible.

by some doctors for several other conditions, including ulcerative colitis, irritable bowel syndrome (p.) and chronic constipation.

The FDA has endorsed faecal therapy, and has elevated faeces to the status of a drug, insisting that the process should be tightly controlled, and donors rigorously screened. There has been much discussion about the useful life of the donated material: some clinicians argue that it must be administered fresh - within about six extracorporeal hours - otherwise the bacteria will have died. There are also divergent schools of thought on whether the dose should be introduced into the upper section of the colon, rather than the lower end; and some practitioners have urged the use in some patients of a nasal tube to deliver it into the small intestine.* It appears in any event that faecal therapy is now firmly established, and benefits, most of its recipients.

The search for new antibiotics from soil (and other) bacteria has been depressingly fruitless in the last two decades, but it has delivered the occasional unanticipated gift. In 1965, when optimism was high and the search was at its most active, a group of Canadian workers brought back a sample of soil from Easter Island (although a plaque on a building at the site commemorates in Portuguese a group of Brazilian scientists as the initial discoverers; whatever the truth of the matter, it was researchers in Montreal who published the first scientific study). The bacterium was a new *Streptomyces* species, *Streptomyces hygroscopicus*, and in 1975 the Canadians in the Ayerst Research Laboratories (part of the Wyeth pharmaceutical concern) published their first paper, reporting the isolation of an active principle with powerful antifungal properties. It was especially active against *Candida albicans*, which is responsible for unpleasant infections of the mouth and the genital tract. The compound, one of the macrolide class of antibiotics found in other *Streptomyces*, was given the name rapamycin from Rapa Nui, the name of the indigenous people for

---

* It is now known that distinct populations of the vast variety of microbial species inhabit different regions of the gut (a type of segregation also observed in other human tissues). The study of the properties of gut microbes – which species are a threat to health, and which a benefit, with perhaps clinical potential - constitute a highly active area of research.

their island. It was animal tests that appeared initially to extinguish all hopes that rapamycin would become a useful drug, for it suppressed the function of the immune system in mice. But this was also the period in which organ transplantation was developing into a life-saving, if not yet an altogether routine procedure, and immunosuppression was the key to the prevention of rejection. Wyeth (swallowed by Pfizer a few years later in 2005) marketed sirolimus for immunosuppressant use under the name of Remune. (The company was accused of illegally promoting off-label* uses for their Remune, and of attempting to bribe doctors to change their prescribing preferences from other immunosuppressants to Remune.) The drug is now know to act by blocking the action of a group of enzymes bound up in the function of central players in the immune system, the T and B cells. Further research exposed new and remarkable properties of repamycin, now renamed sirolimus. It turned out to prevent cell division, which immediately suggested a possible anti-cancer activity. Odder yet, the mice in which the drug was tested, lived longer than the controls by an average of about 30% from the start of treatment. Sirolimus has been introduced for the treatment of some cancers, and its action in increasing longevity has excited high interest among researchers engaged in the study of ageing. After the discovery of the drug a search began for other immunosuppressants from different species of *Streptomyces*. Perhaps the most successful was found in 1984 by Japanese researchers. It was named tacrolimus or fujimycin, and as Prograf, and under other trade names, seems not to lead the market.

An important departure was the creation of the first totally synthetic antibiotics – antibiotics not derived from a living organism. These are the quinolones (from the name of the parent compound). The story began, as so often, with a happy accident. An unsuccessful attempt at a synthesis of the antimalarial, chloroquine by a chemist, George Lesher at the Stirling Laboratories in Albany in New York State, generated a mysterious by-product. Lesher investigated the structure and properties of this substance,

---

* 'Off-label' is the term for a use of a drug other than that intended by the FDA, or equivalent body, and - in principle - the manufacturer. Doctors are permitted to prescribe drugs for off-label applications, but for manufacturers promotion for any such purposes is illegal.

which was given the name, nalidixic acid. He showed it to be a member of a class of compounds called quinolones. When tested, it was shown to have rather weak antibiotic properties against Gram-negative bacteria. It came into limited use for treating urinary tract infections, but more importantly, was the starting point for the synthesis of numerous derivatives - probably now more than a hundred. Those that proved highly valuable broad-spectrum antibiotics were the fluoroquinolones, containing fluorine atoms. (The element, fluorine is the first member of the group of halogens, of which chlorine, bromine and iodine are the succeeding members.) The most potent is *Ciprofloxacin.* This is now one of the primary weapons available to clinicians grappling with refractory infections. Another related compound is linezolid (Zyvox), the use of which is limited by its huge cost. There are now four generations of fluoroquinolone drugs, and the quest continues.

Many more antibiotics of high potency have been discovered, but are too toxic – carcinogenic for instance, or destructive to the liver, kidneys or bone marrow - to use in human patients. An ugly episode developed from one of these, trovafloxacin. Marketed by Pfizer as Trovan, it was the focus of high hopes. It was an inhibitor of enzymes that alter the twist of the DNA helix, called gyrase and topoisomerase, (the latter is also the target of some agents of cancer chemotherapy [p., f.n.]). The first and only clinical trial of trovafloxacin was carried out during a calamitous bacterial meningitis epidemic in Nigeria in 1996, which killed some 12,000 people. The patients consisted of 200 children, half of whom received Trovan, and the other half ceftriaxone, an established cephalosporin-group antibiotic, and the standard treatment for meningococcus infections. The outcome was that five children in the first group and six in the second died, and others may have been left with permanent injury. (An ironical twist was that a Médecins sans Frontières team was treating children at the same time in the same primitive hospital in the town of Kano.) An inquiry revealed that neither the children nor their families had been informed that they were being subjected to an experimental trial, nor was informed consent sought. Worse, the control antibiotic, ceftriaxone had been administered at a third of the normal, approved dose.* On the scant evidence, there was nothing to indicate that the drug performed any better than the older alternative against the meningococci, but in 1998 the FDA licensed its use against a list of infections. However only a year later it was withdrawn from use, except for patients in hospitals and nursing homes, who were critically ill. The reason was high liver toxicity, and in due course it was withdrawn altogether in America and in Europe.

Doctors may now be faced at times with the option of taking a chance with a highly toxic, discarded compound, in the hope that it will cure the infection before it kills the patient. A well-known example is polymyxin (discovered as long ago as 1947 in two laboratories in the U.S.) Also called colistin, it is a polypeptide (p.), produced by a bacterium (*Bacillus polymyxa*), and is highly effective against the most dangerous Gram-negative bacteria, such as *Klebsiella* and *Pseudomonas*, but inflicts damage on the kidneys, and is used as a last resort and with extreme caution. The search for new antibiotics is now being sponsored by governments, but the situation is critical. As matters stand, the death toll from antibiotic-resistant infections, since the first appearance of MRSA in 1998, runs into some tens of thousands in Europe alone. It has overtaken by far the mortality from AIDS (p.) and is approaching that of road deaths. Even the prophylactic use of antibiotics in surgery has become a hazard. There is a real fear that we may return to the pre-penicillin era of septic wards filled with dying and infectious patients, young and old.

---

* The outcome was embarrassing for Pfizer. The leader of the trial produced a letter of exculpation, which proved to have been forged. A long series of legal actions began, initiated by patients' families and by the Nigerian government, which referred to 'an illegal trial of an unregulated drug'. When the case came to court in the U.S. Pfizer's first defence was that informed consent was not a requirement in African countries. To the obvious charge that the ceftriaxone dose had been deliberately reduced to bias the comparison between the two antibiotics in favour of Troman (a practice apparently not unknown in clinical trials [p.]), Pfizer responded that the purpose had been to spare the children pain from repeat injections. Pfizer did not yield easily, and the legal bickering went on for many years, and may not be concluded even now. Nevertheless, Pfizer settle with the families out of court for a total of $75 million, subject to a confidentiality agreement.

An oddity, which appeared to hold high promise, but is now remembered only as a mere biological curiosity, came to light in 1986. The African clawed-toed frog, *Xenopus laevis* has been an important laboratory animal, because the female is an abundant source of oocytes (egg cells). Into these eggs can be injected biological molecules, such as a messenger RNA (the bearer of the genetic message from DNA to the machinery of protein production), and developments within the oocyte can be studied. The removal of the oocytes from the frog is a simple operation, the incision can then be closed, and the animal allowed to recover. This procedure has been performed in hundreds of laboratories, but only one scientist asked a question that might have occurred to any of them. Michael Zasloff, a researcher at the National Institutes of Health in Bethesda, Maryland, observed that the wounds of the postoperative frogs, returned to the dirty, turbid and certainly not sterile water of the tank in which they lived never became infected. Nor indeed had the surgery been conducted under sterile conditions. Did the frog then possess a material that repelled pathogens? Zasloff examined the skin of the frogs, and found that it did indeed contain such a substance. He isolated two closely similar peptides of twenty-three amino acids, which prevented the growth of a variety of species of bacteria, notably the generally refractory Gram-negative ones, and also several single-cell parasites. Zasloff called the peptides *magainins*, not from a Latin or Greek stem as is customary, but from the Hebrew word for a shield. Zasloff conducted a historical search, and discovered that ChineseChinese was an ancient Chinese remedy for the treatment of wound infections. Later studies showed that the skin of frogs would yield many other biologically active substances. Yet the magainins have never received approval for clinical use, because of suspicions of carcinogenic properties, and it appears as though they may be destined for oblivion, so far at least as clinical applications go.

Virus contra bacterium

The increasingly acute problem of resistance revived interest among some microbiologists in a largely forgotten corner of the subject. Bacteriophages ('bacteria eaters', from the Greek) are viruses that lyse (burst) bacteria.

They were first seen, though not identified, by an English doctor and bacteriologist, Frederick (1877-1950) before the First World War. He was exercised by the contamination of smallpox vaccine preparations with staphylococci, and began to investigate their nature and provenance. He isolated the bacteria, cultured them on agar, and observed that small transparent, 'glassy' patches formed in the bacterial colonies where the bacteria had clearly lysed. He lifted some of these patches of dead bacteria off the agar, applied them to new bacterial cultures, and saw that these too were lysing. Something in the glassy patches was killing the staphylococci. Twort then made a further discovery: the killer agent passed through a porcelain filter, which strained out bacteria. Twort guessed that it was an enzyme contained in the bacteria, and lethal to them only when liberated into the surrounding medium. The inference was a reasonable one, since viruses had not yet been discovered and were too small to be seen in the light microscope. They had indeed to await invention of the electron microscope before they could be seen (p.). Twort's report, published in *The Lancet* in 1915, fell on deaf ears. He went off to serve as medical officer in the army, and by the time he returned to St. Thomas's Hospital in London further enlightenment had come from another quarter.

Félix d'Herelle (1873-1949) was born in Montreal to French parents, but when his father died young the mother returned to Paris with her two young sons. Education after the lycée was beyond the family's means, and so d'Herelle could only indulge his interest in biology in solitude. A restless spirit, he wandered for some years through many countries, and while returning from South America had his first experience of infectious disease: yellow fever broke out on board ship, and took the lives of several passengers. The young man apparently decided at that moment to dedicate himself to microbiology. Back in Paris, with still no opportunities for formal study, he decided, at the age of 24, to try his luck once more in Canada. There he was offered a biological project, and since it involved a problem in fermentation, the subject pioneered by d'Herelle's idol, Louis Pasteur, he seized the opportunity. There was at the time a glut of maple syrup on the market, and the idea was to turn the excess into an alcoholic drink, a brandy. D'Herelle showed his skill in developing methods of fermentation and distillation, and the *eau de vie* achieved some popularity even in France. But d'Herelle never settled down in one place for long. He worked for two years, making use of his newly acquired skills, as a bacteriologist in a hospital in Guatemala City, and then in Mexico. Then followed his next major scientific undertaking, which was in pest control, especially of locusts, which he pursued in Argentina and then in Algeria. He returned to France in time for the start of the Great War, and went to work in a treatment centre for sick and wounded soldiers in a Parisian suburb. It was there that he made his great discovery. Dysentery was a major problem in the trenches, and vaccine treatment presented problems. One difficulty was that there were several strains, and even species, of the genus of *Shigella* bacteria. D'Herelle went to work culturing these bacteria from the faeces of affected patients, and he soon found a new and particularly virulent strain. In pursuit of its toxin, he examined the filtrate of the bacterial culture and found that it had strong lytic activity against the bacteria from which it had been separated. Since the lysis agent passed through a filter of the kind used by bacteriologists, such as Twort, to retain bacteria, it was clearly not a bacterium, and since the activity reappeared in filtrates of new cultures it seemed to have the ability to reproduce itself. D'Herelle inferred that, though obviously small and, as he supposed, little larger than the protein, albumin, it was nevertheless microbial. That d'Herelle and Twort had independent;y discovered the same thing was proved by the noted Belgian microbiologist, André Gratia (p.), but it was d'Herelle who coined the catchy name, bacteriophage, bacteria eater.

In 1917 d'Herelle had published a short account of his observations under the title, 'On an invisible microbe antagonistic to dysentery bacilli'. A little later he found that the bacteriophages appeared in the faeces only when the disease was on the wane, and therefore they might be killing the bacteria inside the patient. With the end of the war, d'Herelle was now released from his work on vaccines and was able to devote himself to the further study of his bacteriophages. By this time he had a position as assistant (unpaid) at the Pasteur Institute, and he was able to conduct some animal experiments to learn more about the properties of the phages (as they came to be called). His publications began to attract attention, and some of his colleagues at the Pasteur Institute and workers in other laboratories entered the field, and controversies ensued. In particular many, led by the distinguished Belgian microbiologist, Jules Bordet, refused to believe that the bacteriophages were biological entities, capable of reproduction. In some laboratories there were difficulties in reproducing d'Herelle's results because, as became clear only much later, there are forms of bacteriophages that do not lyse bacteria, are in fact dormant. We know now that these 'temperate bacteriophages' integrate their DNA into that of the bacteria, but do not reproduce or incommode the host. Nevertheless d'Herelle had already tried his preparations on children suffering from dysentery, not before he himself swallowing some of the culture and also gave some to his wife and children. There had been no noticeable effect, and he reported remarkable recoveries among the children, and later also adult patients. Ever restless he travelled to Egypt, India and French Indochina, where there were cholera epidemics, collecting samples of faeces from the sick and dying, preparing phages and mounting a campaign to treat sufferers.*

To demonstrate that the bacteriophage was a particle and Bordet was wrong, d'Herelle performed a classic experiment. He made successive dilutions of a bacteriophage preparation and found that at one part in 10^{10}, that is a ten-billionfold dilution, there was still activity against bacteria, but after a further tenfold dilution the activity vanished. Moreover, when a quantity of the limiting dilution of 10^{10} was added to a series of bacterial culture samples, all of identical volume, there was lysis in some, but not in others. The inference was that some of the set of the added volumes of the bacteriophage dilution contained one phage (or perhaps two or three) and others none. The probability of finding no particle in a sample volume of such a dilute solution, and of finding two or three and so on, can be easily calculated. (The probabilities follow what is known to statisticians as a Poisson distribution.) D'Herelle enhanced the impact of his paper by noting that he had shown his results to Albert Einstein, no less, who was

---

* The reported successes attracted wide attention. D'Herelle's name became known, and even made a fictional appearance. Sinclair Lewis's spirited novel of science, *Arrowsmith*, published in 1925 to critical acclaim. The story is set in the Rockefeller Institute (now University), thinly disguised as the McGurk Institute. Lewis received much help from a microbiologist at the Rockefeller, Paul de Kruif, who afterwards turned writer himself. Martin Arrowsmith is a young scientist who makes a great discovery - the bacteriophage - only to learn from a colleague that he is too late, for d'Herelle's paper has just been published.

regarded by then as an oracle, and who had endorsed d'Herelle's conclusion that the phage was indeed particulate. Bordet and the other sceptics were thus vanquished. Recognition now came to d'Herelle, in the form of medals, honorary degrees, and in 1926 the offer of a professorial chair at Yale University, which he hesitantly accepted. It was not a success: he had no patience with teaching, and he was unwilling to give up his constant urge to travel, and after three uneasy years he returned to Europe, but not to Paris. As for Towrt, his role in the story was overshadowed by that of d'Herelle, but there is no doubt that he found and published the bacteriophage phenomenon first.

Eleven years before, at the Pasteur Institute, d'Herelle had struck up a friendship with a visitor from Georgia, Georgiy Eliava. Now, in 1933, Eliava invited him to the institute that he had established in Tbilisi (or Tiflis, as it then was). D'Herelle, it seems, was drawn, as many scientists were at this period, to communism, and indeed went so far as to dedicate one of his books on bacteriophages to Stalin. Eliava's institute became a leading centre of bacteriophage research. It was generously supported at a time when science was much in favour in the Soviet Union, and d'Herelle was offered a professorship and excellent facilities for research. This still left him time to direct at a distance a commercial operation, which he had set up in Paris. The thrust of the Tiflis institute's work was the practical therapeutic application of bacteriophages, and for a time all went well. But Eliava, a free spirit, had already fallen foul of the First Secretary of the Georgian Communist Party, the notorious Lavrentiy Beria, and was arrested. He was lucky to be released, but in 1937 at the height of Stalin's Great Terror disaster struck again. Eliava was accused of deliberately infecting children with pathogenic bacteria, and condemned as 'an enemy of the people'. He was arrested and shot. D'Herelle thought it prudent to make a quick departure. The institute in Tiflis survived the demise of its founder, and indeed stimulated the founding of new phage laboratories at several centres in the Soviet Union. D'Herelle's services were recognised, and he was invested with the Order of the Red Star. He did not return to Tiflis, but remained for the rest of his life in Paris, where an institute dedicated to bacteriophage research was created for him. His view of the nature of the phage was finally and definitively vindicated in 1941 by one of the first successes of the new technique of electron microscopy, which came to fruition in Germany in 1940. The images showed small particles attached to the outer surfaces of bacteria, in preparation for entry. D'Herelle's interest never wavered. He remained as combative as ever and wrote copiously about bacteriophages, about history and about the nature of scientific progress. He died in 1949. A large part of his legacy has been the dominance that bacteriophages assumed in the rise of the dazzling new discipline of molecular biology in the years after the Second World War. The study of their genetics brought new insights into the fundamental processes of life, along with a crop of Nobel Prizes.

Wither the bacteriophage?

But what of their practical uses? Reports of the effectiveness of bacteriophage therapy against dysentery, typhoid, cholera and other infections came in from researchers in many countries throughout the 1930s, but there seem to have been no large or rigorous clinical trials. Indian scientists have long conjectured that the reason why the many thousands who come to bathe in the Ganges, and even drink its cadaver-laden waters around the burning-ghats of Varanasi, do not (it is said) fall sick is that the river teems with bacteriophages. A number of pharmaceutical companies took an interest, and in 1942 the U.S. National Research Council funded a research programme, headed by the distinguished microbiologist, René Dubos (p.) at the Rockefeller Institute in New York. In Tbilisi the Eliava Institute, as it became after Stalin's death, remained (and remains) a major focus of bacteriophage research, and receives patients from many countries. Bacteriophage treatment is said to have saved thousands of lives on the eastern battlefields during World War II. The science journalist, Thomas Häusler has unearthed papers published during that war in a journal with the unpropitious title of *Der Militärartzt* (The Army Doctor) an account of a bacteriophage production facility at the Behring Works. The product, called *polyfagin*, was intended to treat dysentery, the complaint so prevalent among soldiers in the unpleasant conditions of Eastern front. And yet in Western Europe and the United States bacteriophages faded from the medical literature. The main reason was probably the spectacular success of the antibiotics, but with the emergence of resistance a degree of interest returned. The bacteriophages have certain obvious advantages in the fight against bacterial infections. Unlike most antibiotics they are devoid of toxicity; they are 'natural' agents, which have existed in the environment for perhaps two billion years without causing any known harm to multicellular organisms such as ourselves; for bacteria of every species that has been examined with this in mind, there are bacteriophages with the power to kill them; and whereas bacteria can mutate to evade their enemies, such as antibiotics, so can bacteriophages mutate to re-establish their potency.

What then are the disadvantages? One is that bacteriophages are in general rapidly eliminated from the body by the macrophages – large cells in the circulation and tissues that engulf and destroy alien elements. Mutant phages can be isolated however by successive passages through a human or an animal, selecting at every stage those with the longest survival. Not only that, but the methods of genetic engineering – the manipulation of the genes of an organism – can be easily applied to bacteriophages to induce desirable properties. It would even be possible to arm a phage with the means (enzymes) to penetrate the walls of different strains of their bacterial host, thereby forestalling the survival of a resistant mutant. The reason why phage therapy has been pursued so half-heartedly is not connected to scientific difficulties but to money. Because bacteriophages exist in nature (and even the concept of their clinical application dates from as long ago as 1917) they cannot be patented, and therefore no project to develop a therapy will find financial backers; and because the phages mutate rapidly, and preparations will in general contain a variety of mutants, they cannot be defined as 'pure'. Indeed the common practice in Georgia and elsewhere in Eastern Europe seems to be to use a mixture of phage species to give as broad a specificity as possible. In neither case would such preparations be acceptable to the national drug agencies, which will authorise only pure, homogeneous substances for clinical use. Nonetheless a few intrepid biotechnology companies are engaging in bacteriophage research, and the ominous problem of antibiotic resistance may yet determine that the time of the bacteriophage has come. In Russia and its eastern European neighbours bacteriophages retained their place in the pharmacies, and seem still to be popular, sold in the form of pills, draughts and ointments.

Chapter 12

VIRUSES: BEYOND THE
REACH OF ANTIBIOTICS

What appeared, and for half a century indeed almost was, the end of
bacterial diseases did not extend to the viruses. Viral diseases rank among
the worst of all human woes. They include poliomyelitis (polio), smallpox,
rabies, hepatitis and influenza. This last, as is well-known, killed more
people in the great epidemic of 1919 than died in the Great War. Doctors
were at a loss what to do. Hurried and unsuccessful attempts were made to
produce a vaccine, and certainly the vaccines against other diseases, such
as rabies or smallpox, were ineffective. In Britain doctors tried morphine in
prune syrup, or potassium permanganate solution (a common antiseptic) as
a gargle; an iodine inhalant was another futile prescription, as were friar's
balsam and purgatives, let alone the inevitable mercury compounds as a
last resort. There was also a compound patented as Yadil, a quack nostrum,
widely sold. (The advertisers invented a scientific-sounding name for its
content, but it seems in reality to have been a common disinfectant.)
Nothing availed, and flu remains a problem to this day, although of

course vaccines exist, and give partial protection.* More recently, terrifying new viral diseases with hideous symptoms, culminating most often in death have appeared, such as Ebola virus and Marburg disease. Viruses eluded the best efforts of the great 19th century bacteriologist to track them down. The agents of the diseases were invisible, and they passed through the filters used to separate bacteria from the liquid in which they swam. Pasteur guessed that they might be much smaller than bacteria, and therefore below the resolving power of his microscope, and it was, as we have seen, only when electron microscopes became available to biologists that viruses could actually be observed. Before that, in 1935 Wendell Stanley in California had purified a virus for the first time, and prepared crystals. It was a plant pathogen, tobacco mosaic virus, and his report was greeted with general derision. (By 1946, when he received the Nobel Prize, scientific opinion had relented.)

It was many more years before the first anti-viral agents were synthesised. Before that a vaccine was the only way to combat, or more especially prevent, viral diseases (and before that there were only the practitioners who, at various times and in various places, swore by oil of scorpions, crabs' eyes and fifty millipedes taken twice daily in water). The method was first practised in some middle-eastern countries, and especially in Turkey, and was known as variolation (from the Latin, *varus*, a pustule),

---

* The problem with flu vaccines is that the virus, like many others, undergoes rapid spontaneous mutation, more so than most bacteria, and so new strains spring up to evade the vaccine. The hope is always to find a vaccine target – a structural element in one of the proteins that make up the virus that cannot mutate without disabling its function.

and was brought back to England by the redoubtable Lady Mary Wortley Montague (1689-1762)*, wife of His Majesty's

Ambassador to the Sublime Porte. There she observed how variolation was carried out, and was so impressed by the results that she had her young son variolated, and later, after her return to England, where smallpox was rampant, her daughter. The method was to inject by way of a scratch some fluid taken from one of the smallpox blisters that would later turn into a pockmark. But the sample was taken from someone infected by a mild strain of the virus, and therefore not seriously ill. The fluid would be carried in a nutshell and administered to the children in tiny quantities by women skilled in the practice. There was certainly the hazard of inducing lethal disease, which happened in an estimated 3% of variolated children, but in a time of epidemic posed a ten-times smaller risk than the disease caught in the normal way. In England there was much hostility, some of it religious, but most of it to the very notion of injecting children with the essence of the dread disease. It was only when the Royal family was persuaded to allow their children to be variolated that many patriotic English relented.

An advance came a few years later in 1796. Edward Jenner (1749-1823), a country doctor in Gloucestershire had made a curious observation: no matter how great the toll of smallpox in the population, it seemed never to affect the milkmaids on the local farms. Jenner's brilliant inference was that they were perhaps protected by frequent exposure to cowpox, which caused nothing more than a transient rash and a mild rise in temperature. The fact is that the cowpox virus is sufficiently close to smallpox in its composition that it allows the recipient to generate antibodies effective

---

* Lady Mary, a famous beauty born into an aristocratic family, was also witty, clever and determined. She was a feminist, and became a target of savage mockery by Alexander Pope. She had exchanged letters with him, but the friendship had soured, it was said because the deformed, dwarfish Pope had proposed marriage to her and she had laughed in his face. Lady Mary's brother died of smallpox, which she herself also contracted. She survived, though marked by the disease, which at the time had an incidence of some 10%, with a mortality of up to 40%. In Turkey she learned the language and wrote entertaining letters to friends later published, adverting to Muslim culture and the customs of the people.

against the smallpox virus, whenever it should invade. So that year Jenner tried his audacious experiment. He injected an eight-year-old boy with cowpox, followed six weeks later by matter from a smallpox pustule of a patient in the throes of the disease. The boy did not develop smallpox, so was evidently immune. A further exposure after an interval of some months also produced no disease. There were several more such experiments before Jenner published his results. Unlike the poor reception that variolation had received from the English public, Jenner's discovery was met with almost universal acclaim, and he was voted a reward of £10,000 – an enormous sum – by Parliament.*

Vaccination – the term was coined in Jenner's honour by Pasteur, from the Latin *vacca*, a cow – quickly supplanted variolation, and the incidence of smallpox in the western world fell abruptly.

In the 20th century, when the nature of viruses became clear, new and more rational methods of vaccine preparation came into use. The scheme, prefigured by Pasteur and by Ehrlich in their work on bacteria, was to immunise with a 'disabled' virus, rendered harmless by either of two strategies. The virus could be 'attenuated', that is to say grossly enfeebled in its effects on its victim, by repeated passage from one cell culture to another. Or the virus could be killed by exposure to heat, destructive enzymes or chemicals. With skill and luck such treatment would leave some components (proteins) of the virus undamaged, to the extent at least that they would elicit an immune response in a recipient, with the production of antibodies against the intact 'live' virus. The most celebrated result of researches along these lines was the production of a poliomyelitis (polio) vaccine, which eradicated the disease almost totally. The route to an effective and harmless vaccine was not without its vicissitudes. The key to the eventual outcome was the invention in 1947 by John Enders and

---

* Jenner was equally fêted in other countries. At the height of the Napoleonic wars Jenner begged the Emperor directly to release two Englishmen, friends of Jenner's, held in captivity in France. Napoleon, it was said, had reacted to Jenner's appeal with the words (though no doubt in French): 'Jenner! Ah, one can deny nothing to this man', and the captives were released and allowed to return to England. Jenner apparently also secured the release of several other prisoners.

his colleagues at the Harvard Children's Hospital in Boston of a way to prepare quantities of the virus by *in-vitro* culture. Enders had used human embryo tissue to cultivate the mumps virus – a major technical advance in virus research. The next step was to extend the technique to other pathogenic viruses, and in the course of this a happy chance discovery occurred: Enders's associate, Thomas Weller was making efforts to culture the chickenpox (varicella) virus in embryonic animal lung tissue. He had set up a series of tubes in an experiment, and found that he had a few more tubes than samples of infected tissue. So as not to waste the few residual tubes of culture he searched among his stocks and found some mouse brains infected with polio. It was these, but not the varicella samples that grew, and a new era in polio research began. Enders, Weller and another of their colleagues, Frederick Robbins shared the 1954 Nobel Prize for physiology or medicine for their work on viruses.

Several laboratories quickly entered the chase for a polio vaccine. In 1949 Jonas Salk (1914-1995), a doctor and microbiologist at the University of Pittsburgh set about generating a vaccine from a killed polio virus. The virus was isolated from a culture in embryo tissue, and was killed by prolonged incubation with formaldehyde (formalin). Salk would have been uncomfortably aware of the debacle which had attended two attempts nearly twenty years earlier to create a polio vaccine. No purified virus had yet been isolated, and the two laboratories concerned used ground-up infected animal tissue, such as the spinal cord of a monkey, as the starting material. The researchers had tried it on themselves with no apparent ill-effects, and then on children. In the one case many of the 3000 or so children in the trial had suffered allergic reactions, but at least no polio (though also no benefit in terms of antibody production). In the other trial several cases of paralysis and nine deaths were reported. Salk therefore proceeded with caution. He tested the preparations for any residual trace of live virus, and finding none, injected a group of children who had already had the disease. The vaccine engendered an increase in the level of anti-polio virus antibodies in the blood. Thus encouraged, Salk tried it on a small group of other children, and when the results proved satisfactory, he felt able to proceed to a full-scale clinical trial. In 1954 some 440,000 children were injected with the vaccine and another 210,000, the control group, received a placebo. By then it had been discovered that there were three strains of polio virus (mutants) in the population, which responded variously to different vaccine preparations. The Salk vaccine offered upwards of 60% protection against polio caused by one variant, and 90% or better against the other two. And so in 1955 a nationwide campaign of vaccination began in the United States, and Salk was the man of the moment. The intention was to inoculate 9 million children with vaccine provided by many suppliers, but almost immediately there was a hitch: reports came in from California of children struck down with paralytic polio following inoculation. The problem was traced to serum preparations from one laboratory, and after an interval for reflection, the programme continues with no further alarms. The method was safe.

Meanwhile work had been continuing on attenuated virus in several centres, including the Lederle Laboratories, where an immigrant Polish doctor and scientist (and also a musician, a graduate of the Warsaw Conservatoire) held sway, Hilary Koprowski (1918-2013) developed the method of multiple passage. The virus was passaged (to use the technical term) through a sequence of animal cells to allow it to mutate into a harmless form, incubating each time under conditions known to favour rapid mutation. An extract of the infected material from, say, a mouse brain, is cultured in a second mouse brain, that from the second in a third, and so on. After seven such passages, Koprowski established that the resulting material had no discernible pathological properties. It was then passed through several rats to make sure, and was finally adjudged safe. Injected into an eight-year-old boy, it caused no symptoms. An equally active laboratory was that of Albert Sabin (1906-1993), another emigré from Poland. Sabin had a burning conviction that an attenuated-virus vaccine would be far superior to the chemically killed alternative. Moreover, he appeared to be driven by a hatred for his competitor, Jonas Salk, which expressed itself in public brawls at conferences. Sabin proceeded much as Koprowski had been doing, using monkey kidney cells to grow the virus. He was a skilled operator, with successful vaccines against two other viruses to his name, but by 1956 there was competition, and several preparations of attenuated vaccines were spilling out of laboratories. Sabin's emerged as the most potent, but because of the uncritical adulation surrounding

Salk there was difficulty in finding parents willing to volunteer their children for clinical trials of something new, untried, and as it appeared, unnecessary. Sabin's solution was to conduct his trials in a country that polio vaccination had not reached, in fact Russia. After three years Sabin had data from more than 4 million vaccinations, showing excellent results. The attenuated vaccine gave high protection, and had other advantages besides: it remained longer in the body, and most importantly, it could be administered by mouth, for it could survive and propagate in the gut tissue, and continue to generate antibodies. Yet for two decades the Salk vaccine was officially preferred in the United States, and was distributed throughout the world. Eventually its use waned as Sabin's vaccine became increasingly favoured. By the end of the 20th century the Salk vaccine had vanished from the scene. This would have been a satisfaction to Albert Sabin, but Salk has a tangible memorial, the Salk Institute in California, one of today's leading centres of biomedical science.

Chemicals and viruses

In 1988 George Hitchings, Gertrude Elion and Sir James Black (p.) shoock hands with the King of Sweden and received their gold Nobel Prize medals. Hitchings and Elion had worked together for many years. They were chemists, while Black was a pharmacologist. All had done most of their important work in industrial laboratories, but Black's interests and style had been quite different from those of the other two. George Hitchings (1905-1998) was a virtuoso chemist, a graduate of the University of Washington, and of Harvard Medical School, where he gained his Ph.D. After a period in academic research, Hitchings broke away and headed for the world of industry. From his youth he adulated Pasteur, and was moved by the ambition to pursue research with a directly useful aim. In 1942 he joined the Burroughs Wellcome Laboratories in New York State as head (and sole member) of the biochemistry department. There, two years later, he was joined by a talented organic chemist, Elvira Falco, and after another two years by Gertrude Elion. A few more chemists joined, but the group remained small, and it was Hitchings and Gertrude Elion who formed almost from the outset a perfect scientific partnership.

Gertrude Elion (1918-1999) was born in New York to a Russian mother and a Lithuanian dentist father. A bright child, she was much affected by the death from cancer of a beloved grandfather, and settled on a career in science, so that she could help to alleviate disease. At Hunter College in Manhattan she read chemistry. But the union card for entry into an academic career was (and is) a Ph.D., and at the time there were few graduate opportunities for women. Gertrude Elion temporised and became a schoolteacher, while working in the evenings towards an M.Sc. degree at New York University. Then she enrolled at Brooklyn Polytechnic, hoping to continue to a Ph.D., working at her research project at night while supporting herself by a daytime job in a commercial laboratory, analysing pickles, mayonnaises, and the like. The plan failed, when the Polytechnic rescinded its part-time Ph.D. programme. Then in 1944 the opportunity presented itself to join George Hitchings as an assistant at Burroughs Wellcome. And so Gertrude Elion stayed unanointed until – by then a Nobel Laureate - three universities conferred honorary doctorates on her. She remained at Burroughs Wellcome until her retirement when she was in her seventies.

The year before her arrival at Burroughs Wellcome Oswald Avery and his colleagues at the Rockefeller Institute had proved that DNA was the genetic material, its chemical composition, with its two purines, A and G, and two pyrimidines, C and T (p.), having been already established. Hitchings and Elion absorbed this information and reasoned that if bacteria and viruses reproduced at such great rates compared to any host organism then any compound that could interrupt the process of

DNA replication might arrest an infection*, or indeed a fast-growing cancer. Pursuing this logic, they set about synthesising a series of purine derivatives – analogues of the purine bases of DNA. It proved a rich vein. Several of the new compounds did indeed impede the growth of selected bacteria by blocking the action of enzymes involved in the synthesis of DNA. Not only, in fact, did they stop replication of the bacteria, but equally that of cells in animals, including of course people. From 1947 onwards the most promising of the new compounds were sent for clinical evaluation to the Sloan-Kettering Institute in New York. One of the first, 2,6-diaminopurine (the carbon-nitrogen rings of purine with two amino groups, $-NH_2$, attached) was tried on patients with acute leukaemia in the Sloan-Kettering Memorial Hospital, attached to the Institute, and was found in many cases to cause remission of the disease. Later Hitchings and Elion hit on a more dependable drug against some forms of leukaemia, 6-mercaptopurine – purine with an attached sulphur atom – which became a standard treatment. A succession of new drugs issued from the Burroughs Wellcome laboratory. Azathioprine, another purine derivative, turned out to be a powerful immunosuppressant, used to prevent rejection of transplanted organs by the recipient's immune system. Allopurinol was found to intervene in another purine-linked metabolic process, the formation of uric acid - a purine derivative, which in gout sufferers (p.) accumulates in the form of needle-like crystals in the joints; allopurinol

---

* Viruses function quite differently from bacteria. A virus is not a free-living organism. It cannot reproduce outside the cell that it invades. The virus has its own genome, which is made in some cases of DNA, in others of the closely related nucleic acid, RNA, which differs from DNA in only one atom in each nucleotide sugar unit, and one more oxygen atom in the sugar units. The nucleic acid is surrounded and protected by a protein coat. Once it has entered the cell, the virus hijacks the host's reproductive machinery, and uses it to copy its own nucleic acid, and express the proteins encoded by it. It can thus reproduce itself many times over. The newly formed viruses then burst out of the cell, which is destroyed in the process, and go on to invade other cells. The bacteriophages (p.), viruses that infect bacteria, act differently in that instead of entering the bacterium, they attach themselves to the outer surface and inject their nucleic acid, as if through a syringe. The nucleic acid is then replicated and the genes that it contains are expressed (translated into the proteins that they encode), all by the machinery of the host cell. The bacterium fills up with the newly created viruses, bursts and releases its contents.

became at once the sovereign treatment for the disease. And later Gertrude Elion made yet another purine derivative, acyclovir (trade name, Zovirax), active against the herpes virus. This became the first successful treatment therefore for genital herpes, and indeed the first synthetic antiviral agent of any consequence. Its discovery set off a search for compounds with activity against more lethal viruses, leading eventually to azidothymidine, AZT, a derivative of thymine, another of the four bases that go to make up DNA, and the first effective drug against AIDS. A great number of antiviral agents have since been developed (see p.), and AIDS especially is no longer a terminal disease. Even so, many viruses remain obstinately impervious to all new compounds that science has been able to direct at them.

Fighting the fungus: the mouldy maladies

The fungi are a vast group of organisms, some large, some microscopic, and certain of the small ones prey on man. The fungi are not equipped for an independent existence. Mushrooms, for instance, have no chlorophyll, and so cannot use sunlight to make their own nutrients, as green plants do. Mushrooms and the other fungi must therefore live entirely off their environment. They may be *saprophytic*, that is feed off dead and decaying vegetable or animal matter, or they can be *parasitic*, and some are *symbionts*, which co-exist with another organism, exchanging essential materials in a manner profitable to both. A variety of human diseases are caused by fungi – not happily by any that resemble mushrooms, but by microscopic species. Fungal diseases are only rarely life-threatening. (Ergot, which causes 'St. Anthony's Fire', engenders gangrene in the limbs, and was common in the Middle Ages (p.), is an exception, but it does not attack humans or animals directly; it infects wheat and secretes a toxin, which does the damage. Most of the fungi that infect man result in often distressing and unsightly skin conditions. Some others take root in the lung, and others again in the mucous membranes. Most dangerous are infections in people with impaired immune defences, such as victims of AIDS, or those who have undergone intensive chemotherapy, and immunosuppressed organ recipients. Among the most common fungal diseases (or mycoses, as they are known to professionals) are athlete's foot (which came to Europe from

Southeast Asia during the peak of the colonial period in the 19th century) and ringworm.

It was a remarkable Italian polymath, Agostino Bassi (1773-1856) who first recognised a fungal pathology. His indeed was the earliest demonstration of a micro-organism as an infectious agent, more than thirty years ahead of Koch and Pasteur. Bassi was the scion of a landed family in Lodi in northern Italy. He studied law and became active in the local government, in which he occupied a variety of important offices. But his special interest was in agriculture, and he also had a passion for entomology. He was a man of great intellectual curiosity with a penetrating intelligence. He took up sheep-breeding, on which he published a monograph, and he followed that with studies of cheese and of wine production, on both of which he wrote popular manuals. In about 1807 his attention was drawn, as Pasteur's was to be a half-century later, to a disease that was threatening to annihilate the local silkworm industry. He searched for evidence that the condition, known as *calcinaccio* – calcification – also known as muscardine, was generated spontaneously in the worms, according to the prevalent doctrine. But this was not what Bassi found, and in the course of a study, which occupied much of his time over a period of thirty years, he found the true cause. He first discovered that silkworms isolated in clean conditions did not develop the disease: it had to be brought by an external agency. Dead silkworms most often displayed a white encrustation on the outside, and if not on the outside, then on the inside. When Bassi took a little of this deposit on the tip of a needle and introduced it into a healthy worm the infection quickly developed. Bassi had a good microscope, and was able to show that the white substance consisted of fungi, similar in appearance to *Botrytis allii*. This fungus, related to the 'noble rot' of grapes, which produces sweet wines of France, causes a less desirable rot in onion stems. The silk-worm fungus could also be seen to produce spores, the 'seeds' by which fungi, in general, multiply. Bassi drew up a list of conditions for preventing the incidence of muscardine – disinfecting the silkworm nurseries, maintaining rigorously clean and uncrowded work spaces, insisting on the hygiene of the workers, and especially watching for and destroying any infected worms. In 1834 Bassi presented his results and conclusions before a committee of the faculty at the University of Pavia, and he followed this a year later with two detailed publications. He ran into quite violent opposition from the upholders of the ancient theory of spontaneous generation, but a minority of more open-minded spirits accepted Bassi's conclusions, and followed his precepts. Bassi suggested with remarkable prescience that many human diseases, from cholera and typhus to syphilis, would turn out also to be caused by micro-organisms. It was only, of course, after Bassi's death that his sirmise was proved correct.

In 1841, six years after the appearance of Bassi's papers, a transmissible human skin condition was simultaneously discovered by two doctors, one in Berlin, the other in Paris. David Gruby, who was born in Hungary, studied in Vienna and settled in Paris. Was a well-known specialist in parasitic diseases, and it was ringworm tat he first identified as a fungus. He showed that a sample scraped from the skin of a patient could infect healthy volunteers, of whom he himself was the first. Among his later discoveries was the yeast-like agent of candidiasis, *Candida albicans*. (Long recognised as a cause of genital and mouth infections, it has more recently been identified as an accompanying hazard of cosmetic tongue piercing.) Gruby, as well as the co-discoverer of fungal disease, the Berlin professor, Johann Lukas Schönlein, and several others advanced the state of knowledge of fungal diseases, but could do little for the victims. It was to be no less than a century and a half before the first antifungal remedy became available. Harold Raistrick, while still an outstanding chemistry student at Leeds University, had been drawn especially to the chemistry of natural products. After Leeds, he honed his skills in Cambridge under Frederick Gowland Hopkins (p.). Chief among Raistrick's interests then and later was the chemistry of fungi. In 1929 he was appointed to a chair of chemistry at London University, tenable at the London School of Hygiene and Tropical Medicine. Among several lines of research that he developed in his small department was the attempt to isolate penicillin. He made, as already related (p.), some progress, but assured that penicillin would never amount to anything useful, he turned his attention to other fungal metabolites, among which was one sent to him in 1939 from the Oxford laboratory. It had been isolated from another *Penicillium* mould, *Penicillium griseofulvum*, and was unusual in that it contained a chlorine atom. Raistrick did not test the compound, which was given the name, griseofulvin, for antibacterial activity, but he did show in 1946 that it was identical to an extract prepared by chemists at ICI from another *Penicillium* mould, *Penicillium janczewskii*. This came from a patch of land in Devon, Wareham Heath, which had first caught the attention of the workers at the ICI laboratory because pine trees planted there some years before had all died; and secondly there was a strange absence of soil bacteria. Moreover, fungi growing on the Heath developed curiously deformed hyphae, the long branched filaments tubes by which the organism propagates.

Raistrick was a consultant to ICI, and provided the chemists, who were on the search for new antibiotics, with a large number of mould extracts that he had accumulated over the years. It turned out that several *Penicillium* moulds contained, in greater or lesser amounts, the 'curling factor' responsible for deforming the fungal hyphae. It was in the end the ICI chemists who determined its structure and in 1952 brought off a synthesis. The substance – griseofulvin - had no appreciable antibiotic activity, but it was a powerful fungicide, which ICI hoped would prove useful in agriculture. The synthesis was arduous however, and the product too expensive to compete with sprays then in use, and so griseofulvin was shelved. It was only five years later that some veterinarians thought to test it against fungal infections in farm animals. It cured ringworm, and in 1959 its efficacy against human ringworm and other fungal skin infections had been demonstrated, and pharmaceutical companies strove to develop procedures for culturing the mould and extracting the griseofulvin. It was the first effective fungicide for human use, and is still prescribed, taken by mouth, for some conditions, although it has been largely replaced by nystatin, and more especially amphotericin B. These too arrived in the 1950s.

Nystatin came from a species of streptomyces - yet another of the seemingly inexhaustible genus of soil bacteria, so profitably hunted down by Waksman and his successors. It was discovered by two highly accomplished American women ('maiden ladies' according to the social usage of the time), Elizabeth Lee Hazen (1885-1975) and Rachel Fuller Brown (1898-1980), both in the employ of the New York State Department of Public Health. Elizabeth Hazen was a microbiologist, who had studied biology in her home State at the Mississippi University for Women, and had progressed by painful degrees, for women had limited opportunities for advancement, to a Ph.D. at Columbia University in New York. In time she achieved an appointment at the Division of Laboratories and Research in New York City. The search for antibiotics was in full swing, and Elizabeth Hazen joined it. So it was that while visiting a family friend who owned a dairy farm she examined the soil for promising bacteria, and found one that proved to have remarkable fungicidal properties when tested *in vitro*. The bacterium was given the name, *Streptomyces noursei*, in homage to Mr Nourse, the owner of the dairy farm. The laboratory director decided that attempts must be made to isolate the active substance, and this would demand specialist chemical skills. He put Elizabeth Hazen in touch with Rachel Brown in the Public Health Department's laboratories in distant up-state Albany. Rachel Brown had grown up in Massachusetts in straitened circumstances, the child of an abandoned mother. A relative helped her to enter Mount Holyoke College to read history, but she was soon captivated by chemistry. After graduating she taught science in schools, but eventually managed to enrol for a research degree in the illustrious chemistry department of the University of Chicago. She was hard-up throughout this time, and having submitted her Ph.D. thesis, she was forced to leave to earn a living without waiting for the oral examination. (It was only some years later that she was awarded the degree.) Although the two women seldom met, and the cultures prepared by Dr Hazen were despatched by post in pickling jars, the collaboration bore fruit. The first name given to the fungicide was Fungicidin, but this was found to have been already applied to something else, and so Hazen and Brown chose to call it nystatin, for New York State. The patent was allocated in 1957, long after the discovery and development of the drug to the pharmaceutical company of E.R. Squibb and Sons, and garnered huge profits in royalties to the two discoverers, which they passed to a fund, dedicated to the furtherance of research.

Nystatin, marketed as Nystan, relieved much misery, yet it was a far from perfect drug, for it had minimal solubility in water, and was not absorbed in the gut; it had bad effects on the skin when injected, so had to be applied to the surface in a formulation with detergent. Its action in this form was slow, but watery suspensions were (and are) used orally for mouth infections. Nystatin is still in use, especially for that purpose and against vaginal infections. Moreover, Squibb (later Bristol-Myers Squibb) knew as soon as the properties of nystatin had been analysed what to do next. Even before they had brought nystatin into large-scale production they were already screening huge numbers of soil bacteria from around the world for the previously hidden fungicidal character, hoping for a compound with better properties, especially solubility. In 1953 the effort was rewarded when preparation M 4575 showed spectacular antifungal activity, not only *in vitro*, but also in infected mice and rats, even in the form of a highly impure solution. The bacterium came from soil brought from the Orinoco River basin in Venezuels. The 'active principle' turned out to contain two compounds, very complex members of the chemical class known as polyenes, to which nystatin also belongs. But all was not as it seemed: when tested in dogs and then in patients it had little effect, for again it was not absorbed through the gut, as it had been in the rodents. The well-proven strategy of introducing chemical modifications could not be pursued, because the exact structural formula resisted all attempts at analysis, let alone synthesis. Strenuous efforts at least produced a formulation, involving the preparation of complexes with bile salts (simple natural substances with detergent properties that emulsify fats in the body), which could be injected. The two active substances, called amphotericin A and amphotericin B were separated, and the second of these was found to have much superior activity. Eventually a strain of the bacterium was generated which secreted only this form. Amphotericin B was, and remains a less than ideal drug, for it has to be administered under rigorously controlled conditions, but it generated rich rewards for Squibb after their many years of research. It is still the best antifungal drug available to dermatologists in an age in which AIDS and other conditions that undermine the immune system leave many patients vulnerable to distressing, and even lethal fungal infections. The search for something better continues.

Chapter 13

'WHERE THE HORMONES THERE MOAN I'

So wrote Aldous Huxley's hero in his novel, *Point Counterpoint*, which implies that the hormones had a place in the dinner-table conversation of the 1920s. The term was coined in 1906, from the Greek *hormeo*, 'I excite', by the English physiologist, Ernest Starling. With his colleague William Bayliss, he had found that substances released from glands travel in the bloodstream, each to its own target organ, which it goads into action. The existence of messenger substances that shuttled around the body switching metabolic reactions on and off according to demand had been intuited a half-century earlier by Claude Bernard. In the ensuing years fragmentary experimental evidence came to light, notably the observation in 1856 by Charles Édouard Brown-Séquard (whom we will encounter again shortly) that extirpation of the adrenal gland, which lies (as its name from the Latin implies) close to the kidneys, was fatal to animals. He inferred that a secretion of the gland performed some essential function elsewhere in the body. In 1904 Starling made this remarkably discerning pronouncement in one of the Royal Society's prize lectures: 'If the control of the different functions of the body be largely determined by the production of definite chemical substances within the body, the discovery of the nature of these substances will enable us to interpose at any desired phase in these functions and so to acquire an absolute control over the workings of the human body. Such a control is the goal of medical science,' A century on, and although medical science has taken great strides, it has still not arrived at this consummation. The path has been tortuous and strewn with rocks.

The broken shield

The first hormone to be identified derived from the thyroid gland. That iodine and its compounds could eliminate goitre had been known since early in the 19th century (p.). The connection was also made between goitre and cretinism, a retardation of children's development, both mental and physical. The onset of the effects of iodine deficiency in adults is a general wasting condition, marked also by loss of body heat, and is called myxoedema. The thyroid gland, situated at the base of the neck takes it name from the Greek for a shield, which describes its shape. In the 7th century B.C. the Chinese physicians treated goitrous patients by giving them a sheep's thyroid to eat (as an alternative perhaps to sponges or seaweed if they were far from the sea). Galen was aware of the thyroid, and speculated that it exuded a throat lubricant. The doctor and anatomist, Thomas Wharton of St. Thomas's Hospital in London, writing in 1656, suggested that one of its functions was 'to fill the neck and make it shapely'. The importance of the thyroid for the maintenance of life was not demonstrated until the 19th century when Moritz Schiff (1822-1896), working in Berne, found that dogs died when surgically deprived of their thyroid glands.' He then grafted the pieces of the gland into the abdominal cavity of such thyroidectomised dogs, which enabled them to live for some time. This was a highly significant result, for it showed that the thyroid functioned irrespectively of where it was positioned in the body, and could

---

* Schiff was clearly a remarkable man. He was born un Frankfurt, studied medicine in Göttingen, and physiology with two great masters, Müller in Berlin and Magendie in Paris. He had been active in liberal politics, and this led to his exclusion from Göttingen University, which had appointed him a *Privatdozent*, or lecturer. He worked briefly in Florence, and then, having been chased out by the anti-vivisection movement, in Geneva. He eventually found a safe haven in Berne. His persecution in Florence was particularly unjust, for he was probably the first prominent physiologist to argue for the humane treatment of laboratory animals, and to insist that vivisection should be performed under anaesthesia.

418

therefore be inferred to release some life-giving essence. Schiff also showed that thyroid extracts could preserve life. Eager doctors in Berne tried to persuade Schiff to inject ground thyroid glands into human subjects, but he demurred, and the first such experimental treatment was left to a doctor in Edinburgh.

How the thyroid functioned was not at all clear, but it was evident at least that it required iodine to do its work – a fact repeatedly rediscovered throughout the 19th century, and just as often disputed or qualified, with the result that much suffering was allowed to continue, and many died who might have lived. We know now that the gland is the regulator of the body's overall metabolism. With a malfunctioning thyroid we become sluggish and tired, and if this happens during pregnancy or infancy, whether through a genetic defect or an insufficiency of iodine intake, the child will grow up stunted and mentally retarded. If the thyroid is hyperactive the metabolic rate runs out of control, and all manner of symptoms from weight loss to agitation and depression appear. This condition is also known as thyrotoxicosis, for at too high concentration the secretions of the thyroid become toxic. Hyperthyroidism is relatively rare, and is constitutional, whereas goitre and cretinism were recognised to be a common geographically determined phenomenon. There are descriptions in medieval manuscripts, with their pictures of unfortunate people burdened with monstrous, often pendulous excrescences on their necks. Paracelsus was one who commented on 'Alpine cretinism', and apparently also made the connection between this and goitre. In different parts of the world the condition had different names, 'Derbyshire neck' for example in England. The prevalence of goitre in mountainous regions, where mineral deposits were depleted by glaciers, was noted by writers in Roman and medieval times, Paracelsus included. This was widely

419

attributed to 'stagnant air' in the valleys.* But populations in many low-lying parts of the world were equally badly affected, and the belief that goitre was an infectious condition died hard, even after its cause and cure had been discovered.

Among those who rediscovered the connection of goitre with iodine deficiency was the illustrious French chemist and nutritionist, Jean-Baptiste Boussingault. He reported that widespread goitre in the Andes was linked to a low iodine content in the local salt deposits, and could be cured by adding an iodine compounds to the salt. His paper on the subject, published in 1833, seems to have been generally disregarded. Next, in 1852 another French chemist, Adolphe Chatin made public the results of a series of meticulous analyses of iodine content of waters along the Rhône valley, where some villages were free of goitre and others plagued by it. He extended his work to other sites in Europe, and the correlation was clear, but again excited little interest. (The intelligent suggestion that potassium iodide should be added to cooking salt found no favour until well into the 20th century.) Then in 1873 a doctor in Geneva, Joseph Baillarger, undertook a clinical trial in the Albi region to the south of the city, where the incidence of goitre was high. He arranged for 620 schoolchildren with symptoms of the condition to be administered potassium iodide pills by their teachers. The majority were completely cured, and nearly all the remainder much improved. The waters were muddied however by the gradual recognition that goitre came in two forms. The second and rarer became known as exophthalmic goitre, marked by bulging eyes, accompanied by the symptoms of a hyperactive thyroid, as described above. In many, but not all cases the thyroid was enlarged, generating the

---

* A long letter to the editor of the *Magazine of Natural History* in 1830 by one T.W.D. of Greenwich, was one of many publications that also disputed the theory, and expounded a widely held alternative view. 'I have met with many people of the middle classes', T.W.D. instructs his readers, 'who, in consequence of greater attention to cleanliness, more exercise, a more generous diet, and *using but little of the water*, might be expected to enjoy more robust health, and who constantly inhabit places exposed to the most oppressive atmosphere, without being materially or at all affected, although surrounded by goitre in its most disgusting forms among the lower classes who are dirty, idle and ill fed.' By dismal contrast, 'where the atmosphere is most salubrious and refreshing goitre amongst the lower classes is extremely prevalent.'

familiar swelling on the neck. There were no geographical concentrations of this affliction, and thus it caused confusion. In exophthalmic goitre the hyperactive thyroid proliferates, whereas in the commoner form the inactive or sluggish thyroid grows in the attempt to compensate for the low level of its output of secretions. It was gradually recognised by the more astute physicians among those who made use of iodine treatment that this was at best unhelpful in cases of exophthalmic goitre.

Goitres were occasionally removed surgically – a hazardous procedure before surgeons became more skilled in the late 19th century. The master of the thyroidectomy operation was Theodor Kocher (1841-1917), a native of Berne and a professor at the local university. He was a much-admired surgeon, an exceptionally skilful operator, who had learned his craft in the leading European centres, and introduced important innovations in diverse areas of surgery. Kocher himself performed more than 4000 thyroidectomies, starting in the early 1880s, and his students and followers many more. He believed at this time that the accompanying symptoms of goitre were the result of constriction of the airways, but other than reducing the swelling on the neck, the operation did no more than remove whatever vestigial source of thyroid secretion the patient had left. The consequence was that although the success rate of the operation itself was the highest that had ever been achieved, with a mortality of no more than 0.5%, the distressing symptoms of myxoedema later asserted themselves, the goitre often reappeared, and some patients died. When the deeply conscientious and caring Kocher finally grasped that what his patients were suffering from was a *lack* of thyroid function and not an excess, he was racked with guilt and remorse. But he remained obdurate in his opposition to the use of iodine, which he held to be a dangerous poison. He prescribed instead sheep's thyroid, to be consumed lightly fried. Kocher continued to investigate the anatomy of the thyroid and to improve surgical procedures for excision of tumours, and in 1909 he was rewarded with the Nobel Prize.

Considering the accumulation of evidence over centuries that iodine cured or prevented goitre, and that the disease was associated with the thyroid gland, it seems astonishing in hindsight that nobody thought until about 1890 to see whether the gland contained iodine. This was eventually resolved by Eugen Baumann, professor of chemistry at the University of Freiburg, in the middle of an area in which goitre was abundant. Baumann had been preparing extracts of the gland, but it appears to have been a colleague who suggested he might analyse them for the presence of iodine. The result was startling: the solid material recovered after treating thyroid glands with acid and with the stomach enzyme, pepsin, which digests proteins, contained no less than 19% of iodine by weight. Baumann went on to show that this material caused the regression of goitres in laboratory animals. Baumann also went a step further and prepared from his recovered solid an iodine-containing substance, which he called iodothyronin. This too was highly effective in curing goitre. And still no measures were undertaken by doctors to counter this entirely preventable disease. As late as the start of the 20th century medical textbooks still asserted that goitre was a communicable disease, and that it was linked to poor hygiene. The breakthrough came from the United States, thanks to the persistence of a young doctor, David Marine.

David Marine (1888-1976) grew up on a farm in Maryland, and developed an early interest in zoology, which he studied at university before changing to medicine. Graduating from Johns Hopkins Medical School, he took a position in a hospital in Cleveland, Ohio. The city lay in the very centre of the 'goitre belt', and it was goitre that the young Marine had resolved to study. It was said that he found his direction in research from his encounters with goitrous dogs in the street. He examined their thyroid glands and found that, despite their grossly increased size, they contained very little iodine, compared to the glands of healthy animals. Marine's next discovery was certainly thrust on him fortuitously: he was invited by a local hunting-and-fishing organisation to investigate what was taken to be an epidemic of cancer in fish reared in hatcheries. Marine found that it was not cancer at all, but goitre that was afflicting the fish, and when he inquired into the food on which the fish were reared he quickly saw that it had minimal iodine content. When iodine in the form of potassium iodide was added to the water the swellings disappeared, the fish put on weight and grew fat and healthy. Reinforced in his conviction that the children in the goitre belt must be given iodine as a matter of course, Marine first tried the remedy on a group of children with goitre in his hospital. The success of the treatment, which in truth did little more than confirm what had been done several times in Europe at intervals over a period of almost a century, was insufficient to persuade the authorities in Cleveland to organise a larger trial. Marine had better luck in another town in the same state, Akron. At this stage the entry of the United States into the war in Europe in 1917 intervened. Marine was away on army service for two years, but after his return prophylactic treatment of goitre began in earnest. In the face of continuing scepticism in some corners of the medical profession potassium iodide was added to the waters of the goitre belt. Soon thereafter minute amounts of potassium iodide were added to table salt. When the success of the practice became too obvious to ignore it spread to Europe and beyond, and goitre more or less vanished from the world.

This is not to say that iodine intake will look after all disorders of the thyroid gland. Today goitre through iodine deficiency is almost unknown, but if the gland refuses to manufacture enough thyroid hormone, or the mechanism that controls its release into the bloodstream (which is activated by a so-called releasing factor, thyrotropin, secreted by the pituitary gland), a different treatment is called for. The thyroid hormone, thyroxine was isolated by the American biochemist, Edward Calvin Kendall (1886-1972). Kendall studied chemistry at Columbia University in New York, and began research on the thyroid at St. Luke's Hospital in the city. His biographer relates that when the hospital management sent him a carton of breakfast cereal, with the demand to analyse its composition, he angrily tossed it into the rubbish bin and walked out, never to return. Instead he found a more congenial berth at the Mayo Clinic, a famous centre of research, in Rochester, Minnesota. There in 1911 he set about isolating the 'active principle' (which he realised was not simply iodine) from pig thyroids, and in time he succeeded. He and a group of helpers spent the next ten years trying to determine its structure. He failed. The proposed structure, Kendall decided, must wrong, and a few years later Charles Harington at University College London published the correct formula. By 1925 he and his friend, George Barger, Professor of Chemistry at the University of Edinburgh had effected a total synthesis. The molecule contains four iodine atoms, and it coexists in the thyroid with a small proportion of a more potent version containing only three iodine atoms. It was another two decades before an industrial-scale synthesis was achieved, and thyroxine became widely available.

But what of the hyperactive thyroid and thyrotoxicosis with all its attendant ills? The trail towards a drug began with a paradox. In 1928 Alan Mason Chesney, a professor at the Johns Hopkins Medical School in Baltimore was engaged in studies of syphilis, with rabbits as the experimental animals, when a strange observation came his way: the rabbits were all developing enormous goitrous growths in their necks. Chesney and his group of researchers investigated. They found no shortage of iodine in the rabbits' diets, and no other obvious dietary deficiency, nor was there any sign of an infection. Failing any other explanation, there remained only the diet: the rabbits were being fed on cabbage. Chesney and his colleagues published their conclusion, which was taken up and confirmed in several other laboratories, and especially by David Marine. He extended the observations to other related vegetables of the *Brassica* family and to several animal species. But from one direction came dissent: the laboratory of Henry Dudley Purves in New Zealand could not repeat what the others had observed. Perhaps, Purves thought, the goitrogenic (goitre-inducing) activity might reside in the seeds rather than the leaves, for seeds were commonly the source of toxic or biologically active compounds, especially the sugar-linked glycosides (p.). Different cabbages, differently prepared, might vary in their content of seeds. His guess proved correct. Purves, a researcher of great acuity, chose next to look into the nature of the effect. Administering iodine to the animals did not shrink the goitres, but when the *Brassica* diet was fed to hypophysectomised rats they did not develop goitres. Hypophysectomy means the surgical removal of the pituitary gland (also called the epiphysis), the source of thyrotropin, which turns on the activity of the thyroid. The cabbage-induced goitre must therefore, as Purves deduced, have been a response to the failure of the thyroid to function as it should, for there is a feedback loop which shuts off thyrotropin release when the thyroxine in the blood reaches the required level. But in this form of goitre the thyrotropin does no more than flog a dead horse, for the thyroid fails to produce thyroxine, and the pituitary keeps trying by putting out more thyrotropin. This stimulates growth of the thyroid, but to no useful effect. The condition is called 'compensatory hypertrophy'.

It would have been clear to Purves, to Chesney and to those who saw the reports that if the anti-goitre substance in the cabbage could be isolated it might afford the long-sought treatment for hyperthyroidism. An obvious starting point was to examine the mustard oils found in the seeds of the *Brassica* family. Marine first tested several such oils and drew a blank. He turned next to the cyanide compounds that also lurked in cabbage seeds, and reported that the simplest and least toxic of these, cyanomethane, was anti-goitrogenic, but this turned out to be a mirage. The next clue came a few years later in 1940, when the search for new antibacterial sulpha drugs was at its peak, and an American pharmaceutical company was testing new derivatives in rats. One such, sulphaguanidine was a poor antibacterial agent, but the animal tests revealed a damaging effect on the thyroid. Just as so often before, the activity was a function of a substituent group in the intended drug, and not of the compounds as a whole. Two simple sulphur-containing compounds, thiouracil and thiourea proved equally effective. All had in common that they contained sulphur (implied by the prefix thio), and were related to the sulphur compounds in cabbage, which give it the characteristic smell. Next, in 1941 two workers in an industrial laboratory in Boston were searching for a better rat poison, and found that another familiar sulphur-containing compound, phenylthiourea induced goitres in the animals. This and results from other sources set off a survey of related chemicals that might display the desired properties. The failed rat poison, phenylthiourea was tried on patients with thyrotoxicosis, and then also the still simpler thiourea, which came into wide clinical use.

It turned out, however, that Marine and Purves had both been on the right track in looking to mustard oil and in particular its glycosides for an answer. Edwin Astwood at Tufts University Medical School in Boston conducted a systematic search for anti-goitrous activity in a variety of vegetables and fruits, and eventually found potent activity in the edible part of the swede. The activity was destroyed by cooking, and an extract from the raw root was also inert, but when this was mixed with the macerated flesh the anti-goitrous effect returned. It was clear now that the activity was released through the action of an enzyme. The active product was duly purified, its site of action in blocking the synthesis of thyroxine in the thyroid gland was determined, and Astwood gave the compound the name, goitrin, and its precursor became goitrogen. Thereafter it was left to the pharmaceutical companies to find the most active related compound with the fewest side-effects (which nevertheless remain troubling). Today hyperthyroidism is treated with the sulphur-containing drug, synthesised in 1954 by chemists at University College London, called carbimazole, replacing the cheap but less effective thiourea. Carbimazole is a pro-drug - itself inert, but it converted in the body to the active compound, methimazole. There is, though, another means of dealing with thyrotoxicosis, namely by the use of a radioactive iodine isotope, ^{131}I. This isotope became all too familiar in relation to nuclear reactor accidents. Like the prevailing form of iodine (^{128}I), which is not radioactive, it finds its way to the thyroid gland when it enters the body, and can cause thyroid cancer. The radiation emitted by the radioactive iodine atoms destroys thyroid cells, and this method is often used in preference to drugs, but in rigorously controlled doses, to reduce the mass of the thyroid, and thus its activity.

The sugar disease: a chronicle of acrimony

Doctor Johnson's *Dictionary of the English Language* defines a drug as 'An ingredient used in physick', or alternatively, 'a medicinal simple'. According at least to the first of these definitions, insulin could be classed as a drug, even if it is a natural constituent of the body. The same is true of course of all the other hormones, but the discovery of insulin was arguably the most important single event in the history of medicine. Up to the 1920s a diagnosis of diabetes (more properly diabetes mellitus, to distinguish it from other, and rarer diabetic conditions) meant a wretched and protracted decline and an early death. A doctor hearing the litany of symptoms would glance down at a male patient's shoes, looking for the small white spots of sugar from tiny drops of dried urine. In those less squeamish days the doctor would be expected to make a confirmatory diagnosis by tasting the urine. Diabetes was recognised by its symptoms two millennia or more ago. The body is unable to metabolise its food and convert it into energy, and so begins to waste away. There is a voluminous flow of urine – whence the early English term, 'the pissing disease' – and the victim experiences an unslakable thirst. The intake of carbohydrate cannot be processed it is excreted in the form of glucose, and a violent hunger and craving after carbohydrate ensues. If the patient is allowed to indulge then this the decline merely accelerates with the failure of more bodily functions. So the only alternative course is starvation to prolong life.

The earliest indications of a link between diabetes and the pancreas, an abdominal gland of complex structure, came from evidence of its abnormality, sometimes remarked in autopsies of diabetics. The 19th-century physiologists had found that the pancreas secreted digestive enzymes, and was therefore supposed to have a digestive function. This was true as far as it went, but further enlightenment came much later, and yet again by accident. In 1889 a well-known physiologist, Josef von Mering, professor at the German University of Strassburg, and his junior colleague, Oskar Minkowski, trying to clarify their ideas about the function of the pancreatic digestive enzymes, took out the pancreas of a dog to see what would happen. As Minkowski told it, he noticed that the dog proceeded to urinate frequently and copiously on the floor of the laboratory, and to drink a great deal of water. He further observed flies settling on the puddles, which indicated to him that the dog's urine contained sugar. The dog indeed had diabetes (*Zuckerkrankheit*, sugar disease, in German). The resulting publication was greeted not with acclaim, but with scepticism. In particular, removal of the pancreas was a tricky operation, and the suspicion was that a part of the tissue must have been left behind. Minkowski and von Mering, and workers in a few other centres responded by ligating pancreatic ducts in dogs to induce diabetes, and also relieving the condition in pancreatectomised animals by reintroducing a fragment of pancreas. But interest remained sporadic. It was in general solitary individuals, in some cases medical students, who made attempts to extract an antidiabetic principle from pancreases. There were no less than 22 published reports of partial success, usually in the form of the elimination of glucose from the urine, with or without reversal of diabetic symptoms, in dogs deprived of their pancreas or whose pancreatic ducts had been ligated.

A striking, but transient, advance was achieved by a Berlin doctor, Georg Ludwig Zülzer. It resulted from an experiment designed to test his plausible but incorrect theory that diabetes was caused by an excess of adrenaline (in

American usage, epinephrine). When he injected rabbits with a pancreas extract mixed with adrenaline their blood sugar fell. Encouraged, Zülzer extirpated the pancreas of a dog and found that injections of his preparation depressed the sugar content of the animal's blood and urine. In 1906 he tried his extract on a comatose patient, who was close to death. The man returned to consciousness and his diabetic symptoms receded. It appeared little short of miraculous, but a relapse followed, and Zülzer had no more extract. On the strength of his result Zülzer sought and secured the support of a pharmaceutical company. Schering produced quantities of the extract under the trade name of Aconatol, but this was the zenith of Zülzer's success. The preparations, tested on rabbits, were erratic, and the starting material from abattoirs difficult to come by in sufficient amounts to develop better extraction procedures. Laboratory animals and patients would respond well to the first injection, but were probably sensitised against one or several antigenic substances in the extracts. In any event, further doses engendered serious, life-threatening, side-effects. Zülzer's commercial sponsors lost patience and withdrew their support. He kept trying, but in 1914 on the outbreak of war he was claimed by the army, and published nothing more on diabetes after his return. In 1934 Zülzer, who was Jewish, emigrated to the United States, where he wrote his name Zuelzer. He died in 1949.

The most systematic study before insulin was actually isolated was by a Roumanian professor in the medical school of Bucharest, Nicolae Paulescu, r Paulesco, (1869-1931). In 1916 he had prepared a watery extract of pancreas and injected it into diabetic dogs, causing the relief of the diabetic symptoms. His work was interrupted by the invasion of his country by the Austro-Hungarian armies in 1917, and it was only after the war ended that he was able to begin again. He published four papers on his quite impressive results, all of them on dogs, but he was evidently cautious and had not yet tried his preparation (which he patented) on patients when the Canadians reached the finishing line.

In 1921 John James Rickard Macleod (1876-1935), a Scot, professor of physiology at the University of Toronto was approached by a young surgeon, Frederick Banting. Macleod had done notable work on carbohydrate metabolism, including the study of experimental glycosuria – the excretion of glucose in the urine. Banting (1891-1941) had formulated a theory about the origins of diabetes, and Macleod was an obvious person to whom to apply for help. Banring's idea was that the enzymes produced by the pancreas were the cause of damage to the islet cells, which appeared to produce whatever was responsible for preventing diabetes. The cells occupied the structures known as the islets of Langerhans, discovered in 1869 by a German medical student, Paul Langerhans, and inferred to be the source of this other vital secretion. Banting wanted to tie the ducts supplying the pancreas with blood so as to cause atrophy of the gland. This, he thought, might repress the formation of the enzymes. Macleod listened but was unconvinced. Nevertheless, he offered Banting laboratory space, basic equipment and an allowance of ten dogs. Banting also acquired an assistant, a medical student, with whom his name was to be forever linked. This was Charles Best (1899-1978).

Their first experiment produced an epic result. First Banting and Best performed the duct ligation on a dog, and after some days took out the pancreas, which was indeed considerably atrophied. This they ground up and from the paste they prepared an extract in a salt solution. They injected it into a pancreatectomised dog with diabetes. The dog did not die: its blood sugar and glycosuria fell, and it recovered its vigour, and was kept alive until the supply of extract ran out. Banting appeared to be ignorant of earlier work along the same lines, in particular that of Paulescu, published in French journals. Macleod was guardedly impressed, demanded more experiments, and was finally won over. The next objective, he told Banting, was clear - to isolate the active anti-diabetic substance from the pancreatic juice. Banting too had been hesitant about committing himself to a long and arduous research project in Macleod's department, but was finally persuaded. Macleod and Banting now began to hold frequent discussions on how best to proceed, and on one such occasion a visitor from the University of Alberta happened to be present. This was a young biochemist, James Bertram Collip (1892-1965), with experience in the study of glandular secretions, and Macleod immediately offered him a position.

The work began to make good progress. It soon transpired that Banting's theory, which had been the basis of the project, had been misconceived, for the difficult ligation treatment was unnecessary: the normal, unligated pancreas was just as good a source of the unknown substance as the ligated one, probably in fact better. Banting and Best prepared an extract of a pancreas in a 1:1 alcohol-water mixture, injected it into a pancreatectomised dog, and obtained the desired response, a fall in blood sugar and glycosuria. If the active substance was ever to be purified the procedure would clearly now have to be scaled up, and so cattle pancreases were procured from the local abattoir. Collip extended the observation on dogs to healthy, as well as diabetic rabbits, which manifested a drop in blood sugar to well below normal ('insulin shock'). The time, it was felt, had surely come to try out the cattle pancreas extract on a human patient. Macleod was reluctant, but eventually gave in, and it was agreed that the Professor of Medicine would be asked to select a suitable case. It was a boy of fourteen in the last extremities of diabetes. The extract was prepared by Best and carefully sterilised. Best and Banting both injected a sample into themselves to test for any untoward reaction, and conveyed their solution to the Toronto General Hospital. They instructed the doctor who had been treating the boy on the injection schedule and the time interval to allow before testing the blood sugar level. The outcome was less than dramatic: the blood sugar and glycosuria fell by a quarter but no further, and the trial was abandoned. There was tension between the protagonists and some acrimony, and indeed relations between Banting and Best on the one hand and Macleod and Collip (whom they suspected of trying to hijack the project) on the other had been strained for some time.

Collip had worked ceaselessly to isolate the active principle, and in January 1922 he partly, or as it seemed at the time fully, succeeded. It was no great feat of chemistry, more a tribute to perseverance than any unusual skill. The key was to find the optimal concentration of alcohol (ethanol) in the extraction medium. Proteins are in general insoluble in high concentrations of alcohol. Insulin is a protein, though an unusually small one, and is an exception to this rule. What Collip found was that as he increased the proportion of alcohol all the many proteins in the crude extract progressively precipitated, and could be eliminated, until, when the alcohol concentration reached 90%, the insulin itself finally came out of solution. Collip looked on the insoluble powder and experienced elation. He assayed the product on his rabbits and saw activity of an unprecedented level. (In truth most of the material would still have consisted of impurities, but an appreciable part of it was insulin.)

There now ensued a deplorable scene. There were no witnesses, and we have only the recollections of two of the participants, Banting and Best. (For the full story, see the definitive and highly readable account by Michael Bliss, *The Discovert of Insulin*.) Banting, Best and Collip had agreed that they would function as a team, that anything any one of them discovered would be common property, and that no one of them would claim priority. According to Banting, Collip, who had been growing increasingl, y uncommunicative, came one late afternoon to Banting's small laboratory, and announced

"'Well, fellows, I've got it'.
I turned round and said, 'Fine, congratulations. How did you do it?'
Collip replied, 'I have decided not to tell you'.
His face was white as a sheet. He made as if to go. I grabbed him with one hand by the overcoat where it met at the front and almost lifting him I sat him down hard on the chair. I do not remember all that was said but I remember telling him that it was a good job he was so much smaller – otherwise I would 'knock hell out of him' ….. He told us that he had talked it over with Macleod and that Macleod agreed with him that he should not tell us by what means he had purified the extract."

Best's recollection was that he, Best had been alone in the laboratory when Collip appeared. "He announced to me that he was leaving our group and that he intended to take out a patent in his own name on the improvement of our pancreatic extract. This seemed an extraordinary move to me, so I requested him to wait until Fred Banting appeared, and to make quite sure that he did I closed the door and sat in a chair which I placed against it. …… I will pass over the subsequent events. Banting was thoroughly angry and Collip was fortunate not to be seriously hurt. I was disturbed for fear Banting would do something which we would both tremendously regret later and I can remember restraining Banting with all the force at my command."

Michael Bliss suggests that Macleod and Collip had been incensed by Banting's recent erratic behaviour, when he had made vehement demands for more clinical trials with what they held to be highly impure and questionable material.

Tempers subsided, but the animosities continued to simmer. Collip did not patent his procedure, and when a patent was eventually awarded it was in the names of Collip and Best, and was at once allocated to the University of Toronto. Collip's preparation kept a diabetic dog called Marjorie alive for a record time, and treatment of patients began, with dramatic success and a great fanfare. A paper bearing the names of the four principal contributors to the discovery was published, and galvanised the medical profession around the world. It was in this publication that the name, insulin for the anti-diabetic principle was proposed. (It was suggested by Macleod from the Latin, *insula*, alluding to its source, the pancreatic islet cells.) A desperate clamour now arise for insulin samples to save the lives of the sick and dying, and clearly the demand vastly exceeded the modest capacity of a small university department. After extensive negotiations the rights of commercial exploitation were awarded to the Eli Lilly Company of Indianapolis, a long-established concern with a good record of research. The Eli Lilley chemists developed new procedures for large-scale production, and it was not long before insulin became available to all. It was not until 1926 that John Jacob Abel, a prominent pharmacologist at Johns Hopkins University in Baltimore, crystallised insulin to general disbelief at the time.[*]

---

[*] Nearly all the world's insulin until the last two or three decades was derived from pig pancreas. Pig insulin differs in only one of its 110 amino acids (p.) from the human variety, but this minute change nevertheless created concerns about a possible immune response in some patients. Today pig has been largely supplanted by human insulin, made by recombinant DNA technology in bacteria. Eli Lilly is still one of the two principal suppliers of insulin, and this company and others have developed modified versions, incorporating changes in the amino acid sequence (p.), which act more rapidly.

In 1923 all the bitterness that had divided the Canadian team came to the surface once more, for that year, only months after their triumph, the Royal Swedish Academy awarded the Nobel Prize jointly to Bantin and Macleod. Banting's incontinent hatred for Macleod overflowed. He disparaged Macleod's contribution to the work and announced that he would divide his share of the Nobel Prize money with his friend, Best. Macleod, for his part, also felt that an injustice had been done, and stated in turn that he would divide his share with Collip. Clearly the Nobel committee had had a problem: according to the terms laid down by Alfred Nobel no more than three people may share the Prize, so Collip and Best could not both have been included, and to omit any single one out of the four would have been even more invidious. And what of the earlier researchers in the field, notably perhaps Paulescu and Zülzer? Paulescu might have ruled himself out by reason of his atrocious social and political views, for he was ferociously antisemitic and racist, and held other repellent and bizarre beliefs. (But an eminent Jewish physiologist stated that the recognition of scientific achievements should take no account of personalities, no matter how odious.) In truth the Nobel committee's decision was not unreasonable. The project had been Banting's brainchild – indeed the only one he ever had – and it had been guided throughout by Macleod, even if he never approached the laboratory bench. He had indicated at every stage the best direction the experiments should take, and steered the group away from dead-ends. Yet, because of the obloquy publicly heaped on him by Banting, Macleod's life in Toronto became intolerable, and in 1928 he seized the opportunity to depart for Aberdeen, where he had been elected to the Regius Chair of Physiology. Macleod died in 1936 at the age of fifty-nine.

Charles Best was only twenty-nine when he stepped into Macleod's professorial shoes in Toronto, having first concluded his medical studies. He was deluged with honours, sat on many committees and ran his department efficiently, but made no further significant contributions to science. Collip returned to the University of Alberta, and later moved to McGill University in Montreal as Professor of Biochemistry. There he did important work, especially on hormones from the pituitary gland, including the landmark isolation of ACTH, adrenocorticotropic hormone (p.), used in the treatment of rheumatoid arthritis, asthma and other inflammatory conditions. As for Banting, he was appointed to a research chair in Toronto and was honoured with a knighthood. He assembled a sizeable research group, and attempted to repeat his triumph with insulin by an attack on cancer. But Banting was a one-idea scientist – although that idea can be said to have sufficed - and nothing came of his efforts. He became less abrasive as the years went on, and was reconciled with Collip, though never with Macleod. His personal life was tempestuous. In 1940 when war came Banting wanted to return to the colours, for he had wrought heroically during the First World War as a medical officer, had been wounded and been awarded the military cross. But he was induced to preside over a committee to determine the course of medical research in relation to the war. One night early in 1941, having spent the evening in the company of Collip, Banting boarded a Royal Canadian Air Force plane bound for England. It crashed in Newfoundland, killing all passengers and crew.

The diabetes epidemic: insulin resistance

The discovery of insulin was a momentous event, and it saved countless lives and measureless suffering, and yet it did not solve all the problems associated with diabetes. For one thing, insulin cannot be taken by mouth: it has to be injected, although controlled release by an implanted pump is now an option for some. A greater problem came to light with the discovery that a failure of insulin production by the pancreas is not the only route to diabetes. That is now called type 1 diabetes, but the previously rather rare type 2 diabetes, which results from the inability to utilise insulin, has become, with the increased consumption of sugary foods, a major health problem. In type 2 diabetes a perpetually high level of blood glucose progressively degrades the insulin receptors on the fat cells. The pancreas responds by producing more insulin, but to no or little avail, and a series of evils assail the body. What is needed therefore is an alternative means of reducing the blood sugar. (Weight loss and a Spartan diet are now known, though, to permit regeneration of the receptors in some sufferers from the condition.) The flower, *Galega officinalis*, which appears in the history of folk medicine, contains an alkaloid, galegine, which has a hypoglycaemic (sugar-reducing) effect, but is too toxic to be of much use. Galegine is a derivative of a simple compound, guanidine, which plays a part in normal metabolism. In 1918 a Japanese researcher made a curious discovery: he found that excision of an animal's parathyroid gland (the source of a hormone responsible for regulating the bodily levels of calcium and phosphate) caused guanidine to enter the bloodstream, and the blood sugar to drop concomitantly. Might guanidine then be a cure for diabetes? Alas not, was the answer, for it was too toxic at the concentrations needed. This did however initiate a search for derivatives that might be better tolerated, and several compounds, especially those containing two guanidine groups (bisguanidines), did indeed emerge, and came transiently into clinical use. But all were in greater or lesser degree unsatisfactory by reason of their low level of benign activity or their unacceptable side-effects.

More than two decades passed before new and much better hypoglycaemic compounds became available, although it could have happened much sooner. For in 1921 a pair of chemists at Trinity College Dublin synthesised a guanidine derivative, which was to become known some twenty years later as metformin. In 1929 Karl Slotta (p.) and a colleague in Vienna, studying the control of blood sugar concentration, tried the effect of all the biguanidine derivatives they could assemble on blood sugar levels in rabbits, and found that metformin was much the most potent, and nor did it have any discernible toxicity. Their paper attracted little notice, and metformin was lost to view. The compound was disinterred in the 1940s, thanks to the intervention of a curious figure, Eusebio Garcia, a doctor and researcher in the Philippines. He confirmed the compound's hypoglycaemic activity, but let his enthusiasm run away with him. He used the drug to treat influenza patients during an outbreak in his country (and even gave it the name, fluamine), he convinced himself that it also cured inflammation, and that it was an antibacterial, an antimalarial and even antiviral agent. These were figments, later discredited.

In 1942 Marcel Janbon, professor in the medical faculty of the University of Montpellier, was dealing with an epidemic of bacterial infections. It stemmed from the consumption of spoiled and contaminated food, forced on the local population by the wartime food shortage. He tried treating his patients with a sulphonamide drug supplied by Rhône-Poulenc, 2254 RP. The result was unexpected and distressing. Several of the patients became gravely ill and some died. Baffled by the mysterious affliction, Janbon tried every possible remedy until finally one worked: a glucose injection brought instant recovery. Had the antibacterial cause hypoglycaemia, a catastrophic drop in the blood sugar level? Auguste Loubatières was a physiologist in the medical school with a particular interest in the control of blood sugar, and had been working for some years on a slow-release form of insulin. He proved by administering the sulphonamide to dogs that it did indeed induce a rapid hypoglycaemia. Later he found out the mechanism, which turned out to be a massive stimulation of insulin release. Loubatières's work might have led to a useful treatment for some forms of diabetes, but for whatever reason the idea was never taken up.

It was Garcia's absurd conjectures, published in 1950, that did nonetheless initiate something new, for they caught the attention of a French diabetes specialist, Jean Sterne. Sterne had already done some work on galegine while still a medical student at the Salpetrière hospital in Paris, and was the first doctor to try metformin on patients (in 1953). He was impressed with the results, so much so in fact that he attached himself to a pharmaceutical company, Laboratoires Aron in Paris, which proceeded to develop the drug. It was indeed a remarkable success, not least because, unlike other compounds of the same class, it neither increased the blood pressure nor disturbed the heart rate. Metformin was introduced into clinical practice, first in France, then in 1958 in Britain and other European countries, but only in 1995 in the U.S. Metformin is one of the rare drugs never displaced by anything better in nearly 70 years. It works on a class of fat cell insulin receptors by facilitating the attachment of insulin, and remains to this day the most widely prescribed treatment for type 2 diabetes. It is sometimes given in combination with another medicament, most often one of a totally unrelated chemical kind, pioglitazone. That compound – to chemists a thiazolidinedione – was conceived by the chemists of Takeda Chemical Industries in Osaka, Japan. The company entered the field following the creation of a diabetic mouse strain, on which prospective hypoglycaemic compound could be easily tested. A large number of derivatives were synthesised and tried before pioglitazone, and failed to reach the market by reason of dangerous, most often cardiovascular,00 side-effects. In France pioglitazone was no sooner launched than it was withdrawn because of a suspected tendency to cause bladder cancer, but elsewhere, most often under the trade name, Actos, it has done well. There have nevertheless been accusations of concealment of adverse effects, still unresolved. In the wake of pioglitazone SKF introduced a compound of the same chemical class, said to be some ten times more effective. This was rosiglitazone, about which more later. Other classes of compounds, optimistically offered as anti-diabetic remedies, have come and gone,. There is a depressing history, which takes an oft-repeated course: a much-heralded launch is followed after an interval of a few months or sometimes years by abrupt withdrawal. For the most part, nevertheless, type 2 diabetes is in most cases relatively well controlled.

The fountain of youth: some cures for old age

In June of 1889 Charles-Édouard Brown-Séquard, successor to the great Claude Bernard in the chair of Experimental Medicine at the Collège de France, startled his audience at the Société de Biologie by the tale he told. Brown-Séquard (1817-1894) was a physiologist of high accomplishment in neurobiology and other areas of biological science and medicine. Born on Mauritius to a French mother and an American father, a ship's captain who did not live to see his son, he left the island for Paris at twenty-one to study medicine. He made an early name for himself by his research on the properties of stomach juices when he was still a medical student. He spent a period in England and longer in America. He was for a time a professor at the Medical College of Virginia and then, from 1864 to 1867, at Harvard. In 1869 Brown-Séquard was back in Paris, occupying a professorial chair at the medical school. Finally in 1878, after a second five-year sojourn in the United States, practising medicine, he achieved his apotheosis at the Collège de France. His international reputation was at its zenith: he was a member of the National Academy of Sciences of the United States, a Fellow of the Royal Society, and a member of the Académie des Sciences. He had collected an imposing number of honorary degrees. But he was also in the grip of an obsession.

As a follower of Claude Bernard, Brown-Séquard had long nurtured an interest in 'internal secretions'. He was not the first to pick up the spoor of the sex hormones, for in 1848 Arnold Adolph Berthold, a physiologist at the University of Göttingen had performed a clever experiment. He had excised the testicles from six young cocks, transplanted those of two into their own abdominal cavities, and foreign testicles into two of the others, leaving the remaining pair as eunuchs. These two lost their sexual urge, and their combs shrivelled, whereas the other four birds thrived, with their combs standing proud. The important conclusion was that some secretion was transported through the bloodstream to its site of action. But unhappily an influential colleague, Rudolf Wagner, tried and failed to repeat the experiment, Berthold lost heart, his work was forgotten, and nothing more happened until Brown-Séquard seized the reins forty years later. He, though, had a more grandiose vision, for he was persuaded that a testicular essence was responsible for the preservation of health and vigour. Atrophy of the testes must conversely therefore let loose the dismal agents of decrepitude. It also followed that the vital juices should be conserved. That excessive sexual activity, and in particular masturbation, led to general debility was a widely held opinion, and indeed had a long history. The yoga masters taught that sperm (which they believed to be stored in the base of the skull) contained the essence of bodily virtue and must not be lost. Therefore their adherents had to learn to aspirate their semen back in after the sex act. Brown-Séquard appears to have begun sporadic experiments on the rejuvenation of aged dogs in the late 1850s, but it evidently took him several decades to arrive at the point of decision. He was 72 years old and in failing strength by the time he felt ready to become his own guinea-pig. With the help of his *préparateur*, or assistant, Arsène d'Arsonval* (whom he had inherited from Claude Bernard), he collected testicles of dogs and guinea pigs, ground them up with their

---

* Jacques-Arsène d'Arsonval (1851-1940) was an omnivorous savant, a doctor, physiologist, physicist and inventor. He created devices to facilitate Claude Bernard's physiological measurements, and later invented several instruments that found wide applications in physics, most famously the moving-coil galvanometer for the measurement of small voltages. He made contributions to electrophysiology, and was a pioneer in exploring clinical applications of electricity. He became a member of the Académie des Sciences, and followed his patron, Brown-Séquard into the professorial chair at the Collège de France.

internal fluids, passed the paste through a fine filter to sterilise it, and injected samples of the filtrate under his skin. The effects, after six doses over a period of two weeks, were electrifying. His physical vigour, he told his listeners at the Société de Biologie, had declined markedly over the last ten to twelve years. After one hour on his feet at the laboratory bench, he needed to rest. After working three or four hours, and sometimes indeed only two, he had been overcome by exhaustion and been compelled to take to his bed. He had had difficulty in sleeping. But *now*, after his course of injections, all that had changed. After two treatments and especially after three, he had amazed his assistant by remaining on his feet for hours with no signs of weariness, he could run upstairs without even thinking about it just as in his prime, and his insomnia had vanished. But Brown-Séquard was a rigorous scientist and believed in the measurement of effects, and so he tested his muscular strength with an instrument, a dynamometer, and sure enough, the strength of his forearm had risen prodigiously. Moreover, the ease with which he could evacuate his bowels without resort to a purgative had returned to normal levels, and the trajectory of his urine had likewise increased. He had, in short, been rejuvenated.

This was the beginning of a movement which became known as 'optotherapy', or more generally, 'organotherapy', but it caught on only selectively. Brown-Séquard's lecture was not well received, for the notion of an 'elixir of eternal youth', as the press termed it, sounded as absurd to his more discriminating contemporaries as it does to us today. Yet to be fair, it should be recalled that he did not see his extract as a cure for diseases, among which he included ageing, but more as a means of stimulating the nervous and other organic secretions required to combat these conditions. In a paper in *The Lancet* Brown-Séquard reported the results of experiments by one Dr Variot on 'two old men [sic], one fifty-four, another fifty-six, and a third sixty-eight years old', whose conditions were eased by injections of testicular fluid, even though they were not told what was being done to them. Moreover similar patients experienced no such benefits when treated only with 'simples'. This was the closest approach to a controlled trial of Brown-Séquard's extracts. The public prints took no account of such subtleties in their excited reports of a cure for old age. Under the acerbic heading, *The Pentangle of Rejuvenescence* (the pentangle being the five-pointed star endowed by mystics with magical properties), the *British Medical Journal* commented: 'The statements [Brown-Séquard] made – which have unfortunately attracted a good deal of attention in the public press – recall the wilder imaginings of mediaeval philosophers in search of an *elixir vital*.' Such then was the prevalent view of the profession.

Many among Brown-Séquard's opponents also found the practice of introducing animal materials into the human body repugnant in itself, others an unacceptable exploitation of animals. From Dr Edward Berdoe, a member of an anti-vivisection committee, came a foam-flecked denunciation of Brown-Séquard in the *British Medical Journal*. 'The object of these abominable proceedings', he wrote, 'is to enable broken-down libertines to pursue with renewed vigour the excesses of their youth, to rekindle the dying embers of lust in the debilitated and aged, and to profane the bodies of men which are the temples of God with an elixir drawn from the testicles of dogs and rabbits by a process involving the excruciating torture of the innocent animals'. There was, at the same time, no shortage of credulous or opportunistic doctors, who eagerly embraced Brown-Séquard's theory, and before long reports of amazing revitalisations and cures wrought by testicle preparations came in from around the world. By 1890 an estimated 12,000 doctors were administering such extracts. Brown-Séquard was dismayed. He feared that uncontrolled, incompetently produced material might cause infections and could kill. He and d'Arsonval worked feverishly to make sufficient extract to supply free to responsible users, demanding only reports of the treatment outcomes in return. The nostrum was bottled with a label bearing their names under the rubric, *Laboratoire de Médecine du Collège de France*. According to d'Arsonval, they sacrificed 'a hecatomb of dogs', but there was no hope of keeping up with the demand. Neither would they permit manufacture of the extract for profit, but it was a losing battle. Its author did his best to continue with the research and improve the product and the procedure. Inflammation at the site of the injections drove Brown-Séquard to attempt administration by enema. This, he found, was successful when he tried it on himself, but it required, he thought, a much larger dose to achieve the same result. The rejuvenating effect was in any case beginning to fail, for self-delusion can take one only so far; Brown-Séquard's infirmities reasserted themselves, and four years after his great discovery he was dead.

Brown-Séquard's obituaries sent mixed messages. To one contemporary was attributed the cruel observation, 'Poor Brown-Séquard! He injected himself with testicles, ran upstairs and died at the top'. An obituary in *Nature* was more charitable. It lauded its subject's earlier achievements, and concluded, 'His experimental researches, undertaken in his later days, between 1889 and 1893, to sustain or even renew the vital powers, it is not necessary for us to particularly mention; dreams allowed to a poet are forbidden to the philosopher [the term, 'scientist' was not yet in current use], and time will alone tell whether there be any germ of reason in Brown-Séquard's investigations; if not, they may be forgotten and forgiven.' For all the mockery, the fact remains that Brown-Séquard's eccentric vision of a youth regained initiated, or at least revived, a train of scientific thought. Here (in translation) is a rumination by him and d'Arsonval in a paper published in 1891: 'The question has broadened, and we now believe that it will be possible to employ all the tissues in specific cases as means of treatment, that, in a word, a new therapy has been created in which the medicaments will be products made by different tissues of the organism, that all the cells of an organism are thus linked one [kind] to another by a mechanism other than the nervous system.' This remarkably far-sighted exposition anticipated the birth of the new discipline of endocrinology.

A sequel of sexual exuberance

Whatever informed medical opinion may have concluded about Brown-Séquard's heterodox views, the genie was now out of the bottle. *L'Extrait Brown-Séquardien* soon became available in France and in other countries. *Sequardine* and *Sequardine serum* (which, the label assured the purchaser, 'will bring you relief and restore your health in a permanent way'), took the markets by storm. In 1893 Brown-Séquard had given lectures announcing successful treatments of tuberculosis, diabetes, coughs, heart and kidney disease and sundry nervous disorders by optotherapy with various organ extracts besides testicular fluid. This was all as nothing compared to the curative virtues proclaimed by the advertisers. Most of all, of course, they promised sexual rejuvenation and increased potency. Brown-Séquard's theories undoubtedly also had their followers within the mainstream of the scientific and medical professions. Oskar Zoth (1864-1933) was a mandarin of the Austrian medical establishment, Dean of the Medical Faculty of the University of Graz, and later the University's Rector. He was also a noted Alpinist and a racing cyclist, and he had the idea of using Brown-Séquard's method to improve sportsmen's strength and endurance. In 1923 he and a colleague, a physiological chemist (or as he would now be called, a biochemist), Fritz Pregl (1869-1930) repeatedly injected themselves for a week with a preparation from bull testes, and measured their muscle strength with an instrument built by Pregl (who eventually received a Nobel Prize for his innovations in medical instrumentation). Their publication in 1896 reported an enhancement of muscular performance by up to 50%. This was the start of doping in sport, which was to bring down so much contumely on errant sportsmen a half-century later.

The influence of Brown-Séquard's work extended far beyond the ambitions of sportsmen however. Prospects of rejuvenation captivated a section of the medical profession. It was further stimulated by the well-publicised reports of work by a French surgeon and biologist, working at the Rockefeller Institute in New York, Alexis Carrel (1873-1944). An enigmatic, even sinister figure, Carrel developed methods of uniting severed blood vessels, later an important factor in organ transplantation, and introduced other valuable surgical innovations. For this work he received the Nobel Prize for Physiology or Medicine in 1912. He returned to France to serve as a medical officer in the Great War, after which, back in his Rockefeller laboratory, he began to occupy himself with keeping organs and cells alive in culture media.*

---

* Carrel even worked in association with the famous aviator, Charles Lindberg – a man who shared Carrel's unsavoury political opinions – on the construction of an artificial heart. In 1935 Carrel published a highly popular book, *Man, the Unknown*, about the reform of human society through science along authoritarian lines. World War II found him once again in France, where with the approbation of the Vichy government he set up a foundation with racial overtones, for 'the study of human problems'. He would have been tried as a collaborationist had he not met a timely death.

In the 1920s Carrel described experiments, much admired at the time, that purportedly defined conditions in which cells could be kept alive indefinitely. This, he evidently thought, might lead eventually to an extension of the human lifespan, perhaps even the conquest of death. The subscribers to Brown-Séquard's rejuvenation theory took note. Later workers could not repeat these results, and it appeared that Carrel's laboratory technicians had salted the cultures with fresh cells every so often to ensure that Carrel got the results he desired.

Paris and Vienna became the centres of the rejuvenation movement. Serge-Samuel Voronoff, born in Russia in 1866, found his way to Paris at the age of eighteen. He studied classics at the Sorbonne, and then medicine. After qualifying he set up a practice in Cairo, where he advanced rapidly thanks to his professional and social skills. Before long he had risen to the position of personal physician to the Khedive, and had married the daughter of Ferdinand de Lesseps, the entrepreneur and engineer responsible for the construction of the Suez Canal. (The couple later divorced, and Voronoff married into money a second time.) Returning to Paris in 1910, Voronoff established a surgical practice and began to dabble in organ transplants. He read Carrel's publications and the two men became pen-friends some years before they actually met. Like Carrel, Voronoff joined the French army at the start of the Great War, and served for three years before being invalided out in 1917. Finally, now in his early fifties, he found an academic appointment as head of the Physiological Station of the Collège de France. Now he began his experiments on testis transplants. He reported striking successes almost at once. Senile rams were 'transformed' after grafts of testis slices from young animals. They became frisky and even fathered lambs. The experimental animals were small in number, and there was no untreated control group. Voronoff, who seems to have entertained few doubts of the efficacy of his procedures (and also proved to his satisfaction that castration had the converse effect, engendering enfeeblement and premature senility), could not have known that the grafts would have been rejected in a matter of days. He delivered papers at surgical conferences with mixed reactions, but in this period after the Great War, in which the flower of European youth had perished, talk of rejuvenation and restored fertility found ready listeners.

Voronoff proposed that the testicles of executed felons and of young men who had died should not go to waste, they should be harvested for implantation. This was not altogether a new idea. As early as 1914 a surgeon in Chicago, Dr G. Frank Lydston had implanted in himself the testicle of a freshly deceased young man, and several 'other doctors tried implants, though not perhaps on themselves, in the ensuing years,* inspired probably by the work of Brown-Séquard. Injecting blood under the skin was another custom followed by rejuvenators in the 1920s and 1930s, as was a 'reinvigoration' treatment for decrepit men, consisting of injections of blood taken from the testicle vein of young animals. This last was pronounced highly effective by Charles Richet (1850-1935), one of the founders of immunology and a Nobel Laureate. (There were also advanced societies in which the belief prevailed until quite recently - and perhaps still does - that if an old man slept with a young woman the manifestations of age would be transferred from the one to the other.)

After some years of animal experimentation, Voronoff decided that the time had come to try his luck with human subjects. The testicles were to come from monkeys for reasons of biological relatedness. The technique was to stitch three slices of the donor tissue onto the testicle of the recipient, one monkey supplying several recipients. The first two attempts in 1920 were disastrous: both patients developed serious wound infections, and the grafts had to be extracted. But after that all went swimmingly. Not only Voronoff, but most of his patients also, reported wondrous outcomes, with recovery of sexual vigour and robust health – notwithstanding of course that the grafts would have been almost instantly rejected. It is not out of the question that there might have been some brief effects from residual male hormone in the grafts, but all the fulsome testimonials from Voronoff's patients of the recovery of lost youth would undoubtedly have been the result of a placebo effect. The reports drew little comment from the medical establishment. An exception was an editorial in an American journal in 1926, which declared roundly that Voronoff's procedure was

---

* The macabre practice is all too reminiscent of the medieval (and earlier) belief that drinking the blood of young children would bring renewed youth to the decrepit or life to the dying – an intervention that did not avail Pope Innocent VIII (p.).

useless and even harmful'.* But in the newspapers superlatives proliferated: what Voronoff had wrought must surely herald the postponement and even the conquest of death itself. The man himself told the press in 1927 that 'human life could be extended to 125 years and senile old age practically eliminated'. Voronoff toured the world, speaking on his achievements, a commanding presence on the lecture podium, and in print. He was in general given a hero's reception, (nowhere more so than in Brazil, where the operation became widely practised.) In all, some fifty surgeons around the world seem to have follow Voronoff's teachings, and the demand was such that the establishment of special monkey colonies was proposed. Indeed Voronoff had one of his own in the grounds of a stately mansion, the Château Grimaldi, which he had acquired on the Italian side of the border with France.

The grandeur of Voronoff's ambitions far outstripped his knowledge. His most alarming venture was to transplant monkey ovaries into post-menopausal women, who wished, like their menfolk, to regain their youth. Fortunately few such operations were performed before the grafting craze in general came to an end. The most bizarre adventure was the transplanting of a human ovary – how obtained was unclear, though most probably from the post-mortem room – into a monkey. Voronoff then tried to inseminate the monkey with human sperm, though of course without success. When the story got out it evidently exercised such gruesome fascination that it inspired a novel, published in 1929, by a popular French writer, Félicien Champseul. Its title was *Nora, le Guenon devenu Femme*, (Nora – the name of Voronoff's simian recipient – the monkey who became a woman).

Voronoff, at the height of his fame, had a formidable rival, for in Vienna the prospect and desire for rejuvenation had independently taken hold. But while Voronoff was an upstart with all too little grasp of physiology or of

---

* It may be closer to the truth than they could have known, for the theory is now generally accepted that HIV – human immunodeficiency virus, the cause of AIDS - mutated from a simian counterpart, SIV, which somehow crossed the so-called species barrier. It has indeed been suggested that Voronoff's ill-judged monkey-to-human grafts could have been the primal cause of that leap, and therefore of the AIDS epidemic.

experimental method, Eugen Steinach (1861-1944) should have known better. Steinach had done highly reputable work in endocrinology, and had ascended to the top of the Viennese academic ladder as Professor of Physiology, and Director of the Experimental Zoology Institute, known as the Vivarium. He performed testis graft operations on old rats, and reported spectacular results*, but then he had a better and more profitable idea, which may have been inspired by work published in 1902 by two French anatomists at the University of Nancy. They had ligated (that is tied off) the vas deferens of rabbits - the duct down which the sperm

---

* Worse, Steinach also claimed that ovary grafts in guinea pigs repaired ovaries that had been destroyed by irradiation with X-rays, and that pregnancies was again possible. This was gross self-delusion or – perhaps less likely, considering Steinach's reputation - outright fraud. Steinach involved himself, in fact, in many dubious projects. The Vivarium was a hive of activity, mainly directed at proving the existence of Lamarckian heredity – the inheritance of acquired characteristics. Although in the eyes of the great majority of respectable biologists this doctrine had been laid to rest by Darwin, it had enjoyed something of a revival in the early 20th century. The development was enmeshed with political ideology. During the previous century the great German biologist, August Weissmann had cut the tails off several generations of mice, and shown that their progeny were perfectly well endowed with tails of normal length. The object was probably nothing more than to ridicule the doubters, for, as Julian Huxley observed much later, neither Jewish nor Muslim boys were born without foreskins. Yet in communist thinking the idea that man was the master of his fate, and not the helpless victim of genetic determinism, was highly congenial. This was to lead later to the almost total eclipse of genetics through the influence of the charlatan, Trofim Denisovich Lysenko, throughout the Soviet Union and its imperium. The Vivarium sheltered a number of prominent researchers with communist leanings, the most respected of whom was Paul Kammerer, young, brilliant and personable, and much sought-after in the Viennese *beau monde*. The celebrated *femme fatale,* Alma Mahler, wife to the composer, to the novelist, Franz Werfel and to the architect, Walter Gropius, and mistress to many others, was captivated by Kammerer and assisted him in some of his work. He did many ingenious and exacting experiments, which he thought proved that Lamarckian inheritance had occurred. He was appointed after the Great War to a position at the Soviet Academy of Sciences, but before he could take it up evidence came to light that he had perpetrated a fraud in a critical experiment, and he committed suicide. Steinach had worked with Kammerer on some of the projects. A famous example was to maintain rats at hot temperatures. This, they said, not only changed the structure of their sex organs and increased their procreative activity, but caused these characteristics to be transmitted to their progeny and to later generations.

passes before ejaculation. This, they found, had stimulated the animals' sexual appetite. Steinach saw ligation as a possible means of increasing the blood supply to the testicle. He may also have had in mind the ancient doctrine (see above) that loss of sperm leads to debility, and that conversely its preservation defers ageing. When tested in senile rats, the operation, so Steinach claimed, brought an astonishing transformation: the animals appeared younger and more lively, their coats more silky, and their strength and appetite were restored, their ears pricked up, their eyes shone, and their sexual urge awoke once more. Most miraculously (and improbable), the previously turbid lenses and corneas were now clear and bright. There was of course no control group of rats, which today would have been subjected to a 'sham operation', comprising everything except the actual ligation. And clearly, none of the criteria for rejuvenation could be measured and expressed in numbers. Steinach was evidently convinced nonetheless, and recruited a young urinary surgeon to try the procedure on a man. The operatopn was carried out in November of 1918 on a 'prematurely senile', chronically depressed 43-year-old Viennese coachman. After some three months rejuvenation duly set in (or possibly the coachman recovered from his depression), and at eighteen months he was strong, handsome and full of vigour.

Steinach published a description of the marvel, and around Europe and in the United States doctors woke up to the apparent implications. Between about 1920 and 1935 thousands of Steinach procedures were performed, and most practitioners and patients seem to have been delighted with the recovery of strength and libido. Others were less sure, but in Vienna the enthusiasts far outnumbered the sceptics. Steinach later decided that the ligation of one vas deferens sufficed, and did not make the subject sterile. One disappointed client was Sigmund Freud, who had been an early enthusiast but was now suffering from cancer of the jaw, which was not perceptibly helped. Another was W.B. Yeats, who was treated in London in 1934, towards the end of the Steinach vogue. The surgeon was, it is thought, a fanatical Australian followed of Steinach's, Norman Haire. Yeats, who had been depressed, and had almost stopped writing, emerged from the operation a new man, his poetic inspiration and legendary priapic drive seemingly in place once more. A notorious case was that of a rich, ageing English industrialist, Albert Wilson, who hired the Albert Hall in London with the intention of delivering a lecture to the multitude on 'How I was made twenty years younger', and died only hours before he was due to appear. The pharmacies were engulfed by a tide of patent products, promising Steinach effects without operations. Some contained extracts of animal genitalia, others merely supposed aphrodisiacs; they presumably worked as well as the operation for those who believed.

Voronoff was one who thought Steinach's operation nonsensical, but was of course less objective about his own (which, according, in his turn, to Steinach, was not to be taken seriously). At all events, it was implantation, rather than ligation, that was taken up in the U.S. The most infamous aficionado was the medical superintendent of San Quentin prison outside San Francisco, Dr Leo Stanley. With his captive population of subjects, Stanley was able to experiment at will, starting in the late 1920s, before in fact Voronoff had progressed from animals to humans. Stanley implanted human testicle pieces in the abdomens, not the testicles, of the recipients, and some he injected under the skin with a suspension of pulverised testicular material. He reported cures of senility and improvements in those suffering from a number of ailments in 643 ageing felons. In Europe, following the rise of Voronoff, every country harboured its rejuvenators. One such deserves mention if only because of the large following that he attracted. Francesco Cavazzi of Bologna University asserted that Brown-Séquard and his disciples had all got it wrong. Their testicle extracts, he insisted, neither could nor did contain the vital hormonal essence, which was sent directly into the bloodstream. Cavazzi's own 'hormonal serum' was drawn from the vein leading blood out of the testicles of young mammals – it mattered not which – and he tested its effects on old men in a hospital for the poor in his home city. He claimed great success, but the reception in Italy was hostile. Cavazzi therefore headed for the more receptive climate of Paris, and there too old me were produced for him at the hospice of Ivry-sur-Seine. Again he and well-disposed witnesses saw the marks of old age fall away. The infirm cast off their sticks and hiked several kilometres, which included a stiff climb up to the citadel of Ivry. As judged by their restored sex urge, the trajectory of their urine, the heightened acuity of their eyesight and the strength of their arms, measured with a dynamometer (up from 5 to 25 kilograms), the outcome (with no controls) was a triumph. It was most extravagantly endorsed by the powerful voice of Charles Richet (p.), amplified by his reputation as the discoverer of the immunological phenomenon of anaphylaxis, and his Nobel Prize (awarded in 1913). A paper was read before the *Société de Médecine* to great acclaim, and was accepted unanimously by the committee for publication in its journal. Cavazzi was favoured with a shout of *'Vive l'Italie!'*, and overcome with emotion, he responded with three rousing cries of *'Vive la France!'*.

Far more pernicious were the activities of an outright quack, 'Doc' John Brinkley, who opened a clinic in a small town in Kansas, offering testicular grafts as early as 1918. Brinkley had bought a spurious medical degree from a fly-by-night college, but what he lacked in qualifications he made up for in entrepreneurial talent and audacity. His donor animals were goats, chosen for their well-known procreative capacity, and the dangerous operations were conducted in great numbers on an assembly-line principle. Brinkley built several convalescent centres in the form of luxury hotels, offered a series of pharmaceutical products, and touted for custom by way of his personal radio station. He became enough of a local celebrity to run for State Governor, losing by only a narrow margin. Eventually, after an investigation, Brinkley was driven out of Kansas, but he set up shop again in Arkansas, where he died at an early age before he could bring his efforts there to fruition.

The downfall of Voronoff, his followers and his system came in part from the discovery of the sex hormones in the 1930s and in part from a critical evaluation of the evidence. Voronoff was rich and famous, but he sought still greater riches and wider fame. His experiments with rams persuaded him that his grafting method could improve the quality of livestock. The French government had initiated a programme of sheep rearing in their Algerian colony, and Voronoff believed that he could improve by testicular grafting the yield of wool, and the breeding capacity of the animals. He had also, he thought, revived the performance of an ageing prize bull by the same means. His reputation was such that his claims were scarcely questioned, and he had worked with senior veterinarians, who saw the effects that he saw. But in the veterinary profession there were better scientists, who were unwilling to accept the subjective evaluations of grafting, and set about finding evidence – something that no doctors seemed to have considered doing. Chief among the critics was a veterinary surgeon working in Morocco, Henri Velu, whose grasp of histology – the microscopic study of tissues – was far in advance of Voronoff's cursory and amateurish efforts. Velu performed grafts of testicular tissue according to Voronoff's prescription, and satisfied himself that there was no discernible change in wool yield or in breeding efficiency. Then he examined the tissue at the sites of the grafts in the microscope at different times after their insertion. What he saw, and reported at a meeting of the French Veterinary Academy in 1929, was that no grafted tissue survived more than a few days, and that the supposed residuum of graft cells was nothing more than the animal's own scar tissue. Velu was intemperately attacked by his academic superiors, who had a stake in testicular implantation, but his conclusions were too convincing to disregard. Moreover veterinarians in other countries also undertook investigations on the fate of grafts, which bore out all that Velu had determined. Eventually even some members of the medical profession, particularly in Britain and the United States, stirred themselves and began to question the value of Voronoff's methods, and even Steinach's. And so, as disillusion grew, the ageing roués stayed away, while Voronoff lingered on, still writing and proclaiming the power of the graft. The practice was not totally abandoned, and only gradually faded away. Steinach's fall from favour happened at much the same time, hastened by the rise of the Nazis in Austria, for he was a Jew. After the *Anschluss* – the assimilation of Austria into Germany in 1938 - Steinach was fortunate to escape to Switzerland, his wife having committed suicide. He ended his days there in obscurity, though still apparently full of theories and plans, in 1944 at the age of 83. As for Voronoff, who was also Jewish, he never conceded defeat. There issued from his pen a series of books on grafts, senility and rejuvenation, which continued long after his method had become discredited. (One of the last bore the title, *Du Crétin au Génie.*) He spent much time in Brazil, where he was still held in some esteem. When in 1939 war broke out he returned to his Château, but after Italy declared war on France he fled with his wife, and headed for Spain, and thence for the U.S.. At the end of the war he returned with his wife to France, and died in Paris, largely forgotten, in 1951.

Yet the eclipse of Voronoff and Steinach and all their works was not the end of the quest for enduring youth. A Viennese surgeon continued for a while to satisfy an enduring demand for monkey testis implants until the early stages of the Second World War, when the supply of monkeys dried up. But in the late 1930s a new star was rising in the firmament. A Swiss surgeon, Paul Niehans had been a fervent disciple of Voronoff, and in time broadened the scope of his forerunner's treatments. He transplanted a number of different glands, especially the pituitary, which secretes the hormone releasing factors (p.), which switch on the activities of other glands, and claimed thereby to have cured a number of dire diseases. After exploiting this line of business successfully for some years, he invented something new and hugely lucrative, which he peddled as 'cell therapy'. Instead of organs he implanted cells from a foetal lamb on the basis that they would replace the agents of ageing with those of youth, and would cure diseases, cancer for one. Operating in a private clinic on Lake Geneva, Niehans with his talent for publicity and his charisma, attracted a succession of rich clients (for his treatments were far from cheap). Among his patients were Noel Coward, the Duke and Duchess of Windsor, Emperor Haile Selassie of Ethiopia, and most famously in 1954, Pope Pius XII, seeking evidently to delay the eventual encounter with his superior. The cells would of course have been instantly rejected, but many, perhaps most, of Niehans's credulous patrons reported wonderful results and kept coming. Remarkably, Niehans's clinic has survived, and still offers its 'cell therapy'.

Rejuvenated to death: new rays and their abusers

The dangers of radiations – X-rays and radioactive emanations – discovered at the beginning of the 20th century were slow to be recognised. The early radiographers were particularly at risk, and many died of leukaemia and other malignancies. Plans in the 1960s to put Marie Curie's laboratory notebooks on display in Paris had to be abandoned when it was discovered that they were still so radioactive as to present a danger to the public. Why lethal radiations came to be credited with health-giving, and even rejuvenating properties remains a mystery, but that is what happened.

In 1926 the American geneticist, H.J. Muller discovered that X-rays engendered mutations in fruit flies, but this critical fact probably did not communicate itself to the clinicians. It was, though, at about this time that doctors in Vienna were beginning to try the effects of irradiation with X-rays on old men, and fancying that they were witnessing reversal of ageing.

Not long before, Steinach had exposed young female guinea pigs to X-rays, and was persuaded that the development of secondary sexual characteristics was greatly accelerated. The aforementioned Norman Haire recorded in his book, *Rejuvenation* in 1924 that women 'looked and felt younger' after exposure to X-rays. X-rays were in fact used as a means of sterilisation in Nazi Germany, and before that in the United States during the heyday of the eugenics movement. (Women from what were regarded as families with undesirable heredity were interrogated while unknowingly perched over an X-ray generator.) One of the most reckless experimenters among all the physicians at play in this alluring area of research was the American, Harry Benjamin in New York. Benjamin was an ardent admirer of Steinach, whom he tried without success to lure across the Atlantic. He made such wild claims for the youth-enhancing powers of 'the Steinach', far beyond anything its begetter had claimed, that Steinach was dismayed, and demanded a retraction. Benjamin was not troubled, and he and his followers 'Steinached' at least a thousand American men. He also started to treat women with X-rays at his Life Extension Institute. One highly satisfied patient was a popular novelist of the day, Gertrude Atherton, then aged sixty-six. The novel, based on her experience, *Black Oxen* enjoyed great success, and had as its protagonist a sensationally beautiful woman of thirty, who was in reality fifty-eight. This probably brought many more women to Benjamin's door, eager to be irradiated. It is not recorded how many cases of cancer and sterility resulted from treatment with X-rays, but even by mid-century the extent of the destructive power of the rays was barely acknowledged; witness for instance the X-ray machines installed in many shoe shops, which allowed customers to watch their toes wiggling inside the shoes that they were trying on for size. Benjamin at least had plenty of time to reconsider, for he lived to the age of 101, and towards the end penned an honourable recantation of his theories.

The use of radium as medicine in the early decades of the 20th century had yet more gruesome consequences. Again, a conviction arose, for inscrutable reasons, that radioactivity was in some way healthy. 'Radioactive springs' became popular in health resorts, where the rich would go in summer to 'take the cure', and quacks did good business selling radioactive remedies for a host of diseases. It was the widely-publicised and hideous death of a public figure in America that largely put a stop to the delusion. Eben McBurney Byers was what would now be called a celebrity. Born into wealth and privilege as son of a prominent industrialist, he was handsome and athletic, and gained a reputation at his university, Yale, as a playboy and ladies' man. In 1906 he was the U.S. amateur golf champion, and came close on several other occasions. In 1928 he broke his arm while travelling by train to the annual Harvard-Yale football game. The fracture mended, but the pain lingered. Byers's doctor suggested trying a patent product called Radiothor. This was a solution containing a large amount of a radium salt, made and marketed by one William J. Bailey, a mountebank who laid claim to a medical degree that he did not possess. Radiothor was supposed to alleviate a variety of complaints and to 'stimulate the endocrine system'. Byers was delighted with the effect, for the pain in his arm abated, as it presumably would have done without Radiothor. Indeed he felt invigorated, convinced himself that the medicine was doing him much good, and continued to drink it at the rate of three bottles or so a day. He stopped only when his teeth began to fall out, by which time he had consumed the contents of perhaps two thousand bottles in the space of two years. Then his bones crumbled, he lost most of his jaw, and cracks developed in his skull. Byers died in 1931 and was buried in a coffin with lead shielding. Bailey was never brought to trial, and went on serenely making and selling radioactive products. There were many others on the market, including radioactive toothpaste, radioactive suppositories, radioactive collars, and medicines that guaranteed an end to 'the agonies of rheumatism, neuritis, neuralgia and gout'. These all gradually vanished in the wake of Eben Byers's desperate end.

Enter testosterone

The isolation of an actual sex hormone did not immediately bring about the decline of the rejuvenation craze. New nostrums continued to appear and pass duly into oblivion, but none of them ever caught on to the extent of Voronoff's and Steinach's schemes a decade earlier. There were false starts to the pursuit of sex compounds. In the 1890s a physiologist at the University of St. Petersburg, Alexander von Poehl thought he had the male sex hormone when he discovered crystals in semen. It turned out to be a simple metabo;ite (an amine, given the appropriate name of spermine), which had first been prepared by German chemists some years previously. Von Poehl's conjectures concerning its function in reproduction and development set off a train of experimentation aimed at showing a reviving, or as Brown-Séquard later termed it, a 'dynamogenic' effect on frail old people. Élie Metchnikoff, whose obsessive interest, late in life, was the ageing process (p.), enumerated in his book, *The Prolongation of Life – Optimistic Studies* some improbable outcomes, including the rejuvenation of a woman of ninety-five, who could walk again after injections of spermine, and whose rheumatic pains receded. But spermine, though marketed with some éclat, has no such activity. A good many years passed before the hunt for a male hormone produced a result. Extracts in alcohol or chloroform of testicular tissue, prepared in a number of European laboratories, gave signs of activity when injected into castrated animals, but the results were erratic and weak. There was slightly better progress with ovary extracts containing female hormonal activity, and one dubious preparation was advertised and sold by the Ciba pharmaceutical company in Switzerland in 1913. Then, in the early 1920s Steinach, with two assistants (one of whom, Walter Hohlweg, later became a respected hormone researcher with the Schering company in Germany), came up with an extract of animal ovaries which, they reported, had remarkable reactivating effects on the fecundity of decrepit female rats. It was marketed by Schering under the name of Progynon as a treatment for 'feminine complaints' and also as a rejuvenating agent. Steinach and his American epigone, Harry Benjamin proclaimed its immense benefits for women from seventy to ninety years of age. Benjamin later used Progynon, assisted by X-irradiation of the testicles, to treat at least one trans-sexual male, who wished to become feminised.

Progynon may indeed have contained amounts of one or more hormones, but its composition was undefined, and it certainly would not have satisfied the extravagant claims that were made for it. The first sex hormone to be properly purified in crystalline form (from the urine of pregnant women) was oestrone, one of the so-called oestrogens, which regulate the female reproductive cycle. This remarkable achievement came about simultaneously in two laboratories in 1929, those of Adolf Butenandt[*] in Göttingen and of Edward Doisy in St. Louis[**]. It was an enormous leap forward, for Butenandt guessed from the nature of the crystals that the compound bore a structural similarity to cholesterol, the structure of which had been determined not long before (p.) by Butenadt's mentor, Adolf Windaus. If Butenandt's surmise was correct, then the hormone was a *steroid*, and if it was a steroid then other sex hormones might also be members of the same chemical family. Working on this premise, Butenandt got the structure. In the ensuing years two other oestrogenic hormones, close structurally to oestrone, but much more potent, were isolated. The most important, oestradiol was obtained by Doisy in 1935 from four tons of sows' ovaries from the Chicago stockyards.

---

[*] Adolf Friedrich Johann Butenandt (1903–1995) was an organic chemist, a student of another Nobel Laureate, Adolf Windaus at the University of Marburg. He became a Privatdozent – a lecturer – at Göttingen University, and then, at the age of twenty-eight, Professor of Chemistry at the Technical University of Danzig (now Polish Gdańsk). As his reputation grew he ascended the academic tree to become director of one of the great German state laboratories, the Kaiser-Wilhelm Institute for Biochemistry in Munich. After the Second World War Butenandt was appointed President of the entire Kaiser-Wilhelm organisation, renamed the Max-Planck Society. A relatively late achievement of Butenandt's was the identification and synthesis of the insect hormone, ecdysone, which initiates the metamorphosis of the caterpillar into a butterfly. His reputation was tainted by his membership of the Nazi Party, and his apparently close adherence to the regime throughout its reign.
[**] Edward Adelbert Doisy (1893–1986) was a biochemist who started his career at the University of Illinois, but passed the remainder of his working life, with an interruption for army service in the Great War, at Washington University in St. Louis. In addition to his work on sex hormones, he distinguished himself by his contributions to several other areas of biochemistry, most notably determination of the structure and biological action of vitamin K. For this he shared the Nobel Prize in 1943 with the Danish biochemist, Henrik Dam.

Meanwhile in Breslau, Karl Heinrich Slotta (1895-1987), had returned to the University in 1919 from service in the Great War with a shell splinter lodged in his brain, and was accommodating himself once more to civilian life. Switching his interest from classics to chemistry, he had shown immediate talent for research. He completed his Ph.D., and then, under the influence of his father-in-law, Ludwig Fraenkel, a distinguished gynaecologist, professor at the University Clinic, he had turned his mind to hormones. Fraenkel had a particular interest in the corpus luteum (the 'yellow body'), a transient structure in the ovary, which appears during ovulation and ensures the inception and progress of pregnancy. He divined that this was indeed a gland, and thought that it must produce a hormone. His son-in-law was persuaded to make an attempt to track down and isolate this hypothetical substance, no small task. Slotta and the students he had by then acquired dissected the glands from ovulating sows' ovaries, and after a long siege, prevailed. Within a few months three other laboratories, one of them Butenandt's, also reported isolation of the pregnancy hormone, progesterone.*

The male hormones remained elusive because of their minute concentration in the tissues, and the difficulty of assaying their activity, for without an assay there was no means of tracing the material through the various purification steps. Finally two American workers Fred Koch, Professor of Physiological Chemistry at the University of Chicago and his student Lemuel McGee, found the key: it derived from the observation by Adolphe Berthold nearly a century earlier (p.) that a hormonal secretion injected into a castrated cockerel would cause its deflated comb to rise in the space of a day. The magnitude of this effect could be estimated from the size of the comb's profile. The other critical factor was the discovery that traces of male hormone were excreted in the urine. This was all that Butenandt needed. He set up the cock's-comb assay, using the area of the

---

* That year, 1933, Hitler seized power in Germany, and in 1935 Slotta, who was Aryan but married to a Jewish wife, and also an open opponent of the regime, decamped with his family to Brazil, followed the next year by the Fraenkels. For some years Slotta worked in Brazil, doing research on coffee, and then on snake venoms and their pharmacological properties. In 1956 he found his way to the U.S.A., and passed most of the rest of his long life as a professor at the University of Miami.

comb's silhouette recorded on a photocopier as the quantitative measure of hormonal activity, and he found a source of hormone: 17,000 litres (or nearly 4,000 gallons) of urine donated by two-thousand volunteers in the Berlin police barracks. Butenandt started with an immense chloroform extraction, and continued through a series of purification steps, assaying at each stage with the laboratory cockerels, until finally a few milligrams of crystals of what came to be called androsterone appeared in the solution. Guessing that the hormone was a steroid, like oestrone, Butenandt determined its structure.

Androsterone, it soon transpired, was not the principal male sex hormone. It plays an important part in early development, but by the mid-1930s there were indications that something more potent lurked in extracts from urine and testes. The first suspicions came from a new biological assay. Two American researchers found that the seminal vesicles (the pair of glands that produce a large part of the seminal fluid) of castrated rats were stimulated to grow by the hormonal preparations, and the rate of growth could be measured. This constituted the assay. Ernst Laqueur (1880-1947) was a German chemist, who had qualified as a doctor, and who was buffeted throughout his life by the political upheavals in the first half of the 20th century. In 1905 he was awarded his doctorate by his home university of Breslau, and was offered a position at the University of Halle. His research thrived until the arrival, as head of the department, of one of the more unpleasing figures in the German scientific hierarchy. Emil Abderhalden was a tyrant, something of a charlatan, and, when the opportunity came, a Nazi*. Abderhalden apparently insisted that he alone would determine the direction of Laqueur's work. After a heated quarrel Laqueur resigned his position and left the country. In 1912 he found a berth in Holland at the University of Gröningen, but two years later the Great War erupted, and Laqueur returned to Germany, and enlisted as a medical officer. He served on the western front, was awarded the iron cross first class, and was then transferred to the army gas unit in Berlin to help develop treatments for gassed soldiers. He was eventually discharged and allowed to return to science at the germanicised University of Ghent in occupied Belgium. This could not last, and after the armistice the German members of the Ghent faculty were immediately sacked. Laqueur, who had returned to Germany, was sentenced to death *in absentia* by a Belgian court, probably on the charge of participation in the chemical warfare campaign. In 1920 he returned to Holland as Professor of Pharmacology at the University of Amsterdam.** There he not only began his work on hormones, but also joined with two colleagues to found a pharmaceutical company, Organon. It was to produce hormones on a commercial scale,

---

* Abderhalden peddled a theory based on the supposed existence of enzymes in the blood that conferred protection against foreign invaders, such as bacteria, exactly as antibodies had long been known to do. These enzymes, so Abderhalden claimed, would recognise foetal proteins in women's blood, thus affording an early means of detecting pregnancy. Similarly they would detect cancers long before they revealed themselves in any other way. He later collaborated with concentration-camp doctors, such as the infamous Josef Mengele, who provided him with blood and tissue samples from their victims, because he believed that his 'defence enzymes' exhibited racial variations, and could be used to identify racial origins. Needless to say, all these discoveries were figments, resulting from incompetent experimentation and wishful thinking. Abderhalden acquired considerable power in the German academic communiyu, and was able to persecute those who opposed him. Work on the non-existent enzymes dragged on for another ten years after the war.

** In 1944 history again caught up with Laqueur, for Holland was under German occupation, and Laqueur was a Jew. He was expelled from the university, but he, his wife and one of his two daughters were not further molested, and were probably saved by the German collapse. His other daughter and one of his two sons were arrested and sent to the Belsen-Bergen concentration camp, and survived. His remaining son was allowed his freedom because Laqueur and his wife hit on the ruse of swearing that it was not Laqueur but a true-blooded Aryan who was his real father. Laqueur returned to work in Amsterdam, but died two years later while on holiday in Switzerland.

and develop new compounds with hormonal activity. (Organon is still prominent in the hormone field, but since 2007 as part of the huge Merck concern.)

In 1934 Laqueur examined androsterone preparations from urine and from testes by the seminal vesicle assay in castrated rats. He found that when equal quantities, as measured by the cock's-comb assay, were injected, the testicular extract stimulated the growth of the glands more effectively, by a factor of about 5, than that from urine. The former must then contain a different or additional component, not perceived by the cock's comb, and Laqueur went to work on its isolation. He processed a mass of bulls' testicles and obtained a yield of crystals with unprecedentedly high hormonal activity. Laqueur called the new hormone testosterone. The quantity of material, though, was too small for structural studies, or even trials in human subjects, so the facilities of Organon were mobilised. In a year or so larger quantities of pure material were available, not only from Organon but also from two other pharmaceutical concerns, Schering in Germany and Ciba in Switzerland. This gave Butenandt his chance, and in a matter of months he had determined the structure (which had also been inferred by Laqueur) and achieved a partial synthesis – partial implying that he had not begun from scratch, but from the closely related compound, cholesterol. At almost precisely the same time another organic chemist reported the same synthesis; this was Leopold Ružička**, working at the Technical University (the famous ETH) in Zurich. For this and other important work on steroids the two men shared the Nobel Prize for Chemistry awarded in 1939. (Because the Nobel Committee had incurred the wrath of Adolf Hitler for the reasons related earlier (p.), Butenandt was forbidden to accept the prize, and like Domagk, was able to receive his gold medal at the hands of the King of Sweden only ten years later.)

---

* Leopold (né Lavoslav) Ružička (1887–1976) was born into a poor family in Croatia, studied organic chemistry and obtained his doctorate in Germany at the Technical University of Karlsruhe. He was appointed to a professorial chair at the ETH in Zurich, and became one of the world's leading natural products chemists, active in many areas, notably fragrances and the important class of plant substances, the terpenes, before turning to the steroids.

Once the sex hormones had been isolated and synthesised, and their physiological actions investigated, extravagant expectations arose of what they would do for human health and happiness. Testosterone, we now know, controls the development of the male reproductive tissues, the testes and prostate, and the secondary sexual characteristics, such as muscle bulk, bone density, thick vocal cords, and body hair. It has many other functions in the control of metabolic processes, and in maintaining the integrity of bone and muscle. Women's bodies, too, produce and make use of testosterone and androsterone. Preparations of the hormone still have their place in the clinic in cases of impaired sexual development in the male, which are often associated with an insufficiency of circulating testosterone. It is also prescribed, in association with a hormone of an unrelated kind, human growth hormone, for children with severely retarded growth. One effect of testosterone is to increase the production of red blood cells, and it was accordingly used to treat some forms of anaemia before the primary agent, erythropoietin (also called haemopoietin in English or hemopoietin in American usage) became available. For about two decades after its discovery testosterone was also commonly regarded as a specific for retarding the ageing process. Derivatives (testosterone esters) with a longer survival in the bloodstream were synthesised, and tested in men with failing sexual powers, the decrepit, or those who felt themselves in the throes of an imaginary 'andropause' or male climacteric, the male equivalent of the menopause. From about 1940 courses of treatment were offered in 'rejuvenation clinics'. They consisted of injections of testosterone or derivatives, were called 'Testosterone Replacement Therapy', or 'Total Hormone Replacement Therapy', and preceded the feminine counterpart. (In fact testosterone was given to women, together with female sex hormones to hold the menopause at bay.) Testosterone was also advertised as a 'cure' for homo- and trans-sexuality. And then, of course, there was, and is, the illicit use of anabolic steroids, which include testosterone and androsterone, to improve athletic performance (p.). Anabolism connotes the build-up of tissues, especially muscle, and testosterone, androsterone and many of their synthetic derivatives have this property. They undoubtedly enhance bodily strength and energy output (as does erythropoietin by raising the oxygen-carrying capacity of the blood), at the cost of a range of damaging effects on health.* There was much specious advertising, especially by Schering, who outraged Doisy by invoking his name in support of the spurious claims for their product listed on the label.

Hormones on the loose

Clinicians were all too slow to recognise the dangers in the profligate use of hormones. A case with tragic consequences had its origins in some observations in an unrelated area of medical research. The Courtauld Institute at University College London was a prominent centre of cancer research, led by E.C. (eventually Sir Charles) Dodds. Throughout the 1930s his laboratory had been studying the action of carcinogenic compounds, but Dodds had been struck by a certain resemblance between the structures of a class of carcinogens and those of the steroids, such as oestrone (see p.). And indeed, these carcinogens proved to have distinct oestrogenic activity. A new compound that Dodds wished to test had been synthesised at his request in the laboratory of a leading organic chemist, Sir Robert Robinson in Oxford. It came to be known as diethylstilboestrol, or DES. Even though it did not have the intact characteristic steroid skeleton, it turned out to be highly oestrogenic when tested in rats. The discovery was announced in a brief report in the journal, *Nature* in 1938. It caused an instant stir in clinical (and industrial) circles, for the natural oestrogens were precious and very expensive, while DES was easy to prepared and would therefore be cheap, the more so because – on account of the policy of the Medical Research Council, which had sponsored the research – it was not protected by a patent.

---

* One curious and enduring superstition surrounding androsterone is the belief that it acts as a pheromone – a substance that in minute concentration provokes (subliminally in the human female) powerful sexual attraction. Many animal pheromones are known, but no human version has ever been authenticated. It is also highly unlikely that androsterone, which is not volatile and therefore does not release free molecules into the air, could fulfil such a function. It is nevertheless advertised as a pheromone, usually dissolved in eau de Cologne, and guaranteed to make any nubile women within his aura converge upon the wearer.

But DES also had other and more sinister effects, which soon came to light. In young animals it impeded sexual development and fertility, and in the adults it caused atrophy of the sex organs in the males and of the ovaries in the females. There was also hypertrophy (excessive growth) of the adrenal and pituitary glands. When DES was given to pregnant rats the offspring were similarly affected, especially on reaching sexual maturity. As if this were not enough, DES, Dodds found, was also carcinogenic, as indeed he had anticipated (but so also, in high doses, was oestrone). Interest in this remarkable and multifarious compound spread to other laboratories, one of which discovered yet another unpleasant attribute, namely that it persisted for much longer in the body than oestrone. Connected to this was the property, which it shared with oestrogens, of affecting calcium metabolism. In oestrone this is wholly benign, for it acts (and is prescribed) to regulate calcium assimilation. But with DES the effect runs out of control, and bone deposition does not cease when the treatment is withdrawn.

Despite all the evidence of malign effects in laboratory animals, a clinical trial in American women was carried out and adjudged a success, for it prevented all the unpleasant manifestations of the menopause. More, given in high doses it led to successful pregnancies in women who had suffered repeated miscarriages. When word got out, and stories of a new 'wonder drug' began to circulate in the press, a clamour for DES rose from ageing women and their doctors. The Federal Drug Administration, the FDA, which had been properly cautious, should cease to prevaricate and license DES for immediate use. The animal data, available to all, were disregarded by the majority of doctors, and worst of all finally, by the FDA, which licensed DES in 1941 for treatment of a range of gynaecological woes, complications of pregnancy, menopause symptoms, and as a guard against miscarriages. Gynaecologists hailed DES as the most potent clinical weapon placed into their hands in decades, and one of their number went so far as to propose that it should be given routinely in pregnancy as a prophylactic against miscarriage. Advertising swelled, and grotesque claims were made for the blessings that DES held out for the sick and the whole. Numerous chemical companies were producing the drug; some sent free samples to doctors in the hope that they might try it out off-label for whatever ailment they pleased, and come back for more.

DES remained in use for thirty years before the reports of calamitous effects became too insistent to ignored. The scope of the disaster was compounded by the discovery that DES was a remarkably efficient growth promoter, stimulating muscle accumulation, first in chickens, and then in beef cattle. Stilbosol, as it was called, was injected in massive concentrations, and residues stayed in the meat, so that much of the population was unknowingly dosed with DES over periods of years. Its use was prohibited in 1959, but it was some years before the agricultural industry complied. Nemesis followed in 1971 when a paper from doctors in one of the great Boston hospitals associated with Harvard University reported the results of a study of seven young women who had presented in the preceding years with a vaginal cancer so rare that few oncologists had ever encountered it before. The doctors could only assume that all the patients had been exposed to the same agent. All possibilities, whether of life-style, diet or medication, had been exhausted when an astute patient, a mother, suggested investigating whether the other ailing mothers had, like her, been given DES pills during their pregnancies. It soon emerged that not only mothers, but more especially their children, and possibly even grandchildren, had suffered often distressing and irreversible physical and mental damage from DES. Both boys and girls had distinctive symptoms, for the reproductive organs were most clearly abnormal. Lawsuits continue still.

The fruits of the adrenals

The adrenal glands, which take their name from their location above the kidneys, were first described in the 16th century by the great Italian physician and opponent of Galen, Bartholomeo Eustachio. (Also known as Eustachius, he is commemorated in another of his anatomical discoveries, the eustachian tubes in the ear.) Three centuries on, Thomas Addison (1793-1860), a much-revered doctor at Guy's Hospital in London published in 1855 a remarkable tract on the disease that bears his name. Its title was '*On the Constitutional and Local Effects of Disease of the Suprarenal Capsules*' (another name for the adrenal glands). Addison's disease was also sometimes called 'bronze skin disease', and was at the time a lethal condition. (Among many famous sufferers was President John Kennedy.) Addison showed by meticulous dissections that the condition was associated with – and, Addison surmised, caused by - degeneration of the adrenal glands. What exactly the adrenals did remained a mystery for close on another century. Brown-Séquard of rejuvenation fame showed (see above) that without its adrenal glands, an animal could live for no more than two or three days. Further enlightenment came in 1927 when, following a series of inconclusive studies in several laboratories, a physiologist at the University of Buffalo, Frank Hartman, proved definitively that such adrenalectomised animals could be kept alive for appreciable periods if supplied with an adrenal extract. This proved that the adrenals really were glands, which secreted some material(s) essential for life, and it presented an immediate challenge to physiologically inclined chemists.

The first to take it up was probably Edward Calvin Kendall (1886-1972), the son of a Connecticut dentist, educated at Columbia University in New York, where in 1910 he was awarded his Ph.D. in organic chemistry. He was already leaning towards biochemistry when he joined the Parke Davis Company. There he he was put to work on a project to isolate the active principle in the thyroid gland. Finding the approach unimaginative and his colleagues uncongenial, Kendall left after only five months and returned to New York to set up a biochemistry laboratory at St. Luke's Hospital. This again proved a disappointment, for he had hoped to continue with the work he had begun on the thyroid, but could generate no interest among the clinicians. When, one day, he received a consignment of a breakfast cereal with the instruction to analyse it, he consigned it to the bin and walked out. Next Kendall applied for a position in the biochemistry division of the Mayo Clinic in Rochester, Minnesota, and there he at last found what he wanted. The Mayo was a venerated institution, home to a galaxy of first-rate scientists and clinicians, and it gave him the environment and facilities that he needed. Within a short time he had isolated thyroxine from thyroid glands, although the formula he arrived at was incorrect. He showed at this point the obstinate streak that remained an inseparable part of his personality, and clung to it until he was definitively proved wrong. Another success, though, was the isolation of an important metabolite glutathione, and the determination of its structure.

In 1930 Hartman in Buffalo, with the help of chemists at Princeton, produced a better adrenal extract which could keep adrenalectomised animals alive indefinitely. When this work appeared in print a physician in the Mayo Clinic appeared in Kendall's laboratory and begged him to try to reproduce the result and provide an adrenal extract that could be used to treat patients with Addison's disease. Kendall had recently been exposed to the chemistry of the adrenals because of the presence in the department of an ebullient visitor from Hungary. Albert Szent-Györgyi was on the track of vitamin C (for the isolation of which he was to receive the Nobel Prize some years later), and the adrenal glands were at that time the favoured source of the vitamin. (The goal was in the end achieved when Szent-Györgyi hit on the far more vitamin-rich paprika plant, which was especially plentiful in Hungary). Kendall acceded to the request, but did not mean to confine himself to supplying extracts, successful though they proved to be for the treatment of patients. He would, he decided, isolate the hormone, as he had thyroxine. He was to plough this arduous furrow for more than twenty years.* Kendall was no great chemist, and was ever dependent on the capable and dedicated assistants and collaborators who surrounded him. Most important of all, he had a patron. This was Frank Mann, the head of the division of Experimental Medicine, a highly skilled surgeon who not only performed all the animal experiments, which were such an integral part of Kendall's programme, but also intervened to save

---

* There was something of an interruption in 1941 when the war in Europe was threatening to draw in the United States, and the newly created National Research Council made plans to absorb relevant research into military medicine projects. Kendall was called on to produce adrenal cortex hormones to assist, rather nebulously, the war effort. For a time, indeed, this project was given priority even over the production of penicillin. According to Kendall's biographer, this demand sprang out of rumours that the German regime was importing cattle adrenals in bulk from South America, with the intention of making extracts available to the Luftwaffe, for they were said to increase tolerance to hypoxia – dearth of oxygen. They would thus allow aircrew to operate at higher altitudes than their enemies, and so presumably drop bombs unmolested. Moreover the pharmaceutical companies were insisting that that the hormonal extracts would also be of benefit in mitigating the effects of shock, whether traumatic or surgical, and stress in combat. These canards were discredited, when it was found that the rumours were false, so in 1944 adrenal hormones were adjudged irrelevant to the war effort, and Kendall was allowed to return to his customary routine.

it from being terminated on the many occasions when it seemed to have stalled. The most embarrassing episode had occurred in 1933: Kendall had announced that he now had crystals of active material, but other laboratories, given samples to examine, had failed to find any physiological activity. It required all Mann's diplomatic skills to avert disaster. Kendall's luck changed after he began to receive consignments of adrenal glands from Parke Davis, with whom he entered into an agreement: having prepared his hormonal extract, he would return the adrenalin-rich residue to the company for its own purposes. The much-needed quantities of adrenal extracts sufficed for the treatment of patients in the clinic, as well as for Kendall's fractionations. Finally, beginning in 1935, active crystalline materials began to appear. Kendall was probably the first to recognise that there was not one adrenocortical hormone, but several. (The adrenal cortex is the outer layer of the gland, and the source of the hormones that Kendall was after.) The first to appear he called Compound A, and of the ones that eventually followed, Compounds B, E and F proved to be of interest. But in 1936 word reached Kendall's laboratory that others were in the chase, and that far away in Basel in Switzerland a Polish-born organic chemist, Tadeusz Reichstein was closing in on the quarry. There was consternation in the Mayo Clinic when Reichstein's first paper appeared a few months later.

Tadeusz Reichstein (1897-1996) was the oldest of five sons of a Polish Jewish engineer, who set up a sugar refinery in Kiev, where Tadeusz spent his early years. The eruption in 1905 of murderous pogroms led the family to emigrate to Switzerland. Apart from an unhappy period at a school in Germany, Reichstein spent his long and mainly tranquil life in the family's adoptive country. But the father died young, having lost his business and savings in the Great War, and the family fell on hard times. The immediate consequence was a delayed start to the young Reichstein's career, for having completed a degree in chemical engineering at the ETH, the Technical University in Zurich, he was compelled to take odd jobs to assist the family. As soon as he could he returned to the ETH, and began work towards his doctoral degree in the chemistry department under a German chemist (who was to receive a Nobel Prize much later for his work on polymers), Hermann Staudinger. Reichstein did not much care for the project he had been allocated, and began to spend time in the laboratory of a young assistant professor in the department - none other than Leopold Ružička. Natural-product chemistry held a much greater appeal for Reichstein, and from Ružička he learned many of the techniques, so well indeed that within a short time he had determined the structure of vitamin C. (He gained little credit for this because the English chemist, Norman Haworth achieved the same goal independently, and later shared the Nobel Prize with Albert Szent-Györgyi.) In 1938 Reichstein was offered the newly created position of Professor of Pharmaceutical Chemistry at the University of Basel, where he remained for the rest of his career.

By then Reichstein was well into the analysis of the steroid hormones of the adrenal gland, which he had begun in 1934. His interest had been aroused at that time by the publications of Kendall and the other Americans. Reichstein negotiated support from two pharmaceutical companies, Ciba in Switzerland and Organon in Holland, where Laqueur had established his programme of steroid research. He received a supply of 1000 kg (about one ton) of adrenal glands and began the work of extraction and fractionation. The first essential, as ever, was an assay by which an active compound could be tracked through the purification steps. The best, which consisted in measuring the concentration of nitrogen-containing elements in the blood of dogs, was not available in Basel, but two others were in use in well-disposed laboratories. Reichstein, who was a cheerful and amiable man, had no difficulty in getting help and the assay mainly used involved measuring the response to electrical muscle stimulation of rats injected with the samples. Reichstein began with the 'amorphous fraction' of Kendall – the part that would not crystallise. This turned out to be the first so-called mineralocorticoid, aldosterone – the hormone responsible for controlling the balance of sodium and potassium in the body.* At the outset Reichstein felt sure the hormones were not steroids

---

* The predominant ion inside cells is potassium, and that outside is sodium. Calcium ions, the regulators of many biological processes, are almost entirely outside the cells, and are admitted in very small amounts as required. The membrane that surrounds each cell contains proteins that act as ion pumps, expelling the unwanted and admitting the desired ions. The pumps are fuelled by the universal energy source of life processes, ATP (p.).

because their relative solubilities in different solvents deviated from those of the then known steroids, but once he had begun the chemical degradation experiments - breaking down the compounds into smaller parts, as was the usual way to begin the long process of structure determination, he realised that he had been wrong.

Over the next few years Reichstein and his students and collaborators isolated no less than 29 different steroids, for six of which they found physiological activities. To determine the structures of all 29, Reichstein took a systematic approach. He decided that the methods then available for determining exact structures of organic compounds fell short when it came to such complex molecules, and so he used reagents with known reactivity towards the common groups of atoms to determine which of these groups were attached to the steroid skeleton. By this means the structures could be divined with near-certainty. It was a *tour de force*, which Reichstein followed up with some partial syntheses. The products were designated 'Compound A', and so on, just as Kendall's were, but of course they did not correspond, and there was for a time no little confusion. Reichstein's Compound F*a* was cortisone. Reichstein continued on his path, which became easier when radioactive isotopes[*] came on stream, and it was two visiting English workers, James and Sylvia Tait, who introduced a vastly superior assay technique by which the appearance of the radioactive steroid could be traced in adrenalectomised rats. By this time also samples were being exchanged with the American laboratories to eliminate any residual confusion about their identities.

---

[*] Radioactive tracing changed the practice of biochemistry, physiology and medicine. The incorporation of a small proportion of a radioactive element (most often at the time an isotope of carbon, hydrogen or phosphorus) in a synthetic compound meant that its metabolic fate could be followed in a living organism. A radioactive isotope is essentially identical in its chemistry to the non-radioactive (bulk) form of the same element. (It differs only in the number of neutrons in the atomic nucleus, which does not affect the chemistry.) The minute admixture of the radioactive compound therefore follows the bulk compound through all its migrations and reactions. A radioactive tracer could allow the compound to be detected, and followed through a purification step or a physiological assay. In medicine radioactive tracers became indispensable, for they allowed rates of synthesis, or turnover, or excretion for example, of physiologically important metabolites to be measured. Many disorders can be identified in this way.

The Taits had done still more while working at the Middlesex Hospital in London, and all of it in the evenings and often through the nights. It was only then that James Tait could find time from his duties as a young lecturer in medical physics, and Sylvia (then Simpson) could escape from her labours as a research assistant in another laboratory. Tait's interest, to which he introduced his future wife, lay in the body's sodium, potassium and water balance. The two tried the effects on the regulatory process of fractions from adrenal extracts, administered to adrenalectomised rats, assaying the animals' urine for the concentrations of the ions. In 1951, after three years of nocturnal toil, they had found a steroid preparation with spectacular sodium-retaining activity. They called this substance electrocortin. The head of the department, Sir Charles Dodds was impressed and arranged for the Taits to visit Reichstein's laboratory, where the preparation was duly identified as Kendall's Compound A, or aldosterone, and was synthesised. The Taits' original publication had already by then animated the pharmaceutical companies, for something to supersede digitalis, which had been in use for two centuries (p.) for the treatment of oedema (dropsy) due to an enfeebled heart (congestive heart failure), would be much welcomed. G.D. Searle & Co. in Illinois was in the lead, having started before the structure of androsterone had even been established. The plan was to create a new steroid that would counteract the effect of aldosterone. The assay procedure was to add the trial compound together with aldosterone, and hope for suppression of retention of sodium and therefore also of water. The Searle chemists synthesised more than nine-thousand variants on the steroid structure before one that worked when taken by mouth was found.

Kendall had been struggling all this time to obtain usable amounts of the elusive products, increasingly relying on what was then the small pharmaceutical company of Merck to scale up the preparations. Merck was an enterprising organisation under its enlightened president, George Merck, son of the founder. He had engaged a number of chemists of the highest calibre, notably Max Tishler, the director of drug development, and Lewis Sarett. They both had several impressive accomplishments to their credit, and it was Sarett (1917-1999) who had developed a close relationship with Kendall (based partly on a shared passion for chess). Kendall had made futile attempts to convert his Compound A (which was available in modest quantity) to Compound E, and it was this that he begged Sarett to undertake. The two molecules, Reichstein had shown, differed only by the presence of one hydroxyl (-OH) group in Compound E, but there was no known means of inserting this at the right point of the Compound A structure. Sarett decided there was no option but to take the bull by the horns and synthesise Compound E from the abundantly available steroidal source, deoxycholic acid from ox bile. The synthesis required 36 successive chemical steps, an almost unprecedented achievement, which produced a minuscule amount of pure material. It was too little for practical use, but it did at least confirm Reichstein's inferred structure. Sarett gave it the name, *cortisone*. Max Tishler (1906-1989) now took a hand. Tishler was one of the six sons of poor European immigrants. The father, a cobbler, abandoned the family when Max was only five, and by the time he was twelve the boy was forced to earn money with odd jobs – as baker's assistant, newspaper seller and finally pharmacist's assistant. There he ran errands, delivering medicine to dying victims of the devastating Spanish flu epidemic of 1919. This, it seems, set him on his career path as a pharmaceutical chemist. He won scholarships to Tufts University in Boston, moved to Harvard for his Ph.D. research, and quickly secured a position at Merck in 1937. Tishler was an outstanding organic chemist and a remarkable leader and organiser. Building on Sarett's synthesis, he devised a programme to develop a method that could be adapted to the commercial production of cortisone, for which there was now an eager demand. He divided his forces into six teams, each charged with perfecting a part of the scheme of synthesis. In the end, starting from a steroidal bile salt (a substance involved in the digestion of fats) from ox bile, the best they could do was to bring the number of chemical steps down to 26, but the yield was much improved. This was not the only group to achieve a synthesis of cortisone, for almost simultaneously two much smaller teams - a pair of leading chemists at Harvard, and a remarkable group at Syntex, a minnow of a chemical company in Mexico City - also reported success. Disputes about priority inevitably resulted.

The demand for cortisone later fell off when the side-effects became apparent, although Merck (or Merck, Sharp and Dohme, as it became) remained a major supplier of the drug. But some years before, a professor of chemistry at Pennsylvania State University, Russell Earl Marker (1902-1995) had found a vastly better source of starting material for cortisone synthesis. Marker had been working for some time on plant steroids, and especially on a class called sapogenins, from the soap-like properties of their suspensions in water. Marker had extracted one of these compounds from the giant root of the abundant Mexican yam. The root is toxic, and Marker isolated the toxic principle, diosgenin, and determined its structure. He perceived on contemplating the formula that it should be possible with relative ease to convert the compound into a product of no small interest - the pregnancy hormone, progesterone (which we will come to presently). It was equally amenable, though, to conversion into cortisone, for which it became the world's primary source. Marker – frustrated apparently by his failure to interest any of the major pharmaceutical companies in his discovery - founded a company of his own in Mexico City in 1944. Syntex, against all expectations, attracted a group of brilliant steroid chemists, and became a thriving centre of research on the subject, and most famously in due course on contraception. The company's name is forever associated with the development of the Pill.

The rise and fall of cortisone, the wonder-drug, happened in a space of about three years. Kendall's Compound E had shown highly encouraging results in animal trials, and a perceptive and inquisitive doctor at the Mayo Clinic had been taking a close interest. Philip Showalter Hench (1896-1965) was head of the rheumatology division, and a practitioner therefore in this, one of the least popular of medical specialities, because there was so little that could be done for the patients. Hench had served in the U.S. Army Medical Corps in the Great War, and had signed up when it ended so that he might be enabled to qualify as a doctor, which he did at the University of Pittsburgh. After two years of study in Germany he joined the Mayo Clinic, and proceeded to follow up every possible clue that might lead to a treatment of rheumatoid arthritis. He had become friendly with Kendall, and followed his work on the adrenal hormones closely. In 1944 the two men decided that the time had come to try an extract from the adrenal cortex in patients. Four were selected, but the results were disappointing. Then World War II intervened. Kendall was for a time drawn into the war effort, and Hench was recalled to the colours. It was only in 1948, after Hench had returned to the clinic, that the next human trial was undertaken. Hench had a rationale. He had observed that victims of rheumatic arthritis who happened to develop jaundice as a result of liver disease (most commonly obstruction of the bile ducts because of gall-stones, or hepatitis) experienced a remission of pain, which would last for some weeks after the jaundice had vanished. Was rheumatic disease perhaps caused by deficiency of something normally supplied in the bile? Hench knew that the active constituents of bile, the bile acids, were steroids. It seemed logical therefore to try bile acids and other steroidal compounds on the patients There were other clues, notably reports that rheumatic and other inflammatory symptoms, including asthma, often abated in pregnancy, when the concentrations of steroid hormones in the circulation rise to high levels. Similar remission of symptoms had been noted after surgery, when the body was suffused with complex anaesthetic compounds. Hench tried bile salts (sodium deoxycholate in particular) and whole ox bile by mouth, by injection and by stomach tube on volunteers among his patients, but to no avail. Kendall's steroids were something else to try, considering especially their manifold physiological effects in animals. Hench had a patient, a young woman in a dire state, crippled by rheumatoid arthritis, and in constant pain. She was the first patient ever successfully treated for rheumatic arthritis, and what a brilliant success it must have seemed!

Hench had found no way to help the woman beyond prescribing the standard analgesics. He now approached Kendall for a sample of his Compound E. Kendall had none to give, but he offered to write to his friend Sarett at Merck for help. A package arrived by post and Hench at once gave his patient a dose by injection. Neither this, nor the second dose the following day had any effect, but on the third day the woman's pain faded and she was suddenly able to stand and to walk almost normally. It was startling, a true prodigy. Trials on a few more patients confirmed the result, but there was little more material, and Hench remained cautious. He also knew that a hyperactive adrenal – something that developed in cases of a local cancer – led to Cushing's disease, named after the great American surgeon, Harvey Cushing, bringing with it a range of serious symptoms. Hench doubted whether Compound E – cortisone – would turn out to be a cure for rheumatic disease, rather than a palliative with a powerful but transient action, but when he reported the results at an open meeting in the Mayo Clinic the effect was electrifying. Soon word of the discovery got out and there was an immediate outcry from doctors and in the press for cortisone to be made available. The pharmaceutical companies responded with strenuous efforts to meet the demand for cortisone, which was also found effective in other inflammatory conditions besides rheumatoid arthritis. It was soon hailed, as so often under similar circumstances before, as a panaceas.

In the midst of all this euphoria the Royal Swedish Academy took a hand, and awarded the well-earned 1950 Nobel Prize for Physiology or Medicine to Reichstein, Kendall and Hench. The discoveries of the adrenal steroid hormones were indeed enormously important, and yet it was not long before the limitations began to show themselves, as Hench had foreseen. Among the most obvious was an elevated blood pressure, leading to kidney failure, damage to the eyes, degradation of connective tissue, psychiatric disturbances, and most of all, disruption of the electrolyte balance, that is to say diminution of potassium and increase in sodium ion concentration, leading to accumulation of water, which is responsible for the swelling of tissues, and the familiar 'moon-face' appearance of patients taking high and regular doses. The medical journals warned against indiscriminate use of cortisone and related steroids, and accusations flew of suppression of reports of adverse effects. From the pharmaceutical companies came counter-accusations tof exaggeration and alarmism. The industry hastened nevertheless to develop analogues of cortisone and other adrenocortical steroids with greater potency and reduced side-effects, and prednisolone, dexamethasone and many others are now indispensable for the treatment of a wide range of conditions. For Kendall all the high hopes of curing rheumatic disease once and for all had been dashed though. On reaching retirement age in 1951, by now one of the country's most celebrated scientists, Kendall was appointed Visiting Professor at Princeton University, and there he devoted himself to the search for a non-steroidal cure. He did not find it, but kept trying until his death. Hench died at 69, still in harness as a physician at the Mayo Clinic. As for Reichstein, he continued his work on steroids, but eventually retired and passed his serene old age in pursuit of his second passion, botany. He reserved his greatest enthusiasm for ferns, on which he became a leading expert with many publications to his name. He died in Basel at 99.

The Pill

At around the same time as cortisone entered the public consciousness the search for an oral contraceptive was gaining momentum. The action, so far as the chemistry was concerned was hottest in two places, Mexico City, host to little Syntex, and Skokie, Illinois, the home of one of the mightiest pharmaceutical concern, G.D. Searle and Company. But the impetus for a campaign to turn the vision of a contraceptive pill into reality came from a reproductive physiologist, working in at a small independent research centre, the Worcester Foundation for Experimental Biology in Shrewsbury, Massachusetts. Gregory Pincus (1903-1967), with his friend from student days, Hudson Hoagland, had founded the organisation in 1944. Pincus already had a considerable reputation in the field of steroids, especially in relation to reproduction, for in 1939 he had achieved artificial insemination of rabbits. He had been exerting himself to raise funds for research into contraception when in 1951 he encountered the formidable Margaret Sanger, suffragette and proselytiser for family planning. Thirty years earlier she had established what became the Planned Parenthood Federation of America, with a series of clinics around the land, staffed by women doctors. Margaret Sanger and Pincus made common cause, and she was able to persuade Katherine McCormick, a feminist and philanthropist of like mind, to donate a modest sum of money to get the work started. Pincus, who was a consultant for G.D. Searle, also managed to interest the company in the problem. Yet the North American drug industry was wary of any direct involvement in contraception, for fear that the inescapable antagonism of the Catholic Church might act adversely on sales of its existing products.

The Syntex management in Mexico had no such qualms. Their chief chemist, the Hungarian, George Rosenkranz, an expert on steroids, initiated a programme of synthesis, based on progesterone as the natural lead compound. As its name implies, progesterone is a promoter of gestation. The train of reasoning extends back to the year 1921 and the place, Innsbruck in Austria. Ludwig Haberlandt (1885-1932) was a doctor and professor of physiology at the local university. His interest was mammalian reproduction, a field in which he made a number of important advances, relating especially to the function of a hitherto disregarded organ in the uterus. The corpus luteum – the yellow body – is a transient structure, which has the role of furnishing the uterus with the anatomical demands for implantation of the fertilised egg, the first step in the process of gestation. It does this by continuously secreting progesterone and some other hormones. When the egg is unfertilised the corpus luteum breaks down and vanishes in about two weeks, but it remains in place if the egg is fertilised, all the time emitting progesterone until the placenta is formed. The progesterone acts, depending on the circumstances, to initiate menstruation, or to prevent a second and untimely insemination. In this sense it is a kind of contraceptive, and Haberlandt proved as much by grafting the ovary of one pregnant rabbit into another. The notion that progesterone had the makings of a contraceptive, that it was indeed 'nature's contraceptive', took root in Haberlandt's mind, and he went so far as to develop a preparation, which he asked a Hungarian chemical company to produce, giving it the name, Infecundin. It appears not to have made any great impression, but in his unshakably Catholic homeland it attracted a torrent of vituperation for his presumption in seeking to interfere in God's design. Haberlandt became the target of hostility and ridicule from his colleagues, and in 1932, at the age of 47, he committed suicide.

Yet Haberlandt's work lived on, and progesterone gradually came into use for the contrary purpose - to treat irregularities and other anomalies of the menstrual cycle, often thereby restoring fertility. One of the physicians who led the way was a distinguished gynaecologist, a professor at Harvard Medical School, John Rock, and it was Rock to whom Pincus turned for the evaluation of progesterone and its derivatives as possible contraceptives. Pincus had already confirmed Haberlandt's observation that progesterone prevented the fertilisation of rabbits. In human subjects, though, the hormone, even in huge (and expensive) doses, had only the most tenuous contraceptive effect when taken by mouth, and did little better by injection. An active derivative was clearly needed, and it was soon established at what points in the structure changes could be made without annihilating the progesteral potency. The task of creating derivatives to test for oral contraceptive activity was one for specialist steroid chemists. Pincus had by now convinced Searle to take progesterone seriously, if only for dealing with menstrual problems, and in their chief chemist, the Polish-born Frank Colton they had the right specialist. Syntex, for its part, had a steroid virtuoso in Carl Djerassi, an immigrant from Vienna, and it was he who, with his colleague George Rosenkranz, and his Mexican student, Luis Miramontes, reached the objective first, though only just.

Djerassi had a stroke of luck on the way: adhering to the dictum of a well-known American organic chemist that a year in the laboratory can often save an hour in the library, he did a search of the chemical literature, which disclosed that a German group at the Schering laboratories in Berlin had examined the effects of an unusual substituent (an acetylene group, $-C\equiv CH$) at a point in the structures of the male sex hormone, testosterone. This had engendered a startling degree of progesterone-like (that is to say female) hormonal activity. An analogous substitution in an oestrogen derivative boosted its oestrogenic (p.) activity. This, combined with structural innovations of his own, led Djerassi and his colleagues to the synthesis in 1952 of the compound that was to become for a time the most widely used oral contraceptive, norethindrone. One year later Colton made a similar compound, norethynodrel, with similar activity, and then another. All three were made available to Pincus and Rock to try out for their efficacy in women, following animal testing. Pincus decided to concentrate on norethynodrel, perhaps because of his close association with Searle. Human testing was done, then and later, in Puerto Rico, and subsequent trials were also conducted on equally deprived populations, in Haiti and Mexico. It appeared that the drug was fully effective in preventing pregnancies, but there were reports of occasional side-effects, mainly blood clots, and one fatality was recorded. Towards the end of 1956 Rock and Pincus discovered that their preparation contained an impurity. This was an oestrogenic compound, a residual intermediate in the synthesis that had not been eliminated. But comparisons with the purified product convinced Rock that the impurity was actually beneficial, in that it reduced bleeding,

The following year the FDA bestowed its blessing on the mixed preparation, but only for the treatment of menstrual disorders, and it reached the market under the trade name of Enovid (in Britain, Enavid). This was the start of combination treatment, which is still widely favoured. Thus Enovid was later sold in combination with an oestrogen called mestranol. Soon after the introduction of Enovid there was a mysterious epidemic in America of menstrual complaints: women had discovered that their doctors would prescribe the drug off-label for use as a contraceptive. The doses needed for this purpose were in fact much lower, but Searle were unable to persuade the FDA to approve its use in that form, and by implication for that purpose, for another two years. To issue a licence for a chemical contraceptive was not in fact a trivial matter. An act of Congress, the Comstock Act, restricted the use of contraception, the Pope (Pius XII) having pronounced that only what was then called 'the rhythm method' was permitted to Catholics. H.L. Mencken quipped that they were forbidden to make use of chemistry or physics, but recourse to mathematics was allowed. Rock, moreover, was an observing Catholic, but he was a highly principled man, who had seen the suffering that repeated pregnancies and large families inflicted on poor mothers, and he acknowledged the need for contraception. He hit on an argument that allowed him to appease his conscience, and he felt could be put before the Vatican. He proposed a schedule whereby the pill would be taken for three weeks only, and then withdrawn for one week to allow menstruation. Thus the pill could be regarded as no more than an extension of the rhythm method. (Despite much agonising successive pontiffs have still not agreed to Rock's proposal.) A further stumbling block was the eruption of the thalidomide disaster in Europe and elsewhere (p.), which shook public confidence in pharmaceutical products. But the tide could not be stemmed. The industry eyed the prospects of profits on a vast scale, and suddenly many companies crowded into the field with progesterone analogues of their own. The FDA eventually conceded that the Pill was safe, and side-effects few. Soon there were many combination pills to choose from, and also stand-alone products. Both kinds have their advantages and disadvantages, but in 1988 Searle withdrew their

Enovid-Mestranol pill from the market, and all other pills containing high proportions of oestrogenic compounds also disappeared, but the Pill is here to stay, essentially in the form that the pioneers of the early 1950s conceived. A footnote to the story was the introduction of mixed oestrogen-progesterone preparations in hormone replacement therapy (HRT), with the aim of preventing (or delaying) the onset of the menopause in middle-aged women.

The isolation of the progesterone receptor in the late 1970s gave the French endocrinologist, Émile-Étienne Baulieu the idea that an antagonist of the receptor, which would prevent the uptake, and therefore the physiological action, of progesterone in a pregnant woman, should result in an abortion. Baulieu was a consultant to what was then the second-largest French pharmaceutical company, Roussel-Uclaf, and at his urging one of the company's chemists, Georges Teltsch set about preparing a range of progesterone analogues, which might be expected to bind tightly to the receptor, so as to exclude progesterone itself. With the compound RU38486, later shortened to the more catchy RU486, he succeeded (and indeed later more such compounds followed). In 1980 the compound was given the name mifepristone, later marketed as Mifegyne. It was tested in the Cantonal Hospital in Geneva, and was an instant success, permitting rapid non-invasive abortions. Mifegyne was licensed first in Britain, in 1991, in France in 1998, and in other European countries and the U.S. in 2000. It was to be used as an abortifacient for women up to two-months pregnant, and in cases of more advanced pregnancy when clinically necessary. The course of Mifagyne did not run altogether smoothly, for there was, not surprisingly, an outcry from the Church and from many political parties and individuals, doctors among them. (In 2000 the British Journal, *Catholic Medical Quarterly* ran an article with the lurid title, 'Mifogyne – the Pill of Cain.) Worse for Roussel-Uclaf, the company was in impending danger of being swallowed by the German Hoechst, which already had a controlling share. The Hoechst board was against abortion, and after a struggle Roussel-Uclaf threw in the towel, gave away their stocks of Mifagyne, and stopped its manufacture, which now happens elsewhere around the world. It was discovered that the compound and various of its analogues are also strong inhibitors of another important steroid receptor. The glucocorticoid receptor occurs in several variant forms in most of the body's cells, and is involved in gene regulation and other processes inseparable from life. The RU486 family of compounds are finding applications in the treatment of a number of diseases, including cancers. As for Roussel-Uclaf, it did not fare well in the belly of Hoechst, and eventually after a succession of other cannibalistic events became a minor element of the huge Bayer concern.

A shot of adrenaline

The steroids were not the only, nor for that matter the first hormones yielded up by the adrenal glands, for the year 1894 saw one of the critical revelations in the long history of biology. It came about in a curious way. George Oliver (1841-1915) was a doctor practising in the genteel spa town of Harrogate in Yorkshire, with a penchant for scientific experimentation. He was in fact no mere provincial GP, for he had won prizes as a medical student in London, had done eye-catching research, and had written several books. One of these was a standard treatise on blood pressure, in which he stressed the importance of measuring it as an aid to diagnosis. Oliver was also a gadgeteer, who built apparatus in his home. One of his creations was a device for determining the diameter, and therefore also the swelling or constriction, of the radial artery in the arm. Oliver, who treated his family as convenient experimental animals, must have been reading about the apparent importance for life of the adrenal gland, and was inspired to test a preparation from animal adrenals, procured from the local butcher. He tried samples of this on his young son, and observed that the boy's radial artery contracted. How the solution was administered is not recorded, but if by injection it must have been a weak preparation, for otherwise the boy might have died; if by mouth then little active material, but perhaps just enough, would have survived exposure to the enzymes in the digestive tract. At all events, Oliver thought the effect remarkable enough to approach the Professor of Physiology at University College,

London, the redoubtable Sir Edward Sharpey-Schafer (1850-1935) (at that time though merely Professor Schäfer).*

According to his own account, Oliver travelled to London to tell Sharpey-Schafer about his discovery, bearing a supply of adrenal extract, and inveigled himself into Sharpey-Schafer's laboratory, where the great man was occupied in measuring the blood pressure of an anaesthetised dog. This would have entailed the use of a long tube filled with mercury connected to an artery. The professor was in no mood to be interrupted, but Oliver persisted, mentioning perhaps a common devotion to William Sharpey, who had taught them both. (Oliver later endowed an annual lecture, the Sharpey-Oliver lecture, as an act of piety.) Finally, at all events, Sharpey-Schafer, having concluded his own experiment, agreed to inject some of Oliver's extract into the dog's artery. The effect was startling: the vessel contracted, causing the blood pressure to shoot up so violently that, according to one report at least, the mercury leapt to the top of the tube. Oliver and Sharpey-Schafer gave a presentation of their results, which caused great excitement among physiologists and physicians.

---

* Edward Albert Schäfer was the son of a Hamburg businessman who had emigrated to England. Entering University College in London to study medicine, the young man won high acclaim, and soon after qualifying was appointed an assistant professor in the College, and not long after that, Professor of Physiology. At the age of 28 he was elected a Fellow of the Royal Society, and many honours followed, including a knighthood and the presidency of the British Medical Association. In 1899 he left University College for the University of Edinburgh, where he remained until retiring in 1933, two year before his death. As a medical student the young Schafer had become a protégé of his teacher, William Sharpey, and in 1918 he coupled Sharpey's name to his own, and also discarded his umlaut to re-emerge as Sharpey-Schafer. This may perhaps have been, partly at least, a belated reaction to the violent anti-German agitations in Britain during the First World War, when anyone or anything with a German-sounding name (a dachshund for example) might be physically attacked, when the Battenbergs became Mountbattens, too late for Admiral Lord Louis Battenberg, the First Sea Lord, who was summarily sacked. Of Sharpey-Schafer's patriotism there can be little doubt, for his two sons both gave their lives in the war. He himself merely said that he had wanted William Sharpey's name to be commemorated in his own.

A search at once began for the active principle in the adrenal extract. The year after the experiment in London a cardiologist in Kraków, Napoleon Cybulski and his colleague, Władysław Szymonowicz independently made the same discovery, giving the active substance the name, nadnerczyna, from the Polish for the adrenals (which, needless to say, did not catch on). Cybulski made some attempts to isolate it, but success came four years later, and in America. John Jacob Abel (1857-1938) was the country's leading pharmacologist. He had begun his working life as a schoolteacher and soon headmaster, but spending his spare moments in various laboratories, he acquired a taste for research, and enrolled as a science student at the University of Michigan. Like many American pharmacologists of his generation, he then spent three years in Europe, much of the time at the University of Strassburg, where the great Schmiedeberg (p.) presided, and where he received his doctoral degree in medicine. After that he returned to his alma mater as a professor, but stayed only two years before accepting an invitation from the new medical school at Johns Hopkins University in Baltimore. There, as Professor of Pharmacology, he remained to the end of his life. Abel established at Johns Hopkins the foremost school of pharmacology in the country. He gained a high reputation both as researcher and teacher, and was much revered by the many disciples he sent out into the world to found their own research schools.

Like many other physiologists and pharmacologists Abel was excited by the startling discovery in London, and threw himself into the chase after the active principle. It took him several years before he had a potent but still impure preparation of what he called epinephrine, and still longer to determine, as he thought, its structure. Others, too, were in the race, and in Strassburg an Austrian doctor and biochemist, Otto von Fürth made a crude preparation, which the ubiquitous Hoechst concern took up and marketed in 1897 under the name of Suprarenin (suprarenal glands being another name for the adrenals). Abel was robbed. He was approached by a shrewd industrial chemist, then active in New York, Jokichi Takamine (1854-1922), to whom he divulged the entire hard-won preparative process from the glands to the semi-pure adrenaline. Takamine had studied chemistry and engineering in Tokyo, and had embarked on a career in agricultural products. He had pursued further studies in brewing in Glasgow, at the University and at Anderson's College (now the University of Strathclyde). Back in Japan he had isolated an enzyme involved in the breakdown of starch, still known as Taka-diastase. He touted this as an aid to digestion, and in this guise it was taken up by the Parke Davis company, and achieved enormous popularity in the U.S., where Takamine now betook himself. He married an American wife and remained in the country for the rest of his life. A true entrepreneur, Takamine took up brewing, and produced a successful whisky. He was soon rich enough to establish his own pharmaceutical company in New York, and soon he founded a second in Clifton, New Jersey. He engaged an able young chemist, Keizo Uenaka, who set about reproducing the preparative process that Abel had shown to Takamine in such unstinting detail. One night in the laboratory in New York, Uenaka, who had found a means of preventing the degradation of the rather unstable adrenaline, obtained a crop of crystals. It was Takamine, however, who took out a patent (later unsuccessfully challenged on the grounds that it was a naturally occurring substance, and Uenaka and Takamine had in any case been led by earlier work), and Parke Davis eagerly undertook to produce and market the compound.*

Abel was understandably bitter at what he saw as a betrayal of his collegial openness. He had not in fact quite isolated adrenaline. A critical step in the preparation was a chemical modification, which permitted efficient solvent extraction, namely the introduction of benzoyl groups, which contain a benzene ring (p.). Finally these groups had to be stripped off by another chemical reaction. Abel believed he had achieved this, but in reality one, more stably attached than the others, had remained. Uenaka and Takamine had done better, and removed all three. Abel had been

---

* Adrenaline/epinephrine made Takamine even richer. He used his wealth to create the Sankyo Pharmaceutical Company in Japan, and in New York the International Takamine Fermentation Company. These were followed by the Takamine Laboratory in New Jersey. The Emperor of Japan conferred one of the country's highest orders of chivalry on Takamine, who devoted much of the rest of his life to furthering relations between Japan and the United States. He founded a friendship society and also the Nippon Club of New York, and when the great park in the Potomac Tidal Basin was being planned he contributed a gift of 2000 cherry trees, which are still the pride of Washington.

deceived because the monobenzoyl derivative was physiologically active. He continued to insist that Takamine's crystalline preparation was still not pure, and in this he was vindicated only years later, when it was discovered to contain a small admixture of the close chemical relative, noradrenaline (norepinephrine in the American usage); this has similar physiological activity, and is produced by the adrenal gland, but also, unlike adrenaline, in nerve endings. The correct formula of adrenaline was determined by a Parke Davis chemist, Thomas Aldridge. Adrenaline is a relatively simple compound, but the first attempts at synthesis were attended by difficulties, finally overcome in 1906 by the head of the chemistry division at Hoechst, Friedrich Stolz, and synthetic adrenaline immediately went into production. This was the first hormone to be synthesised in the laboratory. And yet, weight for weight, the pure synthetic material was still only half as active as the crystals prepared from the adrenal glands. The problem was solved by Stolz's junior colleague, Franz Flächner, who had assisted in the structure determination. It was a question of chirality* – the functional difference between two states of mirror-image symmetry - a common, almost universal, problem in the chemistry of compounds made by living organisms. The argument about whether it should be called adrenaline (even adrenalin) or epinephrine rumbles along even to this day, but its discovery was one of the milestones in the advance of modern medicine. In its obituary notice ten years later of George Oliver, who had discovered its existence in the still mysterious adrenal gland, the *British Medical Journal* averred that adrenaline was 'one of the greatest boons to

---

* Organic chemistry is the chemistry of carbon. A carbon atom can bond to four atoms, which may be carbon, or commonly hydrogen, nitrogen or oxygen (as well as some others). If now four different atoms or groups of atoms, *a*, *b*, *c* and *d*, say, are attached to one carbon, then if one of these is exchanged with one of the others, the resulting structure becomes a mirror image of the previous. Now whatever the molecule interacts with – a receptor in a cell, or an enzyme for instance – that target will also have its own asymmetry, and will in general recognise only one of the two possible mirror-image forms of the metabolite or drug, or will at least interact more strongly with the one than with the other. An accompanying phenomenon of mirror asymmetry is *optical activity*, the property of rotating the plane of polarised light in a clockwise or anticlockwise direction. This is explained on p. f.n. The link between mirror-image asymmetry and rotation of the plane of polaris'tion was made by Pasteur in one of the great flashes of insight in the history of science.

suffering humanity'. It immediately transformed the practice of surgery, for its action in constricting the blood vessels allowed haemorrhages to be suppressed or prevented, and pain to be reduced. In dentistry it was (and still is) added to the anaesthetics, such as Novocaine, also called procaine (another Hoechst product). Adrenaline also found applications in other branches of medicine, in obstetrics, cardiology for instant treatment of heart attacks, and in the treatment of asthma and other allergic states, since it also acts to dilate the airways. Many pharmaceutical companies began to make analogues of adrenaline, or other compounds with one or other of the activities of the parent substance, hoping for instance for longer-lasting action, or for bronchodilating activity without any alarming effect on blood pressure. Many such were synthesised and sold to the public, some benign and some dangerous. Isoprenaline, also known as isoproterenol, caused many deaths (3000, it is thought, in the U.K.) when applied as a spray against bronchial spasms, but is still occasionally deployed, now that the hazards and the conditions for its safe use have been defined.

Chapter 14

CANCER: THE LAST FRONTIER

It is doubtful whether any of the vast number of 'cures' for cancer offered to its victims before the late 19th century could have done them much good. Skin ulcerations, probably cancerous, have a place in the Ebers Papyrus of around 1500 B.C. (p.), which suggested the application of arsenical salves. The supposed virtues of arsenic found an echo in the writings of Avicenna at the end of the first millennium A.D. (p.), and again in those of the French surgeon, Guy de Chauliac (p.). In the interim some of the Roman physicians were anointing diseased skin with coal tar, which, closer to our time, was shown to be rich in carcinogens. (Even early in the 19th century the prevalence of scrotal cancer among the small boys who swept the chimneys was an acknowledged scandal.) The treatment must have remained in vogue, for Ambroise Paré (p.) inveighed against it in the 16th century, but failed to put an end to its use. By the early part of the 19th century many of the leading physicians had their own prescriptions, some toxic plant products, others caustic substances, such as potassium hydroxide (caustic potash), silver nitrate or zinc chloride, applied externally, introduced through the nether orifices, or swallowed. This would have done little but exacerbate the patient's pain. On the other hand, improvements in surgical technique did lead to some successes: no-one who has read it will ever forget Fanny Burney's chill`ing account of her mastectomy, with no anaesthetic, in 1811, but she lived for another twenty-nine years to the respectable age of 86.

New directions

In the last decade of the 19th century a new glimmer of light appeared on the clinical horizon. William Bradley Coley (1862-1936), having graduated in 1888 from Harvard Medical School with high distinction, was appointed orthopaedic surgeon at the New York Cancer Hospital (the progenitor of the Memorial Sloan-Kettering Cancer Center). One of his first patients was a young woman who was experiencing increasingly severe pain in her hand. Coley, and a more experienced orthopaedist whom he consulted diagnosed a local infection, but the pain became intolerable and spread. Too late Coley sent a bone biopsy to the pathologist, who identified a sarcoma – a cancer that affects connective tissue and bone. It was an unusual position for this kind of tumour and a rare type of cancer (a Ewing's sarcoma), and Coley – though not his senior colleague - was inexperienced. Coley amputated the lower arm, but it did not slow the spread of the cancer. New tumours appeared by the day, and Coley, who had formed a close bond with his patient, could do no more than administer morphine and watch her die. The experience haunted him for the rest of his days, and it drove him to divert as much time as he could spare from surgery to research on cancer.

Coley began to read deeply and to examine the hospital case reports. Among the ninety or so sarcoma patients who had been treated he found one arresting report. Six years before, a house-painter, a German immigrant, had been operated on for an advanced sarcoma behind his left ear. The cancer had spread, and after another three operations, which had left an open wound that would not heal, the case was adjudged hopeless. But then the patient developed erysipelas, an infection of the skin and lymphatic glands, known to the ancients (pp.), and formerly called *ignis sacer*, the sacred (or St. Anthony's) fire. It is most likely to affect the sick, especially those with an enfeebled immune system. It is caused by the bacterium, *Streptococcus pyogenes*, and before the era of antibiotics it killed one in ten of those it infected. It was also the most common infection in surgical wounds. The case notes that Coley had found revealed that as the infection flared up the surgical wound began to heal, and the cancer to regress. After a short time all trace of the sarcoma had vanished, and so too had the patient after his discharge. Coley decided that the final outcome had to be established, and he resolved to find the patient. He knew only the name, and that he would have a prominent scar below his ear, but he surmised that, if still alive, he would be plying his trade on the lower East Side, where he had lived before entering the hospital, and where indeed most German immigrants were concentrated. After a door-to-door search among the tenements lasting several weeks Coley, remarkably, found the man. Mr Stein was well, and free of cancer, as an examination back at the hospital confirmed.

This was not in fact the first observation of tumour regression in the wake of an infection. Pasteur, Koch and von Behring had all alluded to such a phenomenon, and even a century earlier a French physician had mentioned it in a monograph on tumours. Several reports had however also appeared much closer to Coley's time. Anton Checkhov, who worked as a doctor in remote parts of Russia, including the island of Sakhalin, was one who remarked on it in his diary, although this may not have come Coley's way. In 1867 Sir James Paget, surgeon, inter alia, to Queen Victoria, made reference to unaccountable regressions, and that same year a more explicit report emerged from Germany. Wilhelm Busch was a highly respected surgeon, a professor at the University of Bonn. The case he described was that of a young woman with a sarcoma on her neck, which had grown to an enormous size, threatening her airways and preventing her from closing one eye. Busch evidently reacted as Coley had done to his young patient, and resorted to a new and desperate measure. He had at the same time another patient with erysipelas, from whom he took a cotton swab, which he then applied directly to his sarcoma patient's tumour, having first burned away a patch of skin on its surface. A high fever quickly developed, and the tumour began to soften and shrink. But the patient was weak, complications supervened, her temperature fell, and the tumour again grew. Busch could do no more, and the patient presumably died. It was a remarkable experiment nonetheless. In 1882 another German clinician, Friedrich Fehleisen in Würzburg tried his hand at a similar treatment: he injected an erysipelas culture into the primary tumour of a woman with multiple sarcoma, and again there was rapid and startling regression. The eventual outcome is not recorded in his short publication, but he was sufficiently encouraged that he tried the method on more patients with various cancers, having also carried out successful tests on animals. The results with patients were variable, and the hazards of induced erysipelas infection probably unacceptable. Fehleisen's procedure fell into disrepute., but a few years later another German physician, P. Bruns tried again, apparently with some success, and he surveyed the various attempts made up to 1888 in a paper published in that year with the title (in translation) of 'Healing effect of erysipelas infection on tumours'.

It was against this background, which he must have ingested during his literature search, that Coley set out on his risky and exacting path. In 1891 he infected a patient with a *Streptomyces pyogenes* culture for the first time. Coley's superiors were reluctant to allow this lethal agent to be deliberately loosed in their wards, and so the patient, again a poor immigrant, terminally ill with an inoperable throat cancer, was taken back to his tenement flat and treated there. The patient proved remarkably resistant to the bacterium, and it was only after a series of injections over a period of six months that the infection finally took hold. Once it did, the effects were dramatic. Tumour tissue flowed from the unhealed surgical wound, the swelling subsided in a matter of days, and the wound healed. Soon the patient was considered cured. He returned to his original home in Italy and lived for another eight years, but the cause of his eventual death could not be determined. Coley did his best to standardise his culture – 'Colwy's Toxin', as it came to be called - and he also made what appeared to be an improvement. *Serratia marsescens* is a pink bacterium, commonly associated with urinary tract infections. In 1890 a bacteriologist at the Pasteur Institute in Paris published a paper reporting that when *Serratia* were added to a *Streptococcus* culture its virulence was enormously enhanced. Coley took advantage of this discovery, and henceforth Coley's Toxin contained an admixture of *Serratia marcescens* (which is confusingly also known as *Bacillus prodigiosus*). Coley treated many patients *in extremis*, and of the first twelve two died of erysipelas. This, as much as the advent in 1901 of X-rays as a means of treating solid tumours, turned Coley's chief, the medical director of what was by then the Memorial Sloan-Kettering Cancer Center, James Ewing against Coley's method, and a strong personal animus developed between the two men. Ewing, who was totally wedded to radiation therapy, had the upper hand, and even though Coley was the highly-regarded head of bone surgery, he was impeded at every turn. It was only after Ewing's death in 1915 that Coley was free to do as he wished. He had, some years before, fallen to cogitating on the mechanism of the erysipelas effect. He suspected that a 'factor' secreted by the bacteria must be responsible, and that perhaps therefore the dangers of the infection could be bypassed by using killed bacteria or an extract derived from them. This was indeed the case, and Coley's Toxin was henceforth prepared on this basis.

Coley treated more than a thousand patients with the toxins, which in 1899 the pharmaceutical company, Parke Davis had begun to manufacture commercially. The treatment was taken up in several countries, but medical opinion was sharply divided. In 1894 the organ of the U.S. medical profession, the *Journal of the American Medical Association*, thunderously denounced Coley's Toxins as a delusion. There was certainly scope for criticism: Coley had never attempted to arrange controlled trials of his procedure, statistics were sketchy, and there had been inadequate follow-up of the supposedly cured patients. Yet this does not entirely explain the rather abrupt fall of the toxins from favour. The cynically minded might conjecture that the activity of the giant pharmaceutical companies in promoting their technologically more imposing, and a thousand times more expensive medicines, might have played a part. Coley never lost faith, and asserted the superiority of his approach up to his death in 1936. Interest dwindled nonetheless, and in 1952 Parke Davis, the main supplier of Coley's brew, took it off the market. But interest has never entirely vanished, and received new impetus from the research and writings of Coley's daughter, Helen Coley Nauts, a respected oncologist, who assembled an impressive amount of historical data on the many patients treated and outcomes. Coley's work can be seen as foreshadowing the advent of immunotherapy, which is now at the forefront of cancer treatment and research.

Coley's work had a strange resonance in Soviet Russia in the period immediately after the Second World War. The episode was referred to as 'the KR Affair' after the name of the principal protagonists, Nina Kliueva, an established researcher at the Soviet Academy of Sciences in Moscow, and her husband, Gregorii Roskin, a professor at Moscow University. Roskin was apparently drawn to the notion that powerful toxins secreted by parasites, responsible for serious diseases, might selectively attack cancers. The idea was not new, and at the time there was much interest in the supposed curative properties of infectious agents generally. A major influence was the purported success achieved by a professor at the medical school in Vienna, Julius Wagner-Jauregg*, who was honoured with the Nobel Prize for a method of curing advanced neurosyphilis ('general paralysis of the insane', as it was called) by infecting his patients with malaria. This sprang from the old theory of 'pyrotherapy', which posited that diseases could be driven out by increasing the body temperature, and of course attacks of malaria induced high fevers. The method was fairly widely adopted, though with questionable results. Whatever the inspiration, it took Roskin ten years from the time he started his research, including a five-year interruption by war, to convince himself that he really had a cure for cancer. He and his wife, Kliueva, who had joined in the work, reported in the Russian scientific literature in 1945 that when tumour-bearing mice were injected with an extract of either live or killed trypanosomes (the agents of the tropical disease also known as sleeping sickness) their tumours regressed. Some time later the method was tried on human patients, with (reportedly) excellent results. News of this triumph of Soviet scientific dominance broke in the Russian press and was received with wide acclamation. *Pravda*, the Party newspaper hailed the achievement and its architects, Roskin and Kliueva were invested with honours, including the Stalin Prize, and invited to appear on the huge podium at the Mayday parade through Moscow alongside the members of the politburo.

---

* Wagner-Jauregg (1857-1940) was a deeply unpleasant man. An intolerant and domineering man, he specialised in psychiatry, a fashionable occupation at the time, and especially in Vienna. He succeeded Krafft-Ebing (the man who introduced the concepts of sadism and masochism into psychiatry) at the University of Graz, and rose from there to the directorship of the Psychiatric and Neurological Clinic at the medical school in Vienna. His famous experiments with malaria were published in 1917. Wagner-Jauregg, joined the Nazi party at its inception, swallowed the doctrines of 'racial hygiene', and became violently antisemitic, going so far as to divorce his Jewish wife. University departments and streets were named after him.

The cancer cure from Russia was equally widely and uncritically reported elsewhere, and the predictable demand arose from doctors and patients, especially in America, for access to the therapeutic material. The U.S. Ambassador in Moscow was instructed in 1946 by his masters in Washington to intercede with the regime for a sample of the KR, as it was now termed. This was linked to a proposal of collaboration from the U.S. Surgeon-General: a visit to Moscow of a small, select group of American cancer specialists would allow a valuable exchange of knowledge and experience between American and Soviet experts. In the U.S.S.R. paranoia reigned. Why should the fruits of Soviet genius be delivered to the enemy in the West? On the other hand, the prestige accruing from a Russian cancer cure would be overwhelming. One commentator called it 'a medical atom bomb'. Roskin and Kliueva seized the opportunity, and approached the powerful Andrei Zhdanov, the cultural commissar, with a demand for better support for their research. For were they to go on working on a shoestring, as they had been, then the Americans, with their superior facilities, would assuredly overtake them, and the Soviet lead would be very quickly dissipated. This was the way the scientists and technologists on both sides of the Cold-War divide coaxed funding out of their governments, and it worked again for KR. The appeal, expedited by the Minister of Health, reached the bureaucratic and political pinnacle, the Central Committee, and Stalin personally signed the order releasing of huge funds, with the promise of a new building, for the research. Now came the next question: would permission be granted for the sample of material to be delivered to the U.S. Surgeon-General? The Soviet bureaucracy ground slowly as the favourable recommendation from the Ministry worked its way up to politburo level. Finally the Secretary of the Academy of Medical Sciences, Vasilii Parin, who had flown to New York bearing a precious package, marked 'Russian cancer cure', and a copy of a book, *Biotherapy of Malignant Tumours*, just published by the two scientists, received an affirmative answer. But the very next day the unhappy Parin, having carried out his instructions, received a second cable, informing him that his superiors had changed their minds: on no account was he to give the Americans anything at all. Stalin, it seemed, had abruptly repudiated all notions of scientific and technical collaboration with the West. This new doctrine of isolation was even to extend even to English-language editions of Russian scientific journals.

Kliueva was summoned to an audience with Zhdanov, who berated her for handing Soviet secrets to the Americans, and Stalin himself wanted to know whether the information that had been divulged would make it possible for outsiders to steal the invention. (Kliueva reassured him.) Shortly after this, events took a more unpleasant turn. Kliueva and Roskin were hauled before a so-called Honour Court, a relic from Tsarist times resurrected as a means of publicly humiliating political delinquents. Confronted by an audience of 1,500 of their scientific and medical confrères, the two were charged with complicity in 'anti-state' and 'anti-patriotic' activities, perpetrated by the Minister of Public Health (now sacked), and the 'criminal acts' of the American spy, Parin. Roskin and Kliueva got off lightly: they were found guilty and severely reprimanded, but not otherwise punished, and they were allowed to continue their work unmolested. Parin vanished into the Gulag. The message was clear: anyone found trafficking with scientists in the West would be in big trouble. Kliueva and Roskin were saved because they were regarded as too valuable to sacrifice. (A film was even being made in which the heroes were based on them.) According to the historian, Nikolai Krementsov, who has written an authoritative account of the KR affair, the upheaval was almost certainly orchestrated by Molotov and Zhdanov to serve as a lesson to others, who might feel inclined to transgress. The malign shadow of Trofim Lysenko, the charlatan agronomist, who had Stalin's ear, and was responsible for the eclipse of biology throughout the Soviet imperium in a welter of ideology, quackery and fraud, could also be detected in the background, although his influence was by then in decline.

The KR partnership did not have long to bask in Stalin's approbation in the lavish new Laboratory for Experimental Biotherapy. Oncologists and other doctors had long nursed doubts about the efficacy of the KR method, and towards the end of 1947 Kliueva's report of progress to the Academy of Medical Sciences drew sharp criticism. A committee was appointed to visit the laboratory and examine both the laboratory techniques and the clinical results. The members stayed for a month and produced a damning 600-page report. They had found, they stated, not one convincing cure or amelioration of a cancer case; they could not accept the 'positive evaluation' of the method. But yet they recommended that the research continue, so that a firm conclusion could be reached. The Academy acceded, but withdrew one-third of the laboratory space from the project and made it available for other work. The next inspection led to a report running to over 1,000 pages, and ought to have been the *coup de grâce*. KR, it concluded, 'does not cure cancer in any form or at any stage'; the expenditure of 19,175,900 roubles on the laboratory between 1946 and 1950 was 'not justified by its scientific and clinical work'; and Klieuva and Roskin should be dismissed.*

And yet it was still not the end for the resourceful couple, for it was not in the Academy's power to close a laboratory, especially one that had been sanctioned by Stalin in person. The Council of Ministers, when approached by the Academy, merely demanded that the research be 'reorganised', and that Roskin and Kliueva should continue with work on KR (presumably on the grounds that the Party, and Stalin in particular, never made mistakes), though on a reduced scale. Kliueva appealed once again to the Party with absurd promises of an imminent breakthrough, but this time the Deputy Prime Minister consulted the President of the Academy about the veracity of the claims, and the game was up. Kliueva and Roskin were dismissed, but it was even then by no means the end of their activities. For one thing they both held other posts, Kliueva in the microbiology department of one of the Moscow medical schools, her husband as head of the histology department at Moscow University. Kliueva moved to a vaccine and serum laboratory, of which she became the head, and both she and Roskin occupied themselves quietly with less flamboyant projects. Then in 1953 Stalin died, and the two applied once again to be given the facilities to resume work on KR. This was curtly refused, and they were cold-shouldered by the medical and scientific establishment. And even then it was still not over, for in 1957 Roskin received a communication from Professor Coudert of the University of Lyon Medical School, and the industrialist, Charles Mérieux, who had founded the company that later became Pasteur-Mérieux, informing Roslin that they had launched a project to revive KR, now called Cruzin (from the Latin name of the trypanosome, *Trypanosoma cruzei*), or in Russian Krutzin (incorporating

---

* The figures and quotations are taken from Nikolai Krementsov's book, *The Cure, A Story of Cancer and Politics from the Annals of the cold War.*

the name of KR). With the support of the indestructible Parin, who had emerged from the Gulag during the thaw after Stalin's death and was once more Secretary of the Academy, Kluieva and Roskin applied yet again for support. This time the Council of Ministers instructed the Academy that KR should be disinterred.

Coudert and Mérieux confirmed the discredited KR results, and the British Pergamon Press (the brainchild of Captain Robert Maxwell) published a translation of *Biotherapy of Malignant Tumours*. The drug was marketed in France under a new name, Trypanosa, but sank without trace. Neither did Kliueva and Roskin get any further. He died in 1964 at the age of 71, she in 1971 at 72. Equally fruitless had been attempts to achieve cures with KR in the United States and other countries, although there were scattered reports of success, not however in any convincing controlled trials. Kliueva and Roskin were not charlatans, and the likelihood is that there were some positive results in animal experiments, amidst the self-deception. But for clinical trials reproducible and in principle pure material is needed, and purification of the cultured product would have been very difficult with the fractionation methods then available. Contamination with alien proteins would have presented the danger of immune reactions, including death from anaphylaxis (p.). There were indeed innumerable attempts, both before and after the KR affair and Coley's work, at treating cancers with various kinds of infections, and many tantalising indications of remissions. With the growth of knowledge about the immune system and the control of cellular processes by signalling molecules (p.), a rationale has evolved for the efficacy of such treatments. When the body is under stress cells release compounds called cytokines. They may be small molecules or proteins, such as tumour necrosis factor (TNF). These substances can have a variety of effects, which include the generation of fever and stimulation of the immune system. The consequence can be an assault on a tumour, but tumours are of many kinds, and express a great range of antigens, and so these effects are generally uncertain. Immunological treatments of tumours are today much more scientific and refined, as will appear.

Chemotherapy ascendant

The notion of treating cancers with toxic chemicals was first properly formulated by Paul Ehrlich. At that time arsenicals, in particular Fowler's solution (p.) and potassium arsenite, were being given to cancer patients (and to others) by some doctors, and were said to have had a modest effect on the progress of leukaemia. Ehrlich's experiments with dyes (pp.) had shown him that chemical compounds could discriminate between tissues of different types. Why then should it not be possible to find compounds that would preferentially interact with, and perhaps destroy tumour cells without destroying the normal tissue surrounding them? With this in mind, Ehrlich tried the effects of a series of simple toxic compounds on normal cells, which for the most part they killed. He apparently thought that one of them, ethyleneimine held some promise, but left no record of having pursued the matter further, probably because he had become preoccupied with curing syphilis.

It was only many years later, shortly after the beginning of the Second World War, that more important advances in cancer treatment came about. Mustard gases were developed by both sides in the First World War, and caused many deaths and terrible and lasting injuries. Some 1.2 million soldiers were exposed to gases of one kind or another, and three-quarters of them died. Mustard gases were less lethal than chlorine and phosgene, with about 4% fatalities mong those exposed, but the injuries of the survivors were exceedingly painful and often irreparable. Autopsies by German army doctors and an American group at the University of Pennsylvania revealed that one of the effects of the mustard gases then deployed, mainly sulphur mustard (chemical name 1,5-dichloro-3-thiopentane, but often called yperite on account of its use by the British in the battle of Ypres in Belgium) was to eliminate the white cells from the blood and from the bone marrow, in which they are formed. This discovery gave birth to the notion that good might come from evil if such a compound could suppress the proliferation of white cells in leukaemia, or of the white cells of the immune system, the lymphocytes, in lymphomas. (In diseases such as Hodgkin's lymphoma the cancerous lymphocytes travel through the bloodstream, spreading the disease, and the uncontrolled multitudes can cluster together locally to form tumours.) Precisely how the mustard gases exerted their effects was obscure, but what these compounds have in common is high chemical reactivity as alkylating agents, that is to say they introduce alkyl groups, consisting of carbon and hydrogen, into the compounds that they attack. With the approach of World War II the fear of gas warfare provoked a spate of research on mustard gases (as well as nerve gases and other such weapons forbidden by the Geneva Convention). In the United States programmes concerned with delivering and combatting poison gases and treating casualties were started at several centres. Among them was including Yale University, where two distinguished pharmacologists, Alfred Gilman and Louis Goodman were in charge.

Sulphur mustards had been replaced by then with more effective nitrogen mustards, and the first task to which Gilman and Goodman applied themselves was to determine whether these acted similarly on the white blood cells. Animal experiments showed that this was so, but Gilman and Goodman made a further important observation: the nitrogen mustard, absorbed through the skin, killed many cells, but acted most destructively on those that were rapidly dividing. These included the bone marrow cells, as expected, but also those in the lymph glands. Now of course the chief characteristic of cancer is uncontrolled cell division. It was a short step then to try the effect of the agents on implanted tumours in mice, and there was indeed an instant and dramatic effect. The year was 1942, and Gilman and Goodman prevailed on a surgeon in the local hospital, Gustav Lindskog to try the drug on a patient. There were at the time three nitrogen mustards, simple compounds, all closely related; they were designated HN1, HN2 and HN3. It was HN3 that Lindskog administered by injection to a patient dying from an aggressive lymphoma. The improvement in his condition was as startling as that in the mice: within two days his tumours had started to soften and shrink, and within two weeks they had vanished. The miracle, though, was short-lived, for in a matter of weeks the tumours reappeared, and further courses of treatment failed to contain the progress of the cancer. A further six patients were treated with similar results. At much the same time trials on larger numbers of incurable patients were organised in other centres, using HN2 and HN3, and the outcomes were always much the same, although some partial longer-term regressions were reported. This was the beginning of a systematic exploration of chemotherapy, although wartime security dictated that the work could be published only in 1946, the year after the war had ended. (HN2, known as mustine, or under the trade name, Mustagen, remained in routine use in the chemotherapy of some cancers until only a few years ago.)

While Gilman, Goodman and their colleagues were experimenting with nitrogen mustards the war impinged again on cancer research. On the evening of 2nd December 1943 the Germans launched an air attack on the harbour of Bari in the heel of Italy. The commander of the Royal Air Force responsible for the defence of the area had made the disastrous calculation that the Germans had no aircraft available for such an exploit, and surprise was total. The bombers' target was the cluster of thirty supply ships loaded with materiel for the American and British armies advancing slowly northwards through Italy. Among them was the American ship, the *SS John Harvey*, carrying a consignment of mustard gas shells. Hitler had apparently been persuaded that the use of gas would be highly imprudent by reason of the much greater capacity of the Allies to wage a chemical war; nor were the Allies intending to use gas unless the Germans did so first. The German bombers had an essentially undefended and floodlit target, for unloading was in progress. The ammunition ships were struck and exploded, and so did the *John Harvey*, which had caught fire, killing all on board. The shells also exploded and the gas mixed with the oil already covering the surface of the water. An odour of garlic penetrated the atmosphere. The survivors rescued from the water and many civilians on the land began to experience breathing difficulties and fading vision, sinking blood-pressure and painful excrescences on their skin. Some died immediately, and eighty-three by the end of the month. The Allied Governments, anxious to avoid offering the Germans a propaganda coup, would not divulge the nature of the cargo on the *John Harvey*, which probably delayed the efforts of the doctors to find the right treatment for the injured.

It was an American army medical officer, Lieutenant-Colonel Stewart Alexander, sent to Bari five days after the attack to take charge, who eventually deduced that the cause was a chemical agent, despite the hot denials of the local military authorities. The nature of the burns on the corpses left no room for doubt that a chemical agent had been responsible, and the distribution of the bodies fished out of the harbour pointed to the *John Harvey* as the epicentre of the disaster. And finally an unexploded gas shell was retrieved from the water and found to be of American manufacture. At that stage, and all too late, the military had no choice but to confess that the *John Harvey* had indeed been carrying a massive cargo of mustard gas. The proportion of fatalities among those in the vicinity was far greater than from the clouds of gas that had enveloped the trenches in 1916, because of the enormous local concentrations in the air and especially in the oil films on the water's surface. Alexander established that the most conspicuous effect of the gas, apart from the skin lesions, was again the rapid destruction of the white blood cells, first the lymphocytes (essential elements of the immune system), and then all the other types, platelets (p.) and the rest. The potential that chemicals of this kind might have for the treatment of blood cancers could scarcely escape the notice of the few doctors who had not been excluded because of the stringent secrecy that continued to surround war gases. One of them was a powerful figure, Cornelius Rhoads, seconded to the Army Chemical Warfare Service as head of its medical division, from his position as director of the Memorial Hospital in New York**. Rhoads was impressed by what he read in Alexander's report on the Bari casualties, and threw his weight behind the proposal by Goodman and Gilman after the war for clinical trials on patients with white-cell cancers. The result was that in 1949 HN2, or mustin became the first synthetic anti-cancer drug to be approved in the U.S. for clinical use.

---

* Cornelius Packard Rhoads (1898-1959) was a pathologist specialising in cancer. In 1931 he became embroiled in a notorious controversy. That year he had travelled to Puerto Rico as member of a commission set up by the Rockefeller Foundation, a charity, to study the prevalence of anaemia in the population. One night he had emerged, apparently drunk, from a social function, and found that his car had been vandalised. Back in the laboratory he had written a letter addressed to a friend in Boston, which he incautiously left on his desk where it was seen by a technician, who made copies and sent them to the leader of the Puerto Rico nationalist parliamentary party. The substance of the letter was a denunciation of all things Puerto Rican, beginning: 'The Puerto Ricans are the dirtiest, laziest, most degenerate and thievish race of men ever to inhabit this sphere', and it concluded, 'What the island needs is not public health work but a tidal wave or something to totally exterminate the population. I have done my best to further the extermination by killing off eight and transplanting cancer cells into several more'. You might think that this could have been intended only as a rather tasteless joke, but the politician who received the copies did not waste the opportunity, and passed the rest to several newspapers and embassies, to the League of Nations, the Vatican, the Panamerican Union and the American Civil Liberties Union. The story was picked up by *Time* magazine, where it appeared under the title, 'Puerto Ricochet'. The Governor of the island had no option but to institute an inquiry, and the Rockefeller Foundation followed suit. Rhoads told them that it had indeed been meant as a private joke, written, he said, for his own diversion with no intention of actually posting it. The inquiries found no evidence that Rhoads had either killed anyone, or injected them with cancer cells. It was undoubtedly a joke, and nothing more was said about it when Rhoads returned to the Rockefeller Institute, where he had his laboratory. It did not impede his career, for in 1929 he was appointed director of the Memorial Hospital, and then the founding director of the Sloan-Kettering Cancer Center to which the hospital was attached. That year, 1949, he appeared again on the cover of *Time*, lauded for his achievements in cancer research. Yet from time to time after his death, the Puerto Rico episode has been rediscovered and disinterred for political effect, until finally in 2002, under pressure from the Puerto Rican government, the American Association of Cancer Research expunged Rhoads's name from the Cornelius P. Rhoads Scientific Achievement Award, which is now nameless.

When the outcome of the disseminated clinical trials was published, it set off a search by academic and industrial laboratories for new and better anti-cancer agents, though mainly based on variants of the original nitrogen mustards. The challenge was to find compounds with an enhanced capacity to penetrate into the tissues, combined with low general toxicity. From this intensive, though somewhat random search emerged several compounds which came into clinical use, with names like chlorambucil and melphalan. The best, synthesised in 1956 by chemists in a German company of modest size, ASTA-Werke in Bielefeld, was cyclophosphamide (trade names, Endoxan, Cytoxan amongst others). The decision had been taken taken by the ASTA management in 1952 to direct the bulk of the company's effort to the development of cancer drugs, and the head of pharmacological research, a doctor and chemist, Norbert Brock had settled on the plan to produce a prodrug (p.). Cyclophosphamide was indeed one of the first examples of such a compound actually designed as such.

A prodrug, also known as a 'latent drug', is a compound that is itself inactive, but is converted by an enzyme residing in the cancerous tissue to the active drug. This scheme has the advantage that the prodrug, which has intrinsically negligible chemical reactivity, and therefore (in principle at least) minimal toxicity against biological tissues generally, should be far less likely to evoke unpleasant side-effects. There would also be good hopes that the range of cancers against which it was found effective would be high. Brock and his colleagues decided that nitrogen mustards were ideal candidates for conversion into prodrugs, for it was clear what certain parts of the structure were essential for their action, and also that it should be a relatively simple matter to mask them chemically. The plan worked. The new compound proved highly effective against tumours in mice and rats. It was only later that its precise mode of action was established. The nitrogen mustard released *in situ* attacks not only the cell's DNA but also the enzyme that replicates the DNA. The initial expectation was that cyclophosphamide would be especially useful for the treatment of prostate cancer. But perversely, although it was found to be effective against many malignancies, prostate cancer was not one of them. Nor was cyclophosphamide entirely without side-effects, but it is still in use, and it also found an unexpected application in the treatment of rheumatic diseases. The success of cyclophosphamide set off a search for other masked nitrogen mustards, and for a wider range of prodrugs, of which many are now available.

Precious metal to precious drug

Platinum is a valuable metal because of its scarcity and its great chemical resistance. It is hard to oxidise and does not dissolve in acids other than aqua regia, the mixture of nitric and hydrochloric acids, so named by the alchemists for its ability to dissolve gold, the royal metal. Because of these attributes platinum, one of the group of elements referred to as the 'noble metals', finds many uses in the laboratory in situations that demand resistance to heat or corrosive substances. One such application is in electrodes, for in an electrolysis cell, in which an electric current passes between two electrodes, a positive (anode) and a negative (cathode), immersed in a salt solution, which conducts electricity, chemistry occurs at both electrodes. Hydrogen (H^+) ions (acid) are generated at one electrode, and hydroxyl (OH^-) ions (alkali) at the other. In addition the ions or other substances in the solution may undergo oxidation at the anode or the opposite – reduction – at the cathode.[*]

In 1964 a biophysicist at Michigan State University, Barnett Rosenberg was examining the effects of an electric current on the growth of bacteria. Accounts differ as to details, and particularly purpose behind the experiments, but they all agree that the result was a total surprise. According to some accounts, Rosenberg had been struck by the visual resemblance of a dividing chromosome to the outline created by iron filings clustering around the poles of a magnet, and had the wild notion that an electric current might interfere with the process in the cell. Rosenberg himself, writing many years after the event, remembered it differently: he cogitated that an electric current might well do something to DNA - which after all was a highly electrostatically charged structure, surrounded by a

---

[*] This is the basis of electroplatinmg, when for instance silver, the reduction product of a salt such as silver nitrate is deposited on an electrode consisting of the object to be plated.

cloud of ions of the opposite charge and to its function, during for instance the separation of the two strands of the double-helix. This was a rational enough conjecture, but in essence it was a simple matter of curiosity to see what would happen. Another version has it that Rosenberg's laboratory was engaged in the search for a quick, cheap and reliable method of sterilising clinical and laboratory equipment. All that would be needed, supposing that the electric current killed bacteria, would be to pass such a current through a salt solution in the vessel to be sterilised.

Whatever the reason, the upshot was momentous. The bacterium Rosenberg chose for his investigations was *Escherichia coli*, which lives in great abundance in the gut, and has been for many years the favoured experimental system for a limitless range of genetic and biochemical research. It is an undemanding organism, easy to grow, and far better understood than any other. Rosenberg's experiment was quite rudimentary. He could follow the rate of multiplication or the killing of the bacteria in a culture by observing the rise or fall in turbidity (haziness) when he applied an alternating voltage across two electrodes, each consisting of a platinum wire, which would resist the action of the corrosive electrode products. What the research assistant who was carrying out the experiments found was something unexpected and unprecedented: passage of a low alternating current through the culture did indeed alter the turbidity, but not in a manner indicative of cell destruction. On examining the *E. coli* in the culture suspension under the microscope she saw that they had aggregated in long chains of around 300 individuals. In the sense that all the aggregated bacteria had also stopped dividing, it appeared that the solution must be sterile.

This was sufficiently odd to heighten Rosenberg's curiosity, and drive him to continue the experiments. It seems to have been the technician, Loretta van Camp who first wondered whether it might not have been the platinum rather than the current that had stopped multiplication and brought about the formation of bacterial filaments. Perhaps, after all, the metal was not as resistant to the electrode products as everyone had supposed, and perhaps it had given rise to a minute amount of a platinum salt in the solution? To test this possibility the researchers added fresh bacteria to a culture that had been subjected to electrolysis before hand, and indeed the same phenomena resulted – cessation of growth and filament formation. Loretta van Camp could find only one platinum compound on the laboratory's reagent shelves, and when she dissolved a little of this in the culture medium the bacteria died without forming any filaments. But then luck smiled again: when the culture medium containing the dissolved platinum salt, a chloride in which the metal is in its tetravalent state (that is bonded to four other atoms, all of them in this case chlorine) was left standing on the laboratory bench in bright light it was slowly converted by a photochemical (that is, light-induced) reaction into a compound in which the metal is divalent (linked to only two chlorine atoms). The *E. coli* in this solution formed a fine crop of filaments.

Rosenberg now sought help from the chemists, who provided him with samples of a range of platinum compounds. Most were active. One that was later found stable and highly potent in its bacteriostatic effect is properly called *cis*-diamminedichloroplatinum (II), but it is now famous in the cancer clinic as cisplatin. This compound had in fact been synthesised in 1844 by an Italian chemist, Michele Peyrone, and was known as Peyrone's salt. (Its formula was not determined until 1893 by one of the great inorganic chemists, the German, Alfred Werner.). Rosenberg's persistence was to pay off abundantly, for it also struck him that what his compounds did to bacteria they might conceivably do to other rapidly dividing cells, that is to say tumours. He approached the National Cancer Institute in Bethesda, and both cell-culture and animal tests demonstrated an astonishing anti-tumour activity. It cured mice with lethal tumours within two weeks, and the response of human patients was deemed highly encouraging. It was nevertheless eighteen years before, in 1979, the FDA gave cisplatin its full approval, although it had come into clinical use in the early 1970s for the treatment of a number of cancers. Cisplatin was found especially effective against the deadliest of malignancies, ovarian and testicular cancers, and is still a front-line therapy. The unpredictable result of Barnett Rosenberg's curiosity has saved untold thousands of lives, a lesson to the funding agencies, who increasingly direct their support to what is now called 'translational' (meaning applied) research, at the expense of the merely curiosity-inspired. Since that time a number of variants, such as carboplatin and oxaliplatin, have been developed in the hope of minimising side-effects, mainly kidney damage. This can fortunately be much reduced by flushing the patient through with large volumes of water, so that lingering residues of drug are eliminated in the urine.

A curious circumstance arose at about the time that cisplatin was discovered. A series of compounds, all closely related, were rationally designed by researchers at the Imperial Cancer Research Fund Laboratories in London to contain a metal atom. These, it was hoped would inhibit the action of an enzyme thought to be involved in tumour formation. All were inactive save one, and that one turned out to be the only member of the series that did not retain the metal atom. The reason was that a reaction which formed part of the synthesis had behaved anomalously and given an unforeseen product. This compound became the lead for a useful drug, used in treating a form of leukaemia and some other cancers. It was called rasoxane, or Razoxin, and appears to be still in occasional use.

Hormone, sex and breast

Following the discoveries by Laqueur, Butenandt and others (Chapter), interest awoke, after a long period of stasis, in the relation of hormones to cancer. There were some encouraging results from attempts to treat enlarged prostate glands with female hormones. Charles Brenton Huggins (1901-1997) was a Canadian urinogenital surgeon working at the University of Chicago. His chief interest was research, particularly into the function of the prostate. In the course of his investigations he made an accidental discovery. It occurred while he was examining the effects of testosterone on prostate secretions in castrated dogs. Like us, dogs often develop prostate cancer in old age, and what Huggins observed was that such tumours shrank following castration, whether by the knife or chemically induced by diethylstilboestrol (p.), the synthetic analogue of the female sex hormone, oestrone. In 1941, after more animal experiments, Huggins tried the hormone on patients with advanced prostate cancers. The results were strikingly successful, with tumour regression and relief of symptoms. Castration by whatever means immediately became the preferred method of treating advanced prostate cancer. For this work Huggins received the Nobel Prize in 1966.

Huggins's success led to a search for hormonal therapies of other cancers, and diethylstilboestrol was found to be effective in some cases of breast cancer. The sketchy evidence that certain cancers appeared to be hormone-dependent was to have important therapeutic repercussions. As early as 1896 George Beatson, a surgeon in Glasgow had noticed that women with breast cancer whose ovaries he had extirpated experienced shrinkage of their tumours. This seems to have attracted little attention, but Huggins a half-century later, made a similar observation - that surgical removal of the adrenal glands (p.), which control the release of the sex hormones, also retarded the growth of breast tumours. It took a further two decades before the first really satisfactory drug against breast cancer, free from unsupportable side-effects, became available to oncologists. It worked by blocking the access of oestrogen to its target, and it came about – yet again - quite fortuitously. At the beginning of the 1950s, when steroid chemists were busy synthesising oestrogen analogues, the vision of huge profits appeared before the eyes of some pharmaceutical companies, in the form of a morning-after contraceptive pill. At the ICI laboratories at Alderley Park in the north of England the division of reproductive research was led by a respected endocrinologist, Arthur Walpole. By this time the existence of receptors for biochemical 'messengers' was an accepted fact, and the plan was to find a compound that would compete with the natural substance, oestrogen, by binding with greater avidity to its receptor. It would be in effect a key that fitted into the lock but would not turn it, and would thus obstruct the entry of the real working key. Many compounds were screened for anti-oestrogen activity, until one, synthesised by Walpole's chemist colleague, Dora Richardson, designated ICI 46,474, was found to have an unexpected and interesting property: tested in mice, it acted as an oestrogen – it turned the key. Might it not in that case be put to the opposite use to that for which it had been designed? Could it be developed as a fertility pill instead of a contraceptive? But then it was tested in rats, and the result was once more the inverse: it prevented ovulation. How then would it perform in humans?

At this stage ICI applied for a patent with broad scope: Walpole knew about the effects of some oestrogen antagonists on certain cancers, so the new compound might not only control the hormonal state in humans and animals, it might also prove effective in the treatment of tumours, especially of the breast[*], and (an additional onion in the stew) might reduce high cholesterol levels. The patent was approved (though not in the U.S., where another twenty years would pass before the FDA gave the drug the green light. Walpole initiated assays for anti-tumour activity, which gave positive, though less than dramatic results. The most encouraging aspect up to this point was that ICI 46,474 had no discernible side-effects, a most unusual attribute. By now it was 1972, and clinical trials on women with advanced breast cancer were finally arranged at two cancer hospitals. The results were again positive, but only moderately so. Thereupon the ICI management decided to abandon the project. Walpole objected and threatened that if he were prevented from continuing the work he would take early retirement.

There was evidently an uneasy accommodation. In the face of a reluctant management Walpole enlisted the help of a pharmacologist, Craig Jordan, on whose Ph.D. thesis he had been an examiner, and who was now working in the U.S. Jordan managed to isolate the oestrogen receptor and he showed that ICI 46,474, now given the name, tamoxifen, bound avidly to it. Most important was the discovery that only one class of breast cancers were oestrogen-dependent, namely the 70% or so in which oestrogen receptors are generated in the breast. In the remainder of cases tamoxifen is ineffective, which accounted for the ambiguous trial results. Clinical studies to define suitable patients, the best drug regimes and the advantages of simultaneously giving other drugs, made tamoxifen the most valuable known weapon against breast cancer of its time. It was later found to be a prodrug, converted in the cell to a hydroxylated (that is a hydroxyl-, or –OH-containing) active form. Unlike nearly all cancer drugs,

---

[*] Cancers commonly have many of the characteristics of the tissues in which they reside. Breast cancers are an example. Hormones are messenger molecules that switch metabolic processes on or off when they bind to their receptors. A hormone therefore migrates to locations rich in receptors, which recognise and take up that hormone, for where there are no receptors there is nothing to detain the hormone. Oestrogen is no exception. It has (in most women) receptors in the breast, and so also does a breast tumour. When an oestrogen molecule binds to a receptor it delivers the message for the cell to divide, and so oestrogen will cause a breast tumour to undergo cell division and growth.

tamoxifen does not destroy the malignant cells. Instead it prevents them from dividing – in effect paralyses them. It is therefore called an oncostatic. It has no toxicity, but in blocking the access of oestrogen to its receptors it engenders menopausal appearances, while paradoxically at the same time exerting its other effect of enhancing fertility. For all that, tamoxifen has saved thousands of lives and is still one of the most extensively used drugs. Because of its lack of toxicity it can be taken for years and is even used prophylactically by women at the highest risk of developing breast cancer. Several related compounds are also in use. Tamoxifen is often described as the first 'targeted' drug, that is to say designed to home onto a defined target, in this case the oestrogen receptor. Targeted therapy, made possible by an increasingly comprehensive understanding of the function of cells, is today a central feature of drug development.

By the time tamoxifen, under a variety of trade names, had come into common use, another important fact had come to light. The existence of a ubiquitous enzyme, aromatase was inferred from evidence, accumulated over two decades, that the male hormone, androgen is converted in the adrenals and elsewhere into the female oestrogen. Steroid chemists managed to produce preparations of increasing quality of aromatase in the mid-1970s. Knowing now the structural change that the enzyme catalysed in generating the female from the male hormone, chemists could embark on the rational, structure-based design of inhibitors of the enzyme, and to test them on the steroid preparations. Several compounds were found to work, and were assayed for toxicity and therapeutic effect. The resulting drugs are now among the most important in the armoury, but their value extends only to breast cancers in postmenopausal women. The reason is that before the menopause the primary sources of oestrogen are the ovaries, whereas after the menopause this shifts to the breast and other (including fatty) tissues. So in the older population there is no aromatase in the breast to be inhibited. Aromatase inhibitors are now used in conjunction with tamoxifen and its relatives (notably raloxifene (Evista), which has even fewer uncomfortableeffects, and is given to women whose menopause is behind them˙). The outcome of all the laborious research is that a large proportion of breast cancers are now curable.

Marmite and other drugs: new directions

In 1930 a remarkable English doctor, Lucy Wills travelled to India at the request of another redoubtable woman, the head of the Indian Medical Service, Dr Margaret Balfour. The problem Lucy Wills, at the time a pathologist at the Royal Free Hospital in London, was being asked to investigate was the incidence of severe anaemia among pregnant women working in textile factories. Seven years before there had been a landmark discovery in the study of anaemias. The cause of pernicious anaemia had been uncovered as a result of the curious tastes of a patient in Boston and the persistence of his doctor, William Murphy. A diagnosis of pernicious anaemia was invariably a sentence of death, when Dr Murphy, who ministered to the Irish community in the city, discovered that one of his patients, who should have been dead, was hanging on. Murphy questioned the man about his lifestyle and dietary habits, and learned that he was very fond of liver. Murphy tried a liver diet on other of his patients with pernicious anaemia, but with no effect, so he returned to question the original patient further, and elicited the additional information that the man had a curious addiction: he liked the liver raw. This was the key to the treatment of the disease. Murphy forced raw liver on his patients and cured them. He then approached a Gorge Minot, a doctor at Harvard Medical School for help, and together they extended the observations and prepared a highly active liver extract, which infallibly cured the disease. Murphy and Minot presented their results at a conference in 1926 to

---

˙ Raloxifene likewise acts on oestrogen receptors. It is one of the class of drugs, of which tamoxifen is the archetype, that now go under the American name of selective (o)estrogen receptor modulators (SERMs), recommended only for women post-menopause. Besides diminishing the incidence of breast and uterine cancer in such women, it acts on bone, and retards osteoporosis. It was approved by the FDA for this purpose in 2006, and is now widely used in many countries. A general problem in the development of drugs of this kind is that the oestrogen receptors in these tissues differ subtly from each other and from those in the breast. And so a single compound will not generally serve for all purposes.

general astonishment and acclaim The outcome of their work was the discovery of vitamin B_{12}, and in 1934 a well-deserved Nobel Prize, shared by both men and George Whipple, a professor at Johns Hopkins University in Baltimore, who had found that dogs, rendered anaemic by bleeding, recovered if fed a diet of red meat or, best of all, liver.

Lucy Wills knew about pernicious anaemia, and it was clear to her that it was not the disease afflicting the textile workers; nonetheless, the liver diet had to be tried as the first step. It worked to a small yet undeniable degree, but an extract that would have contained the active substance (vitamin B_{12}) in sufficient amount and more, was inert. Lucy Wills proceeded to search for other sources of nutrients, which might contain whatever it was that, as she surmised, was vestigially present in liver. What she found was Marmite. Marmite, for those who don't know it, is a thick dark brown pungent yeast extract, familiar only to the British. It is cheap, and was the solution to the problem – the cause and cure of Wills anaemia as it came to be called - of the Indian women. Lucy Wills knew that she had discovered a new vitamin, and went on to prepare enriched extracts. She proved that a dearth led to anaemia in rats, which was quickly cured by her extracts. It was to be another ten years before chemists at the Lederle Laboratories in America isolated the pure vitamin – folic acid – from spinach leaves, and determine its structure. Folate deficiency is the commonest nutritional disorder, and the cause of neurological damage in the foetuses of mothers suffering from it. Folic acid or its salt, sodium folate, is now added in trace amounts to bread. It plays an essential part, as we now know, in the synthesis of the nitrogenous bases that make up the structure of DNA, whence the connection to cancer, first made in 1941.

Richard Lewisohn (1875-1964) was a German surgeon, who emigrated to the United States just before the Great War, and passed his career at the Mt. Sinai Hospital in New York. His most famous contribution to research was to develop an anticoagulant that allowed blood banks for the fist time to store blood for weeks, rather than days. On reaching the age of retirement for surgeons Lewisohn set off in a new direction: he set up a cancer research laboratory, and with a small group of assistants he began a search for anti-tumour agents. He had apparently been struck by the rarity of cancers in the spleen, and had fallen to wondering whether something in the tissue had a protective influence. He found that an extract of mouse spleens indeed caused marked retardation of tumour growth when injected into tumour-bearing mice. But the volumes of curative extracts that could be collected were far too small for extensive trials, much less for any hope of isolating an active constituent, and so Lewisohn decided to conduct a survey of natural metabolic substances that might be involved growth. This was probably the beginning of the quest for a metabolic therapy of cancers. Lewisohn and his group began with the B family of water-soluble vitamins, and in 1941 seemed to have struck gold with a yeast extract, which caused regressions of a sarcoma and a breast cancer in a sizeable proportion of the thousands of sick mice. Barley seed extracts proved comparably effective. This was promising enough to require independent confirmation, which Lewisohn entrusted to a research group at the Memorial Hospital, two miles downtown. Their results, using their own extracts, were uniformly negative. There was no obvious explanation, and the resulting consternation can be imagined. Lewisohn kept trying. He conjectured that the constituent in the yeast and barley, which had worked for him, was folic acid, and so he turned to the Lederle Laboratories for help.

Lederle's lead in this area of research was due to one man, a doctor and highly accomplished organic chemist, Yellapragada SubbaRow (1895-1948). SubbaRow was born into an impoverished Brahmin family in Madras (Chennai), had studied at the medical school in the city, and then, for want of anything better, had taught at a college of Ayurvedic medicine. In 1922 he had taken the hopeful step of migrating to Boston in the hope of finding a research position. This proved remarkably difficult in the temper of the time, but SubbaRow did finally locate a laboratory that would accept him as a Ph.D. student. For survival he relied on a meagre income from work as a night porter at one of the Harvard hospitals. SubbaRow quickly put his stamp on biochemistry by devising a sensitive method for determining phosphorus concentrations in biological tissues, which bears his name and still has a place in the textbooks. Diffident and retiring, SubbaRow made little attempt to promote his work, and others accordingly took most of the credit, including his first research supervisor.

George Hitchings (p.) wrote that SubbaRow had published so little of his work that it was only years later that much of it was rediscovered by others. He managed to secure a toehold on the academic ladder as an assistant professor, but the turning-point in his fortunes came when he joined Lederle as head of research. Very soon a stream of important research in a surprising number of therapeutic areas began to flow from his initiatives. The purification of folic acid in 1944 was one, followed by the determination of its structure and the synthesis of a series of important derivatives.

But the course of discovery did not run smooth. Folic acid was difficult to produced in sufficient amounts from the known sources, and the Lederle team, searching for something better, thought they had found it in a growth factor of milk bacteria. *Lactobacillus casei* could be grown in bulk, and the factor was identified as folic acid. A sample was sent to Lewisohn, and assays in tumour-bearing mice were wholly gratifying: folic acid appeared to cure cancer, or at least cause the regression of tumours. Yet this was all counter-intuitive all along, for if folic acid was required for cell division, then why would it inhibit tumour growth, which after all was a matter of the acceleration of that very process? Nevertheless, Lederle, now in possession of the folic acid structure, set about making derivatives in the hope as usual of finding some that worked even better than the parent compound. Then SubbaRow and his assistants found the answer to the paradox: the bacterial product was not folic acid, but a derivative, and this same derivative was present as an impurity in all the genuine folic acid preparations. It was, moreover, an antagonist of folic acid, which bound strongly to the folic acid receptor in the tumour cells, and prevented the folic acid from exerting its growth-inducing activity.

The discovery came too late to avert a near-calamity, for in 1946 a paediatric oncologist at the Children's Hospital in Boston, one of the famous clinical institutions associated with Harvard University, had also conceived the idea of trying the action of folic acid on cancers. He was Sidney Farber (1903-1973), trained as a pathologist, but obsessively dedicated by then to the treatment of children with leukaemias – much the most common cancers of early childhood, and one he found so harrowing to cope with. Farber was an imperious figure, elegant and courtly, but with an unwavering sense of mission. It was he who, with the support of the Variety Club of New England, a fraternity of performing artists devoted to charitable works, raised funds for the establishment of the Children's Cancer Research Foundation. Farber and the President of the Variety Club plucked the heartstrings of the local population by an emotional television and radio campaign, with a winsome boy representing the dying children (for they had at that time little hope of a lasting cure). The stars of the local baseball team played their part, and were shown visiting Jimmy, as he was re-christened for the purpose, for Farber was ever scrupulous in protecting his patients' privacy. (Jimmy's real name, Einar Gustavson, emerged only forty years later, when he reappeared, a truck driver in his early sixties). Thus, and with further stout help from the philanthropist, Mary Lasker, was the Jimmy Fund brought into existence, and indissolubly linked with the name of Doctor Farber, venerated as the saviour of the children in Boston and far beyond.

But in 1946 Farber was still an almost unknown pathologist with a vocation. He was aware of the seemingly successful results with folic acid in mice, and had decided to try it on children with acute leukaemia for whom little else could be done. He had made the acquaintance of SubbaRow, when the reticent Indian was working at the Children's Hospital, and now approached him at the Lederle Laboratories for samples of folic acid and its analogues. The first dose was given to a single young girl, and then a small group of other children were injected. The result was a swift acceleration of the leukaemic symptoms, with an almost instant and steep rise in the production of white blood cells. Farber feared that he had killed his patients, but desperate measures eventually brought them all back from the brink. The doctors on the governing body of the Children's Hospital were infuriated by what they regarded as Farber's reckless experiment on patients, and issued a severe reprimand. If folic acid actually stimulated the production of white cells, then perhaps what was wanted was a folic acid antagonist. The concept of antagonists in the form of derivatives or analogues of the agent itself, which would block its access to its site of action, was then in the air. It had been ventilated in 1946 in a long review paper by an American pharmaceutical chemist,

Richard Roblin. In this remarkably prescient discourse he envisaged a receptor to which the antagonist – a term he seems in this context to have introduced – would bind tightly to the receptor without activating the normal consequences (the' jammed lock' concept, referred to above [p.]). Farber knew SubbaRow, and learned of the latest discoveries at Lederle, in particular that the bacterial product, which had been taken for folic acid, contained an antagonistic derivative. Folic acid belongs to a class of compounds called pterins; it is pteroylglutamic acid (a pterin nucleus coupled to glutamic acid, one of the twenty amino acids of which proteins are made), whereas the bacterial product was pteroyltriglutamic acid – a pterin nucleus with three glutamic acids attached.

Farber begged a sample of this teropterin, as it was now called, synthesised by SubbaRow, along with the pteroyldiglutamic acid, or diopterin, with two glutamic acids, and tried it on his children. It had no effect, but at least did not aggravate the disease. The Lederle chemists pressed on, and in 1947 prepared a version of folic acid containing an amino ($-NH_2$) group. This aminopterin was the breakthrough: when Farber gave it to his children their white cell count fell to practically normal levels. Two years later another derivative, amethopterin, with an additional methyl ($-CH_3$) group, followed. It had lower toxicity and similar activity. Called methotrexate, it became the primary drug of choice for the treatment of leukaemias. The problem was that if even a few abnormal white cells remained the leukaemia would reassert itself, and Farber insisted on lengthy courses of treatment, which were hard on the patients, but some at least were cured. The search for better metabolic agents to combat leukaemias was now in full spate. Farber had approached other laboratories for new compounds that he could try. One was that of Selman Waksman (p.), for Farber felt that antibiotics too should be tested against cancers, and indeed actinomycins from various strains of bacteria had been found to reduce tumours in mice. Many of these preparations were mixtures, but one of Waksman's strains produced a pure compound, which he called actinomycin D. This had astonishingly high anti-cancer activity in mice, and Farber immediately began a trial in leukaemic children. It had no effect at all, and was abandoned. The disappointment was great, but was mitigated by results on other cancers: Wilms tumour of the kidney, most often found in children, responded dramatically. Previously fatal, it is now treatable with actinomycin D (also called dactinomycin), combined with radiation. Here then was yet another highly beneficial chance discovery. But Farber's disappointing experience with actinomycin D had a second happy consequence, indicating once again the truth of the dictum that id you do nothing, nothing will happen, while if you do something, something will happen, but not what you expected; for the failure of the drug to act in leukaemia stimulated a search for further *Streptomycin* compounds that might do better. A species of *Streptomycin* examined in an industrial laboratory in Milan produced several active molecules, especially doxorubicin, given the trade name, Adriamycin. This has excellent activity against a range of cancers, and occupies an important place in chemotherapeutic arsenal, but it is highly toxic, most of all against the heart, and is used cautiously, and in combination with other agents.

Cancer can arise from a spontaneous mutation, by damage to the cell's DNA by radiation, such as X-rays, by damage to the DNA or the metabolic machinery by a chemical (a carcinogen), or it can be caused by one of many species of virus. But viruses can also help a tissue mount a defence against cancer. This phenomenon was first observed by two Japanese workers, Yasu-ichi Nagano and Yasuhiko Kojima, at the University of Tokyo. Their results were published in French in a rather obscure journal in 1954, and attracted little attention. Alick Isaacs, a South-African, and Jean Lindenmann, a Swiss, virologists at the National Institute for Medical Research in London, were unaware of that work when they published similar, but more comprehensive observations in 1957. What they found was that influenza virus, rendered inactive by heating, suppressed the multiplication of active influenza virus in a tissue (in their case the thin layer of cells under the shell of a chicken egg). The development of the infection was interrupted, Isaacs and Lindenmann discovered, by a protein secreted by the cells. They called it *interferon*. We now know that there are actually a number of interferons, and that they can oppose the spread through the body of many pathological intruders – not only viruses, but also bacteria, parasites and cancer cells. The interferons are actually glycoproteins – proteins with attached sugar groups - which are formed and excreted by a dying infected cell. They bind to the surfaces of surrounding cells and set in motion a highly complex series of events in the cells' interiors, all inimical to a takeover by the pathogen. Interferons also stimulate the action of certain components of the immune system, which then mount a further attack on the intruders. The discovery caused no little excitement and generated high expectations of a long-sought treatment for viral diseases, but the hopes were only partly fulfilled. In the first place, producing an interferon by isolation from a cell culture is costly and inefficient. It was only in 1980 that an interferon gene was successfully cloned, so that the protein could be made in bulk from the gene introduced into a bacterium. But the interferons are not highly effective against every kind of parasitic cell, but they were found useful for controlling infections by hepatitis viruses. Nevertheless, interferons are widely used in cancer therapy, though only for a limited range of tumours against which they are effective, and generally in combinations with other anti-cancer agents.

Mutation of cancers: combination therapies

The Lederle chemists were not the only seekers after an anti-folate drug. At Burroughs Wellcome in Tuckahoe, not far from New York City, George Hitchings and his group (p.) were thinking along similar lines, and it was Elvira Falco who in 1947 synthesised a chlorine-containing folic acid analogue. When tested by the oncologists at the Sloan-Kettering Institute, it displayed strong inhibitory activity against folic acid, and started another drive for new therapeutic anti-folates. It was also at Burroughs Wellcome that Gertrude Elion put forward the principle of combination therapy. It was based on the dispiriting observation that all the known anti-cancer agents brought about remissions but seldom cures, for too often the cancer returned after an interval, and this time it responded less well to the drug that had caused the remission. At this stage there was little more that doctors could do. What could be the basis of this universal phenomenon? What rendered a tumour progressively less susceptible to a seemingly effective drug? The analogy to antibiotic resistance of bacteria (p.) was not slow to suggest itself. If, like bacteria, rapidly dividing cancer cells are subject to occasional random mutation, then a large population of such cells will eventually generate one or two that are resistant to the drug.

These will multiply undisturbed by the drug when all the original drug-sensitive cells have been killed.** The eventual development of resistance against a new drug is guaranteed. But suppose now that the oncologist has two drugs capable of killing the cells of a given tumour, but with different targets in those cells. If, for illustration, that there is one resistant cell in one billion. It will remain after the course of chemotherapy is finished, and will suffice to regenerate the tumour, but now in resistant form. But if the second drug, with comparable efficacy, is given at the same time, the probability that there will be a doubly-mutated cell, resistant to both drugs becomes one in a billion billion - effectively zero. This is the principle of combination therapy, just as applied in the treatment of infections by antibiotics (p.). Put another way, it is unlikely that a particular strain of malignant cells, resistant to a drug, will also be resistant to a different drug with a quite different mode of action in the cell, and therefore the more drugs, each with a different target, are given to the patient the less likely it becomes that any viable mutant cancer cells will remain.

That, at all events, is the theory. The greatest snag is that each drug has its own range of side-effects, and the combination may therefore be devastating to an already weak patient. Sidney Farber, the doyen of paediatric cancer, and especially leukaemia specialists, refused to inflict such suffering on his patients. His strategy was to use more than one drug, but to use them serially. Meanwhile, he made clear, the search for the single ideal drug must continue. The consequence was that most of his patients gained a period of healthy life, but then in most cases the

---

* Mutations, it should be noted, can occur spontaneously, without the intervention of a mutagenic chemical or radiation. They result from the occasional glitch in the mechanism of copying of the cell's DNA. Now, only a small proportions of the human genome – our total DNA – consists of genes or elements active in controlling those genes. Therefore most mutations will have no effect at all. But if the mutation is in a gene the result will most often be the conversion of one base in the DNA into another, and therefore in general replacement of the corresponding amino acid in the protein that the gene specifies by a different amino acid. Often the protein will tolerate the substitution, and mutation will again be harmless. But if it strikes in a vital part of the protein structure such an outcome is less likely. If then that protein is an enzyme for example and the substitution changes the specificity of its action, this could be enough to allow the cell to evade the attention of the anti-cancer drug.

cancer returned, the second time fatally. In the mid-1950s two doctors, recently arrived at the National Cancer Institute in Bethesda, resolved to deal with the problems of combination therapy. Their names were Emil Frei and Emil Freireich*, and the patients were children with leukaemia, mainly the deadly AAL, or acute lymphoblastic leukaemia. Around that time new drugs were becoming available. The most interesting were two related plant products derived from the roots and leaves of a flower, the Madagascar periwinkle, *Vinca rosea*, later, at the whim of the botanist, renamed *Vinca catharanthus*. The periwinkle had been used in the folk medicine of tropical countries for centuries for the treatment of various afflictions, including diabetes (against which it would have been largely, if not wholly ineffective). In the early 1950s a Canadian doctor, Clark Noble was told by a patient from Jamaica of the matchless anti-diabetic properties of an infusion of the periwinkle leaves, and was presented with a handful of the leaves in an envelope., to whom he passed the sample. Noble knew about diabetes. He had been a prominent member of the team in Toronto that discovered insulin, but he had retired from research, and was in no position to undertake an investigation. He did however have a brother, Robert, an endocrinologist at the University of Western Ontario, to whom he passed the sample.

Robert Noble looked at the effect of an extract on blood sugar levels in rats, and saw no change. It remained unchanged when the extract was injected into the peritoneum (the body cavity), but after a time the animals died of what proved to be infections. Noble investigated further and found that the rats were almost devoid of white blood cells and therefore of immunological resistance to bacteria. This was interesting enough to merit further study, and Noble and a chemical colleague, Charles Beer isolated the active principle, later given the name, vinblastine, which they asked an oncologist in the local cancer institute to test on rodents with leukaemia. The result was dramatic: the animals were cured. The first human trials took place in a hospital in Toronto, with equally gratifying results. But in the interim Noble and Beer had presented their data at a meeting in

---

* Freireich recalled his displeasure when, on arriving in Bethesda to take up his new appointment, he found that his name on the name-plate on the door of his office had been carelessly truncated, and read, Dr Emil Frei.

New York, and there discovered that a group of workers at Eli Lilley, led by Gordon Svoboda had been proceeding along exactly the same limes, and had simultaneously arrived at the same conclusion. They had indeed found that their preparations caused regression of leukaemia and several solid tumours in rodents. It was adopted for human use under the name of Velban. Further investigation of the vinca root turned up a huge range of different alkaloids, and out of this cornucopia the Eli Lilley chemists isolated one with a structure differing only slightly from that of vinblastine. Its activity against leukaemia was also similar, but more powerful. It was given the name, vincristine.

We now know that the two vinca alkaloids work by preventing cell division (mitosis). They do this by disabling a protein that forms a component of the machinery (the mitotic spindle), which pulls the two progeny cells apart. The drugs therefore fall into the class of 'spindle poisons', and are both fearsomely toxic, so have to be used with caution. A few years after their discovery another spindle poison – this time not an alkaloid - came to light. It came from the roots of a common American plant, the May apple tree. An infusion was used by the North American Indians as a purgative, and was taken up by physicians in parts of the country during the early 19th century. The extract was caustic and highly irritating, and found another use in burning off warts. It was a doctor in Ohio who made an active preparation and sent to the nascent William Merrell company in Cincinnati. Merrell sold it as a cure for warts from the mid-19th century. Because warts were (incorrectly) regarded as skin tumours, the active ingredient, called podophyllotoxin, from the Latin name of the tree, was tried by dermatologists, with some success, as a remedy for skin cancers. Derivatives, developed later to eliminate the irritant properties, are now used.

Another anti-cancer drug arrived from a quite different direction. In 1943, it may be recalled, Kendall had injected tumour-bearing mice with large doses of cortisone (p.), and had recorded some regression of the tumours. Others had obtained similar results, and Sidney Farber had seen transient remission of leukaemia in children given steroids of one sort or another, but especially the pituitary hormone, ACTH (p.). In 1950 a chemist, Arthur Nobile at the U.S. branch of the Schering company had created a derivative of cortisone with better activity than the parent compound; prednisone was in fact no more than cortisone deprived of two hydrogen atoms, but it took Nobile another four years to hit on a commercially viable way to prepare the substance – by exposing the cortisone to a culture of a bacterium capable of effecting the required oxidation. It was later discovered that prednisone was a prodrug, which was converted in the liver to prednisolone. Prednisolone thereupon supplanted prednisone for therapeutic use. Both caused regression, as ever transient, of leukaemia and other cancers.

There was yet another drug, one of a quite different nature, which had largely fallen into disuse, but was resurrected when combination therapy came into its own. Asparaginase is an enzyme that digests the amino acid – one of the twenty that go to make up proteins – asparagine. The anti-cancer effect of asparaginase had once again been discovered by pure accident. In 1953 an endocrinologist at New York Hospital by the name of John Kidd was studying the effects of blood serum (the transparent liquid in which the blood cells are bathed) on lymphoid tumours (malignancies of the immune system arising in the lymph nodes) in mice, and found that their growth was strongly inhibited by guinea pig serum. Why he tried a variety of sera is unclear, but in any case, neither rabbit nor horse serum had any effect on the tumours. This led Kidd to a search for information about the composition of the sera of different animals, which for the most part are all very similar. He found a work from 1922, which had recorded that guinea pig serum alone of all the many surveyed contained asparaginase. Why it is only the guinea pig that finds a use for asparaginase in its blood is a mystery, but Kidd inferred, quite correctly as it turned out, that asparaginase must be the constituent of the animal's serum responsible for the tumour regression. Now asparagine is one of the so-called non-essential amino acid, which means that we do not need to take it in with our food because (by contrast with the essential amino acids) we synthesise our own. But the tumour cells, Kidd further determined, have lost the ability to make their own asparagine, and this is their Achilles' heel, for if they are not supplied with asparagine they make no protein and die. They get their asparagine from the blood, but if it contains asparaginase the supply is destroyed. Treatment of leukaemias with asparaginase did indeed cause regression, and the usual optimism. Asparagine could be derived from certain bacteria, which were easily cultured, but because of its relatively low activity, the transience of its efficacy, and as ever, side-effects, it soon fell out of favour, until reintroduced as a component in the combination formula.

Let's return now to the National Cancer Institute and to Freireich and Frei, grappling with the intractable problems of how to treat children with ALL. Committed to combination therapy, they assimilated vincristine into their collection of anti-leukaemic agents, and also prednisolone and asparaginase. The first combination Frei and Freirich tried was methotrexate (also called amethopterin) with 6-mercaptopurine, and to these they then added vincristine and prednisone. The mixture went under the acronym of VAMP. Each of these four substances alone would have been enough to tax the weakened constitution of a gravely sick child, if not to fell an ox. Certainly the majority of paediatric cancer specialists denounced the proposed treatment as insane, if not positively criminal, and the consortium of oncologists that Frei and Freireich had themselves brought into being refused to approve it. It was indeed a hazardous course, and for two years it teetered on a knife-edge between triumph and catastrophe. The distinguished haematologist, David Nathan, who was then a junior doctor recruited to the study, has described in an absorbing book, *The Cancer Treatment Revolution* the hideous effects of the drugs on the young patients, and the debates that surrounded the treatment. He found dealing with the children under the combination regime too harrowing, and asked to be released from the study. After the first treatments the condition of the children worsened and they appeared close to death, as their bone marrow, their gut and their nervous systems were progressively poisoned. But just when all seemed lost a gradual recovery began, normal white cell precursors reappeared in the bone marrow, the leukaemia cells vanished, and some at least of the children seemed to have been fully cured. There was exultation as those children were discharged. Frei and Freireich pressed on, adding another two drugs to the combination. One was asparaginase, the other cytosine arabinoside (Cytosar), synthesised by chemists at the University of California in Berkeley, is another derivative of one of the four DNA bases, following the principle devised by Gertrude Elion and George Hitchings (p.),.

The cures turned into yet another mirage. Just as the principle of combination therapy was gaining acceptance, and the sceptics were beginning to waver, the patients' symptoms returned, and this time there was no remission when the treatment was repeated. There was renewed condemnation of combination therapy and its perpetrators, and cries of 'I told you so'. Frei and Freireich discovered the reason for the recurrence, and it was shocking: the cerebrospinal fluid, the liquid that fills the centre of the spinal cord and the hollows of the brain, was seething with leukaemia cells. They had somehow penetrated the blood-brain barrier, which isolates the brain from the circulation. The idea that a few cancer cells may lie concealed in some bodily crevice after an apparently rigorous treatment has eliminated all that can be seen had in fact been aired by a colleague of Frei and Freireich's at the National Cancer Institute. Min Chiu Li was a Chinese physician who had arrived in the U.S. in 1947, and been marooned there by the revolution in his home country. Li was a notoriously contentious character, with a short temper and an annoying habit of being right. He discovered among other things a marker for a cancer of pregnant women, choriocarcinoma. The tumour arises in the placenta, metastisises very rapidly, and quickly kills. The marker was a peptide hormone (p.), chorionic gonadotropin in the urine. Li showed first that choriocarcinoma responds very well to methotrexate, although in advanced cases a combination therapy is needed. But the revolutionary discovery was the persistence of gonadotropin in the urine in many instances after an apparently total elimination of tumour cells. Li inferred that cryptic tumour cells still lurked somewhere undetected, and would cause the cancer to erupt once more. He therefore continued giving his patients high doses of chemotherapy until there was no more of the marker in the urine. For insisting on this apparently unnecessary procedure, with its unpleasant and dangerous side-effects, Li attracted much opprobrium, but he was proved correct, and choriocarcinoma became the first great and indisputable victory for cancer chemotherapy.

Freireich and Frei took heart from Li's discovery, but theirs was a harder nut to crack, for there were no drugs that would cross the blood-brain barrier. They therefore saw no option but to use radiation therapy to target the leukaemia cells in the children's brains, and even advocated prophylactic radiation along with the combination therapy. This again roused the ire of paediatricians and oncologists, but it did greatly reduce the recurrence of the leukaemia, and an increasing number of children, and later adults, were fully cured. And so combination therapy became the new orthodoxy. And yet there were some conscientious doctors who would not countenance it, the most prominent of whom was Sidney Farber. Farber remained unwilling to subject his patients to such pain and stress. David Nathan, by then head of haematology at the Children's Hospital in Boston, felt he must confront Farber, and he has given a memorable account in his book of the encounter, and of the great man's dreadful wrath when Nathan told him that he would no longer refer children with leukaemia to Farber at the Jimmy Fund. Farber died soon after, having in effect recommended the arch-proponent of combination therapy, Emil Frei to succeed him. It was a poignant confession that he, Farber, had been wrong, but could still not bring himself to inflict the inescapable suffering on his children. As time went on new, more effective and somewhat less toxic reagents were developed, treatment regimes were refined, and means were found of mitigating the distress caused to the patients, who are now more likely than not to return to the world cured.

The principle of combination therapy was of course soon applied to most other cancers, besides childhood leukaemias. Breast cancers, for example, were treated before the advent of tamoxifen with fearsome cocktails of toxic drugs. One mixture favoured by oncologists for at least a decade went under the acronym, CMFVP, and contained cyclophosphamide, methotrexate, and fluorouracil (a pyrimidine base of RNA, bearing an atom of the ferociously reactive element, fluorine: the compound inhibits DNA synthesis, and acts most effectively on the rapidly dividing tumour cells); and finally there were vincristine and prednisolone. There was often a mere hair's breadth between elimination of the cancer and the endurance of the patient, challenged by the deadly effects of this and similar drug brews. As the poet of an earlier age, Matthew Prior had it,

> Cured yesterday of my disease,
> I died today of my physician.

In some cases the destruction by the drugs of the bone marrow, in which the blood cells are made, necessitated a bone-marrow transplant from a donor if the cured patient was to live. These heroic measures progressively gave place in the 1970s and 1980s to the much better tolerated hormone therapy, at least in the majority of women who had oestrogen receptors in their breasts (p.), and as we will shortly see, by Taxol.

The happy trees

In 1960 the United States Department of Agriculture (the USDA) launched an ambitious programme. The idea was to screen the widest possible range of plants for compounds with medicinal properties. By the time the Department wearied of the task in 1981, having by then entered into an agreement with the National Cancer Institute, its staff had sampled some 114,000 plants, in addition to about 16,000 animal samples. This colossal effort produced only one drug of any consequence, but that drug was a winner. The central personalities in its development was an organic chemist, Monroe Eliot Wall (1916-2002), a man with many achievements in the branch of science known as natural-products chemistry, which reached its apogee in the period from about the mid-19th to the mid-20th century. Wall spent his entire career in the search for substances that would be of direct medical value, and by the time he was drawn into the USDA's project he had already devoted some years to the study of a tree prized in Chinese folk medicine as the source of a treatment for cancer. From this tree, which bears the name, *Camptotheca acuminata*, but is known to the Chinese as the 'Happy Tree', Wall extracted a compound which he called camptothecin, and the structure of which he later determined. He sent samples of the extract to a friend, a prominent chemist, Jonathan Hartwell, head of a department at the National Cancer Institute. There it had been found to possess powerful inhibitory activity against cancer cells, but to Wall's frustration the USDA, of which he was an employee, was apathetic; their primary objective at that moment was to find a plant steroid that could be easily converted into cortisone. He therefore left to join a recently founded visionary organisation located in North Carolina, the Research Triangle Park, as head of the Natural Products

Division. From there he pursued his collaborations with Hartwell, who could provide materials and carry out biological testing. Camptothecin did eventually enter into clinical use, but its scope was limited by both its very low solubility and the side-effects that it provoked. Over the next years, derivatives with more accommodating properties were synthesised, and retain a place in chemotherapy of various cancers. The mechanism of action of camptothecin, later elucidated, is quite different from that of other anti-cancer agents then known, for it impeded the action of an enzyme that had not yet been discovered, an d essential for the process of DNA replication.*

Another anti-cancer agent surfaced at about the same time. One day in 1962 a botanist, who had been despatched to Oregon in the northwest to collect plant samples, took his axe to an unprepossessing tree, the Pacific yew, *Taxus brevifolia*, filled a bag with samples of its needles, twigs and bark, and sent the dried material to the USDA laboratories, where Wall was then still working. The extract was found to have anti-cancer activity when tested against a cell line in culture. This was the beginning of a bumpy twenty-year journey to the most profitable cancer drug to date. Wall and his colleague, Mansukh Wali at Research Triangle Park set about the task of tracking down the active ingredient in the bark. It was 1965 before they had a promising extract, labelled K172, which they sent to the National Cancer Institute for biological testing. The results caused a great

---

* The enzyme is called topoisomerase 1. When cells divide the DNA in the chromosomes must replicate itself. This involves the formation of a new double helix by the addition of successive nucleotides (p.), while the parent helix unwinds. At the Y-shaped 'replication fork', as it is called, which travels down the length of the DNA as replication advances, the double helix has to deform – to over-wind. Imagine two identical lengths of string twisted about each other to form a double helix: when the twist is increased the double helix twists on itself, forming supercoils. In real DNA the strain of supercoiling (over-winding) must be released to allow copying, by introducing a cut in one strand, and this is accomplished by the topoisomerase. If the stress is not released the process grinds to a halt, and cell division is stalled. The camptothecin binds tightly to the topoisomerase, and prevents it from attaching to the DNA. (In certain situations in the cell, a secondary twist can also occur in the opposite sense to the twist of the primary helix. To relieve such under-winding also demands a topoisomerase.)

stir: the extract had prodigious activity against a wide variety of tumours. But the active material in the Pacific yew bark was sparse, and the trees had to be cut down and stripped before it could be extracted. The remedy, assuming it worked in human patients, would be dismayingly expensive. After two more years of exacting toil to improve the extraction process Wall announced the results at a meeting of the American Chemical Society in 1967. The paper on taxol – the name the material was given, after that of the tree – excited much interest. The National Cancer Institute organised the collection of more material – 1200 kilograms of bark, which produced 28 kilograms of crude extract. It took until 1971 to determine the structure of Taxol, which turned out forbiddingly complex; a total synthesis, it was clear, would never generate commercial quantities of material. The best hope would be to produce an active fragment of the molecule, or to find a more abundant source in a related plant.

At this point interest apparently waned, and taxol lay fallow for another five years, when further tests revealed that the extract was highly effective in killing melanoma cells, which are responsible for the deadly skin cancer, and also cells from a form of lung cancer. Then Susan Horwitz, a pharmacologist at the Albert Einstein Medical College in New York, begged the National Cancer Institute for some taxol, and made good use of it. For in 1979 she published a paper in which its mode of action was laid bare. Taxol bound with high affinity to microtubules, filaments essential for many processes in the cell, including cell division. Microtubules are made up of a protein called tubulin. Many molecules of this protein assemble end-to-end to form the long tubular filaments, and these can grow or shorten in response to the demands of the cell. Attachment of taxol freezes the microtubules in the assembled state, and prevents them from functioning. Understanding the mechanism of action of a biologically active substance is always a stimulus to more extensive studies, and additional encouragement came from the discovery of a solvent system for this very refractory compound – a castor oil preparation, mixed with alcohol.

Several laboratories now began to search for taxol or similar compounds in plants related to the Pacific yew. A French chemist, Pierre Potier found a species of yew growing in profusion near his laboratory, producing masses of needles. These, Potier found, contained a taxol precursor that could be converted to taxol with reasonable yield. This then would be a continuing source of the drug. Some American laboratories meanwhile, with the backing of the National Cancer Institute (NCI), were attempting other partial syntheses of taxol. A total synthesis was in fact achieved, but the complexity of the structure demanded many successive chemical steps, which precluded its commercial use. What was needed was a starting compound, not so far distant in structure from taxol that it could not be converted to taxol or a functional relative. First to succeed in this was a group at Florida State University in Tallahassee under Robert Holton, although the yield of the product was low. At this point a disgruntled NCI, which had been rapped on the knuckles for inefficient use of money on the taxol project, opted for Holton over Potier, but decided that the time had come to deliver the problem of yield into the hands of industry. But the industrialists showed little appetite for the task, until finally Bristol-Myers Squibb agreed to take it on. By this time the generic name of the drug had been changed: it was henceforth to be called *paclitaxel*. Clinical trials had begun four years earlier, and not before time, in 1984. Paclitaxel, now marketed once more under the trade name of Taxol, emerged in due course as a highly effective drug against types of breast cancer and, among several others, ovarian cancer, for which it remains, despite severe side-effects, the most important treatment.

In 1993 there came a final twist to the story. That year there appeared a paper by a group of researchers at Montana State University, showing that paclitaxel is not a product of the yew tree at all: it is made by a fungus, *Taxomyces andrianae*, living harmlessly within the tree. The following year another publication from the same source reported that the corresponding species of fungus, specific to the Himalayan yew produced larger amounts of paclitaxel than its American relative. A long search turned up many such fungi, which inhabit the various species of yew and produce paclitaxel. One of them is even a Penicillium - *Penicillium raistrickii* (named in honour of Harold Raistrick [p.] the mould chemist, who gave up on penicillin). So now much of the world's paclitaxel is manufactured by an American biotechnology company with a fermentation plant in Germany; the drug is isolates from cultures of cells of a yew species, laced with the fungus, all grown in huge fermentation vats.

Mantraps on the path of progress: quackery revives

Medical science has never succeeded in shaking off its disreputable companion, marching ever just behind. Quackery has advanced by learning the language of modern science, and it preys most profitably on those who suffer from the most feared conditions, not least cancer. There is no doubt that many purported cures have been (and are still being) urged in good faith by zealots on the fringes of the healing profession. There are fashionable doctors who will offer to analyse a sample of a patient's hair, diagnose the problem as an insufficiency of cobalt or copper in the diet and prescribe accordingly. The shadow of the Abrams box (p.) hangs over such proceedings. An episode of egregious quackery, which took in many doctors and patients, erupted in the United States in 1949. A Serbian doctor, Stefan Durovič and his entrepreneurial brother, Marko arrived in Chicago from Argentina, bringing with them a treatment for hypertension, derived from cattle blood. He presented himself at the University of Illinois, and was referred to a member of the faculty, Andrew Conway Ivy. Ivy was a prominent doctor and physiologist. Vice-President of the University, and former President of the American Physiological Society, he had served as the American Medical Association's representative at the Nuremberg trials of the Nazi doctors in 1946.

Durovič, it turned out, had more to offer than the hypertension drug: he had a treatment for cancer, likewise derived from cattle blood, but from animals that had been inoculated with a species of *Actinomyces* bacteria (p.). This product was called *Krebiozen* (*Krebs* is the German for cancer), and its inventor claimed to have tested it on cancerous cats and dogs, of which more than half had been cured. Ivy was impressed, and with material his visitor gave him, he performed animal trials, and, having tested it on himself for toxicity, tried it on human patients. So convinced was Ivy of the efficacy of the mysterious substance that he allowed himself to be appointed President of the Krebiozen Research Foundation, established in 1951 by the Durovič brothers. Krebiozen quickly became news and attracted a number of prominent personages, including a Senator. But trials organised by the American Medical Association in several clinics did not support the claims. Worse, the FDA analysed a sample provided by Durovič, and found it to contain nothing but a common metabolic substance, an amino acid, creatine, dissolved in mineral oil. When other samples, sold commercially, were examined they did not even have creatine. Patients were being charged a hefty price for bottles of mineral oil. Durovič was arraigned for tax fraud and left the country in haste, but Ivy did not lose faith and in 1959 marketed his own brand of Krebiozen, under the name, Carcalon. But in the face of universally unfavourable reports confidence collapsed, and so did Ivy's reputation. Krebiozen lingered on for many years, and is still advertised to this day.

But perhaps the most enduring quack cure for cancer emerged from a curious but passionately held theory of its genesis. John Beard (1858-1924) was an embryologist at Edinburgh University who conceived the idea that all forms of cancer (which as we now know, encompasses a wide range of disparate diseases) have a common origin. In 1902 he unveiled his theory in a publication with the title, *The unitarian trophoblastic theory of cancer*, which he followed up with several more papers, and, in 1911, a book. The trophoblast is a tissue associated with the placenta in pregnant women (or animals), which gives rise to several metabolites including a steroid hormone. Beard's theory was that cells from the trophoblast could pass into the circulation of mother and foetus and initiate tumour formation unless they were destroyed by proteolytic enzymes – enzymes that digest proteins. He had in mind two well-studies enzymes generated in the pancreas, trypsin and chymotrypsin. Women constitutionally short of these natural molecules, and their offspring, were most prone to cancer, and should be treated with trypsin or chymotrypsin. Beard attracted a certain following, and belief in enzyme treatment of cancer survives in some quarters even now.

One doctor who was drawn to this idea was an American, Ernst Theodor Krebs (1876-1970). A shifty character, he concocted and sold early in his career a syrup containing an extract of a plant supposedly used in the medicine of an Indian tribe in Nevada, where he practised. He claimed that it would cure the deadly influenza, which was decimating the population in 1918, and also asthma and other bronchial complaints. The claims were found to be fraudulent by the FDA, and the existing stocks were impounded and destroyed. This did not stop Krebs from furtively peddling his nostrum, which found favour amongst the gullible for many more years. He also made a living on the side analysing contraband liquor for the poisonous wood alcohol, and in the course of this activity made the useful discovery that adding bitter apricot kernels helped the flavour of inferior bourbon whisky. This evidently led to a new brainwave: the kernels, which contained a substance called amygdalin (isolated a century earlier by Robiquet in France from almond kernels [p.]), Krebs realised, could be put to other uses. In accordance with Beard's cancer theory he had been treating patients with chymotrypsin. This may have given him the idea that amygdalin, which is broken down by chymotrypsin into glucose, benzaldehyde – a compound with a strong almond taste and smell – and hydrocyanic acid, could make a convincing anti-cancer nostrum, on the grounds that it would kill tumour cells by releasing hydrocyanic (prussic) acid. This sales pitch demanded the additional invalid hypothesis that tumour cells are exceptionally rich in enzymes like chymotrypsin.

In any event, Krebs presented the amygdalin extract to the world as pangamic acid, and later as vitamin B_{15}. Krebs claimed that he had successfully tested it on cancer patients, but had kept no records. By then he had been joined in California by his equally unscrupulous son, Ernst Theodor Krebs, Jr (1911-1996). Krebs, Jr was always known, like his father, as 'Dr Krebs', although he had no doctoral qualification, other than an honorary degree from the now defunct American Christian College of Tulsa in Oklahoma, an unaccredited institution with no science courses. He had in fact enrolled as a medical student in the Hahnemann Medical College, a homeopathic institution in Philadelphia, but had been thrown out. After further attempts in other colleges around the country he eventually obtained a B.Sc. degree in biochemistry at the University of Illinois, but for the sake of appearances promoted himself to Ph.D. The main contribution of Krebs *fils* was to improve the extraction from apricot kernels and to invent a name for the medicine – Laetrile (an acronym of the long structural name of amygdalin). But also, in 1945, Krebs, Jr established the John Beard Memorial Foundation to carry out research and disseminate the creed. Father and son, with the aid of another shady friend, elaborated Beard's trophoblast theory, and got papers describing their version of Beard's theory and experiments into print. By a legalistic device the Krebs Research Laboratories evaded the FDA and produced Laetrile for marketing by an outlet down the coast in Pasadena. Anxious cancer patients in their hundreds, and too often their physicians, snapped up Laetrile samples, and reports of great results began to flow in. In 1953 the California Cancer Commission, an arm of the State Medical Association requested samples of the wonder drug for clinical trials, but Krebs Jr was willing to cooperate only on his own terms, in particular that he himself would be allowed to nominate a doctor to lead the investigation. This was obviously unacceptable, but the Cancer Commission found another way: they procured Laterile sufficient for animal tests from the FDA, and duly found that it had no detectable effect on the progression of tumours in mice. Nor did the available records from hospitals of cancer patients treated with Laetrile afford evidence of any positive outcome. The Commission's report was unequivocal: Laetrile was useless.

The verdict merely spurred the Krebs to yet greater efforts to promote their discovery and louder proclamations of its virtues. They were willing to take on the FDA, which had reacted sluggishly, but from 1960 started impounding shipments. The usual assertions now began to fly from the Krebs and their growing band of supporters: the trials were flawed, and the medical and pharmaceutical establishment was out to prevent outsiders with heterodox views from intruding on their territory. That same year the Krebs found a powerful patron. Andrew McNaughton was a well-connected Canadian entrepreneur and arms dealer, who saw opportunities in Laetrile. He set up a company, Biozymes International Ltd in Montreal, and proceeded to manufacture Laetrile and sell it around the world. Within a short time it had been administered to many thousands of cancer sufferers, and testimonials of pain assuaged and lives saved streamed in from patients and doctors. NcNaughton agitated for FDA approval, though without success, but patients formed their own organisations, most notably the International Association of Cancer Victims and Friends, demanding that the life-saving remedy should be made freely available. A particularly enthusiastic and effective evangelist for Laetrile was a doctor in San Francisco, John Richardson, who joined the fray soon after meeting the younger Krebs in 1971 and became famous and rich from treating not only cancer patients but also those he thought were heading for the disease – afflicted in his terminology with 'preclinical syndrome'. In 1972 he was arrested for breaching the State laws relating to treatment of cancer, but the case against him failed on technical grounds. The dramatic arrest attracted the attention of the extreme right-wing John Birch Society with its obsession with citizens' rights, and became something of a political *cause célèbre*. (In the following years Richardson had another two brushes with the law, and finally in 1976 his licence to practice medicine in the State of California was revoked, and he spent the rest of his colourful career in Mexico.)

The debate and the legal battles raged throughout the 1960s and 1970s. Eventually, after some vicissitudes, and apparently positive results with Laetrile in laboratory experiments from one respectable source, various clinical trials were conducted, and gave uniformly negative results by all criteria. The Laetrile aficionados squirmed: the results were biased, the amygdalin had been of inferior quality, the remedy should have been administered with chymotrypsin or other substances. One doctor even argued that research on gravely ill patients was unethical, and the testimony of doctors who had had success with the treatment, and that of their patients had already provided evidence enough of cures. The lawyers engaged to defend Laetrile also tried to make a case for citizens' freedom to choose to take a drug, whether effective or not. The case came before the Congressional Subcommittee on Health, chaired by Senator Edward Kennedy, which was battered by the impassioned rhetoric of the Laetrile supporters, and wilted under the impact. The founder of one of the many groups formed to champion the medicine, a political extremist of the far-right, addressed the committee in threatening terms: 'Rest assured, gentlemen, that the people demand Laetrile', and would get it whether 'Big Brother' wanted or not. But at long last, in 1980, more than three decades after Laetrile made its first appearance a thoroughgoing clinical trial was organised. Results from four of the most important cancer centres in the country came up with the expected result: Laetrile had no effect on the progression of cancer or on any of its symptoms, whether given alone or in conjunction with other substances. A little later animal experiments disclosed that the theory on which the purported efficacy of Laetrile was based, the release of cyanide in tumour cells, was false. Ernst Krebs Jr had countered the earlier negative results with the fanciful assertion that Laetrile was a vitamin - vitamin B_{17} in fact – the lack of which leads to cancer. It had of course none of the defining attributes of a vitamin, and the idea met with appropriate ridicule. In the end Laetrile was banned and its manufacturers prosecuted. Production moved mainly to Mexico, where it continues still. Krebs *père* and *fils*, still have the posthumous adulation of their adherents, who regard them as traduced and victimised geniuses, Nobel Laureates *manqué*. Huge numbers of cancer victims, running probably well into six figures, have placed their hopes in Laetrile over the years, and continue to do so. It is offered on the Internet, and stands as a monument to human weakness and credulity.

The coming of targeted therapy: the age of Gleevec

The history of targeted cancer therapy properly begins in 1909 when Peyton Rous, a doctor and oncologist at the Rockefeller Institute, as it then was, in New York was moved to investigate an outbreak of a disease that was killing the chickens on a poultry farm. The mysterious disease was especially remarkable in that it was clearly a cancer, a sarcoma (p.), yet was equally clearly infectious. Rous extracted a fluid - highly infectious - from the tumours, and set about fractionating it. After a succession of filtrations he was left with a clear liquid, which contained no cells, bacteria or any other microscopic matter, yet retained high infectivity. Rous could only conclude that the carcinogenic agent was a virus.* This Rous sarcoma virus,

---

* No-one had at that time actually seen a virus, because viruses are too small to show up in a light microscope. To perceive the physical form of a virus scientists had to await the invention of the electron microscope (p.), but the existence of viruses was first established in 1892. In that year a Russian botanist, Dmitri Iosifovich Ivanofsky, charged with finding the cause of the disease that was devastating the tobacco plants in the Ukraine, proved that the infectious agent was invisible and passed through the filters used to separate out bacteria. In 1898 Ivanofsky's conclusions were confirmed by a Dutch scientist, Marinus Beijerinck, who coined the word, 'virus'. The tobacco mosaic virus was an object of much research during the next century, and, as already related (p.) was first observed in the electron microscope by Wendell Stanley at the Rockefeller Institute in 1935.

as it came to be known, or RSV, excited no interest among oncologists. The few who read the report in 1911 scoffed at the idea, and Rous's case was not helped by his obdurate insistence that *all* cancers were caused by viruses. But RSV did at least become an object of curiosity to virologists, and was indeed the first of several cancer viruses (also called oncoviruses) that came to light in later years. It was to be nearly six decades after Rous's discovery before advances in biochemistry caught up with his inference that viruses could cause cancer.

The first important fact to emerge about the nature of RSV was that it is an RNA virus. All viruses have their own genetic material, which may be DNA or its cousin, RNA (p.), and once in the cell, the virus subverts the cell's synthetic machinery to make the proteins encoded by the viral genes. They combine to build more finished viruses, which then burst out of the cell and invade other cells in the vicinity. It was an Italian virologist, Renato Dulbecco, transplanted from Turin to California, who found that cancer viruses, such as RSV, take command of their host cell in much more radical style by infiltrating its very genome. They stitch their genes into the DNA of the host cell, causing it thereby to lose control over its reproductive cycle, so that it divides unchecked, and passes on this behaviour to its progeny, which are therefore now all cancer cells. This was a startling and enormously important discovery, but now the increasing number of researchers studying RSV were confronted with a paradox: the genes in all cells in all autonomous organisms are made of DNA, and to translate a genetic message into protein the DNA must first be copied into RNA (messenger RNA), which is then read off by the protein synthesising machinery. This sequence of events – simply stated, DNA makes RNA, which makes protein – was laid down as an immutable principle of life by Francis Crick, the man who did more than anyone since Darwin to change the face of biology. He called this rule the 'Central Dogma', and no one doubted its validity. How then were genes embedded in the RNA of the RSV copied into the DNA of the chicken cell genome? The answer emerged in1970 from two American laboratories simultaneously, those of Howard Temin at the University of Wisconsin and of David Baltimore at the Massachusetts Institute of Technology. The virus circumvents the Central Dogma by making an enzyme that runs the system in reverse and copies RNA into DNA. It is called *reverse transcriptase*, and for its discovery – initially met with scepticism, since it appeared so improbable - Temin, Baltimore and Temin's former patron, Dulbecco were rewarded with the Nobel Prize in 1975.

In 1970, hard on the discovery of reverse transcriptase, a graduate student at the University of California in Berkeley, Steven Martin, was adding chemical mutagens to RSV to find out which of its genes was responsible for transforming normal into malignant chicken cells. He found the answer, and something more – a mutant of the virus that survived and reproduced in the host cell, but did not cause cancer. But then je found that this held only if the infected chicken cells were grown in a dish at normal physiological temperature. The mutant virus did, though, transform the same cells at a lower growth temperature. The mutant virus, then, was perfectly capable of functioning, with the one curious proviso, that it would effect malignant transformation of its host only at reduced temperature. The inference was obvious, at least to those who have lived with proteins): the protein encoded by the mutated gene (which was not implicated in the growth process), was structurally enfeebled, and would not tolerate any but a low temperature. (This is a common enough effect in mutant proteins, and in fact all proteins become inactivated at some temperature, high or low, depending on their structure.) The discovery of the cancer-bearing gene led immediately to the next question: what was the product of that gene? What enzyme, in other words, did it encode? The answer was not long in coming: the enzyme, solely responsible for causing such mayhem in the cell, was a *protein kinase*.

There are many kinases in our cells, and what they all do is to attach to selected proteins at a particular site in the structure a phosphoryl group ($-PO_3^-$, a phosphorus atom with three attached oxygens and a negative charge). This *phosphorylation* is an on-switch in many enzymes, which then go to work on their substrates, most often other proteins, and continue to work until the phosphoryl group is split off by another enzyme, called a phosphatase. Kinases control an immense range of metabolic reactions and cellular processes, such as cell division. The gene that Martin found, designated the *src* gene, was the first *oncogene* to be discovered. An oncogene, as the name implies, is one that can cause cancer, and the product of the *src* gene is a particular kinase, called a tyrosine kinase (because tyrosine is the amino acid in the target protein that it phosphorylates). Clearly this particular phosphorylation was aberrant, not permitted to any kinase in the uninfected cells, and its effect was to override the off-switch in an enzyme that directs cell division. The next great leap was made in 1976 by Harold Varmus and Michael Bishop, virologists at the San Francisco campus of the University of California. It was they and a few associates who determined that the DNA of a normal healthy chicken contains the very same kinase gene, though with small differences. The only explanation is that, over evolutionary time, the virus assimilated, and modified the gene of its habitual host, the chicken. Such gene transfer proved to be a widespread event in the co-existence of animals of different species (our own included). Yet the chicken does not generally develop cancer, and this holds also for other animals, and humans, all of whom possess closely related forms of the *src* gene. Varmus and Bishop dubbed such genes (of which, as was later found, there are many scattered throughout the genome) *proto-oncogenes*, and for their work they were awarded the Nobel Prize in 1989 (Peyton Rous having been similarly honoured in 1966, at the age of eighty-five, fifty-five years after he made his discovery). The impact of these discoveries was profound, and it redirected thinking in the cancer field, for it had until then been taken as axiomatic that cancer could result only from the influence of some external agency, whereas it was now clear that our cells carried within them the seeds of their own destruction. But what did the oncogenes actually do?

The *src* gene product, the tyrosine kinase, performs essential functions in the cell, but our DNA is prey to frequent and random mutations (see p.). These are most often harmless, but far less likely to be so when they strike the *src* gene, or any other of the many proto-oncogenes littering the genome. For the enzymes expressed (in the jargon) by these genes are commonly involved in such processes as DNA-copying or cell division.

Thus, if the substitution of one amino acid for another in the sequence,* engendered by the mutation, should disable the enzyme's 'brake' cancer is apt to result. In some cases the problem arises not from a single-nucleotide mutation in the DNA but from a chromosomal anomaly, seen in the cells of patients with a form of leukaemia (chronic myelogenous leukaemia, CML). In man the DNA, and thus the genes, are distributed among 23 chromosome pairs (one from each parent), residing in the cell nucleus. The classic exemplar is the so-called Philadelphia chromosome, from the city in which it was discovered in 1960. The chromosomes can exchange elements of DNA, and in rare cases chromosomes may fracture and a piece of one may unite with another chromosome. In the Philadelphia translocation, as it is called, a fragment from the end of chromosome 22 has broken away and united with the tip of chromosome 9. By malign chance the join in the new chromosome brings into apposition the genes for two separate tyrosine kinases, which give rise to a hyperactive fusion protein (two proteins joined together). This hybrid 'superkinase' resists the normal off-switch mechanism, and works relentlessly, replicating the genome over and over again. The cells proceed to divide without cease, and either one of two forms of leukaemia, most often chronic myeloid leukaemia (CML), ensues.

The point of this long preamble should now become clear, for we have entered the realm of a new pharmacology. It was the first time that a target of therapeutic intervention – a particular molecule – was in plain view. If a compound could be found that would bind to tyrosine kinase and jam its action, then perhaps the accelerating cancer could be brought to a halt. One protein kinase inhibitor was already known by 1977, an antibiotic, staurosporine, extracted from a species of *Actinomyces*, but found too

---

* The genetic code is a triplet code, that is to say three successive nucleotides (p.) in the DNA chain specify one of the twenty amino acids found in proteins. So for instance the triplet (called a codon) ATG specifies the amino acid methionine. If now there is a mutation in that triplet, changing it from ATG to ACG, the amino acid, threonine will now appear in the position in the protein sequence previously occupied by methionine. This may (or may not) alter the protein's structure. It may completely annihilating the function of the protein, or perhaps cause some more subtle change, such as disabling a structural feature, which allows the molecule to switch between its active and dormant states; then the signal normally exercised by phosphorylation or dephosphorylation would not work.

promiscuous in its targets to be useful: interfering with all the myriad metabolic processes involving one or other of the dozens of kinases in the body would cause mayhem in the cells. To find a selective inhibitor, which would attack only the one kinase responsible for CML would be a tall order. Two researchers at the Ciba-Geigy laboratories in Switzerland, Nicholas Lydon and Alex Matter were undaunted. The amino acid sequences of several of the kinases recognised at the time they set out on the chase in 1984 revealed the positions of the site of enzymic action - the active site (or active centre), as biochemists call it. As expected, all were similar, but there were small differences, according to the substrate protein on which the enzyme worked. By this time the synthesis of proteins in bacteria, or where this failed, in cultures of other types of cell, was almost routine, and so a piece of the tyrosine kinase enzyme containing the active site could be made in quantity. The plan then was to test a range of compounds on the activity of the enzyme thus prepared.

The procedure was little different from the time-honoured routine on which the pharmacologists of fifty years earlier had relied. Start with a known kinase inhibitor, however unspecific, such as staurosporine, and the handful of other compounds discovered in the intervening years to possess an anti-kinase activity, and synthesise modified versions, based on enlightened guesses. After nearly a decade of patient synthesis and assaying, a class of compounds, the phenylaminopyrimidines, was found to have the right sort of promise. Other research groups in the pharmaceutical industry and in university departments helped in the effort, and one discovered that a substitution at one point in the structure of the 'lead compound' eliminated the inhibitory activity of a large family of kinases. The end product was imatinib. It stopped the activity of the fused kinase in the cells of people with the Philadelphia chromosome. Prolonged animal and clinical testing satisfied all parties that side-effects were few, and the cures achieved of CML remarkable and lasting. In 2001 the drug was approved by the FDA, and marketed under the trade name of Gleevec, or Glevec in Europe. Moreover, some other cancers, notably the previously intractable gastrointestinal stromal tumour, or GIST, also responded to Gleevec. This, though was by no means the end of the road, for it soon transpired that advanced CML was often refractory to Gleevec, because the continuous mutation of the cancer cells would throw up a resistant mutant. A demand therefore arose for variants of the drug that could be given in combination therapies, and so the research continues, with the aid now of new technologies (p.). Gleevec remains nonetheless one of the great successes of rational targeted oncology research.

Chapter 15

CANS'T THOU NOT MINISTER TO A MIND DISEASED?

Man has known mood-changing plant preparations since ancient times. There was the opium poppy, and its relatives, such as hemp and jimsonweed; there were the plants of the *Solenaceae* family, which includes the deadly nightshade (*Belladonna*), the mandrake and henbane; and then there were those that produced cannabis and marijuana; in South America there was mescaline from the peyote cactus and cocaine from the coca plant; and always there was alcohol. Plant preparations, such as hyoscyamine (p.) - marketed in 1839 by Merck in Germany, and known in the U.S. as scopolamine - from some *Solenaceae*, were used to induce torpor or sleep, to deaden pain, or to induce euphoria. Hallucinogenic mushrooms, of which there are two important groups - the so-called 'magic mushrooms', which contain the hallucinogen, psilocybin, and the many *Amanita* species, such as the fly agaric, *Amanita muscaria* – were used in religious ceremonies in many ancient societies. In some cultures, as in Siberia, they served an important social role. In medieval France they were regarded as the property of the local nobility, and the broth prepared from them was served at table on special occasions. The active hallucinogenic component of fly agaric, an alkaloid called muscimol, was discovered to pass out of the body unchanged in the urine, which was accordingly collected, since the mushrooms were scarce, and would often be sent down as a treat for the vassals. All these mushrooms were in greater or lesser degree toxic, and the most potent, *Amanita phalloides*, the poison cap, was a notorious means of murder in ancient Rome and elsewhere. A staple of ancient Indian medicine was the snakeroot, *Rauwolfia serpentina*, named after the 16th-century German traveller and botanist, Leonhart Rauwolf. It served many purposes: it soothed troublesome babies, acted as a sedative and narcotic for the treatment of insomnia, and calmed the uncontrollably manic. It was not until the 1940s that Indian doctors, notably Rustom Jal Vakil in Bombay, who carried out an extensive controlled trial, demonstrated that it also reduced blood pressure. Thus it came into use as an effective treatment for chronic hypertension. Several active constituents were identified by Indian chemists, but purification proved difficult, and it was not until 1951 that the most interesting, with good hypotensive (blood-pressure lowering), and incidentally, strong sedative properties, was isolated. This was *reserpine* and it was purified in the Ciba laboratories in Basel, and sold as a treatment for hypertension, and put on the market in 1953 as Serpasil.

Chemistry of the mind: the coming of barbiturates

The options for treating psychological and neurological disorders remained very limited until well into the 20th century. Up to then then the 'lunatic asylums', as they were known to the Victorians, were hellholes, in which inmates were made to suffer the utmost brutality, and where treatments, such as immersion in cold water, were still often practised*. A notable early advance in treatment was the introduction of chloral hydrate, a simple compound, first synthesised in 1832 by the great German chemist, Justus von Liebig (p.). Because it could be broken down in the test-tube by alkali into its component parts, one of them chloroform, the idea arose in the mind of a leading pharmacologist of the day, Emil Buchheim, that this reaction might happen in the blood of people suffering from diseases, associated (wrongly) with excessive alkalinity. (This could never happen in the very mildly alkaline state that the blood could attain.) Moreover, thought Buchheim, chloroform is known to decompose under certain conditions to yield hydrochloric acid. (This happens on exposure, for instance, to ultraviolet light, but is hardly conceivable in the blood.) Then the hydrochloric acid would neutralise the blood alkali, and all would be well. Pursuing this comprehensively erroneous train of argument, Buchheim decided to examine what effect chloral hydrate might have on the human body, so swallowed a stiff draught, and persuaded some students to do the same. All sank into a deep slumber, and on waking, Buchheim

---

* To take just one example of the bizarre practices with which the mentally sick were tormented almost within living memory, Henry Andrews Cotton, the medical director of the New Jersey Lunatic Asylum in the U.S. in the second and third decades of the 20th century, conceived the theory that the universal cause of madness was a bacterial infection. This could come from rotten teeth, and other sites in the body, such as tonsils and abdominal organs, especially the colon. He pursued his idea to its logical end: if extracting the patient's teeth did not result in the return of sanity – and indeed one might have supposed it to have the opposite effect – Cotton would proceed to the tonsils or to extirpation of the colon. Many patients are said to have died, for operating procedures were primitive. Cotton was widely admired within his profession for the depth and originality of his insights, and when he died in 1933 there were many fulsome tributes to his achievements. He may have been inspired by the work of his near-contemporary, the London surgeon, Sir William Arbuthnot Lane, who promulgated the doctrine that most disease was engendered by toxins – 'ptomaines' – lurking in the colon, a consequence of infrequent evacuation. For many years he treated the most fundamental affliction, constipation, by cutting out the colon. Not long after Cotton's heyday fashions took a new turn, with the introduction of the frontal lobotomy operation, performed by an implement resembling an ice-pick, designed to sever the frontal lobes of the brain. It calmed unmanageable patients, but at terrible cost. The Portuguese surgeon, Egas Moniz was awarded the Nobel Prize in 1949 for this innovation.

abandoned his. theory and the study of chloral hydrate. Eight years elapsed before, in 1869, Oscar Liebreich, a young lecturer at the medical school of Munich University arrived by similar reasoning to Buchheim's at a different conclusion – that chloral hydrate might generate chloroform in the blood and cause anaesthesia. After animal experiments, which appeared to support his conjecture, Liebreich undertook human trials. He described his results in a book on '*Chloral hydrate, a new hypnotic*', in which he also discussed side-effects and hazards. And so the compound became at once the most widely used sleeping draught and treatment for difficult psychotic patients. It is by no means devoid of side-effects, especially an undesirable influence on the heart.

Another simple compound, acetaldehyde, which is an oxidation product of ethanol (the alcohol we drink), was investigated during the 19th century as a possible hypnotic or sedative, but its irritant properties precluded its clinical use. It had, though, long been known that acetaldehyde molecules can easily be made to associate with each in rings of three to form paraldehyde. This compound is relatively devoid of irritant action, but has a repellent taste. Its physiological properties were studied in the mid-19th century by Buchheim's protégé, the great pharmacologist,

Oswald Schmiedeberg*. The result was that paraldehyde came into use as a hypnotic, but was found most useful for the control of epileptic seizures. It is still used for that purpose even now, commonly administered by enema. Many related compounds were synthesised and tried out. Some found enthusiastic champions, but all turned out to have drawbacks, some were lethal and none endured. Bromides – sodium and potassium bromide (p.) – remained a stand-by for the treatment of agitated and psychotic patients and epileptics. Army recruits, experiencing stress and anxiety, have as is well-known, tended to put down their unaccustomed loss of libido to the potassium bromide, that someone has always seen being shovelled from sacks into the tea. Bromides have the merits of cheapness and tolerable safety, and probably still find applications today.

The paucity of safe and effective treatments for mental conditions led to an eager run on the new hypnotic, barbital, synthesised in 1864 by Adolph von Baeyer. It was a new kind of ring compound, which he called barbituric acid. (How he chose this name is unclear, but various legends sprang up around it – that it was to honour an elusive inamorata named Barbara; that he caroused in his favourite beer-house to celebrate his discovery, in the

---

* Johann Ernst Oswald Schmiedeberg (1838-1921), commonly referred to as 'the father of pharmacology', passed his childhood and early career in Dorpat, which is now Tartu in Estonia. He worked with Buchheim on the metabolism of chloroform, which formed the substance of his doctoral thesis. He was offered a faculty position, his research thrived and his reputation grew. In 1872 he was called to a professorial chair at the University of Strassburg, as Strasbourg had become after the German victory in the Franco-Prussian war two years before. Schmiedeberg built up a distinguished school of pharmacology, and remained in Strassburg until 1919, when the city reverted to French Strasbourg following the German defeat. The remaining German faculty members were expelled, abandoning all their belongings. The ageing Schmiedeberg was found by a friend, a professor of theology at the University, waiting disconsolately at the railway station to board a train for Germany. He was clutching a bundle of paper – the manuscript of his final publication on the action of digitalis – in fear that it would be taken from him by the soldiers searching the departing Germans. The theologian took the bundle, promising to get it to the old man in Baden Baden, where he would take refuge with his old friend, Bernhard Naunyn. (Their names have remained linked in the name of the journal, which they had founded many years before the, *Naunyn-Schmiedeberg's Archinen für Pharmacoloiey*). Schmiedeberg died shortly after the paper was published.

company of officers of the local artillery regiment, of which St. Barbara was the patron; what is not in dispute is that the name incorporates that of a Barbara and uric acid, which was the starting point of the synthesis.) At all events, the compound was found to have no discernible physiological properties. All the same, some thirty years later an eminent pharmacologist, then at the University of Halle, Joseph von Mering (1849-1907) (whom we have already met [p.]), decided that any new class of compounds needed to be properly investigated for pharmacological activity. Moreover, contemplation of two or three hypnotic compounds then known led him to speculate that a pair of ethyl groups (C_2H_5-) attached to a single carbon atom in the ring structure might hold the key to hypnotic activity. This wild conjecture had no substance, but it brought about one of the major revolutions in clinical practice. Von Mering was fortunate to have a friend from student days, who happened to be (apart from von Baeyer, whose assistant he had been) the most celebrated organic chemist in the land, probably indeed the world. This was Emil Fischer (1852-1919), professor in Berlin, who found a way to prepare diethylbarbituric acid. Fischer and von Mering could actually have saved themselves the trouble had they been acquainted with the literature, for two German chemists had reported its synthesis ten years before. (This is yet another illustration of the principle, well-known to students of chemistry, that six months in the laboratory can often save a half-hour in the library.)

Animal experiments by Fischer and a nephew revealed that diethylbarbituric acid had powerful hypnotic properties, and a report was published by Fischer and von Mering in 1903, in which the name, veronal first appeared. (There is again doubt about its origin: one version has it that von Mering was on holiday in Verona when he received the news from Fischer, but according to another, Fischer took it from the Latin, *verus*, the truth, on the grounds that it was a true hypnotic. Before long the drug had shown its potency, however loosely defined, when tested on patients with serious psychotic and neurotic conditions, associated with sleep disorders, and also in the treatment of epilepsy. It was both a sedative (tranquiliser) and a hypnotic, and one use was therefore in the 'sleep cure' favoured by a fashionable school of psychiatrists for dealing with severely psychotic patients.* In addition to all that, it was the first injectable anaesthetic.

Both Fischer and von Mering had close connections with the firm of Bayer, and it was there that further tests were carried out, and production of veronal began in 1904. In 1917, the year after the United States entered the Great War, Abbott Laboratories in Chicago breached the Bayer patent under the terms of the Trading with the Enemy act, passed by Congress that year, which allowed German products to be impounded as war booty. Abbott developed and improved the synthesis of the drug, and also gave it their own name, barbital, whereas in Europe it became barbitone. The enormous success of barbitone/barbital started a headlong rush by pharmaceutical companies around the world to produce 'me-too' variants. In the end a prodigious number, amounting to some 2,500 or even more, were synthesised. But the most successful was one of the twenty or so prepared by Fischer himself, which was marketed by Bayer under the name of Luminal, and later became more familiar as phenobarbitone. It proved especially effective in diminishing the frequency and severity of epileptic seizures. Other leading products were the fast-acting and rapidly eliminated butabarbitone, and a widely used surgical anaesthetic, pentobarbitone, or Nembutal.

It was, alas, all too soon that the drawbacks of the barbiturates began to show themselves. They were depressants of the central nervous system, but worse, they were addictive, and the serious social consequences of dependency became apparent. The drugs were cheap and were prescribed, and in places bought over the counter, all in huge amounts well into the mid-1950s. Apart from the major dependency problem, with its attendant risk of accidental overdoses, they became the favoured means of suicide, especially among the rich. It seems not unlikely that both Emil Fischer and von Mering may have fallen victim to their own discovery. A half century later, amylobarbitone, also known as Amytal, acquired an evil reputation as a 'truth drug' or 'truth serum', favoured by many unsavoury regimes, with dubious results, for the interrogation of political prisoners. (Scopolamine, which is hyoscine [p.], found a like application.)

---

* Also known as 'deep-sleep therapy', it consisted essentially in drugging psychotic subjects with heavy doses of barbiturates. After some patients died the practice fell into disrepute and was discontinued.

Amphetamine, LSD, hallucinations and addictions

Even at the height of their popularity as sleeping pills, the barbiturates did little for more serious conditions. A measure of the despair to which doctors in mental hospitals were driven in their efforts to cope with violently psychotic and schizophrenic patients can be gleaned from the eagerness with which so many of them seized on the promise of insulin shock. In 1933 Manfred Sakel, an Austrian doctor, was working in Berlin. While at the Psychiatric Hospital in Vienna he had tried to induce hunger in a severely schizophrenic patients, who was refusing food, by way of an insulin injection to lower his blood sugar level. Sakel noticed with surprise that the patient became less agitated. Small insulin doses appeared to Sakel to exert this effect on schizophrenics consistently. In Berlin he tried larger doses on both schizophrenics and morphine addicts, suppressing the blood sugar to the point that the patient became comatose. The ultimate effect, as long as the doctor was skilful and the patient survived, was beneficial, and Sakel's insulin-induced coma treatment was widely adopted to treat severe cases, most of all in the United States. It was an exceedingly unpleasant procedure, probably rationalised, at least partly, by the notion that insulin, discovered not very long before, had broad life-enhancing properties. Such heroic measures reflected the dearth of options open to neurologists.

In 1937 a child psychiatrist, Charles Bradley, director of a children's psychiatric hospital in Providence, Rhode Island, made an accidental discovery (like almost every other in his discipline throughout the ensuing decades). But Bradley's was to resonate around the Werstern world. Amphetamine is a compound closely related to ephedrine, the active constituent of the Chinese *Ephedra* plant (p.). Ephedrine was first synthesised unintentionally in 1887 in Berlin by a Romanian Ph.D. student trying to make a different compound, while almost at the same time a Japanese worker purified the substance from the plant. In 1910 Henry Dale and the organic chemist, George Barger in London (p.) took a close look at amphetamine. They determined that it bore a resemblance to adrenaline in both structure and physiological properties, but did not pursue the matter further. The spotlight now shifts to Los Angeles, where in 1927 an English organic chemist, Gordon Alles, not long out of the

California Institute of Technology with a Ph.D., found employment with an allergologist, who had a small private laboratory. Alles's assigned task was to synthesise compounds for the treatment of asthma, to replace ephedrine, which his employer had been prescribing, but which was scarce and expensive. In short order Alles brought off an economical synthesis of amphetamine, probably knowing nothing of the previous German work. He was disappointed to find that his product did nothing for the asthma patients, but all the same, he tried it on himself, and was gratified by the variety of physiological and psychological phenomena that it evoked – a rise in blood pressure, dilation of the pupils, an accelerated heart rate, a loss of appetite, on the one hand, and a sense of heightened awareness and well-being on the other. But best of all, it could free a blocked nose. (It was Alles who coined the name, amphetamine for the compound had previously been known as phenisopropylamine.)

Alles's next move was to approach the Californian pharmaceutical company, Smith, Kline and French (SKF), and persuade the managenevt to take an interest in the compound. It had scant success until 1932, when the company reformulated it as an inhalant for stopped noses. It was soon selling well over the counter under the name of Benzedrine. Alles went on to show that only one of the two optical isomers – the mirror-image forms (p.) – generated by his synthesis expressed the activity; this was the dextro- or D-isomer, for which SKF coined the name, Dexedrine. It also then turned out that a derivative bearing a methyl ($-CH_3$) group in the ring system, had a much enhanced potency. This became known to its adherents as Speed, and its crystalline hydrochloride salt as crystal meth. Alles continued to develop derivatives of amphetamine and various hallucinogens for SKF. He had taken out a patent on his original product, which he allocated to SKF with a highly profitable royalty agreement, and he became rich. He died in 1963 at the age of sixty-one, so was spared the full realisation of what he had wrought.

We return now to Charles Bradley, the paediatric psychiatrist in his children's clinic. Bradley noticed that when he administered Benzedrine to a child in the manner intended by the manufacturers it appeared to cause a brightening of the patient's disposition, and he decided to investigate.

He selected thirty of his captive children, seemingly at random, observed them for a week, then dosed them with Benzedrine for a second week, and finally kept them under observation without further medication for a third week. The results were, Bradley thought, 'spectacular'. During the second week of the trial half the children showed a striking improvement in in their school work with heightened interest, while half of the 'behaviour problem' children became 'emotionally subdued', though with no loss of interest in their surroundings. SKF realised that they were on to a good thing, and within a short time Benzedrine pills ('bennies') were being consumed in the United States and around the world for endurance, intellectual performance and soon for pleasure. Amphetamine, Dexedrine and another derivative, methamphetamine were given to soldiers during World War II to counter fatigue. These free issues afterwards flooded the market with dire consequences, for they were addictive, and taken in large doses, caused hallucinations and often other unpleasant, and in some cases irreversible effects.* The remaining legitimate use for amphetamines is in treating narcolepsy, a sleep disorder, which causes the narcoleptic subject to fall suddenly asleep at any time, however inappropriate. The use of Benzedrine and related compounds to the detriment of mental and physical health has never really ceased, despite all warnings.

The emptying of the psychiatric wards

In the mid-20th century some gleams of hope flickered on the neuropsychiatric horizon. A glimpse of what the future might hold came in the shape of a publication in 1954. Its author was Nathan Kline, a clinical psychiatrist in New York. Kline had begun two years before to investigate the effects, first of Rauwolfia, and then of reserpine preparations, on schizophrenic patients, and noted that most became more tranquil and less hostile. His publication proved, for good or ill, a turning-point in the treatment of the condition, and it made Kline famous. At almost the same

---

* Yet it has to be said that some users were able to control the effects. The great (and eccentric) Hungarian mathematician, Paul Erdös, took Benzedrine daily until he died to sharpen his concentration and mental staying-power, and remained productive into his eighties in a profession in which creativity is generally attributed to the young.

time, at the U.S. National Institutes of Health, an experimental study was in progress on the effects of Rauwolfia on 'chemical events inside the brain. A small group of researchers from three countries, led by an eminent pharmacologist, Bernard Brodie (1907-1989), found that when rabbits were dosed with reserpine they became torpid, and the secretion of a chemical in their brains, serotonin rose. The higher the reserpine dose the greater the amount of serotonin released. Serotonin had already been conjecturally linked to the control of mood. In their paper, published in 1955, Brodie and his colleagues made the following suggestion: 'It is conceivable that the beneficial effects of reserpine in mental disturbances results from the liberation of serotonin'. This, the first link between biochemistry and the state of the mind, marked the start of a new departure in brain research.

While all this was unfolding across the Atlantic, something new was simmering in France that would transform the treatment of mental illness. Most of all, it would largely empty the grim mental hospitals in which patients could languish all their lives, sometimes in seclusion or physically restrained, and made to endure the torments of electroconvulsive therapy, if not the assaults of surgeons practising the dehumanising and discredited frontal lobotomy operation. From about 1933 the prodigious team of chemists at Rhône-Poulenc (p.) had been on the trail of anti-histamine drugs, to mitigate such conditions as hay-fever and asthma. The first was discovered by Daniel Bovet (p.), and he and his colleagues went on to create several more, notably Benadryl, Antergan and Neo-Antergan. (We will come to these later [p.].) Then in 1947, another Rhône-Poulenc chemist, Paul Charpentier came up with a compound of a different kind: RP4560 belonged to a class called the phenothiazines, and had excellent anti-histamine activity with minimal toxicity. But in animal tests a wholly unexpected side-effect revealed itself: the animals became torpid from even the smallest dose.* The Rhône-Poulenc directorate had no wish to embroil itself in the alien area of psychopharmacology, but the observation came to the attention of a doctor in Paris, Henri Laborit. Laborit (1914-1995) was an outsider. Born in Hanoi in what was then French Indo-China, the son of a colonial army doctor, he followed his father into the profession,

---

* Promethazine (Phenergan) is still widely used, though predominantly to suppress motion sickness.

served in the French army in North-Africa and then in the Navy during the Second World War (when he spent long hours in the water after his ship was sunk during the Dunkirk evacuation). His experiences on the field of battle sparked an interest in the mechanism and management of pain. He developed a curious theory of pain and stress relief, believing that a drug acting on the central nervous system could bring a patient into a state of 'artificial hibernation', free of pain and anxiety. He referred to this as 'sedation without narcosis'. It would, he thought, also avert the dangers of the drop (or in some cases the rise) in blood pressure during major operations. The term for the type of drug that he was after is an anxiolytic, literally an anxiety solvent.

By good fortune, Laborit, who had been posted to a military outpost in Tunisia, was transferred at the right time to Paris, where he was given facilities at the Val-de-Grâce military hospital. There he organised a series of seminars, and on one such occasion made the acquaintance of a young anaesthetist and surgeon, Pierre Huguenard (1924-2006). They became friends, and Huguenard began to experiment with 'lytic cocktails' of drugs that might both repress patients' agitation, and stabilise their blood pressure. It was Huguenard who first tried promethazine, as Charpentier's new compound was called, on a patient. It was a woman of the *haut monde*, determined to have a cosmetic operation on her nose, but terrified nonetheless of the bloody ordeal, which she would have to endure under local anaesthetic, since the procedure obviously precluded the use of an anaesthetic mask. Huguenard began by dropping into her nose a mixture of promethazine and pethidine, a local anaethetic, not long available. He was surprised to see his agitated patient become suddenly tranquil, and apparently quite indifferent to her circumstances. She heard the impact of the hammer, which broke her nose, but met it with composure.

Laborit and Huguenard thereupon embarked on a more comprehensive study of the effects of RP4560 on human subjects, but Laborit, who worried about some untoward effects of high doses, and wanted a faster-acting substance, also begged Charpentier to make more and better derivatives. Charpentier complied, and it was one of this next series, synthesised at the end of 1950, that would change history. Tested on rats in the Rhône-Poulenc laboratories, modest doses of the compound induced an indifference to electric shocks in the otherwise perfectly alert animals. Laborit and Huguenard began trials of the new material on surgical patients at the Val-de-Grâce hospital. They gave it intravenously, together with the routinely used pethidine, and it more than fulfilled all expectations. The patients became calm and felt reassured, their blood pressure remained stable, and their temperature under anaesthesia fell from the normal 37 to 33-35°C (from 98.4 to 91.5-95°F), which fitted gratifyingly with Laborit's theory of 'hibernation'. The drug was also an aid to analgesia, for it it hastened the action of anaesthetics when given in mixtures, and it suppressed vomiting. Because of the broad scope of its action, Laborit suggested Largactil (*large* – broad in French – action) as the name of the drug, which in America was eventually registered as Thorazine, but is better known universally as *chlorpromazine*. His hibernation theory also impelled Laborit to embed anaesthetised patients in ice-packs, but this had no discernible effect, and indeed the theory had no physiological basis.

The bearing that the new tranquilliser might have on the treatment of psychiatric patients could scarcely be overlooked, nor was it lost on Laborit, and he and Huguenard indicated as much in their first publication. Almost immediately the psychiatrists at the Val-de-Grâce tried the drug on patients receiving sleep therapy, though in a mixture with conventional preparations, and reported on its advantageous effects. The first systematic trial was undertaken on a cohort of 38 psychotic patients at the Hôpital Sainte-Anne, the largest psychiatric hospital in the city, and also a teaching hospital attached to the University. In the rancorous dispute dragging on at the time between the psychoanalysts and the psychiatrists, wedded to therapy by means of drugs, the institution was fully aligned with the latter school. Pierre Deniker, who had charge of one of the wards, had read the work of Laborit and Huguenard, and approached Rhône-Poulenc for a sample of RP4560. He and the autocratic director of the hospital, Jean Delay (whose name appeared on all publications of work performed by his staff) gave the patients the drug by itself, and reported the outcome at a French Congress of Psychiatry and Neurology in 1952. They followed this by a series of publications in the leading French medical journals, starting in 1954. The results had been startling. Even violent patients, seen as hopeless cases, destined to remain immured for life, recovered, and many could be discharged. Deniker did more: he treated patients suffering from various types of mental disturbances with chlorpromazine with equally gratifying outcomes. He also, albeit accidentally, disproved Laborit's hypothermia theory: the hospital pharmacy was unable to keep pace with the demand for ice-packs, and so Deniker was forced to dispense with them, with, as it turned out, no detriment to the efficacy of the treatment.

In 1954 Deniker travelled to Canada to expound the wonders of chlorpromazine to the local practitioners. The news quickly spread to the U.S., where it was received within weeks of Kline's revelations on the efficacy of reserpine. In Montreal a German psychiatrist, who had trained in Berlin, had emigrated in 1937, and was himself a depressive, read a report in a French journal about the new drug that had emerged from Rhône-Poulenc. Heinz Edgar Lehmann went into action at once, and set up the first clinical trial on a group of 70 severely afflicted schizophrenics, depressives and assorted psychotics. His report on the results came at almost the same time as Deniker's talk in 1954. It told that after a week nearly all the subjects were almost unrecognisably improved. Even so, it was some time before psychiatrists were fully persuaded, and a problem that persisted was the high cost of chlorpromazine compared to reserpine. But once set in motion, the chlorpromazine bandwagon could not be held back. In time the drug, marketed in America by Smith, Kline and French, as Thorazine, all but replaced reserpine, which in addition to its lower potency has a more complex structure, and was thus a more difficult proposition for organic chemists to modify. Chlorpromazine and its relatives dominated the market for treatment of schizophrenic, and for psychotic patients generally, for some twenty years, certainly one of the great clinical advances of the 20th century. Its magnitude was obvious to all who worked in mental hospitals, and even passers-by at the Hôpital Sainte-Anne noticed that the perpetual din of manic and schizophrenic patients in the wards had abated. Of the main protagonists in the story, five - Laborit, Deniker, Lehmann and also Kline and Robert Noce, another American clinician who contributed to the formulation of chlorpromazine therapy - received the highly coveted American Lasker Award for advances in clinical research. But some of them caught the scent of something bigger; for did the discovery not merit the highest accolade of all, the Nobel Prize? Delay too craved recognition, and he at least left to psychiatric posterity a new word, *neuroleptic*, for a drug that acts to alter for the better any psychotic state.* There was some ugly bickering: Deniker made clear his belief that he was owed greater recognition, and Laborit, too, was aggrieved, and evidently died an embittered man. Perhaps in retrospect the action of chlorpromazine on psychoses should not have been quite so surprising, for another phenothiazine is methylene blue, Paul Ehrlich's favourite dye, which in those remote days had been tried as a treatment. Its modest success had not sufficed to stimulate further efforts. At all events, it is beyond doubt that chlorpromazine reduced mightily the sum of human suffering. It has even been described as a landmark in human history. In the decade beginning with its introduction into the clinic, some 50 million people made use of the drug.

At much the same time other chance discoveries – if discoveries they were – caught the attention of psychiatrists. Isoniazid, the first successful synthetic compound for treatment of tuberculosis (p.), was found by two doctors at the Sea View Hospital on Staten Island in New York to have a generally euphoric effect on the patients. This went, the physicians thought, beyond mere relief at the abatement of the disease. They tried the drug on patients with severe depression, and especially those with what is now called bipolar disorder; they showed, the doctors thought, a marked improvement. Iproniazid, a modified version of isoniazid, did even better, and with the advocacy of the ubiquitous Nathan Kline, came into wide use. For a while it did good service for the treatment of both depression and tuberculosis, but in 1961 it was withdrawn, following repeated reports of liver damage. Both drugs were in any case supplanted by imipramine, which was developed at the start of the 1950s as an antihistamine. Since antihistamines had produced such abundant rewards in the treatment of

---

* Delay appears to have been generally unpopular. Jean Thuillier, a member of the team at the Hôpital Sainte-Anne, recounted in a book, written some 25 years later in 1980, that during the student riots in Paris in 1968 Delay, as one of the undeserving *patrons*, became a target, and his office was pillaged.

psychoses, the Swiss Geigy (later Novartis) company began a hopeful search through the large number of such compounds that they had prepared and for various reasons shelved. Among them was one, designated G22355, which had a structure quite similar to that of chlorpromazine. Along with an assortment of other substances, it was given to several local psychiatrists to test.

One of them was Roland Kuhn, who finding as the others presumably also had, that the compound had no beneficial properties when tested on schizophrenics, in fact aggravated their symptoms, nevertheless persisted. For he thought, as nobody else had, that it seemed to ease the condition of a number of severely depressed subjects. He went on to test it on some hundreds of mental patients, and concluded that it worked extremely well on a subset – on those whose depression was accompanied by movement abnormalities. For this reason, when it came on stream in 1958, it offered no serious competition to the other antidepressants (a term apparently first used by Kuhn), which were then entering the market. It was a popular drug nonetheless, and must have given a further impetus to the chase after other antihistamines with unpredictable neuropsychiatric actions. The continuing search threw up several such compounds with interesting properties, real or imagined, and some reached the clinics, either transiently or – like Eli Lilley's sleeping pill, Sominex, and the all-purpose headache and flu medicine, Tylenol – for the long haul. The irony is that the undoubtedly sincere labours of Kuhn and so many other psychiatrists were in the main, if not entirely, built on sand, as we shall see.

The advent of chlorpromazine had in any event set off a frenzied search by other pharmaceutical companies for equally effective ('me-too') tranquilizers, and many variants were produced, some of which found applications in the treatment of other conditions, such as Parkinson's disease. The Rhône-Poulenc chemists, never idle, came up with prochlorperazine, which appeared under many trade names, such as Stemetil and Compazine. As a tranquilliser it was pronounced ten times more powerful than chlorpromazine. It also had anti-emetic properties, and was (and is) an excellent suppressor of travel sickness. It was tried out on French soldiers for that purpose, but was quickly abandoned when the men were seen to sink down and refuse to take any interest in what went on around them. It had other side-effects in addition, particularly the muscle stiffness and tremors that were also manifested by some patients given high doses of chlorpromazine. These effects were reminiscent of the symptoms of Parkinson's disease, and were seen as a further incentive to develop alternative drugs.

Among the thousands of synthetic products made and tested for tranquilliser activity, some of which entered clinical practice, one emerged supreme. It was not a phenothiazine, but a distant relative of the opioid analgesic, pethidine. Its creator was a Belgian chemist, Paul Janssen, who ran his own company, founded originally by his father. In 1957 he was searching, not for a tranquilliser but for an analgesic to improve on pethidine in speed of response and potency. His idea was to make the molecule more hydrophobic (p.), so that it would more rapidly traverse the fatty nerve sheath. The new product, norpethidine was indeed an improvement, though not for the reason Janssen supposed. He continued to tinker with the structure, taking it in new directions, and he found answering changes in activity. Finally he generated a compound, R1625, which had truly remarkable physiological properties. It engendered a catatonic state in laboratory rats, deeper than that produced by chlorpromazine. It nullified the stimulatory effects of amphetamines (p.), which were then much favoured by sportsmen, by soldiers and pilots and others needing to resist sleep and maintain alertness (as well, of course, as many pleasure seekers). Janssen asked to have his compound evaluated by the staff of a mental hospital in Liège, but they took an interest only when the deranged son of one of the doctors suffered a mental collapse and failed to respond to the usual drugs. The R1625 effected an immediate and startling improvement, and thereafter tests on schizophrenic and other patients showed the drug to surpass all other tranquillisers in its potency, for it was some 100 times more effective weight for weight than chlorpromazine, and low in side-effects. This drug is *haloperidol*, also known by the trade name of Haldol. It was quickly adopted throughout Europe, but in the United States FDA approbation came only after ten years.

The manic marvel

Perhaps the most remarkable and unanticipated coup in the history of neuropharmacology came in 1948, five years before chlorpromazine from an improbable quarter. Lithium is the third-lightest element, a metal belonging to the same group in the Periodic Table as sodium and potassium, and the salts of these elements are all similar in their chemical attributes. There was no logical sequence by which the pharmacological effect of lithium salts could have been divined, and their discovery was an inspired accident. John Frederick Joseph Cade (1912-1980) was an Australian psychiatrist in a small mental hospital in Melbourne when the story began to unfold. The son of a doctor, he had qualified in Melbourne and specialised in psychiatry, when at the outbreak of World War II, he joined the army as a surgeon, and was posted to Singapore. He was there when it was overrun by the Japanese and spent the next three years in the notorious Changi jail. In 1945 he returned to Melbourne, and after a period of recuperation took up a position in the Bundoora Repatriation Mental Hospital. In between treating his patients he set up a rudimentary research laboratory in a derelict kitchen. His odd idea was that manic depression – what is now called bipolar disease – might be the result of a toxin produced in the body. The thinking behind this fancy was that thyrotoxicosis, the condition caused by excess output of thyroid hormone (p.), leads to a mentally excited state, not unlike that seen in the manic phase of Cade's patients. Were it so, the substance might be excreted in the urine, as many extraneous toxins also are. To test this exceedingly long shot Cade collected urine samples from depressives and normal control subjects, and injected them into guinea pigs. The animals sickened, regardless of the origin of the urine that they had received, but Cade was not discouraged, and tried another curious experiment. For no very obvious reason he tried urea, the main waste-product in the urine, extracted from the urine samples. This the guinea pigs did not tolerate at all, and they all died, presumably of kidney failure.

Cade pressed on. His next thought was to try uric acid. This is a compound related to urea, and a metabolic product, excreted in the urine. A too high concentration of uric acid in the blood is associated with gout. Some animals, particularly birds, excrete uric acid as the metabolic end-product instead of urea. The concentration of uric acid can never approach that of urea because its solubility is low. As an acid, however, it can form salts and some of these are much more soluble. A search in the chemical literature revealed to Cade that the lithium salt, lithium urate was one that had the desired property. Lithium, moreover, was cheap. Administered in moderate quantity it seemed to do the guinea pigs no harm, and in fact diminished the malign effects of urea. Cade found that the normally agitated guinea pigs became calmer and more tolerant of the hypodermic. This was probably due to nothing more than toxicity. All the same, it was at this point that Cade ceased groping for inspiration, and did a control. He had treated his guinea pigs with two new substances, uric acid and lithium, and it was not out of the question that it was the lithium and not the uric acid that was responsible for the effect. Cade found some lithium carbonate and experienced his eureka moment. He did not dissemble: 'that' he later wrote, 'is how lithium came into the story'. It is unlikely that Cade knew of the scattered reports of dubious validity from the 19th century and earlier, of the clinical uses of lithium; he would not have thought to scan the obscure journals in which they appeared, even if he had had access to them.

At all events, he tried lithium carbonate and lithium citrate on a few of his most intractable patients, who made an astonishing recovery. Cade was cautious and warned against possible side-effects, but his report in the *Australian Journal of Medicine* in 1949 stirred up no little local interest. Another Melbourne psychiatrist, together with a physiologist, conducted a trial on 100 patients in mental clinics with excellent results on manic depressives. More such revelations followed, but doctors around the world really took notice only when a Danish doctor, Mogens Schou repeated the Australian observations and published a comprehensive study. But then came reports, mainly from the U.S., of serious side-effects and a number of deaths from heart and kidney failure. Moreover, lithium held no attraction for the pharmaceutical companies because, as natural substances, lithium salts could not be patented, and so was not properly advertised or distributed.

In the U.S. the use of lithium was banned, and remained unavailable to mental patients until 1970. It had emerged, however, that the victims were people with heart disease, and it turned out that the dangers had been greatly exaggerated. Analyses of lithium concentrations in the blood were belatedly conducted, and schedules for safe doses, including maintenance doses, were worked out. It was seen as a tragedy that so many desperate, often suicidal patients, especially in America, had for so long been denied relief. Cade had by then moved on to more elevated positions in Melbourne, and later received many prizes and other marks of recognition. They were well deserved, for lithium therapy has arguably done as much to relieve human suffering as any other single drug in the 20th century. A postscript appeared in 2009, when Japanese researchers announced to the world of psychiatry a negative correlation between the incidence of suicides in different parts of a prefecture in their country and the concentration of lithium in the water. These vary with the nature of the rocks, but are always minute compared to the amounts given therapeutically. The authors of the paper suggest that even these small amounts ingested over long periods may exert a neurophysiological effect. While recommending caution and further research, they foresaw the possibility of the addition of lithium salts to the drinking water where the natural concentration is low.

Big Pharma tightens its grip

Mental illness had in general had little attraction for the major pharmaceutical companies until well into the latter part of the 20th century, and then, quite suddenly, it grew to monstrous proportions. The cult of Freud and his followers, and those of his rivals had held sway, and most of their numerous adherents were resolutely hostile to chemical intrusion into the brain, which they guarded as their province. Chlorpromazine and lithium had certainly made a breach in their defences, and the barbiturates had become for many an indispensable adjunct to a good life. The revolution was initiated, thanks to a mixture of chance and astuteness, by two central European Jewish emigrés, running from the Nazis just before World War II. The director of one of the great American museums commented at this time that 'Hitler shakes the tree and I collect the apples'. So it worked for the American pharmaceutical companies.

Frank Milan Berger (1913-2008) was born in Pilsen, now Plzeň in the Czech Republic, which was at the time a part of the Austro-Hungarian empire. His father was German, his mother French. He qualified as a doctor at the Charles University in Prague, worked for a while on a research project to treat gonorrhoea with oestrogen, and then took up a position as a bacteriologist in the Czechoslovak Institute of Health. He had been there only a few months when the German army marched into the country, and he departed hastily for England. There he was instantly interned as an enemy alien. He ministered to his fellow-inmates as a doctor until his release, when he was allowed to join the chemical company, British Drug Houses (BDH), which was working for the Government, and return to his calling as a bacteriologist. The task to which he was assigned was to develop a means of preserving the penicillin then being urgently manufactured in quantity. The problem was contamination with Gram-negative bacteria (p.), which were not susceptible to penicillin, and in fact produced their own means of destroying it – an enzyme, penicillinase. The antiseptic then added to penicillin solutions to avert such contamination was unreliable, and Berger was searching for a similar but better compound, lacking toxicity, to add to the penicillin preparations. One that he tried became known as mephensin, and displayed an unexpected effect when tested for toxicity in mice and guinea pigs: the animals became motionless, and entered a trance-like state, while still conscious. Rhesus monkeys, aggressive by nature, became docile and friendly. Berger realised that the chemical was a muscle relaxant, strong enough to engender total inertia. In small doses it appeared merely to render the animals soporific. Berger published a paper on his observations in 1946, and mephensin came into use for the treatment of spasticity and uncontrollable tremors. The next year Berger emigrated to the United States. He went first to a junior faculty position at the University of Rochester Medical School in Minnesota, and after two years, became in 1949 research director of a small pharmaceutical laboratory in New Jersey.

The Wallace Laboratories were a subsidiary of Carter Products, chiefly remembered as manufacturers of Carter's Little Liver Pills, a patent medicine guaranteed to rescue the 'under par and listless' from their miserable state. The pills also had the unusual and impressive property of turning the urine a vivid turquoise. (The manufacturers were later made to delete 'liver' from the name.) Berger seems to have been given a free hand, and he began by recruiting an able organic chemist, Bernard Ludwig. Berger's objective was to find a better soporific or anxiolytic than mephensin, which was short-acting, and after synthesising and testing well over a thousand compounds, he and Ludwig struck gold. The product was meprobamate, more familiarly known by its trade name, *Miltown*. It was also licensed to Wyeth Laboratories, who marketed it under the name of *Equanil*. It was tested on a hundred assorted patients in mental hospitals in Mississippi, of whom a few were adjudged totally cured of their afflictions, and most of the rest much, or a little, improved. Miltown gained FDA approval in 1955, but initially there was little response from the profession or enthusiasm within the company.

Berger, though, had worked up an evangelical fervour over the exceptional benison that his drug would confer on an anxiety-ridden population. It would, he believed, allay suffering and spread contentment, and his protestations won the company over. Up to then a very proper caution had prevailed about the possible consequences of prescribing drugs that tampered with the workings of the brain, except in seriously ill patients. Now Berger and his company got their way, thanks in part, at least, to a *coup de théâtre* that he himself devised: he organised the shooting of a film, showing rhesus monkeys before and after – aggressive, then placid and finally relaxing amicably. It was shown to assemblies of doctors, and made an instant impression, helped probably by growing unease about the addictive properties of the barbiturates then coming to light. Another step, taken apparently at the urging of Nathan Kline (p.), was to brand the drug, not as a sedative but as a tranquilliser, then a new concept, though essentially a distinction without a difference. Miltown was launched with a gigantic advertising campaign, and its success was stupendous. By 1956 an estimated one American in twenty was taking the drug. It made appearances in films, books, songs and stories, and the manufacturers were unable to keep pace with the demand. Notices reading 'Out of Miltown – more Tomorrow' appeared in the windows of chemists' shops, or sometimes, 'We have Miltown'. The main consumers were women, and so fashion accoutrements appeared in the jewellers' shops, such as signet rings to contain a single pill, and pill boxes, encrusted with precious stones. There were even Miltown cocktails, consisting of Martinis into which pills were dropped. Miltown was a new phenomenon in medical and social history.

The noses of the pharmaceutical companies, twitching in the wind, caught the scent of profits on an unprecedented scale. There had been several accidental discoveries before meprobamate, which had not been exploited. One had emerged from a search for an antimalarial, another was a derivative of thiamine (vitamin B_1), and yet another (given the provocative name of Oblivon) came out of a steroid investigation. But, following the rise of Miltown, meprobamate progeny were being synthesised in profusion, none apparently offering any great advantages over Miltown itself. Some came from Berger's laboratory, offered as muscle relaxants, and he created a number of other profitable products, without ever recapturing anything like his first grand coup. Miltown was thought to be non-addictive, but this was shown in time to be a misapprehension. Its primacy did not, in any case, survive the emergence of another class of tranquillisers, the diazepines in 1960. They arose out of yet another chance observation.

Leo Henryk Sternbach (1908-2005) was born, like Frank Berger, in an outpost of the Austro-Hungarian empire, Abbazia (Opatia in what is now independent Croatia). Having, as a boy, helped out in his father's pharmacy, he went on to study chemistry, and took his doctoral degree at the Jagiellonian University in Kraków. He had a penchant for organic synthesis and wrote his thesis on an unexplored class of compounds to which he was to return later. Hounded out of Poland by antisemitism, he worked briefly in Vienna, then in Zurich at the famous technical university, the ETH. Then in 1940 he took a position at one of the world's great pharmaceutical concerns, Hoffmann-La Roche in Basel. The following year most of Europe had been overrun by Germany, and there were fears that Switzerland might be next. The company took the admirably enlightened course of sending its Jewish employees to its American branch at Nutley, New Jersey, and there Sternbach took root, and remained to the end of his long and illustrious career. The company had begun, in the wake of chlorpromazine, to consider entering the field of psychoactive drugs. Sternbach took up the challenge, and decided in the first place to investigate some new tricyclic molecules (those containing three carbon and nitrogen rings) - like chlorpromazine in fact. His thoughts turned to compounds of a ring system with which he was familiar from his days in Kraków – the quinazolones – and to what substituent groups in the rings might exert an interesting influence. But by then the management was having second thoughts, and Sternbach was told to abandon this line of research, and take up another project. He chose nevertheless to continue pursuing his tricyclics in spare moments, and he synthesised forty or so compounds of the quinazolone series. Animal tests yielded no worthwhile activity from any of them, but then came the first stroke of good fortune. One of the forty-some compounds had been forgotten, and eighteen months after these events, a research assistant, clearing up the laboratory detritus, found it and instead of throwing it away, asked Sternbach whether it should be discarded or sent for testing. After a pause for thought, Sternbach decided that it might as well be tested like all the others. The report came back from the head of the pharmacology section: the compound had powerful tranquillising activity in mice, much like Berger's meprobamate, though better. It turned out also to be an anxiolytic and a muscle relaxant, all with a very low level of toxicity and little in the way of detectable side-effects.

The new substance created no little excitement, and also posed a question: why, if all the other compounds based on the same ring system had no measurable physiological activity, was this solitary specimen so different? Sternbach returned to the chemistry, and quickly discovered that the molecule was not a quinazolone at all. The particular substituent in one of the rings had been the cause of an unsuspected reaction, which converted one of the three six-atom rings to a ring of seven atoms – a seven-sided polygon. It was the first ever member of a new series, a benzodiazepine, and in 1960 chlordiazepoxide was granted FDA approval, and thudded onto the market as *Librium*. There can be few parallels for the luck that accompanied so momentous a discovery – one man's decision to trust his instinct and persist with his plan, contrary to the wishes of his employers; the wholly accidental emergence of a new and seemingly improbable class of compounds; and finally the chance recovery of a forgotten synthetic product, and its reprieve from the rubbish-bin.

Sternbach immediately set about determining whether the complex structure, accidentally generated, could be simplified, and its properties improved. It took him only a year to produce a simpler and much more potent derivative, diazepam, known as *Valium*. Like Librium its side-effects appeared few and its toxicity minimal. (This was emphatically demonstrated when President Reagan's security adviser, Robert McFarlane attempted suicide, following the exposure of the infamous Iran-Contra arms scandal in 1986. He ingested two dozen Valium pills, and sank into a refreshing slumber, from which he awoke some days later, well rested and restored to a more optimistic frame of mind.) Valium quickly became the most widely prescribed drug in the country, and soon the world. It maintained that position from 1969 until 1982, and at its peak of popularity more than 2.3 billion pills were gulped in a single year in America alone. Indeed, about a quarter of the country's citizens were popping Valium. It was "Mother's little helper", and an estimated one in five American women became users. Its unprecedented success set off a frantic search after more benzodiazepines, with advantages, real and imaginary. Thousands were synthesised, but Sternbach maintained his lead with fluorazepam, known as Dalmaine. nitrazepam, or Mogadon, and several others. Many benzodiazepam tranquillisers (minor tranquillisers, as they are now termed) are in abundant use still. Leo Sternbach rose through the Hoffmann-La Roche hierarchy, but never entirely abandoned the laboratory bench until his retirement, nor did he deviate from his principle of himself sampling all promising compounds that he had synthesised. Among a series of other achievements he brought off the first commercial synthesis of the vitamin, biotin. An amiable, undemanding and contented man, he never made money from his many discoveries, and sold his patents for Librium and Valium to the company for $1 apiece. Sternbach was still visiting the laboratory daily when he was well over ninety years old.

Valium became the most profitable drug in the world. In the United States its sale price was twenty times the manufacturing cost, and it made many billions of dollars for the company. It was advertised to doctors and to the public with unparalleled abandon. The fair wind that it enjoyed was reinforced by the waning of Miltown. With the rise of more rigorous, placebo-controlled clinical trials, and a more scientific formulation of criteria for the actions of psychoactive drugs generally, criticism of Miltown had grown. An influential paper published in 1971 by two American psychiatrists at the Montefiore Hospital in New York was a death-blow: meprobamate, they asserted, 'is no less toxic and no more effective in reducing anxiety than a barbiturate such as phenobarbital' (by then fallen out of favour). And they concluded in damning fashion, 'the history of the tranquillizer meprobamate illustrates how factors other than scientific evidence may determine patterns of physicians' drug use. Forceful advertising and publicity; an attitude of general optimism, and uncontrolled studies with favourable results combined to elevate meprobamate to the position of America's magical cure-all tranquillizer. This drug remains in wide use despite a large body of sound scientific data that questions its efficacy'.

The words still resonate.

It was some time before it dawned on doctors that dependence and abuse of the diazepines, Valium in particular, were becoming a pressing problem, and that the drug was often taken in excess, and also used for pleasure. In 2003 the *New Yorker* magazine ran an article about a party at the Nutley laboratories to commemorate the fortieth birthday of Valium, and incidentally the ninety-fifth of Leo Sternbach. He opined, according to the *New Yorker*, that "It's a very good drug. It has pleasant side effects. It's quite a good sleeping drug, too. That's why it's abused". And then he added: "My wife doesn't let me take it".

Hoffmann-La Roche evidently took fright at the alarming reports of dependency, and the Basel myrmidons were set the task in the early 1970s of finding an antidote for a benzodiazepine overdose. They had no success, but then in 1979, when they had long abandoned the search, they accidentally found what they had originally wanted. They had still at that stage been trying to synthesise new benzodiazepams with more restricted effects than those of Valium and the others. It was one of the new compounds that reversed the deep torpor induced by a Valium overdose. It acted by competing with the established drugs on their receptor (p.), and went under the name of flumazenil, sold as Anexate, Lenexate or in America as Romazicon.

Meanwhile in the 1960s another psychoactive drug had crept into the pharmacopoeia in the wake of a new malady – attention deficit hyperactive disorder, or ADHD. That there are people who incline to restlessness and find difficulty in concentrating has been intermittently remarked on by doctors since at least the 18th century. In the mid-20th century ambitious parents in the prosperous western societies came to see such tendencies in their offspring as an actual disease. The drug companies were not slow to see a gap in the market. Methylphenidate was first synthesised as long ago as 1944 by a chemist in the Swiss Ciba company (which is now Novartis), but a decade seems to have elapsed before its potential was recognised. The chemist responsible for the compound had a wife called Rita, and when in 1954 its stimulant character came to light he would give her a little to boost her energy. He named the substance *Ritalin*. It had effects that pleased the consumers: it raised alertness and held back fatigue, and since only trivial side-effects could be found, it was held to be safer than alternatives, such as amphetamine. The FDA made only one condition: Ritalin must not be given to children under the age of six, for how could one know whether the drug might not have some long-term effect on brain development? Intensive advertising engendered a belief that Ritalin should be used to assuage everyday domestic miseries – tensions in the home, irritations at work, the trials of commuting, the 'empty-nest' effect, and so on. Side-effects inevitably began to show themselves, the more so when consumers, especially the young, discovered its recreational possibilities, and took it regularly and in large quantities, as they had previously taken Benzedrine (p.). The debate about the wisdom of consuming Ritalin without restrictions, and especially of using it to tame unruly children, has never abated.

Ritalin has competition. Adderall is a 'cognitive enhancer', popular with students and with workers in occupations demanding alertness over long stretches - commodity traders no doubt, for example. It is a mixture of amphetamine enantiomers (p.), and therefore of quite ancient lineage. Like Ritalin, it is not licensed for the its most common uses, for which it is procured off-label. Adderall is sold in a fast- and a slow-release form. A more sophisticated drug was developed in France in the late 1970s. Its begetter, Michel Jouvet (b. 1926), is a retired professor at the University of Lyon, noted for his studies on sleep, and still immersed in research on the subject. He was trying the effects on animals of a series of compounds, which he hoped might lead to a treatment for narcolepsy (p.), a condition defined by a tendency to fall suddenly asleep at any time of day. Jouvet found what he wanted, and began to treat patients with the new product, adrafinil in 1986. Continuing research brought to light a better compound, the active metabolite of adrafinil, a prodrug. This was called modafinil, and Jouvet approached Laboratoires Lafon in Paris, who agreed to produce the drug under the trade name of Modiodal, bringing it into clinical use in 1994. Four years later Lafon licensed their product to an American company, Cephalon (which eventually bought Lafon). It was approved by the FDA as a treatment for narcolepsy, 'shift-work disorder', sleep apnoea (interruption of normal breathing), and other sleep-related problems. Modafinil was reborn as Provigil, in which guise it has penetrated into the sleep-deprived professions, but more especially into universities and even schools as a stimulant and 'cognitive enhancer'. One neurologist in the U.S. has termed this 'cosmetic neurology'. Side-effects of taking, or as some would say, abusing these compounds have been reported, ranging from heart problems to addiction. Yet they seem to be here to stay, and surveys in the U.S. have revealed that in some seats of learning as many as one in three students use cognitive enhancers. Social observers have also described a new craze among adolescents: 'pill parties' consist in swallowing handfuls of randomly mixed pills taken from a bowl, and awaiting developments.

New generation: hopes and illusions

In the 1970s the strategy of antipsychotic drug research underwent a change. It became less reliant on random exploration of promising classes of compounds, and increasingly informed by discoveries in brain biochemistry. The compounds generated in the 1950s are referred to now (though some experts regard this as a distinction without a difference) as 'first generation', or 'typical' antipsychotics, and those that progressively displaced them are 'second generation' or 'atypical' antipsychotics (or if not antipsychotics, then neuroleptics, from the Greek stem, meaning to seize the neurones). Conversely the relation between drugs and their receptors in the brain seemed to offer new insights into the complexities of brain function. In reality the waters were a little more muddy than the triumphalism of the pharmaceutical companies, and of many of their academic consultants made it appear. The revolution can be said to have begun with the discovery of acetylcholine (p.), and it took flight with the uncovering of a profusion of other neurotransmitters, all with their cognate receptors.* The ramifications appeared endless. Even acetylcholine has more than a single receptor: there are two classes, called muscarinic and nicotinic receptors, named after the substances first found to block their action - muscarine, the toxin of the *Amanita* mushroom in the one case, and nicotine derivatives in the other. Some neurotransmitters are excitatory, that is to say they cause the target cell at the synapse to 'fire', while others are 'inhibitory', and quench such a process. The neurotransmitters that

---

* We need here a rudimentary picture of how the system operates. A neurone, or nerve cell, of which there are many billions in the brain, comprises a long filament (axon), a globular 'cell body', which contains the metabolic machinery, and emanating from the axon, a large number of fine, branched threads called dendrites. (The term alludes to the branches and twigs of a tree.) Through these dendrites the neurone forms contacts with other neurones in a vast network through which chemical signals pass continuously back and forth. Some emit and some receive. This traffic occurs at the synapses, where pairs of dendrites meet. The synapse (as previously outlined [p.] in relation to the neuromuscular junction) is a minute cleft between the two partners, and the signal – a neurotransmitter substance – passes in tiny packets from the emitter to the receiver, where it is taken up by receptors, which recognise the particular neurotransmitter. The signal is conveyed into the axon, and, when it has done its work, the surplus neurotransmitter is eliminated, generally by an enzyme.

largely control brain function are *monoamines* – quite simple compounds containing a single amino (-NH$_2$) group. The ones that matter most in relation to psychoactive drugs are dopamine, adrenaline (epinephrine in American usage), noradrenaline (norepinephrine) and serotonin, all found in the 1950s to be regulators of brain functions.

It was already known by the early years of that decade that victims of Parkinson's disease had an abnormally low concentration of one particular monoamine, dopamine in a part of the brain (the basal ganglia) in which this chemical is mainly concentrated. The Parkinson's-like manifestations engendered by high doses of chlorpromazine or reserpine therefore gave rise to the conjecture that the drugs might perhaps interact in some way with the dopamine pool. A Swedish pharmacologist, Arvid Carlsson (b. 1923) at the University of Göteborg found in 1957 that while reserpine did indeed lower the dopamine concentration in the brains of laboratory rats, chlorpromazine had no such effect. Carlsson did not abandon the theory, but measured the metabolic breakdown products of the dopamine, excreted in the rats' urine, and found that the amounts went up in animals given chlorpromazine. Was the drug then perhaps an *agonist* (the opposite in pharmacospeak of an antagonist), and forcing the brain to secrete an excess of dopamine? So whereas reserpine impeded dopamine release from the nerve terminal, chlorpromazine blocked the access of the dopamine to its receptor. With the dopamine prevented from doing its work, the dopamine-secreting cells would receive the false message that there was an insufficiency of dopamine, and they must therefore make more. The two drugs were therefore achieving the same end in contrary ways. This was a notable intellectual leap, and Carlsson's results also implied that dopamine was a neurotransmitter, a conclusion strongly resisted, even ridiculed, by the physiology establishment of the time, led by Sir Henry Dale. Carlsson recalled in his Nobel Lecture – he shared the Prize with two American neurobiologists in 2000 – that when he reported his results at a meeting in London in 1960, it was as though he had not spoken; he was simply ignored. In the event Carlsson did a great deal more, and in particular made a huge contribution to the understanding and treatment of Parkinson's disease, as will be seen.

Clozapine (commercially known by many names, most commonly Clozaril) is often seen as the first of the 'atypical' drugs, in the sense that it exhibits a specific preference for one neurotransmitter receptor, and therefore represses primarily the action of that neurotransmitter, serotonin. It crept into use in Europe in the early 1960s, produced by Sandoz in Switzerland, although it had first been synthesised some years before, but not subjected to controlled trials until 1972. It was found to have remarkable efficacy in eliminating the delusions and hallucinations of schizophrenia, and was enthusiastically deployed by psychiatrists for that purpose. Then a dismaying side-effect made itself known. The drug prevented the production of granulocytes, a type of white blood cell with an important role in countering infections. A report came from Finland that a group of patients on clozapine had been struck down by infections, and several had died. The drug was abruptly withdrawn, but not forgotten, for some schizophrenic patients became resistant to the alternatives, and more than ten years later it was reinstated. It is given to severely affected patients. The granulocyte count in their blood is monitored, and the drug dose regulated accordingly. It is more effective than any of the older ('typical') drugs, and apart from the loss of granulocytes, there are fewer side-effects than manifested by chlorpromazine and its direct successors, such as haloperidol and fluphenazine. Needless to say, the efficacy of clozapine set off an intense search after similar compounds that would control schizophrenia, while eschewing its one major drawback. The quest was greatly helped by the development of an *in-vitro* assay that allowed binding to different receptors to be measured on brain extracts*. This and other technical advances disclosed that many drugs were not specific, or had only a weak preference, for a particular receptor. Thus clozapine bound strongly to the serotonin receptor, but also, though to a lesser extent, to the dopamine receptor. And then it transpired that there was

---

* The technique was developed by Solomon Snyder, a brain researcher at Johns Hopkins University in Baltimore. Macerated brain tissue contains intact synapses, which can be partly purified, encased in microscopic membrane bubbles (synaptosomes). Radioactively labelled drugs can then be assayed for their ability to bind to the synapses. The strength of binding can be determined, and also exactly how effective the compound is in displacing another drug already bound, for instance in the living animal before it was killed.

not just one, dopamine receptors, but several, labelled D_1, D_2, D_3 and so on, all with different affinities for particular drugs. From these new revelations came compounds of greater specificity and, it was proclaimed, fewer unwanted effects. Eli Lilly scored a notable success with olanzapine, which as Zyprexa became the sovereign anti-schizophrenia medication, and one of the most profitable drugs of all time. It is also popular in the form of Symbiax, a mixture with fluoxetine (Paxil). Yet Zyprexa too has had its vicissitudes, culminating in some 18,000 out-of-court settlements, on account of its tendency to cause obesity, with the ills that stem from it. There were also reports that it could *induce* schizophrenia-like symptom in people who did not have the condition. Then there was Pfizer's sertraline, commonly known as Lustral, an SSRI (see below) introduced in 1991, and found effective for 'panic disorder', but later stated by the FDA to be only marginally better than a placebo. Many other psychoactive drugs were launched, none without their problems, as will appear.

Many of the leading brain researchers, including Carlsson, learned the exacting analytical skills that made possible the untangling of the biochemical action of psychoactive drugs, while working at the National Institutes of Health near Washington. Most sat at the feet of one of its most prominent pioneers, Bernard Brodie (1907-1989). It was Brodie and his associates and disciples who discriminated between the various neurotransmitter-controlled circuits in the brain. The new data made sense, at least in principle, of the actions of a number of the established psychotropic drugs. To begin with there were the amphetamines (p.), such as amphetamine itself, or the much more powerful methamphetamine. Animal experiments revealed that the primary function of these drugs is to provoke a surge of dopamine into the synapses. But nothing is ever quite what it seems when one is dealing with an organ of such impenetrable complexity*. Secondary effects must also be at work; for one thing, the irrigation of synapses happens almost immediately after the drug enters the body, while the psychological effects develop on a much slower time-scale. There are evidently therefore longer-term reactions in the brain contingent on the continuing saturation of receptors.

Next came the revelation that iproniazid (Marsilid) worked by inactivating an enzyme, monoamine oxidase. Its function is to destroy (by oxidation, as the name implies) the monoamine neurotransmitters. Any neurotransmitter must be eliminated when it has carried out its mission, for otherwise stimulation would never cease. The drug can, on the other hand, overcome a pathological insufficiency of the neurotransmitter. Other monoamine oxidase inhibitors came into use later, but all had their drawbacks. One of the most widely used, an amphetamine compound, tranylcypromine (Parnate or Jatosom) was developed by Smith, Kline and French, as it then was, in 1960; its most curious and if disregarded, dangerous side-effect is the 'cheese effect' - a reaction with a simple metabolite, abundant in well-matured cheeses and in yeast extracts, such as Marmite, which leads to a sudden and violent rise in blood pressure, and caused some deaths (though too few to cause the withdrawal of the drug from the market).

The most illustrious of Brodie's many protégés who rose to eminence was Julius Axelrod (1912-2004). Born to Polish Jewishimmigtants in New York, Axelrod, like so many ambitious but indigent young people from that milieu, studied at City College for a degree in chemistry. His wish was to become a doctor, but he was rejected by a succession of medical

---

* A well-known parable encapsulates the kind of ambiguity that dogs the study of systems made up of so many interdependent components. Imagine a biologist setting out to determine the relation between how far an insect can jump and the number of its legs. He raps the bench on which the creature is sitting; it jumps, he takes his tape-measure and records the length of the jump. Then he cuts off one of the creature's legs, and repeats the experiment. This continues until the insect has only one leg remaining: it jumps, though not very far. He cuts off the last leg, and raps the table repeatedly, but the insect does not move, and so he writes in his notebook: 'Loss of last leg destroys the hearing'. By purely logical criteria this is a perfectly rational conclusion, and it has parallels in drug – and perhaps especially psychopharmalogical - research.

schools (from which he received apologies following his apotheosis as a Nobel Laureate in 1970), and had to settle for a laboratory technician job at New York University. After that he worked at the city's public health laboratories, analysing food additives, and eventually found his way to Bernard Brodie, then working in a university hospital. (By this time the young recruit bore the scars of battle, for he had lost an eye in a laboratory explosion and acquired his trademark black eye-patch.) Under Brodie's benign guidance, Axelrod finally found his avocation. He did notable work on drug metabolism, took a master's degree, and in 1935 entered the National Institutes of Health. It was not until 1954 that he achieved a Ph.D., having taken time out at George Washington University for the purpose. Axelrod did much important work, amongst other things on the diurnal sleep cycle, controlled by the pineal gland in the brain, but his Nobel Prize was the reward for a discovery about neurotransmitter function. What he found was a truly astonishing phenomenon: first he uncovered another enzyme, which inactivated the neurotransmitter, noradrenaline. (It is called catecholamine-O-methyltransferase, or COMT). This was, at first sight, the terminator of noradrenaline action, but it was only a part of the story. For Axelrod then uncovered a quite unexpected mechanism: most of the noradrenaline released into the narrow space (the synaptic cleft) between the two nerve terminals is retrieved by proteins on the surface of the terminal from which it had escaped.

The discovery of this process, called 're-uptake', initiated a search for a drug that might block the mechanism. Imipramine, it soon turned out, was that drug. This was the first of the famous *tricyclic antidepressants*, so called because the core of the chemical structure comprises three rings of carbon and nitrogen atoms fused together. Imipramine was found actually to be a prodrug (p.), chemically converted in the liver to the active compound. This compound, desipramine became the preferred drug. Neither is a highly specific reagent, for both inhibit re-uptake of all three monoamines, dopamine, noradrenaline and serotonin, though predominantly that of noradrenaline. They are therefore sometimes referred to in the trade as 'dirty' drugs. The road to more specific compounds that would bind to only one type of receptor was tortuous, and full of potholes. An antidepressant drug made by Merck in 1961 was re-evaluated, and found to block re-uptake of noradrenaline and serotonin (though not dopamine). This compound, amitryptiline was further discovered to undergo a chemical change in the liver to one that impeded only noradrenaline uptake. It found uses as an antidepressant, and as a treatment for ADHD (p.) and some other conditions, but it has unpleasant side-effects, which included severe constipation. The last of the major tricyclic series of antidepressants, which was also considered the best, was clomiprazine, brought out by Geigy (which became Novartis). Most commonly known as Anafranil, it is still prescribed.

Worse problems than constipation followed the introduction of the first antidepressant explicitly described as a selective serotonin re-uptake inhibitor, or *SSRI*. Arvid Carlsson, searching through antihistamines, so many of which had turned out to be golden eggs from the one goose, came upon bromphaniramine. This was one of several closely related compounds, including chlorphaniramine, from which it differed only in the substitution of a bromine for a chlorine atom. All were sold over the counter as antihistamines (used to ease the symptoms of the common cold, hay-fever and the like). But this antihistamine had been reported to possess antidepressant properties. Carlsson investigated, and found that it inhibited re-uptake of noradrenaline and serotonin. Working at the time for the Swedish pharmaceutical company, Astra, he was able to launch a programme aimed at finding the most specific and active derivative for clinical use. The search resulted in zimelidine (Zelmid, soon to be licensed to Merck in the U.S.), which was indeed an SSRI. It was hailed as a highly effective antidepressant, also cure for narcolepsy.

Zimelidine was the first of the many explicit SSRI antidepressants to reach the market in 1982, but it did not last long. Within a few months reports began to come in of serious side-effects in a small minority of patients. The worst was a devastating neurological disease, Guillain-Barré syndrome, marked by paralysis of involuntary muscles, including those that control breathing, and there were a number of deaths. An increase in suicides among depressed patients was also reported. It was enough to ensure the drug's hurried withdrawal. But Carlsson and Astra kept trying, and soon came up with alaprocate. This too ran into trouble, for there were indications of destruction of the cells in the bone marrow, responsible for producing blood cells. Astra had not been the only players in the game: a French chemist, Gérard Le Fur, working in the small though highly productive company, Fourneau Frères, subsumed within the medium-sized Pharmuca (all soon to be absorbed by the giant, Rhône-Poulenc), had created indalpine, sold in France as Upstène), some years earlier. It reached the market soon after zimelidine, beginning in France, and quickly reaching the rest of the western world, to great éclat. But yet again, there were a few cases of a dangerous side-effect, the elimination of a class of white blood cells with a function in the immune system. And so in 1985 indalpine followed zimelidine into oblivion.

In the event it was the Duphar Laboratories in Weesp in Belgium from which emerged fluvoxamide, known as Luvox, approved in most European countries in 1983 and 1984, though only much later in the U.S. It derived again from an antihistamine (tripellamine), as also did a product that came soon after from a Danish organisation, the Lundbeck Foundation. Citalpram, or Celexa was one of a large series of compounds synthesised by an exceptional young organic chemist, Klaus Peter Bøgensø. The drug was highly successful. (When, much later, in 2002, the patent expired Bøgensø managed to extend its profitable life, for the compound was a mixture of two enantiomers (p.), only one of which was active. He separated this from its inert companion, and this product gained FDA approval as escitalipram.) Thusantidepressant followed antidepressant, and some remained in use, especially for the most serious cases. Some also found other applications, on- and off-label. There were more mishaps, as new SSRIs and noradrenaline and dopamine reuptake inhibitors displayed unsupportable side-effects, and yet the demand for such drugs remaoned insatiable. The dam was soon to break.

The antidepressant industry had been given its special impetus in 1965, when Joseph Schildkraut, a professor of psychiatry at Harvard,* published the paper in which he formulated his 'chemical imbalance' hypothesis of psychiatric disorders. It was predicated on a conjecture – that a deficiency or excess of one or other neurotransmitter in the brain was the cause of, and its correction the cure for, all such states. A mysterious allure also attached itself to serotonin in particular as the key to physical and spiritual wellbeing, whence the vertiginous rise of the SSRIs. Yet the industry was initially slow to mobilise. With Astra and Merck's Zelmid still threatening, before its eclipse, to annex the market in antidepressants, the other major drug companies were cautious. So when David Wong, a pharmacologist with Eli Lilley, starting yet again from an antihistamine, found a new SSRI with a high degree of specificity, and only a weak secondary effect on noradrenaline re-uptake, the management hesitated. Compound LY110141 had surfaced in the course of a search by a colleague, an organic chemist, Bryan Molloy for an antihistamine derivative devoid of antihistamine properties. Such a substance, he conjectured, might be more likely to be a good antidepressant. Taking advantage of an antihistamine risk-benefit balance analysis, he settled on diphenhydramine, which had the desired properties, and made many derivatives, only one of which appeared interesting in tests in mice. It was in fact a moderately effective noradrenaline re-uptake inhibitor (NRI). This compound never entered into clinical use, but by now SSRIs had become all the rage in brain research, and Wong, the pharmacologist, decided on a comprehensive survey of Molloy's numerous compounds for re-uptake activity of any kind. From this there emerged in 1972 one compound with potent and quite specific activity against serotonin re-uptake. It was called fluoxetine, and appeared highly promising. Eli Lilley were hesitant, in view probably of what had gone before, but eventually overcame their doubts, and in

---

* Another influential promoter of psychopharmacology in the U.S. was a psychiatrist, Frank J. Ayd. His most notable achievement was to recognise the value of chloramphenicol (Thorazine) for treating schizophrenia, and he was the first practitioner in the country to prescribe it. Of his fifty-some books the one that made the greatest impact was *Recognizing the Depressed Patient*, published in 1961. It contained information and commendations of antidepressants. Merck bought 50,000 copies of the book, and sent them out to all the known general practitioners.

1977 the drug was given the name, *Prozac.* That year it appeared in the pharmacies of some European countries, but it was another ten years before the FDA gave its approval, and it was launched in the U.S.A. with huge ceremony. In Germany it was never granted a licence, on the grounds that the benefit-risk balance was too unfavourable, and thus it was entirely unsuitable as a treatment for depression. The German health officials were right, but it is estimated that some 50 million people use, or have used the drug. In the U.S. and in Britain measurable concentrations have even been found in the drinking water.

The commercial success of Prozac was stupendous, but by no means without obstacles. It was considered initially to be a tranquilliser, destined to supplant Valium, which had become less popular by reason of its addictive character. But since it appeared to exert a good effect in the early trials, Prozac was also recommended as an antidepressant, good for dispirited adults, and even as time went on (though against medical advice) young children; for them there were peppermint-flavoured preparations. Among its advantages over other SSRIs was that it did not, or so it was claimed, make the user fat and sluggish. The use of the elixir quickly widened, to embrace the treatment of compulsive-movement disorder and ADHD; it has even been given to manic patients, and before long it was another of 'mother's little helpers'. And then there was the voice of Authority.

The bible for American psychiatrists, and also for many in other countries, is a wrist-breaking volume with the forbidding title, *Diagnostic and Statistical Manual of Mental Disorders,* the DSM. It made its first appearance in 1952, and new editions followed at diminishing intervals, the DSM-V, in 2012. (The cost has risen with the bulk, and sales now greatly enrich the parent organisation, the American Psychiatric Association.) As in the Soviet Encyclopaedia in its day, the truth undergoes transformations from edition to edition. The major upheaval had come in 1980 with the emergence of DSM-III. Its compilation had been entrusted to to a controversial New York psychiatrist, Robert Spitzer, who assembled a team of like-minded associates, with the aim of bringing about a revolution in psychiatric practice. Freudian psychoanalytic principles and similar aberrations, as Spitzer evidently saw it, were to be toppled from their dominant position, and supplanted by drug therapy. In this he largely achieved, but not without acrimony. A striking feature of the ensuing editiions has been the proliferation of mental disorders, of which DSM-V recognises more than 350 – up from 112 in 1994 and 265 in 1980[*]. Each is characterised by nine symptoms, and if a patient is adjudged to display any five out of these nine the diagnosis is secure. The symptoms include such revealing attributes as feeling low, bearing grudges, smoking, and the like.[**] Now, if such character traits as 'shyness', 'social anxiety disorder', and 'hoarding disorder' ('persistent difficulty discarding or parting with possessions, regardless of actual value') are classified as illnesses, it is scarcely surprising that a drug like Prozac can be prescribed to mitigate any of life's irritations. In most cases prescriptions have been written, not by psychiatrists, but by general practitioners who have also often obliged parents, displeased by their children's behaviour or performance at school, or who believe them to be depressed. Long before all this Carl Gustav Jung was quoted as announcing in a rare moment of self-revelation, "Show me a sane man, and I will cure him for you".

---

[*] The European counterpart of the DSM, the psychiatry section of the International Classification of Diseases (IDC), which has reached its tenth edition (IDC 10), has moved in the same direction, although much more hesitantly than the DSM. Neither do its compilers appear to have such close links to the pharmaceutical industry as their American confrères (see below).

[**] It is only fair to add that psychiatrists are by no means unanimous in their attitude towards this trend, and some denounced it in uncompromising terms from the outset. A commentary in the *British Medical Journal* on the DSM-V suggests that new classifications are apt to turn the grief of bereavement, for example, into a pathological state, and that the recommended reduction in the number of diagnostic criteria for psychotic states may further encourage a process of 'epidemiological inflation'. The authors are most of all concerned at the dangers that enthusiastic drug treatment of such ill-defined conditions as 'Disruptive Mood Dysregulation' and 'Attenuated Psychosis Syndrome' (not to mention ADD) may represent to the most vulnerable - very young and the very old. They also identify a rather alarming dilution of the impeccable principle laid down in DSM-IV that 'Neither deviant behaviour (e.g., political, religious, or sexual) nor conflicts that are primarily between the individual and society are mental disorders, unless the deviance or conflict is a symptom of dysfunction in the individual'

Prozac was in fact the only antidepressant considered effective in children (odd, if we are to believe that, in common with all other SSRIs, it raises the serotonin concentration in the brain). Occasional side-effects were reported - insomnia, stomach upsets, loss of libido, and then more alarmingly, suicidal inclinations, often in children. Causality was however endlessly disputed, despite an expensive legal settlement over a case involving a series of murders, followed by the suicide of the perpetrator. Cases of birth defects have also been linked to the drug, which now comes with a warning that it should be avoided by pregnant women. A wider concern is with drug's efficacy. In clinical trials it has not always done particularly well, relative to placebos, and the outcome of meta-analyses (analyses of several independent trials in different places) have been less than spectacular, although many consumers have obviously benefited, or believed that they had, which may amount to the same thing. More of this, however, presently.

The drug companies too, of course, have not been backward in the invention of new diseases to match their drugs.* Pre-menstrual tension, a recognisable complaint, undoubtedly caused by shifts in hormonal balance, was elevated to a syndrome, so PMT became PMS. A few American psychiatrists then came up with a variant, to which they gave the name, pre-menstrual dysphoric disorder, PMDD. (Dysphoria translates as unpleasantness or malaise, said to afflict a minority of women in greater degree than the others.) This did not meet with a great deal of approval within the profession, but at least one pharmaceutical company, Eli Lilley grasped its promise, and within a short time was cultivating the believers. The company organised a conference to which carefully selected psychiatrists were invited, along with some of its own scientists and representatives of the FDA. The papers given at this meeting were published in an academic journal, and lo! – PMDD was a recognised clinical entity, for which the FDA approved the use of Eli Lilley's fluoxetine, Prozac. It was formulated for PMDD, and a vigorous advertising operation was set in train to persuade American women that what they had taken to be PMS might actually be PMDD, and therefore required a different therapy. The

---

* In the U.S. mood-altering drugs for pets have also blossomed into a major industry. Cat and dog psychiatry is evidently now a veterinary specialism.

European regulatory agency, the EMAA, unlike the FDA, would have none of it. PMDD, it decreed, was not a recognised disease, and needed no special treatment. It also expressed concern that women unnecessarily prescribed fluoxetine would be put at risk of dependence.

After Prozac came paroxetine, which was unveiled in 1992, and became famous as Paxil or (in Europe) Seroxat, and later, after the patent expired, as Capramil, Lustral and more. It originated from SmithKlineBeecham, soon to become GSK, and has been an object of controversy almost from the outset. The main selling points were that the drug had few side-effects, was not toxic and did not cause dependence. The side-effects turned out to be numerous, and worst of all was indeed the addictive character, so that attempts by consumers to come off the drug led to terrifying withdrawal symptoms, culminating in some instances in suicide. In clinical trials on depressed children paroxetine came off no better than a placebo - a result for which a plausible explanation suggests itself (p.). The same was found to hold for adolescents.

Scandal: Big Pharma overreaches itself

In 1994 the FDA gave its blessing to gabapentin, a drug produced by Parke Davis, by then a subsidiary of another old-established company, Warner-Lambert. Gabapentin was developed as an inhibitor of a neurotransmitter, γ(gamma)-aminobutyric acid, or GABA. The drug was licensed for the treatment of epileptic seizures, though only in combination with other anti-seizure medicines. In 2002, under its commercial name of Neurontin, it was additionally approved for treating the pain from shingles. By this time Warner-Lambert, complete with Parke Davis had been engulfed by Pfizer, for whom the drug in its new guise achieved blockbuster status. But all was not as it seemed, for six years earlier, David Franklin, a doctor and employee of the Parke Davis subsidiary of Pfizer, working as a sales representative, brought a legal action, accusing his employers of illegal practices. The substance of the case was that the company had engaged in the illicit procedure of promoting the drug for off-label use. Doctors, as we have seen, can prescribe a drug for anything at all, but such profligacy is not open to the manufacturers. It had involved suborning academic researchers to put their names to ghost-written publications, endorsing a variety of applications for Neurontin. The supposed evidence was based on small and perfunctory trials of no statistical value. Some academics must have had scruples, for Marcia Angell in her book, *The Truth about the Drug Companies*, cites a plaintive note in a report by one of the companies paid to produce the papers commending the drug: 'Our company has draft complete, we just need an author'. The Federal legal authorities took up the case. It emerged in the trial that Parke Davis had bribed doctors to recommend Neurontin to their colleagues for off-label uses with money and trips to sunny places and to the 1996 Olympic Games. Meetings, purportedly arranged by independent bodies were organised for doctors, and Parke Davis staff were distributed around the audience to make suitably enthusiastic remarks about the drug. It transpired in court, as the *New York Times* reported, that doctors were even paid to allow company representatives to sit in on consultations with patients. These ruses were so successful that an estimated 90% of sales were for off-label uses, such as pain, migraines, drug and alcohol withdrawal symptoms, and so on. Dr Franklin, the whistleblower also told the court that what most disturbed him was that doctors had been urged to prescribe the drug in doses much higher than had been approved. The judgement cost Pfizer $430 million, not including payments to patients who sued the company independently, and $26.5 million for Dr Franklin for his pains (permitted by law). Pfizer protested that the illicit activity started (as it did) before they had acquired the offending company, and promised to appeal against the judgement. Gabapentin, also called Neurontin, it seems, is still being prescribed by some American psychiatrists.

The second *cause célèbre* followed not long after. In 2004 the then Attorney General of New York state, Eliot Spitzer sued GSK, accusing the company of failing to disclose unfavourable trial results on the safety of Paxil, and fined the company a rather pitiful $2.5 million.* In Britain the regulatory authority, the MHRA (p.), though widely castigated for indecisiveness, had nonetheless warned doctors a few months earlier against prescribing any of eight antidepressant drugs, SSRIs, NRIs and SNRIs**, including Paxil (Seroxat) for children or adolescents. An epidemiologist in the employ of the FDA urged a similar move but was overruled. The drumbeat became stronger as stricken families won compensation claims against GSK for tragedies imputed, justly or not, to Paxil. The FDA eventually acted, to the extent of imposing a 'black box' requirement on the manufacturer to make clear on the label that the drug was not to be given to anyone under the age of 18. Not only that, but the shadow of thalidomide (p.) also fell over the SSRIs generally, for the bulk of the body's serotonin is elsewhere than in the brain, and has other actions besides mood control, not least, it appears, in foetal development. And indeed, reports appeared of birth defects or convulsions in babies born to mothers who had taken paroxetine during the first three months of pregnancy. The FDA also warned against the hazard of a dangerous lung condition, and ruled that pregnant women were to be denied Paxil. GSK, which had explicitly urged the value of the drug for pregnant women, countered that the risks were outweighed by the peace of mind that it engendered, for depressed women were far more likely to harm the baby by smoking, drinking or drugging themselves in other ways. The argument did not prevail against the strictures of the FDA.

In 2012 GSK's misdemeanours finally caught up with it. The company pleaded guilty before a U.S. Federal court to accusations of 'misbranding' of drugs (which embraces errors of commission and omission in labelling,

---

* The drug had been promoted by an unsparing advertising operation, which had even assured the American public that one in eight of them were in need of treatment, such as only Paxil could provide. Such advertising has long been entrusted to agencies specialising in this type of work, some in fact exclusively for psychotropic drugs. These agencies set out to persuade the populace that 'social anxiety disorder', (which indeed has its place in DSM V catalogue of woes [see above] is a disease requiring treatment.

** SNRIs are another category of antidepressants, the so-called 'specific serotonin-*and*-noradrenaline uptake inhibitors', of which venlafaxine, most commonly offered as Effexor, is the best-known. Since these drugs affect the reuptake of both neurotransmitters, the term 'specific' is, it seems, loosely used here.

such as false claims of efficacy and concealment of risks), failure to divulge unfavourable trial outcomes, and pressuring and bribing doctors. The offences refer to Paxil, Wellbutrin and the asthma drug, Advair (fluticasone [p.]). Paxil and its cousins remain on the market. Unpublished clinical trials of Paxil on children, which GSK were forced by the FDA to open to public view, stirred up a hornet's nest, for it emerged that children taking SSRIs were nearly twice as prone to contemplate suicide as those on placebos. Why were children, whose depression was supposed to be relieved by the drugs, then more suicidally inclined? One psychiatrist had the answer: when depressed patients begin to feel better they recover the strength and resolve needed to commit suicide. GSK, at all events, admitted concealing or obfuscating the disadvantages of their product, and instructing their sales reps to promote its illicit use in adolescents.

The activities of GSK in respect of the other two drugs were of a similar order. Wellbutrin was approved for treating adults with severe depression and for nothing else, but GSK saw to it that it was commended to doctors and public by sales reps and unscrupulous doctors in GSK pay for a wide range of other ailments, real or imagined. The third drug, Advair, which had been approved for severe asthma, but not mild disease, for which other remedies had been judged preferable, was proclaimed the best treatment for any asthma. Mild asthma was dismissed in GSK literature as 'a myth'.* Of the conferences in holiday locations to which GSK brought doctors, one of their number, less easily impressed than most of his confrères seem to have been, wrote, 'The style of the conference would have been suitable for a convention of cosmetics sales reps; this is supposed to be a scientific meeting', and owned that he found the whole affair demeaning. The court, having heard the evidence, imposed a penalty of $3 billion on GSK, a record for a pharmaceutical company. More may follow when legal actions against GSK relating to the diabetes drug, Avandia (p.) have run their course. The sum may appear substantial, but it should be measured against the company's profits of $11.6 billion for Paxil, $10.4 billion for Avandia and $5.9 billion for Wellbutrin. The affair raises many questions about the ethics of the industry, and especially about the relation between the major drug companies and the academic community, senior members

---

* It emerged in the trial that a doctor who acted as host in a widely disseminated radio programme, recommended Wellbutrin in florid terms for treating obesity, sexual inadequacy, ADHD and bulimia. He also instructed his listeners that the drug might offer women 60 orgasms per night. He did not mention, on the other hand, the reward from GSK of $275,000 for his services. Another physician was paid $1.5 million to speak for the drug at conferences over a period of three years. Other doctors were suborned by bribes in the form of a large payment for every talk they gave, proclaiming the virtues of one or other GSK drug, or by trips to luxury resorts and the like. It has to be said that GSK were by no means alone in encouraging doctors to promote their products by generous gifts of vacations and other enticements. What is most striking is the proportion of this largesse that has gone to psychiatrists, and even to their professional bodies, and to mental health charities. Perhaps it is the elusive nature of so many of the disorders that evidently make the psychiatrists a more attractive target than orthopaedists, cardiologists and the rest. Many more psychiatrists also therefore have financial interests in drugs featured in publications in learned journals (which now demand full disclosures of connections with relevant companies). These interests comprise both personal rewards from consultancies and seats on advisory boards, and financial support for laboratories, including salaries for research staff. There have been examples of evasions of full disclosures, punished by the occasional slap on the wrist.

583

of which have been caught up in such corrupt practices as putting their names to ghost-written publications* in academic journals.

The third famous case of a pharmaceutical company brought to book for a deception that cost many lives has already been chronicled (p.). This was Merck's now infamous painkiller, Vioxx – numerically the worst disaster yet.

The end of an era? SSRIs under the microscope

In the first decade of the new millennium in the U.S. about one in twenty men were taking antidepressants, and twice that proportion of women, some 25 million adults in all. A later estimate puts the number of American women on antidepressants at 22% of the adult female population. One can hardly imagine that all this multitude, leading presumably normal lives, earning and spending and doing what people do, can all be clinically

---

* An academic brawl, which illustrates the fraught relations between the industry and a section of the medical research profession, erupted over Paxil in 2011. A professor on the Faculty of the University of Pennsylvania accused academic colleagues of attaching their names as authors to a paper in a medical journal, written by a company paid by GSK. The paper, he said, presented data on the clinical performance of Paxil in an unjustifiably glowing light. The University in the end took no action, but the episode underlined the prevalence of ghost-writing of papers, commissioned by pharmaceutical companies, who select authors, often bound to them by generous consultancies or research funding, to serve as authors. Scandals of this nature were several times exposed, relating in many cases to the evaluation of psychotropic drugs.

depressed.* Arguably worse was the ever-increasing number of children being dosed with antipsychotics. Between the two quinquennia beginning 1993 and 2005 in the U.S. the number of prescriptions of such drugs to children (some aged five or even less) rose by a factor of more than 7 to 1.83 in every 100. These were drugs intended for adult patients with serious conditions, especially schizophrenia and bipolar disorder. A professor of clinical psychiatry at Columbia University in New York has calculated that the great majority of the prescriptions were off-label.

Prescriptions for children, and 13% of those for adolescents conformed to FDA guidelines. In Britain the situation, if not so far advanced (considering that at the last count in 2000, the U.S., with 5% of its population, was consuming 80% of the world's Ritalin) is broadly similar. In 2012 some

---

* The many descriptions of the effects of pathological depression from personal experience exclude any such possibility. The interaction between clinical depression and modern drugs is particularly well illustrated by the account of a writer, Andrew Solomon in the *New Yorker* in 1998, under the title, 'Anatomy of Melancholy' (borrowed from the classical treatise published in 1621 by Robert Burton). Solomon's ordeal began in 1994, and he estimates that his efforts to grapple with his condition by way of drugs and visits to his psychoanalyst cost him $70,000. In his desperation, he took, in various combinations of drugs and doses, Zoloft, Xanax, Paxil, Navane, Valium, Buspar and Wellbutrin. (We have met all these, except Xanax, a benzodiazepine, Navane, a thioxanthene class drug, licensed in 1967 for treatment of schizophrenia, and Buspar, licensed for treatment of 'Generalised Anxiety Disorder'.) How much good this formidable medicine chest did him is impossible to gauge, but the side-effects were appalling, and worse was the 'cold turkey', which took possession of him when he decided to stop all the drugs. After prolonged inability to perform the simplest tasks, tormented by effects ranging from constipation, total loss of libido and insomnia, and flirting with suicide, his condition suddenly abated, and he brought his drug regime under control. He describes the immediate effects of some of the drugs: 'Zoloft', he relates, 'made me feel as though I'd had fifty-five cups of coffee. Paxil gave me diarrhea, but fortunately Xanax, though it made me exhausted, was also constipating. Paxil seemed better than Zoloft, and I soon adjusted to its making me feel as though I'd had eleven cups of coffee – which was definitely better than feeling as though I couldn't brush my own teeth. Only after a year did I discover Effexor [the then recently introduced SNRI (see p.) that on the suggestion of his psychoanalyst he took in three times the normal dose], which made me appreciate that Paxil had been only partly effective.' What Solomon took from this was that different people needed different drug regimes.

15,000 prescriptions for powerful antipsychotic drugs with fearsome side-effects, and intended for sick adults, were written for recipients aged less than 18. A clinical psychiatrist in Britain described this as 'a slow fuse to disaster'. An American psychiatrist thought it 'a national disaster', and opined that the brains of 'millions' of American children had been ruined. The drugs are used mainly for ADHD, or generally unruly behaviour – lapses with which parents in the past were able to cope - and have been described as 'a chemical cosh'. About one in ten male ten-year olds in the U.S. have been branded with a diagnosis of ADHD, and the majority of those receive treatment by pill. That number doubles when the boys enter highschool. British children too are dosed with Ritalin (p.), which is approved for ADHD, or with related drugs, at the rate of 660,000 prescriptions annually. There is even a drug to cure attention deficit** in grown-ups. Eli Lilley's atomoxetine (Strattera), an NRI and failed antidepressant, was approved for the treatment of adults and children, although it had not been tested on children below the age of 6. It was said to be harmless, and inert from the recreational viewpoint, but neither of these claims held up; or at least, reports to the contrary surfaced, and the

---

* Pets have increasingly come in for similar treatment. The causes are aggressive behaviour, anxiety (especially in cats), depression, and in dogs a condition termed 'separation disorder', when the animal sits dolefully by the door all day, waiting for its master or mistress to return from work. It is perhaps not surprising that animals kept in flats in high-rise buildings may be very apt to become, in some sense, psychotic. Since the American pet industry brings in around $50 billion per annum, the pharmaceutical companies have seized the opportunity to offer help to the 80% or so of American dogs, and 50% of cats dosed with medicines. Pfizer have an Animal Health arm, and Eli Lilley a 'companion animal' division. These and similar organisations are regulated by the FDA, with its Center for Veterinary Medicine. Clinical trials, placebo-controlled and double-blinded, are performed on animals (although it is the owners who are blinded, as well as the supervising vets). The most favoured mood-changing medicines are Clomicalm, which is merely the tricyclic antidepressant, clomiprazine (Anafranil to human consumers), and Reconcile, which is fluoxetine, that is to say, Prozac. These medicines come in chewable form with a beef flavour.

** Psychiatrists make a distinction between attention deficit disorder, ADD and ADHD, which it subsumes. ADD is merely ADHD without the H for hyper, devoid, that is, of hyperactivity. The DSM V subdivides ADHD into subtypes, according to subtle differences in behaviour.

British regulatory agency, the MHRA issued warnings in 2006 of reported psychotic symptoms and misuse. Atomoxetine affords another indication of the extent to which a solution is now sought in drugs to the inescapable trials of everyday life.

The question that psychiatrists and other practitioners, nudged along by epidemiologists, are now pondering is whether and to what extent the modern antipsychotics and antidepressants, and especially the SSRIs, NRIs and the like, actually do good. The question has been framed by a number of clinical and academic luminaries, beginning with the very logic behind the principle of these chemicals. Why, during the long years of their ascendency, did no one articulate the obvious paradox: if the conditions that these drugs are meant to treat are real and caused by a want of serotonin or noradrenaline, why was no deficiency of these neurotransmitters ever found in any of the brains of depressives or psychotics? The treatment is rather like infusing blood cells into people who are not anaemic because blood is know to be necessary for health. (The practice, moreover, would be very dangerous). This of course does not impugn any empirical efficacy the drugs might have, though it does undermine – one might say, obliterate - the 'chemical imbalance' theory of brain disorders.

But there are more questions, concerning in particular the validity and the reporting of the clinical trials. Irving Kirsch, a psychology professor at Harvard Medical School and at the University of Hull in England, has set out the case against the antidepressants most lucidly and accessibly in his book, *The Emperor's New Drugs*. The first challenge is to define depression and devise a quantitative measure of its magnitude. This presents greater difficulties than measuring the severity of diabetes, say, or heart disease or inflammation. Psychiatrists in many western countries put their trust in the Hamilton Rating Scale for Depression, which is based on a list of symptoms, such as mood, suicidal disposition, sleep disturbances and so on, all of a distinctly subjective nature. Some professional bodies prefer other types of measure, but they can be expected to embody similar uncertainties. An inescapable complication in drug evaluation is that a proportion of patients who report amelioration of their symptoms would, as psychiatrists concede, have got better without the drug. When the

587

margin of apparent success in a clinical trial is small, as has been generally the case, this will naturally bias the results in favour of the drug. An important criterion of efficacy therefore is what pharmacologists call dose-dependence: alleviation of the condition brought about by the drug must increase with increasing drug concentration. All the SSRIs failed the dose-dependence test: high doses have no greater effect than low. Yet this does not cause the drug to be written off. The drug companies can also argue that an unsuccessful trial was flawed – that the number of participants may have been too small, or it was based on a poorly selected type of patient - too young, too old, too depressed, or insufficiently so, for example.

In recent years trials of antidepressants and of many other types of drugs have been increasingly controlled not by placebos but by another drug - one that has seen a period of untroubled use. This is called an *active comparator trial*, originally introduced on ethical grounds. The argument was that if half the patients in the trial (the placebo group) are denied a treatment for their condition, believed to be effective, even life-saving, then they are being put at indefensible risk. But the comparator trial also gives the pharmaceutical company, if it is running the trial, an opportunity to bias the outcome by choosing as the standard the weakest drug on the market – pitting its horse against the slowest nag in the opposition's stable. Yet it is at first sight remarkable that an active new drug does better in comparator than placebo-controlled trials. Thus if 45% of patients, say, report an improvement in their condition in a placebo-controlled trial, then typically 60% will feel better in a comparator trial. In the last decade or so another variant of trial design has gained ground; this is the *three-arm trial*, in which the new drug is measured against both an established drug and a placebo. Under current procedures laid down for the conduct of clinical trials, as Kirsch explains, the three-arm trial affords a statistical advantage to the pharmaceutical company. This curious circumstance comes about thanks to another criterion for the evaluation of a new drug, the *non-inferiority* principle, which lays down that for approval the drug must merely not be inferior to an existing drug. This means that even if the trial exposes it as no better than the placebo (as has happened with about half of new antidepressants) it still has a chance in the comparator arm. For if it should happily turn out that the old drug is likewise no better than the placebo, then the trial is void by reason of 'assay insensitivity'. But the old drug is respectable because already approved, and so the failure of both does not count against the new drug, which lives to be tested again in another trial. Consider now what constitutes a success in a simple placebo-controlled trial: the drug has to perform better than a placebo, but according to the statistics it has only a 50% chance of surmounting that hurdle. In the three-arm trial, though, it may have the good fortune to be judged against an equally ineffective standard and prevail in the second round, if the first round was a draw (a void assay). This gives it twice the chance of succeeding than in the placebo-only case.

In 2009 a group of researchers in Germany published in *The Lancet* the results of a meta-analysis of 150 'second-generation' antipsychotic drugs. The message was that as a group they were no better than those – the 'first generation' – that had gone before; and when it came to refractory schizophrenia, the one drug that stood out was clozapine, a very old drug indeed (p. Neither the article, nor an editorial commentary suggested that the 'second generation' drugs were useless, but they warned doctors to consider the balance of benefit and harm through side-effects, for each individual patient. They did suggest that it was time to discard the first- and second-generation descriptions, devised by the drug companies to create in the minds of doctors and patients the impression that the older antidepressants were obsolete, and should give place to the newer and vastly more expensive products. Worse was to follow. According to previously undisclosed data extracted by Kirsch, by way of the Freedom of Information Act, from the FDA on clinical trials of six 'new-generation' SSRI antidepressants (including Prozac and Paxil), the placebos were on average 82% as effective as the drug. But, as Kirsch explains, the abiding weakness in clinical trials has been the frequent failure in design of the famous randomised double-blind (p.) placebo-controlled model. Taking account of this, several eminent figures in the field have arrived at the conclusion that the effectiveness of the SSRIs, NRIs, and related drugs may in fact be zero or as near to it as makes no difference, and so a mere chimaera all along. For the explanation of this dramatic conclusion, see Chapter ..., which enlarges on the nature of the placebo effect.

The objurgations of Kirsch and others during the last few years do not *prove* that the antidepressants (and antipsychotics) have no beneficial effects, although it seems clear that such effects are very small. There have indeed been loud counter-arguments – for instance that patients who choose to enter into a clinical trial of a new drug may be atypical – but the evidence appears in general to be what statisticians like to call 'anecdotal' (as opposed to statistical). This is a poor basis for a valid conclusion, since as we have already seen, no end of fulsome testimonials, heaping praises on a drug, can be collected, often imputing miraculous healing virtues to even the most absurd nostrums. But if we accept that there are serious doubts about the benefits of the drugs, is there any evidence that they may be doing actual harm? The drugs were touted as non-addictive, but this has turned out to be untrue. It has proved extremely difficult for those who have taken an antidepressant for long periods to shake off the habit. Metabolic processes are regulated in many cases by feedback loops that maintain the concentrations of metabolites at their correct levels. So, to take a familiar example, when one's blood-sugar level falls a little, a feedback loop causes the pancreas to release insulin; the insulin stimulates sugar release, switching off again when the sugar level has returned to normal. But if a high-sugar diet keeps the blood sugar perpetually high, insulin release continues unchecked, engendering a series of malign consequences; worst of all, the insulin receptors begin to die under the constant stimulation, and because the tissues then fail to respond, the pancreas pumps out more insulin, the vicious cycle accelerates and ends in mayhem.

It is not inconceivable, then, nor does it seem to have been excluded by the evidence, that a brain subjected to a permanent excess of a neurotransmitter, induced by a drug, might react in like manner – by, for instance, atrophy of the receptors for that substance, leading to a vicious cycle of more secretion with less response. There have been reports of structural changes in the brain after prolonged use of antipsychotic drugs. There is yet another source of unease that hangs over re-uptake inhibitors and other psychoactive drugs: the pharmaceutical industry, and indeed leaders of the medical profession, tell us that the age of personalised medicine is fast approaching (Chapter 18). This is inevitably linked to what has been described as the transition from symptom-based to cause-based treatments. For causes of diseases researchers will increasingly look to the genome and the proteome (p.) for anomalies in a protein or in the gene from which it derives. The causes, in this sense, of many diseases have been identified - though seldom so far those of mental diseases. The search for a gene (or genes) associated with schizophrenia has gone on for decades, and succession of reported sighting proved a mirage. Recently more convincing reports of mutations in schizophrenics have appeared, but the disease is (not surprisingly) multigenic, and the difference between a mutation that causes and one that merely 'predisposes' to a condition is often elusive. (So also are the genetics of schizophrenia, considering for instance that if one of a pair of identical twins has the disease, the likelihood that the other will have it also is not 100, but is only around 50%, even if environmental factors are left out of the equation.) What hope then of discovering an organic cause for a 'syndrome' like shyness, or ADHD? This realisation has led some psychiatrists, mainly in Europe, to wonder whether after all the conditions that they treat, even schizophrenia and bipolar disorder, may not be simply a consequence of distressing environmental circumstances. The assault on principles regarded as axioms by a large section of the psychiatric profession is becoming increasingly heated. For the moment the unregenerate school and their patients are winning, judged at least by the inescapable fact that the second-best-selling drug in the U.S., at $14.1 billion per year, is a dopamine agonist called aripiprazole (Abilify or Aripiprex), while number four at $11.6 billion is duloxetine (Cymbalita), an SNRI. (At the top is Nexium for soothing the discomfort of stomach acid [p.]; and at number 3 is the most popular statin, rosuvastatin, or Crestor [p.].)

Dementia: the most elusive quarry

It is now a commonplace that Alzheimer's disease, which (loosely defined) can strike its victims at any age, and other forms of dementia are a huge, intractable and – as the population ages – increasing problem. The treatment options are severely limited. To compensate for the relentless loss of nerve cells in the brain, the best hope is to limit as far as possible the resulting dearth of neurotransmitters, especially acetylcholine. Early attempts to treat the condition with drugs that block acetylcholine receptors were counterproductive, and accelerated, rather than reduced the evanescence of memory. A more promising strategy has been to increase the concentration of what acetylcholine there is in the failing brain by inhibiting acetylcholinesterase, the enzyme that eliminates acetylcholine when it is no longer wanted (p.). There are many compounds that act in this manner, of which the first recorded example was huperzine. Now known as huperzine A, it derives from a plant, which was used for several centuries in Chinese traditional medicine to treat a variety of conditions, including dementia. The first laboratory compound found to block acetylcholinesterase action was physostigmine (p.), synthesised in 1935 by Percy Julian at DePauw University in Indiana. Despite high hopes and widespread use it was found in the end to be of little help to patients by reason of its short lifetime in the body. Many attempts were made to find something better, but most of the products worked feebly at best. More effective was tacrine, the first drug approved by the FDA for treatment of dementias. More commonly known as Cognex, it came to light by accident during a search for antimicrobial agents, initiated by the Australian government at the beginning of World War II. The programme was aborted when penicillin came on stream. But Adrian Albert, the pharmacologist who had synthesised the substance, noticed a strange manifestation: given to anaesthetised animals, it caused a return to consciousness. This stimulated an American physician, William Summers to try it on demented patients. The effect was encouraging, as were the ensuing clinical trials, and tacrine was approved by the FDA for the treatment of Alzheimer disease. Its success was again transient, for approval was revoked after reports of liver damage. Summers insisted that the grounds for the decision were weak, and that a good drug would be wasted, but it was nonetheless consigned to oblivion.

Then in the late 1990s a random survey of compounds of many types by Hachiro Sugimoto and his colleagues at the Eisai Company in Japan threw up a result that yielded an interesting lead compound. By the usual process of modification by trial-and-error a far better compound eventually emerged - E2020, given the name, donepezil. It was effective in boosting the acetylcholine concentration in the brains of rats, and clinical trials were deemed successful in enhancing the cognitive performance of people with Alzheimer disease. The compound was marketed in association with Pfizer under the name of Aricept. It is the most abundantly prescribed drug for the condition, and is said to benefit between 40 and 70% of sufferers. The wide range reflects the inherent uncertainty in quantifying the manifestations of the disease. Another drug, menantine (Ebixa) blocks the receptor of a different neurotransmitter, N-methyl-d-aspartate (NMDA). It has complex and uncertain effects on brain function, and, incautiously used, can damage the nerve cells. Some substances, which have the same kind of action, such as ketamine (p.), have been, or still are used as anaesthetics, and recreationally. Menantine is thought to offer some help in certain cases of Alzheimer disease. There are now more than a hundred drugs said to improve the mental state of patients and slow the progress of dementia. The most widely used is probably still donepezil (Aricept). There has been more than one flash in the pan in recent years. One of the brightest was an antihistamine, developed in Russia in 1983, called latrepirdine. It was reported twenty years later to produce spectacular improvements in the condition of Alzheimer victims, and animal tests purportedly showed a large reduction in the death of brain cells. The drug, given the name, Dimebon, was espoused by Pfizer in association with a smaller company, Medivation, but human trials in the U.S. gave totally negative results, and by 2010 the drug was dead. The problem for researchers hoping at least to mitigate the symptoms of Alzheimer disease is that, like schizophrenia, and indeed the majority of human afflictions, it is a multigenic condition. There is, in other words, no single target for a magic bullet, but several quite disparate metabolic circuits, in which intervention might be profitable. To make matters worse, there are all the genetic differences between populations and individuals that too often provoke different responses to any given drug. But more on that later.

Unforeseen uses: overindulgence and its consequences

The misuse – if that is what it is – of psychotropic drugs extends back through the millennia. The intensely addictive opium and heroin had, as we have seen, medical applicatiions from ancient times, but were also the cause of wars and of countless ruined lives. Hallucinogenic plant extracts were of course used recreationally, ritually, and to some extent medicinally, long before the active constituents were isolated, and their activities quantified. Cannabis, also called marijuana, and the low-grade hemp come from strains of the *Cannabis sativa* plant, which contains many compounds of the class known as cannabinoids. The most active is tetrahydrocannabinol, or THC. It has been estimated that about six in every thousand of the world's population are regular cannabis users. THC and other cannabinoids have a broad range of physiological and psychological effects, and especially after the two optical isomers (p.) of THC were purified in 1964 one of them especially (known to chemists as Δ^9 THC) grew into a useful medicinal item. It is a mild analgesic, and it suppresses nausea and stimulates appetite in patients undergoing chemotherapy for cancers and AIDS. More recently it has been found to moderate the symptoms of multiple sclerosis, and possible applications in the treatment of mental diseases have been explored. The pure isomer has been available for some time, under the name of Marinol. Whether, or to what extent cannabis is addictive has been debated for decades. What seems clear is that it impairs the mental development of children. It is proscribed in many but not all Western countries. Many cannabinoid derivatives have been synthesised and tested for therapeutic potential, but little of lasting interest seems to have resulted.

Acid

In 1938 Albert Hofmann (1906-2008), a Swiss chemist in the Sandoz Laboratories in Basel was exploring the therapeutic possibilities in compounds related to the deadly ergot fungus (p.). Starting from natural ergotamine, he prepared a compound that was to achieve notoriety, lysergic acid diethylamide, or LSD (from the German Lysergsäure diethylamid). Tested on animals, it induced mild agitation, but little else besides uterine contractions. It was thought to offer little promise for further studies, and was forgotten by everyone except, it seems, Hofmann. His thoughts, according to a memoir set down in old age, returned intermittently to his compound, until one day, five years on, in 1943, 'during a creative midday break, the idea came to me in a strange way, once more to synthesise lysergic acid diethylamide for further pharmacological testing'. (Hofmann seems in fact to have had religious convictions and to have believed that an unseen hand was guiding his researches.) 'It was', he continued. 'no more than a hunch! I liked the chemical structure of the substance – which led me to take this unusual step, since compounds as a rule were never handled again, when once discarded'. What happened next is not clear, but Hofmann must have swallowed some of the LSD, it is said through a mouth pipette (a simple glass device for metering out known volumes of liquids, and filled by sucking; mouth pipetting is generally forbidden now by laboratory safety regulations.) Hofmann merely states that 'Although I was accustomed to scrupulously clean work, a trace of the substance must accidentally have entered my body, probably during the purification via recrystallization'. From what one now knows of the dosage required for a significant effect this explanation seems unlikely. Hofmann relates, at all events that he 'was overtaken by a very weird state of consciousness, which today one might call "psychedelic"'.

Hofmann was evidently sufficiently captivated by this experience to do a deliberate experiment on himself. He took one-quarter milligram in water, and within a short time was overcome by dizziness, acute anxiety, distorted vision, a sense of paralysis, and an urge to laugh. At this point he asked his laboratory assistant to escort him home. Travelling by bicycle despite a feeling of immobility, he reached his house, unable to stand, and lying on the couch, was seized by terrifying visions and the illusion that a demon had taken possession of his body. After some hours the aberrations abated, and were replaced by joy at the vivid colours and shimmering shapes now before him. Hofmann had experienced the first 'bad acid trip'. These were all apparitions that Aldous Huxley described in his book, *The Doors of Perception*, and Hofmann was thrilled later to meet Huxley in person, and to compare their experiences. Hofmann's rather lurid, perhaps somewhat embroidered, accounts of the effects that LSD had on him caused a stir in psychiatric circles, and many practitioners began to assess its effects on their patients. It became popular as an adjunct to 'the talking cure', with the special power of releasing memories supposedly buried in the unconscious. It was also held to cure alcohol addiction, and even the early observation of its power to induce uterine contractions in childbirth was briefly put to use. LSD has never quite vanished from psychiatric practice, nor of course from the illicit recreational drug 'counterculture', which reached its peak in the 1960s.

The military and especially the CIA took a deep interest in the substance, and one of its contracted associates, an eccentric psychiatrist, Louis Jolyon ('Jolly') West, who dabbled in such cults as dianetics (the bizarre belief system behind scientology), was the chief protagonist in an infamous episode, when he determined to test the power of LSD to its limit in an animal experiment. With two members of the faculty of the University of Oklahoma, he sought permission to inject an enormous dose of LSD into an elephant in the Oklahoma City zoo. The large African bull element, named Tusko, received the injection by way of a dart in the buttock, and after a short period was seized with convulsions and died. West and his associated wrote a report in a scientific journal, but other scientists expressed doubts about whether it could really have been the LSD or the measures taken to try to revive the animal that actually caused its death.

Angel dust to horse tranquilliser

Many other psychotropic substances came to prominence, for good or ill, in the mid-20th century. One such was phencyclidine, otherwise known as PCP, or angel dust. PCP was synthesised in 1926 by chemists at Parke Davis in Detroit, but the company could not have entertained any great hopes of it, for it was not until 1952 that they thought to patent the compound. The following year, however, it was on sale as Sernyl, to suggest serenity. Sernyl belonged to a curious class of drugs, termed 'dissociative anaesthetics'. They generally block several receptors in the brain, especially the NMDA receptors (p.), and their effect is to throw the patients into a cataleptic state, in which they can see and even swallow, but have no awareness of their surroundings. They experience no pain, but they may have hallucinations and other unpleasant apprehensions as the anaesthesia wears off. Such anaesthetics may be used in minor operations or intrusive examinations. PCP had been tried out on soldiers during World War II well before it became available commercially. After some years of use psychotropic side-effects became increasingly obvious, and PCP was withdrawn, but it had an extended life on the streets, where it did no little damage.

PCP was supplanted by a related derivative, ketamine, another Parke Davis product, with fewer alarming psychotropic side-effects, and an earlier recovery. It was first introduced into veterinary medicine, and was familiarly known as a 'horse tranquilliser'. From 1964 it came into use for human patients as an anaesthetic and sedative. It was valued in emergency medicine, in part because it also dilated the airways. It was used in minor wound surgery during the Vietnam war in the early 1970s, and it seems to have been there that soldiers discovered the relaxation and pleasurable euphoria it engendered when taken on the quiet. It was soon on the streets in the U.S. and elsewhere, but then something even better crept out of the ever-fertile laboratories of the pharmaceutical industry. Quite recently there has been revived interest in ketamine as a possible antidepressant.

That story begins in 1912 when the management of the Merck laboratories in Darmstadt in Germany, which were in hot competition with Bayer in Bavaria, conceived a stratagem. Bayer had produced a profitable haemostatic drug, one that induces clotting of the blood, and stops haemorrhages. It was called Hydrastinine, and derived from a plant. The Merck chemists wanted something equally marketable, and thought that a simple modification of Hydrastinin would enable them to evade the patent constraint. They were after, in short, what has become known in our time as a 'me-too' drug. An able chemist, Anton Köllisch was set to work on the problem, and soon made the simplest possible modification by introducing a methyl group. The methylhydrastinin was tested in animals and then in hospital patients, apparently with success, but Merck did nothing more besides patenting a new route of synthesis, which Köllisch had developed for such derivatives generally. One of several new compounds that his procedure yielded was 3,4-methylenedioxy-N-methylamphetamine, which was given the hardly less memorable commercial name of Methylsafrylamin. Tests showed a relatively high level of toxicity, and Merck gave up. Nevertheless, it remained in the laboratory records like a stone in the shoe for later researchers, and at intervals of a few years they would come back to it, and try more tests. Finally in 1953, when Merck was established as an international company, the compound, more commonly called MDMA, was chosen as one of several to be tested in animals by the U.S. Army for psychological and physiological effects. The results were declassified in 1973, but by then word had got about, and NDMA was already being taken for pleasure. Many psychiatrists took an interest in the substance, and reports of its value in the treatment of psychotic, anxious or otherwise disturbed subjects vary. Certainly there have been strong claims of its effectiveness in treating such conditions when linked to psychoanalysis. A notorious depression sets in as the euphoric effects of the drug fade. Prolonged use is said to cause impaired memory, and excessive doses can result in severe systemic damage of several kinds. It remains a widely used recreational material. The name, originally given to it in California, is ecstasy.

Chapter 16

A GALLIMAUFRY OF HUMAN ILLS AND MODERN COMFORTS

Chemistry and the nerves

While this hectic pursuit of new drugs for the treatment of mental disturbances continued unchecked, relying still on a refined process of trial-and-error, an understanding was taking shape of the biochemistry and physiology of mental illnesses. It was responsible for the next phase in the development of psychopharmacology. To understand where the insights came from we need to return once more to the origins of the science. It was the South- and Central-American Indians who really discovered neurotoxins in preparing arrow poisons from extracts of plants, insects, snakes and frogs (p.). European explorers, soldiers and priests sent back samples, which were described and catalogues in several learned works. In 1751 the great French explorer and savant, Charles Marie de la Condamine came home with preparations of particular interest, above all a substance obtained from species of the liana vine, referred to by the Indians as urari, wouralia or wourari, which to Europeans became curare. It was known to be lethal, causing paralysis of the skeletal muscles, then of the involuntary muscles, including the diaphragm, so that breathing stops and the victim dies. It was nearly a century, however, before in 1841 Claude Bernard, together with a colleague, Bernard Pelouze, became interested in curare.

Bernard, at this time, was starting to concern himself with the workings of the nerves, and he and Pelouze quickly found that a minute amount of curare (an alkaloid) introduced into the blood of a frog caused instant paralysis. In a series of clever experiments Bernard and Pelouze established that both the muscles and the nerves in the paralysed frog were still functional, and thus curare must be blocking the transmission of signals from the nervous system to the muscles. The site of action, in other words, had to be the link between nerve and muscle, the *neuromuscular junction*. It was some years before Bernard published this result, which was to have great clinical repercussions, but he and his student, Magendie (p.) made abundant use of curare in experiments, of a kind later banned in England by Act of Parliament, on paralysed but fully conscious animals. In an experiment regarded as a landmark, an English physiologist kept a curarized donkey alive by ventilation with a bellows through a tracheostomy (a hole in the windpipe) until gradually the effect of the curare wore off.

When the results of Bernard's experiments became known it occurred to some alert doctors that curare, cautiously applied, might be useful in the treatment of uncontrollable tremors or spasms in such conditions as tetanus or epilepsy. This met with only limited success, mainly because of the poor quality of the plant extracts, and the irreproducible nature therefore of different preparations. In time pharmaceutical chemists investigating poisonous plant products came to recognise that that 'curare' was really a catch-all description of a large family of chemically related plant alkaloids. (Arrow poisons from other plants were used, in fact, by tribal hunters in other parts of the world besides South America; the best-known is the *eséré*, extracted from the deadly Calabar bean in West Africa.) Further research was animated by the desire of doctors and surgeons for a reliable muscle relaxant, and the pharmaceutical companies began to listen. Progress was spasmodic until the early 1930s, when an American planter, Richard Gill brought north from Ecuador 26 specimens of different species of poisonous vines. The Squibb company in New Jersey bought most of this material, and in 1935 made available a curare preparation called Intocostrin, cautiously designated an 'unauthorised extract of curare'. This was tried out by surgeons in combination with their usual anaesthetics to great effect. The relaxation of the muscles that it engendered allowed easier access to the target of the operation, and also made the introduction of tubes and instruments into the bodily orifices simpler and safer. It also proved its worth in electroconvulsive therapy, much in vogue for the treatment of psychotic conditions. So fearsome were the convulsions often caused by the treatment that they could lead to the fracture of vertebrae, a risk eliminated by the application of muscle relaxants.

It was also in 1935 that Harold King, a chemist at the National Institute for Medical Research in London (where Henry Dale led a team of researchers studying the mechanism of nerve conduction), begged a sample of South American curare from the British Museum. From it he extracted and purified an alkaloid, which he called *d*-tubocurarine after the bamboo tubes used by the South American Indians to store the poison), and in one of which he had received his sample. (The *d* standing for *dextro*, meaning that a solution of the substance would impart a right-handed rotation to the plane of polarised light; the mirror-image of this configuration would have caused a left-handed rotate, designated *l* for *laevo*. [See p. .]). King also inferred an approximate structure. It was primarily *d*-tubocurarine that so changed the practice of surgery when, some years later, the chemists at Squibb found a process for extracting the same material on a commercial scale. A further series of curare alkaloids were isolated in the succeeding years, notably alcuronium, which largely replaced *d*-tubocurarine. In 1946 the ever-fecund Daniel Bovet and his associated as Rhône-Poulenc synthesised an analogue of *d*-tubocurarine, which he called Flaxedil (while the chemical name was gallamine triethiodide). This has remained a staple in surgery as a means of maintaining muscle relaxation. But the most important outcome of the research on curare over the years was yet to come.

Myasthaenia gravis is a rare disorder, characterised by muscle weakness. The first signs are generally loss of control of the muscles that operate the eyelids and the movements of the eyeball. The muscles of the face are affected, resulting in an altered and expressionless aspect, and also those that control chewing, swallowing and speech, all of which become difficult. The muscles in the limbs cannot sustain prolonged activity, and so the gait is affected. These indications were described by a famous English physician, Thomas Willis in 1671. The condition was familiar to most doctors in the 19th century, and around 1900 it was studied in great detail by a number of specialists, among them a German, Samuel Goldflam, whence it became known as Goldflam's Disease. In 1901 another German, Hermann Oppenheim noted the similarity of the manifestations to the paralysis of the muscles occasioned by curare. There was no meaningful treatment for myasthaenia gravis until, in 1934, a brief report appeared in *The Lancet* by a remarkable woman doctor, Mary Broadfoot Walker (1888-1974), working in a small hospital in London. Born and trained in Scotland, she served in the Royal Army Medical Corps during the Great War, and on her return, became physician in the 'Poor Law Service' at St Alfege Hospital in Greenwich, London. There she was confronted with two myasthaenia gravis patients, and, like Oppenheim, noted the similarity of the condition to curare poisoning. She also knew that victims of curare had been treated with an extract of the Calabar bean, the seed of the plant, *Physostigma venenosum*, native to Calabar in modern Nigeria.

The background was the following: the bean was known to be highly toxic, and was used in Nigeria as an 'ordeal poison' (according to the same principle as the ducking stool in England). Suspected criminals were made to drink an extract of the bean, and were freed if they survived. Death was proof of guilt. The Calabar bean was much prized by the Africans, and difficult for outsiders to obtain, but in 1855, Robert Chritison, the distinguished Professor of Materia Medica in Edinburgh, an authority on poisons, procured a bean from a missionary. Having tried its effect on animals, he took a little himself, and recorded opium-like sensations. Encouraged, he tried a larger dose, with immediate and alarming results. He felt extreme weakness, his pulse and heartbeat became weak and irregular, and it was as well that, on the point of collapse, he found an emetic close at hand – the, presumably soapy, water in which he had just shaved. (Christison gave a vivid account of his experience twenty years later in the *British Medical Journal*.) Christison's protégé and successor in the professorial chair, Thomas Fraser conducted a study of the bean, and isolated the main toxin, which he called eserine after the African name for the bean (p.), but which is now known as *physostigmine*, from its Latin name of the plant. It was Fraser who determined that physostigmine is an antidote for curare poisoning, the first ever discovered (though initially by the Africans). He further showed that it exerted several kinds of effects on the eye when applied as drops. It constricted the pupil, thus acting in opposition to belladonna, of which atropine is the active principle (p.). Most importantly, it causes a reduction in the pressure of the fluid between the lens and the cornea, the aqueous humour, and accordingly came into use as a the first treatment for glaucoma, a cause of blindness occasioned by an elevated pressure. In 1925 Edinburgh chemists determined the structure of physostigmine, and synthesised several analogues, of which one in particular, called neostigmine, turned out to be more potent than the parent compound.

This, then, was the state of knowledge when Mary Walker took note of the symptoms displayed by her myasthaenia gravis patients. In her letter to *The Lancet* in 1935she described the plight of a patient whose eyelid was drooping, as was her jaw, which she had to prop up with her hand in order to eat. Her speech had become slurred and she had difficulty swallowing. After a physostigmine injection there was a distinct improvement. On a second patient Mary Walker tried neostigmine, with still better results. The benefits, though, were transient, and so the patients had to keep receiving the drug. Perhaps because of this drawback, and also its unprepossessing source, the reports aroused little interest, at least until they were confirmed by other doctors, and in 1938 were the subject of a demonstration before the Royal Society of Medicine. Mary Walker, who made a number of other contributions to medical progress, eventually received proper recognition for her work on myasthaenia gravis, which was important not only for the patients, but also because it was the first indication that here was a disease of the neuromuscular junction. When researchers finally understood what they were looking for they discovered that myasthaenia gravis was an autoimmune disease - resulting, that is, from a response of the immune system to one of the victim's own bodily constituents, a protein, which it treated as an interloper, like a virus or bacterium. A search revealed the presence in the blood of patients of antibodies against *acetylcholine receptors*. These had yet to be discovered when Mary Walker was plying her hypodermic syringe in Greenwich.

How then to explain why a neurotoxin – a substance such as physostigmine from the Calabar bean – can neutralise the effect of another neurotoxin, curare from the poisonous vine, or whatever its equivalent might be in the bloodstream of patients with myasthaenia gravis? The answer lies in the workings of the neuromuscular junction. This is the *synapse*, comprising the apposed surfaces of a motor neurone – a nerve fibre which comes from the central nervous system, originating in the spinal cord - and a muscle fibre. Both nerve and muscle cells, like all others, are enveloped in a thin membrane. The question now is how the impulse travelling down the neurone activates the muscle. Is the stimulus electrical? In other words is there a discharge across the tiny gap between the two membranes? Or does a chemical signal pass between them? This 'spark' or 'soup' dichotomy was an issue of passionate, sometimes acrimonious debate, which was resolved by an experiment conducted by Otto Loewi (1873-1961) in 1921. Loewi began life in Germany, but at the time of the critical discovery he held a professorial chair in Vienna.* He had learned how to maintain the excised heart of a frog in a biological solution by electrical stimulation of the attached vagus nerve. When he then discarded the heart, and introduced the freshly excised heart from another frog into the medium, it began to beat without electrical stimulation. Clearly then, stimulation of the first heart had caused the secretion of a substance – *Vagusstoff,* or vagus substance, Loewi called it – which activated the beating of the second heart. This was proof positive of the 'soup' theory of nerve transmission. Seven years earlier, in 1914, the great physiologist, (Sir, as he later became)

---

* The idea of the experiment came to Loewi while lying in bed one night, but when he awoke the next morning it had evaporated from his mind. Loewi spent a tortured day, trying to recollect the revelation, but it was only in the following night that he awoke and found that the idea had returned. This time he scribbled the details on a scrap of paper and went back to sleep. The next day he did the experiment. Loewi was a Jew, and after the *Anschluss* in 1938, when Austria and Germany were merged, he was dismissed from his position and arrested. According to his own account, he had been compiling an important paper on his most recent, as yet unpublished work, and his fear was less for the wellbeing of his wife and family than that if he died in Nazi captivity the results of his work would be lost. He was greatly relieved when he managed to bribe a gaoler to despatch a hurriedly written account of the research to a journal. Loewi succeeded in obtaining a position in England, and later emigrated to New York, where he remained to the end of his career.

Henry Hallett Dale (1875-1968) had, while studying the effects of ergot poisons (p.) extracted from the fungus a substance that contracted a muscle in exactly the same way as electrical excitation. Dale's associate at the Wellcome Physiological Research Laboratories near London was Arthur Ewins (the man who began his distinguished career [p.] as a teen-aged laboratory assistant at the Wellcome labs, and ended up as head of research at the pharmaceutical company, May & Baker). Ewins isolated the active principle and identified it as acetylcholine. This later proved also to be Loewi's *Vagusstoff*, and in 1936 Dale and Loewi shared the Nobel Prize for Physiology or Medicine. Soon after, Loewi added another chapter to the story. For the muscle to keep working it must also be allowed to relax between contractions, and therefore the acetylcholine, having induced the contraction, must depart from the scene. In 1926 Loewi and a collaborator published a paper describing the inactivation of acetylcholine by a heart extract. The extract lost this capacity when heated. The implication (not unexpected) was that it contained an enzyme, an *acetylcholinesterase*, which converted the acetylcholine into an inactive product. In the early 1930s Edgar and Ellen Stedman* at the University of Edinburgh isolated the enzyme from horse blood serum, defined its properties, and showed that what it actually did was to split the acetylcholine into two inactive pieces, choline and acetic acid.

---

* Edgar Stedman (1890-1975) had an unusual start in chemistry. He came from an impoverished background, his father having ben captured in South Africa during the Boer War and never heard from again. The son left school at 14, and found employment in a glass factory, where he developed a fascination with chemistry, and educated himself through evening classes in London. He attracted the attention of George Barger, a well-known natural-products chemist, in whose laboratory he met his wife, the daughter of a labourer. She had achieved a Ph.D., and persuaded Barger to take her future husband as a student. The Stedmans followed Barger to Edinburgh, where he had been appointed professor. There Edgar Stedman completed his own Ph.D. with a thesis on physostigmine, and was eventually appointed lecturer. He and his wife derived the structure of physostigmine, and Stedman and a student, Leslie Easson found that when a part of the molecule was chemically split off (hydrolysed) the activity was lost. This led to the synthesis of a series of compounds containing the lost group, which Stedman guessed encapsulated the activity. One such was miotine, which was used for a time as a miotic – an agent that constricts the pupil of the eye – but was later replaced by the more effective neostigmine.

Henry Dale was responsible for fitting the next piece into the jigsaw. In 1933 the Nazis took power in Germany and immediately promulgated the racial laws. Thus it was that a young German physiologist, Wilhelm Feldberg, like Loewi a Jew, was ejected from his position at the University of Berlin. He was lucky: he managed to gain an interview with a representative of the Rockefeller Foundation, who was at first discouraging, but then, rummaging among his papers, found a note from Dale to look out for a promising young physiologist called Feldberg. And so, Feldberg was able to leave Germany and join Dale's laboratory in London. He immediately showed his mettle by inventing an assay for acetylcholine – a critical step because the minute concentrations of the molecule jn the nervous system precluded its measurement by the chemical methods of analysis then available. Only a biological assay would serve, and Feldberg's was based on the response of the single large neurone of a leech. This made it possible for him and Dale to show that the membrane of the muscle cell at the neuromuscular junction in the tongue of a cat was rich in receptors for acetylcholine. Here, then, was the definitive proof that acetylcholine was indeed the neurotransmitter - the agent that carries the signal from the nervous system to the muscle, directing it to contract. (It was later discovered that there are also other neurotransmitters, as will appear.) The report on this milestone in the history of physiology appeared in print in 1934 at almost exactly the same time as Mary Walker's letter to *The Lancet* on the alleviation of myasthaenia gravis by physostigmine. It was not long before the connection was made.

When the autoimmune nature of the disease was confirmed and antibodies against the acetylcholine receptor were found in the patients' circulation, the inference was obvious: the antibodies bound to, and occluded the acetylcholine receptors, and prevented access of the acetylcholine released from the nerve terminal. The contraction signal from the nerve to the muscle therefore was not delivered. The further inference was that curare acted in the same manner – by blocking the access of acetylcholine to its receptor. But what of Mary Walker's physostigmine? How did it reverse the effects of curare and the symptoms of myasthaenia gravis? The first guess would have been that it somehow increased the supply of acetylcholine so as to overwhelm, in part at least, the blocking action of curare or of the anti-acetylcholine-receptor antibodies. But if it could not somehow stimulate the nerve to emit more acetylcholine, it might instead prevent the existing acetylcholine from being destroyed by the acetylcholinesterase. And that indeed was how it worked: when Edgar Stedman and his collaborators added physostigmine to a preparation of acetylcholinesterase, the enzyme stopped working because the drug had bound to its active centre (p.), and prevented its substrate – the acetylcholine – from getting to it.

Several derivatives of physostigmine, in addition to neostigmine, were developed by pharmaceutical companies to improve on the parent compound and reduce its side-effects, but the most powerful acetylcholinesterase inhibitors have a more baleful history. In the 1930s interest grew in organophosphorus compounds – quite simple organic structures containing phosphorus atoms, and also some that contain fluorine in addition. Their toxicity exceeded any expectations. Some were synthesised with clinical objectives in mind (and indeed one at least was briefly used to treat glaucoma). But for the most part they were developed as plant sprays to kill insect pests, and most of all in Germany, as nerve gases for use in war. The first, secretly created by the Baeyer laboratories, was tabun, and it was followed by the yet more lethal sarin. Bulk production had begun well before World War II, and once the war was in progress, human tests were entrusted to scientists and doctors, mainly on prisoners in a plant in Posen (Poznán) in occupied Poland. The Americans and British responded to the threat of chemical attack with compounds of their own. The nerve gases (in reality liquids, delivered as aerosols) are absorbed through the skin, and there are no effective antidotes. Whereas poison gases of a more primitive kind caused many and terrible casualties in World War I, and were much feared, the nerve gases were never deployed on the battlefields of the Second World War. This was mainly for fear of reprisals in kind, but stocks still exist in many countries today, as events in the Middle East have shown. No compounds of this class or their close relatives have secured any toehold in drug therapy. The closest appears to have been the use of some organophosphates in veterinary medicine against infestations by ticks or other parasites. The compounds are presumably too hazardous for human use.

The final resolution of myasthaenia gravis came only in 1963, thanks to new technology. Two biochemists, Chiang-Chiung Chang and Chen-Yuan Lee at the National University of Taiwan had a particular interest in snake venoms. From the venom of the most poisonous of all reptiles, the multi-banded krait, they isolated two compounds. They called them α- and β-bungarotoxin from the zoological name of the snake (*Bungarus multicinctus*), showed that both were ferociously powerful neurotoxins, and determined that the α-bungarotoxin binds to the acetylcholine receptor at the neuromuscular junction, just like curare. To measure the amount and strength of the binding required the introduction of a radioactive label into the toxin molecules, because only in this way could the binding of minuscule amounts be measured. Chang and Lee thus determined the number of receptor molecules on the muscle side of a neuromuscular junction by counting the radioactive disintegrations from the tightly attached toxin, glued so to speak to the receptors. This was in itself at the time a technical advance, but it also allowed similar measurements to be made on neuromuscular junctions of myasthaenia gravis patients, and, indeed, the number of available, unblocked receptors was much smaller than in normal controls.

There was more, for it transpired that β-bungarotoxin acted in a quite different manner: it prevented the release of acetylcholine from the nerve side of the junction. The acetylcholine is not in fact spat out by the nerve terminal as a spray of single molecules, but rather as packet, wrapped up in a vesicle – a tiny hollow bubble of membrane. This membrane bubble merges with the muscle membrane, releasing its cargo within the muscle cell. The release of the vesicles from the nerve terminal is blocked by the toxin. The snake thus makes sure that if its venom does not paralyse its prey by the first mechanism it has another equally deadly weapon in reserve. So, while α-bungarotoxin (like weaker toxins of other snakes, such as the cobra) imitates curare, β-bungarotoxin resembles in its action another notorious neurotoxin, *botulinum*. Botulinum toxin was identified in 1897 by a Dutch researcher, who named it, and purified it in 1928. It was known from much earlier times as the 'sausage poison', for it was rotten sausages (among other spoiled meats) that laid its victims low. The erudite Dutchman recognised that it was produced by a bacterium, to which he gave the name *Clostridium botulinum*, from the Latin for a sausage, *botulus*, a little bag. Much later analyses revealed that the very dangerous toxin is a mixture of seven related molecular species, three of which function exactly like β-bungarotoxin, by - as Arnold Burgen and his co-workers in Cambridge showed in 1949 - preventing the release of the packets of acetylcholine. Botulinum toxin, like most bacterial products, is relatively easy to produce, for the bacteria can be grown in bulk in culture. It was therefore not long before uses for botulinum toxin were found. It is used locally to treat a variety of distressing muscular anomalies, particularly all manner of uncontrollable spasms of face, eyelids, throat and neck (torticollis, or wryneck); it alleviates the symptoms of cerebral palsy, and affords a means of treating strabismus (squint). The effects are in most cases transient, and so the treatment must be repeated at intervals. It also shuts down the sweat glands in cases of excessive sweating. And today, of course, it is widely used cosmetically (Botox treatment) to smooth out skin folds - to convert, as it were, a prune into a plum. It has also in the past been 'weaponised' for applications in war.

The taming of histamine

We cannot do without histamine, and yet this small, quite simple molecule is the bearer of many of our ills. It commands several essential bodily functions. It is most familiar as the cause of allergic symptoms, such as sneezing and itching in hayfever sufferers. Histamine is released by specialised cells, called mast cells, and it sets off the inflammatory response to undesired external agents. It also has neurotransmitter activity, and, as first revealed in a famous paper by Dale (p.) and Laidlaw in 1910, it stimulates the contraction of smooth muscle. Smooth muscle (as opposed to the striated muscles attached to the bones) controls the pulsations of organs, such as the stomach and gut, the bronchial tubes, and the blood vessels, for it is the active layer of the walls enclosing them. When an allergen – a substance that elicits the distressing effects of allergy, or worse, asthma and even anaphylactic shock (p.) – impinges on susceptible individuals, possessing antibodies (p. against that substance, those antibodies pounce on the intruder. The allergen-antibody complex binds

609

to the mast cells, which thereupon spew out histamine. The histamine attaches itself to receptors on mucous surfaces, and the familiar response is set in train through dilation of local blood vessels, penetration of blood plasma into the tissues, and general disorder.

The discovery of histamine and its significance, set out in a series of classic papers by Henry Dale and his colleagues at the Wellcome Laboratories, spurred the pharmacologists in Europe and America into action, but to little effect. The aim was to discover a histamine antagonist, but the problem, as usual was to find a lead compound, and there was little in the way of clues. It was not until 1936 that there was real progress, and it came, not for the first time, (see Chapter …) from Daniel Bovet and Ernest Fourneau at the Pasteur Institute in Paris. Bovet seized on an observation in one of Dale's papers that the effect of histamine on the contraction of a strip of guinea pig intestine – Dale's standard assay system, which had led him to the identification of histamine in the first place – was marginally reduced by adrenaline. So adrenaline became Bovet's lead compound. Bovet already in fact had some adrenaline analogues that blocked the action of the parent compound. One such, designated F929, was synthesised by the old virtuoso, Ernest Fourneau, and it had a striking effect in the intestine-strip assay. More, it was highly active in the intact guinea pig, which recovered from what should have been a lethal dosf by injection of histamine. Bit F929 failed in humans, for not only was its effect weak but it showed unacceptable toxicity. Bovet continued, and he and a young colleague, Anne-Marie Staub, found that several more derivatives made by Fourneau were effective in man, though were still too toxic for clinical use. At this point the baton passed to the group's commercial collaborators at Rhône-Poulenc, and it was one of their chemists who finally, in 1942, struck gold with phenbenzamine, which came on the market as Antergan. Two years on, Bovet and his friends produced a close relative of that compound, mepyramine, also called pyrilamine, or Neo-Antergan. It was even better and became a universally popular treatment for hayfever and other allergies. Bovet's success and the enormous demand for pills to suppress the symptoms of allergies set off a fierce competition in the pharmaceutical industry worldwide after 'me-too' medications, and soon large numbers of these swamped the market. All were descendants of F929. There was animated debate about whether antihistamines of this sort should be used to treat asthma, and for a while doctors prescribed them for that purpose, but later studies indicated that this was actually a harmful strategy, and the practice was stopped.

Cardiology: a new awakening

James Whyte Black (1924-2010) was a Scot, the fourth of five sons of a mining engineer of modest means. As a boy he had two passionate interests – music and mathematics – but when the time came, he entered St. Andrew's University at the urging of a doctor brother, to study medicine. His talents were recognised, and after graduating he was invited to teach physiology at St. Andrew's, the subject that had caught his imagination. Then came an interlude at the University of Singapore, which offered an income sufficient to discharge his student debts. His research career began on his return to Scotland, where he was offered a position in the physiology department at Glasgow University. There he built up a highly effective research group, and in 1950 started the work that would in time bring him universal acclaim, a knighthood and a Nobel Prize. Black was an exceptionally original thinker, prepared always to question received wisdom. Until then the approach to heart disease caused by constricted arteries, and leading to the distress of angina, was to increase oxygen supply to the heart with a vasodilator, such as nitroglycerine (p.) was held to be. Black thought otherwise. Why not instead reduce the heart's oxygen demand? The actions of adrenaline and noradrenaline (p.) on different physiological functions had presented some paradoxes: their actions appeared to differ according to where they were exerted. In 1948 Raymond Ahlquist at the Medical College of Georgia published – with difficulty, for it was several times rejected by medical journals - a classical paper. It was regarded at the time as controversial, and was for the most part disregarded because its conclusions ran counter to current teaching. Ahlquist had been searching for a drug that would selectively relax smooth muscle, but his observations led him to a resolution of the enigma of the divergent activities exerted by both adrenaline and noradrenaline. There were, he suggested, two types of receptor for the two hormones, and also others related to them, which activated different metabolic processes. Ahlquist called them α and β (alpha and beta) adrenotropic receptors. They are now called α- and β-adrenergic receptors (or adrenoceptors), and each was later discovered to comprise a collection of subtypes. The importance of Ahlquist's work was not lost on James Black, and it determined the direction his research would take.

The α-adrenergic receptors, which are the regulators of smooth muscle relaxation and also contraction, and therefore dilation or constriction of the blood vessels, play a major part in determining blood delivery. The arrival of adrenaline – boosted of course by excitement or stress - has a parallel effect on the heart. It provokes a rise in frequency of contraction of the muscle (an increased heart rate) by binding to β-adrenergic receptors. What Black was after was an antagonist of adrenaline binding, but only to the β-receptor, for the resulting reduction of the heart rate would decrease the consumption of, and therefore demand for oxygen. Several of the major pharmaceutical laboratories had been searching during the previous decade or so for adrenaline antagonists, with mixed success. Many adrenaline analogues had been generated, and some had found their way onto the clinic, but none had any worthwhile effect on the heart, until two chemists at the Eli Lilley company made, as so often, an accidental discovery. They were looking for long-acting smooth-muscle relaxants for use as better bronchodilators for asthma patients. They assayed their compounds on the smooth muscle contained in strips of trachea, pre-treated with pilocarpine (p.), an alkaloid that induced contraction of the muscle. A bronchodilator would reverse the action of the pilocarpine. To economise on assay material the trachea strips would be re-used, but to ensure that they were still functional they were first tested by exposure to adrenaline. This led to the unexpected discovery that exposure to one of the new compounds, dichloroisoproterenol, or DCI, rendered the smooth muscle resistant to adrenaline. When this observation became publicly known in 1957, Neil Moran, a pharmacologist at Emory University in Atlanta thought of trying the compound on the action of the heart. It did indeed appear to block the β-adrenergic receptors, but also induced the known effects associated with adrenaline, and so Eli Lilley lost interest.

Black had by this time left Glasgow for the more affluent environment and freedom from teaching that the Pharmaceutical Division of Imperial Chemical Industries (ICI) at Alderley Park near Manchester afforded him. There, moreover, he had found an exceptional organic chemist, John Stephenson, who, as he later recalled, 'taught me about modern deductive organic chemistry; how to be more than merely curious about a molecule with an interesting biological effect; how to ask questions about it. He converted me to pharmacology'. Black decided that in the hunt for the selective blocking agent, DCI was to be their lead compound, and in 1960 a derivative surfaced, which blocked the β- but not the α-adrenergic receptors. Tested on patients, it eased the agonies of angina and increased the sufferers' capacity for exercise. Black spoke in his Nobel Lecture about his exultation and that of his team at this vindication of their conjectures. But the new compound, pronethanol, did not survive a full clinical trial, for a series of side-effects soon came to the fore, and more extensive animal tests gave evidence of carcinogenicity. It was 1963 before compound ICI 45,520, propanolol came along. This substance showed no carcinogenicity in animals, and remarkably little in the way of side-effects, and it changed the practice of cardiovascular medicine. It was launched in 1964 under the name of Inderal, and did more than lessen the frequency of angina attacks: an evaluation after three years revealed that it reduced deaths from ischaemic heart disease – that is disease caused by impaired blood supply to the heart, due usually to blocked arteries – fourfold. It was also effective in combatting arrhythmia – irregular heartbeat. Propanolol became for a period the world's most widely sold drug, although the FDA in the United States withheld its approval until 1973, a delay that must have cost many lives. Within a few years many new and still better drugs, based on the same principle as propranolol, were on the market.

The rebellious stomach

Stomach disorders have troubled mankind through all of recorded time. In ancient days tthey were commonly treated with earths and clays, such as *terra sigillata* ('sealed earth', now more familiar to potters than to physicians), Armenian bolus and kaolin. These do have the property of absorbing many substances, such as bacterial toxins and intestinal gas. Better for this purpose, and still used, is animal charcoal. A different approach was to take a carbonate, such as natron (sodium carbonate with an admixture of bicarbonate) to neutralise excess acid (for acid was inferred, even as early as 1702 by van Helmont (p.) in his work, *De debribus stomachi*, to be the seat of digestive problems). Calcium carbonate in its many forms, such as limestone or alabaster, would have served equally well. (Pliny recommended powdered corral, which is also calcium carbonate, but obviously harder to come by, so certainly more expensive, and therefore probably regarded as superior.) Powdered metals, including iron and lead, were recommended by some physicians and healers. These and many other inorganic materials were the best that medicine had to offer for millennia.

The 19th century was, in the prosperous nations of the west at least, the age of dyspepsia. The word has largely fallen out of use. One talks now of indigestion, or if one is a physician, of *gastroesophogal reflux disorder*. Hippocrates is said to have declared that 'bad digestion is the root of all evil', and indeed that 'death sits in the bowels'. Two millennia on literary Victorians gave vivid descriptions of its torments; Thomas Carlyle and Charles Dickens were two who endured the condition for most of their working lives. Henry Lytton Bulwer, diplomat and writer opined that 'Some evils admit of consolations, but there are no comforters for dyspepsia and the toothache'. Dickens's affliction was designated 'nervous dyspepsia', occasioned by overwork and anxiety, and it caused him not only perpetual discomfort but also the embarrassment of breaking wind at both the upper and nether ends. Commonly chronic heartburn and stomach pain were the result of stomach ulcers. That stomach juice resembled car battery acid in strength was established early in the 19th century, and it was not long before the medical profession was unanimous that ulcers were caused by an excess of hydrochloric acid, and that this was commonly linked to stress and ill-temper, or overindulgence in unhealthy foods and alcohol.* The treatment was still to neutralise the superfluous acid with a mildly alkaline reagent, such as sodium bicarbonate, but the intense effervescence could damage the stomach, and its effect in any case was transient. A distraction in 1915 was an allegedly superior therapy conceived by a Chicago doctor, Bertram Sippy. This consisted of drinking a large volume of milk and cream at hourly intervals for ten days. It could then be supplemented by eggs and boiled cereal for a further extended period. This was reported to give some relief, but most patients found it too burdensome, and a number of those who persisted developed

---

* There was a certain amount of evidence for this theory, most famously from the researches of an American army doctor, William Beaumont on his human guinea pig. One night in 1822 Dr Beaumont had been summoned to the aid of a Canadian fur trader, Alexis St. Martin, who had been accidentally shot through the midriff while carousing in a saloon in Michigan. The man was not expected to live, but thanks to Beaumont's ministrations, and against all expectations, the wound healed, leaving however a fistula, which gave access to the interior of the stomach. Beaumont saw an opportunity to make medical history, and drew up an agreement with his patient to feed and pay him in return for, in effect, possession of his stomach. He could introduce fragments of food through the fistula and observe their erosion by the digestive juices, which he had analysed at intervals throughout the digestive process. He also found that when St. Martin became enraged – something to which he was fully entitled – a flow of bile ensued. Moreover, after a rich meal, and an intake of hard liquor, a surge of acid was released. Beaumont wrote a series of papers on his observations, and exhibited his peripatetic stomach at conferences. There was in fact nothing very surprising in what Beaumont was able to report, for animal experiments in the previous century had delivered much the same results, but it nevertheless brought the information to the attention of doctors. Experiments on the digestive process were performed throughout the 19th century. One American doctor even lowered a small silver bucket on a thread down his subjects' gullets and into their stomachs at different times after meals. He would then haul it up and analyse the contents. (Oddly, the American writer and *farceur*, Robert Benchley conceived and practised in the 1950s a jape on this theme, which he obviously thought too outlandish to be believed by any but the simple-minded. When travelling, he would loop a string round his ear with the other end in his mouth. When questioned, as he rarely was, by an inquisitive stranger - for most people who noticed were too discreet to comment - he would reply that he was a doctor from a famous medical school, performing a digestion experiment a silver bucket in his stomach was securattached to the string, and he would haul it up and analyse his stomach juices after ingesting foods of different sorts.)

615

serious kidney disease, a rise in blood alkalinity, or a fall in blood calcium level, with various unpleasant consequences. Sippy's method was hastily abandoned, and sufferers returned to bicarbonate and other antacids, as they are called. Better, less damaging versions were developed over the years. They include magnesium hydroxide, aluminium hydroxide (Gavascon) and bismuth subsalicylate (Pepto-Bismol). These and others fill the pharmacies' shelves in the form of tablets and liquid suspensions. They are a help, especially for trivial upsets, but have undesired effects if taken in excessive amounts, and of course treat symptoms but not causes. A real advance in the treatment of stomach ulcers was a long time coming.

It came from James Black. Restive at the prospect of time spent refining and exploiting a new generation of β-receptor blockers (commonly now referred to as β-blockers), he was already incubating a new project. He had become convinced that the histamine antagonists then in use would turn out to be related to α-receptor blockers. If this were so it might be possible to develop inhibitors of histamine-dependent acid release in the stomach to treat indigestion and stomach ulcers. Thus it was that when in 1964 the head of the pathology division at ICI left for a position at Smith, Kline and French (now GlaxoSmithKline or SK) in Welwyn Garden City near London, Black asked to accompany him. At SKF Black once again built up a skilled and enthusiastic team, and he found especially another first-rate organic chemist, Robin Ganellin, to take the place of ICI's John Stephenson. That histamine elicits secretion of acid in the stomach was well documented. It had been demonstrated in 1920 by a Polish physiologist, Leon Popielski, professor at the University of Lwów (then Austro-Hungarian Lemberg, and now Ukranian Lvív). He had injected histamine into a dog and measured the amount of acid in the animal's stomach, whereas Black and his colleagues assayed acid release by histamine and its analogues in rats.

The plan was to find a histamine analogue that would block the presumptive histidine receptor on the stomach cells, but to find a lead compound was no small challenge. Indeed, it took four years and the synthesis of more than 200 compounds before there was a glimmer of hope - by which time the management had directed Black to abandon the project, but their injunction was disregarded. The substance found by one of Black's team was not primarily an antagonist of histamine activity, but a 'partial agonist,' which initially acted more powerfully on the receptor than histamine itself, and caused an acid surge. Here nonetheless was the long-sought lead compound, and the effects of different substitutions in the structure could now be rationally explored. Relatively quickly, in 1972, an effective histamine antagonist was found. This was burimamide. Yet it was not ideal, because it could be administered only by injection, and so work continued. Gamellin eventually produced metiamide, which worked when taken by mouth, and was much more potent than burimamide. This was still not the end of the road, for human trials exposed a serious side-effect: some patients developed the blood disease, agranulocytosis – the loss of granulocytes (p.) in the blood. Finally, in 1973, came the desired product, which abundantly vindicated Black's faith. It was called cimetidine, and came on the market in Britain 1976 and in the U.S. a year later under the name of Tagamet. Such was the instant demand that the priority became the improvement of the synthesis to permit production on a larger scale. This was achieved in the American laboratories of SKF, and the drug became one of the best-selling pharmaceutical products of all time, and offered tortured humanity at long last an effective treatment for stomach acid and ulcers.

Black had characteristically moved on as soon as the essential discovery had been made, and took up an academic position, as Professor of Pharmacology at University College London. (After four years during which he redirected the teaching of the subject, he moved again, back once more to a pharmaceutical laboratory, as director of Therapeutics at the Wellcome laboratories, and thence after another seven years to King's College London. There he enjoyed several more productive years before his retirement with, by then, a knighthood and the Nobel Prize in Physiology or Medicine for 1988.) Research on histamine receptor blockers did not end at this point. For one thing it had been established that there were four kinds of receptors associated with the multifarious activities of histamine in the body. That in the stomach was designated H_2, and cimetidine reacted only with this one. In 1976 researchers at Glaxo found that variants of cimetidine with one substitution (of an oxygen for a nitrogen in the central ring system) were equally effective, but more specific blockers of the H$_2$ receptor, and had fewer side-effects. One such is ranitidine, known commercially as Zantac, developed in England by David Jack (p.) and his research group at Allen and Hanbury* (subsequently absorbed by Glaxo and then GSK). Ranitidine largely displaced cimetidine from which it was derived, for it was longer-acting and had fewer side-effects. It became until 1989 the world's most widely prescribed drug, until it was in its turn supplanted by AstraZeneca's omeprazole, sold as Prilosec, among other names. Prilosec at its zenith cleared sales of nearly $6 billion per year; for by then - perhaps because of the rise in the U.S. of overindulgence and obesitygastroesophogal reflux disease', or GERD, known in more innocent times as heartburn, was afflicting a large proportion of Americans. Thus the acidity suppressants (proton pump inhibitors) ascended to third in the most widely used categories of drugs, after antipsychotics and statins. They were moreover available over the counter.

Omeprazole became the focus of some skulduggery by AstraZeneca when the patent expired in 2001. The company managed to delay the change to generic status for a while by court actions, but then hit on a new stratagem. Omeprazole is a mixture of equal parts of two enantiomers, a left- and a right-handed form (as most complex synthetic compounds are, unless the trouble is taken to separate the two [p.]), one of which possesses the full physiological activity, while the other is a passenger or perhaps or only slightly active. AstraZeneca separated the isomers, and persuaded the FDA to approve the active form (half of the original Prilosec) as a new drug. It was given the name esomeprazole, put on the market as Nexium. Esomeprazole is of course active, presumably in fact twice as active weight-for-weight as the mixture from which it is derived. A vast advertising campaign ensured that Nexium largely displaced Prilosec as the

---

* Allen and Hanbury was a small, well-respected company, established in London by Quaker owners in 1715. It produced over-the-counter medicinals, such as cod liver oil, but was especially famous for its glycerine black current pastilles, which were immensely popular. There were also many other kinds of pastilles – the genre probably invented by the company – with fruit flavours, some of them medicated. Allen and Hanbury became a force in pharmaceutical research only in the mid-20th century, largely under the influence of David Jack.

most-favoured anti-GERD drug, although the now much cheaper generic omeprazole may be catching up.

In recent years warnings have been issued about the dangers of using proton pump inhibitors for long periods. The stomach, after all, is meant to be strongly acid if it is to fulfil its function of digesting foods. Persistent suppression of the acid-secretion mechanism leads to a reaction involving the formation of more and more acid-secreting cells, and a vicious cycle begins, resulting in dependence on the drugs. A further consequence is that absorption of important nutrients, such as vitamins, is impaired, and is apt to lead in turn to repression of red-blood-cell production and anaemia. Other problems may arise, including an increased risk of colonisation of the stomach by the pathogenic bacterium, *Clostridium difficile* (p.). Omeprazole is nevertheless a valuable medicine, prescribed, often together with antibiotics against *Helicobacter pylori* (see below), as a treatment for stomach ulcers.

The malign life-form lurking in the stomach

One day in 1979 a young doctor, Barry Marshall (b. 1951) at the Royal Perth Hospital in Western Australia, in search of a research project, which would form part of his training, visited a pathologist in the gastroenterology department. The pathologist, Robin Warren (b. 1937) had made a curious observation: he had found that stomach biopsies of patients with persistent inflammation and often ulcers of the stomach seemed nearly always to contain curved elongated bacteria. Warren was able to rule out contamination on the grounds that the bacteria were lodged under the mucous layer covering the stomach lining. He had therefore begun to wonder whether there might be a causal relation between the disease and the bug. Marshall was captivated. He had read the literature of gastroenterology and had found occasional reports of such bacteria in the stomach acid. Indeed there had been recorded sightings from time to time since the previous century, but nobody had tried to culture the bacteria, and the reports had aroused no interest. If gastroenterologists had thought about the question at all they had probably assumed that the bacteria were comensuals – organisms that cohabited with another life-form (in this case man), without bestowing any benefit or causing any harm. Others may have disbelieved the story on the grounds that no bacteria could be expected to live in the corrosively acidic stomach environment. But during the 20ᵗʰ century it became clear that there were species of bacteria that could thrive in the most extreme of conditions, in the Dead Sea, in which the salt concentration was close to saturation, and in hot springs, and the thermal vents in the floor of the Pacific Ocean, where the temperature approaches that of boiling water. Such bacteria are now known as 'extremophiles'.

Marshall, at all events, resolved to dedicate himself to the problem, which he began to study on finding a position in gastroenterology in another teaching hospital in the city, the Fremantle Hospital. His work continued throughout a period in a remote town far north of Perth, and then in what time he could spare from his clinical duties back at the Royal Perth Hospital. The first encouraging sign came in late 1981 when he gave an antibiotic, tetracycline to a patients suffering from an obstinate gastritis. After two weeks of treatment the condition abated. The essential step now was to culture the bacteria, and prove that they were indeed the cause of the illness, in accordance with 'Koch's postulates' (p.), and this turned out to be unusually difficult. Marshall tried many variations of culture media, but to no avail. It was, as so often, an accident that led to success. After repeated disappointments Marshall departed on a four-day break, leaving several abandoned Petri dishes in an incubator in the dark laboratory. On his return he found rich growths of bacterial colonies on the agar. The new species of bacteria grew, it turned out, with exceptional reluctance and so slowly, on any of the culture media. It later appeared that they preferred something altogether richer in the way of protein in the medium. This was something Marshall had not thought to take into account, for he had misidentified the bacteria as belonging to a known species, *Campylobacter jejuni*, similar in appearance, and more than once reported in the stomach, but less fastidious in its demands for nutrients.

This was well and good, but to fulfil Koch's criteria for proving that a micro-organism was the cause of the disease, and not an epiphenomenon, more was needed, and Marshall's attempts to infect animals with preparations of the bacteria persistently failed. Out of patience, Marshall finally decided to perform the critical experiment on himself. He obtained ethical approval from the hospital, but felt it prudent not to divulge his intention to his wife, since the prospect of a gastric ulcer was not an enticing one, and could even be life-threatening. Expecting the onset of gastritis (inflammation of the stomach), and perhaps the appearance of an ulcer in a space of weeks, he swallowed a suspension of the bacteria taken from a patient, and awaited developments. It was only three days before he began to experience stomach discomfort and ferocious halitosis. On the eighth day after taking the dose endoscopy (examination of the stomach by way of a flexible tube with a light and video camera at its end) revealed severe inflammation and damage to the stomach lining, and the presence of a rich culture of the bacteria. After fourteen days, Marshall took antibiotics and the condition eased. It was time to try treating patients with gastritis and some with stomach ulcers in the same manner, with antibiotics. On the way, Marshall had also made another discovery: he found that bismuth compounds, which had been used for two centuries to soothe the distress of gastritis and ulcers (and today most commonly as Pepto-Bismol) inhibited the growth of the bacteria. These compounds give relief, though of short duration. Warren and Marshall reported striking improvements in a large majority of patients treated with antibiotics and bismuth in their clinical trial.

Their publications were met with a mixture of interest and derision, for most doctors knew, or thought they knew, that ulcers, if not gastric distress generally, were caused by stress, excess stomach acid or unsuitable food. The observations were however soon replicated in European, American and Japanese centres, and gradually the sceptics were convinced. An advance was the identification of the bacterium as a hitherto unrecognised species, unrelated to *Campylobacter*. It was given the name *Helicobacter pylori* (*helico* because the electron microscope revealed that it had the form of a corkscrew, or helix, and *pylori* because the infection was concentrated mainly in the pylorus, the channel at the bottom of the stomach, leading to the duodenum). Marshall and Warren were awarded the Nobel Prize in 2005 for their discovery, which was undoubtedly important, although it turned out, as ever, to be less than the whole story. It is still not clear exactly what part *H. pylori* plays in the mechanism (the aetiology in the jargon) of gastritis and the formation of stomach and duodenal ulcers. It is now known that in some parts of the world, depending presumably on diet and other environmental factors, a high proportion of the population are hosts to the bacterium without experiencing any ill-effects. Nevertheless, ulcers are now treated with mixtures of antibiotics, bismuth and an H_2 receptor blocker – one of the successors to James Black's cimetidine.

Thicker than water

Anticoagulants – substances that prevent the clotting of blood – have saved lives without number, and their introduction counts among the most important advances in medical and surgical practice of the 20th century. Anticoagulants are given to victims of heart attacks, strokes, pulmonary and venous blood clots (such as DVT, or deep-vein thrombosis) and atrial fibrillation (a form of arrhythmia, or irregular heart beat), which predisposes to strokes. The sooner the anticoagulant is administered following a heart attack or stroke the better the chances of recovery, but long-term, even lifelong, treatment of people liable to such mishaps is equally important. Anticoagulants are now inseparable from some kinds of surgery, and also from the efficacy of artificial organs. The prodigious use of leeches in medicine to bleed the sick (Chapter 3) must have suggested to the more perceptive practitioners that the creatures possessed the means of preventing the blood that they ingested from clotting. Yet it was only in 1884 that a British doctor John Berry Haycraft, who had dedicated himself to the study of clotting, showed that this was indeed the case. He made a preparation of dried leeches, and showed that it caused blood to remain liquid. He called this preparation hirudin from the Latin name of the leech, *Hirudo*. There are of course many species of leech, but the one most widely used by physicians of the time (as it still is in some specialised areas of surgery) is *Hirudo medcinalis*. Hirudin found applications in research but not in medicine until seventy years later, when a pure anticoagulant material was isolated from the crude extract. But in the meantime there had been progress from other sources.

In 1915 William Henry Howell, professor of physiology at Johns Hopkins University in Baltimore, and an expert on blood clotting, assigned a research project to a second-year medical student, Jay McLean. McLean came from a medical family, and had an ardent ambition to prove himself in research. He saved money to support himself for a year, which he would spend entirely in the laboratory with the firm resolve to make a discovery. With this in mind, he moved from the University of California to Johns Hopkins, a prominent centre of medical research. The clotting process was still veiled in obscurity, and what Howell asked his student to attempt to isolate a clotting agent from a crude extract of brain tissue that had been found to accelerate the clotting process. McLean began by learning enough of the language to read the German literature on the subject, which disclosed that similar extracts from heart and from liver would also assist clotting. He nevertheless chose to follow first the original procedure for making an active preparation from brain. He extracted the dried tissue with ether, and then precipitated a mass of dissolved material by adding ethanol (ordinary alcohol). (The starting material was so malodorous that McLean was banished from lunch with Howell and his colleagues.) The solubility in ether implied that the active substance was fatty in character. McLean confirmed that it lost its potency on storage and exposure to the air, but in addition he found something that had escaped Howell, namely that successive extraction and alcohol precipitation steps yielded less and less activity. So the active material was largely insoluble in alcohol and remained for the most part in the ether. Turning to heart and liver, he noted that the extracts had similar properties to those from brain, the clot-promoting fraction remaining in the ether. It must be, he thought, an unsaturated fatty acid (p.), which lost activity through oxidation by air. But then, in 1916, McLean made his discovery. He had followed the rate at which the clot-inducing activity declined, and was trying to relate it to the rate of oxidation of the fatty substance. But when testing the oldest samples he found not only that the clot-promoting activity had fallen to zero, but that a clot-retarding activity had appeared in the samples, most strongly in those from liver.

McLean did not tell Howell until he had repeated the observation many times, and was convinced it was correct. When told of the result, Howell would not believe it. The only known natural clot-retarding substance was an 'antithrombin' in the blood, and since this was a protein, it could clearly not have entered the ether solution. Nothing McLean promised to persuade Howell to take him seriously. He summoned the laboratory technician, who brought and bled a cat. McLean placed the small vessel of blood on the bench in front of Howell, added a little of his liver extract, stirred, and invited the professor to tell him when it clotted. It did not clot.* McLean departed from protocol, and without apparently tellimg Howell, submitted an account of his work for publication to make sure that he would not be deprived of the credit. A full paper by Howell and McLean followed, which included the first experiment in a living animal, a dog, injected with McLean's preparation. Howell gave the compound the name, heparin (from the Greek for the liver). It was to be some years before heparin became a viable therapeutic proposition. Only in 1935 did a Swedish biochemist determine its structure, which guided the first procedures for producing it (most often from pigs' intestines) in bulk. In 1936 it was made available by a Swedish pharmaceutical company, Vitrum AB, and soon after that by the Connaught Laboratories in Toronto (where Charles Best, one of the co-discoverers of insulin (p.) led the research).

Heparin is a polymer – a long chain of similar chemical units, in this case types of sugar, linked to one another. It occurs in many places in the body. It has a somewhat chequered history on account of impurities that have in the past often accompanied it. In 2008 stocks in America, imported from China, gave rise to a toxic product. The worst effect was a precipitate drop in blood pressure in some patients. A few people died and there were some 800 recorded cases of serious illness. The contaminant turned out to be another naturally occurring polymer, the highly sulphated (containing, that is, a large number of the highly acidic $-SO_3$ groups) chondroitin sulphate. Heparin is also sulphated, although to a much lesser degree, but both variable sulphation and uncertain chain length of different preparations made for erratic activity. Since that time, therefore, polymers of short and fully controlled chain length have often been preferred, because of more

---

* Jay McLean wrote an account of his discovery and of his early career in 1957, stopping short at this point, which was when he fell ill and soon after died. It was published in 1959.

reproducible activity and fewer side-effects. Another version is synthetic, consisting of only five linked sugars. All heparins have to be given by injection, which has the advantage of instantaneous action. But it is an undesirable feature for long-term users, and hardly had heparin come into use than the search was on for an oral anticoagulant.

Clotting, or coagulation, of blood is a process of enormous complexity, encompassed by a large congeries of proteins acting sequentially. Haemophilia is a hereditary disease (which famously plagued Queen Victoria's extended family), caused by the failure of just one link in the chain of events, and is treated by supplying the normal functional form of the defective protein. Different anticoagulants have different targets in the chain of events, the disabling of any one of which amounts to a spanner tossed into the delicate machinery. The first oral anticoagulant acts quite differently therefore from heparin. Like heparin it was not being sought when it was found. Here, according to an account by the principal protagonist, Karl Link, written 25 year later, is how it came about. On an icy Saturday afternoon in February 1933 a Wisconsin cattle farmer appeared at the door of the Biochemistry Building of the University of Wisconsin in Madison. His animals had been dying of haemorrhages, and desperate for advice, he had drive nearly 200 miles (although, according to Link's biographer, the distance had increased and the temperature diminished with the telling) to confront the State Veterinary Officer with the evidence. Finding the office closed, he had accidentally found his way to Link in Biochemistry.

Karl Paul Link (1901-1978) was one of ten children of a German immigrant family. His father was a Lutheran pastor, who encouraged the children's academic ambitions, and Karl was sent to the University of Wisconsin to study chemistry. After a period gaining experience in three leading laboratories in Europe he returned to Madison in 1927 as Assistant Professor, and busied himself with research in plant carbohydrates and plant diseases. Link was not the easiest of colleagues; he was jealous of his standing in relation to others, assertive, and given to fits of temper, which led him once to a brawl with one of his own best students. But he nurtured a long line of outstanding protégés, who went on to distinguished careers. Having inspected the evidence – a dead cow and a milk can containing uncoagulated blood - Link was able to offer the farmer a diagnosis, confirming in fact that of the local vet. The cows had died of 'sweet clover disease'. Sweet clover was the source of hay on which cattle in the region were commonly fed in the winter. It was so-called because it exuded a sweetish scent, reminiscent of vanilla, and in damp conditions, as in the previous summer, it was susceptible to a fungus, which contained a toxin. In 1920, after an exceptionally wet summer, there had been an epidemic of the disease, and it was two veterinary scientists who had independently discovered its source. The toxin prevented clotting, and the cows simply died of an internal haemorrhage, or bled to death when they suffered a scratch, just like a human victim of haemophilia. Link could only advise the farmer to change his surviving animals' feed or to ask for transfusions for those already sick. But Link also decided to find the toxic constituent, and put three of his research students to work on the problem.

Extracting and identifying the active factor was no trivial matter, especially because its solubility in water and other solvents proved to be low. The earlier veterinary workers had tried and failed. Eventually one of Link's students hit on mild alkali as an extracting medium, but the substance was still accompanied by much other soluble material from the hay. It was only in 1939 that a pure crystalline compound was isolated, which had unprecedented anticoagulant activity. The students determined the structure: it was 3,3'-methylene*bis*(4-hydroxycoumarin, or dicumarol for short, a compound prepared by German chemists in 1903. The students were then set the task of synthesising it to show that the laboratory product worked as it should, and as indeed it did. Most importantly, tests on dogs showed that it worked when given by mouth. Next, it was established that its activity was counteracted by vitamin K, one of the components in the clotting cascade that had recently been discovered. This was a major advance, and the clinical potential of the compound was not lost on Link. When the paper by him and his students appeared it at once caught the attention of the cardiologists, and within weeks it had been tested on patients with emboli, and soon secured approval for clinical use. It was marketed as dicoumarol.

Link was still not satisfied. The action was slower than might have been wished, and there were other disadvantages. Then in 1945 Link had a recurrence of tuberculosis, which had first afflicted him as a young man working in Europe, and had confined him for some months to a sanatorium in Switzerland. With the return of the disease he was again forced to stop work at the university, and take shelter in a sanatorium near Madison. There he found the leisure to study the literature and his laboratory records and to cogitate. His next generation of students had in the interim synthesised and tested more than 100 analogues of dicumarol, and his cogitations led him to compound 42 as the most promising. Link and two of his students took out a patent on this substance, and allocated it to the Wisconsin Alumni Research Foundation (WARF), an organisation set up by Harry Steenbock, a professor at the university, whose patent on vitamin D had generated a large income, used to support research. Link called his compound warfarin as a tribute to WARF, and patented it as a rodent poison, for laboratory data had shown it to be particularly potent in that respect. Its translation into the most widely used long-term anticoagulant, as it still is, for vulnerable human patients came about in a curious way: in 1951 a young recruit in the U.S. army made a failed attempt at suicide by taking a large dose of rat poison – warfarin. He apparently suffered no ill-effects, and when Link came to hear of it, he suggested that the lack of toxicity of the compound in the human subject might make it the anticoagulant of choice (although of course there must be a lethal limit somewhere far beyond the clinically effective dose). Warfarin was soon available for clinical use under the name of Coumadin, as it has remained.

New anticoagulants, which work at different points in the clotting cascade, have been developed in recent years, and there are circumstances in which they are preferred to Coumadin. But the oldest of all waited many years before it was identified as such. In 1950 a paper appeared in the *Annals of Western Medicine and Surgery*, an organ of surpassing obscurity, and then another in the *Journal of Insurance Medicine*. The author was Lawrence I. Craven (1883-1956), a general practitioner in the Californian town of Glendale. Dr Craven was a cautious man, and modest to an unusual degree, for had he published his observations in mainstream journals, they would have attracted a great deal more attention than they did. Craven performed minor surgical procedures in his practice, as did many general practitioners at the time. The bulk were the removal of tonsils, as was then highly popular, and adenoids. In 36 years of practice, he wrote, he had performed hundreds of such procedures, only five of them in a hospital. Craven would take out the tonsils in the morning, and by early afternoon the patients would be sent home. In hardly any cases had there been any haemorrhage, but that suddenly changed. In the last six years before Craven wrote his brief reports there had been an alarming incidence of haemorrhages. On searching for any change in the circumstances he found that the start of the episodes coincided with the introduction of a pastille containing aspirin, given to alleviate the postoperative discomfort.

Craven fell to thinking about what a previously unnoticed anticoagulant property of aspirin, if this was indeed responsible, might portend. Might aspirin have the power to prevent the formation of the blood clots that lead to heart attacks and strokes? He had been struck by the rarity of heart attacks in women compared to men. Women, he had noticed, took aspirin frequently. They used it to alleviate headaches and other minor unpleasantness, while men tended to regard a recourse to pills as unmanly. In 1948 Craven decided to put his theory to the test: he persuaded his patients – those between 30 and 90 - to take two aspirin tablets every day. After two years, when he wrote his first paper, he was able to report than none had suffered a heart attack. Over the next two years Craven received letters from several doctors who had seen his report and had tried his treatment on their own patients, and their observations bore out his own. In 1953 he published his third and only other paper, for which he selected yet another recondite periodical, *The Mississippi Medical Journal*. By then there were 1500 men in the trial, and none had suffered a heart attack, though this must have been to some, perhaps minor degree fortuitous. In this report he restricted his recommendation of a small daily dose of aspirin to men aged from 45 to 65, and those who were at risk by reason of obesity or a sedentary life-style. Craven also did a telling experiment to prove to himself that aspirin was indeed an anticoagulant: he swallowed twelve tablets a day for five days, when he experienced frequent and profuse nose-bleeds. Craven's clinical trials were not of course placebo-controlled and blinded, nor would he have been in a position to organise such an undertaking. Craven is now properly remembered for his remarkable perspicuity, not to say diffidence, and he has been vindicated by extensive later research in many famous centres of academic research, which have found out how exactly aspirin intervenes in the clotting process. This simplest of drugs has never been ec, ipsed.

The coming of the clot busters

Another question is what can be done to save someone who has just been smitten with a stroke, thrombosis or heart attack. Warfarin will help to prevent clot formation in people at risk, but when a clot has already formed and the victim been felled by a heart attack or a pulmonary embolism it is far too slow in acting, and even heparin is of limited help. How might a life-endangering blood clot, then, be rapidly dispersed? What is needed is a thrombolytic (also known as a fibrinolytic) agent. A clot consists mainly of the protein, fibrin, a thread-like molecule, which, in the clot, is chemically bonded to several identical molecules – is cross-linked – to form a sticky mass. This much was known in the 19th century, and as we have seen, the process by which it is formed involves many players, acting on each other in sequential manner. In 1933 William Smith Tillett (1892-1974) a doctor and microbiologist, Associate Professor at Johns Hopkins University, where so many medical advances had their origin, made a curious observation, an oddity that most researchers might have disregarded. He was studying the course of streptococcal infections, which at the time were often fatal (and are not to be taken lightly today). One of the defences against some kinds of bacteria is a blood protein, which Tillett had discovered some time before, and named C-reactive protein. Its function is to bind to the surfaces of the bacteria and agglutinate them, that is to say glue them together into a clotted mass and thus inactivate them. The amount of C-reactive protein in the blood increases in response to acute infections by pathogens.

Tillett had added some cultured streptococci, rod-like bacteria, to test tubes containing human plasma, and to others containing serum. Human plasma is the pale yellowish fluid seen above the layer of dense red cells when blood is spun in a centrifuge, or even simply allowed to settle. Plasma has all the proteins required for plotting. Serum is plasma from which the protein, fibrinogen has been removed. Fibrinogen is converted to fibrin in the late stage of clot formation, and so serum cannot clot. Tillett noticed to his surprise that not only the serum but also the plasma to which the streptococci had been added remained free of agglutinated bacteria. This was not what he was looking for, but the inference – that the bacteria were producing an agglutination inhibiting or a dispersant – struck him as too interesting to ignore. He conjectured that fibrinogen night be important in bonding the bacteria just as, on conversion to fibrin, it forms the adhesive in the blood clot. To test his hypothesis he treated some plasma with oxalate, a simple compound that sequesters calcium ions. Without calcium ions blood does not clot. (Thus when blood is taken for diagnostic purposes or for transfusion it is collected in a vessel containing such a substance, although oxalate was later replaced by citrate, and later still by heparin.) If Tillett's theory was correct then adding streptococci, followed by calcium to plasma would not result in an agglutinated mass, for the bacteria would have released their clot-dispersing agent into the solution. A clot formed, and Tillett went away disappointed. But he did not clear away the experiment and left the tubes in their rack on the laboratory bench. A little time later he looked again, and the clot had indeed dissolved, leaving clear liquid plasma. It seemed, then, that the streptococci were secreting the clot-buster, as it came to be called, in response to their contact with fibrinogen. Tillett explored further, and found that the activity was confined to streptococci, and displayed by none of the other pathogens that he went on to test, nor was it common to all streptococci strains. Then he did one more critical experiment: he took blood samples from patients recovering from infection with the most dangerous haemolytic (red-cell bursting) streptococci, and showed that the plasma would not agglutinate added streptococci in the test-tube. This result was published in 1934, and soon after, Tillett and a biochemical colleague isolated the active factor, which they showed to be a protein, and gave it the name, *streptokinase*.

The clinical potential of streptokinase was clear enough to Tillett, but to prepare it in useful quantities and in pure form presented a formidable challenge. It was not until 1947 that Tillett felt able to contemplate trying a preparation on the sick. That year he invited Sol Sherry, a doctor at Temple

University in Philadelphia, to conduct trials on patients with arterial blood clots. The results were initially gratifying, but side-effects soon showed themselves in the form of inflammation, headaches and pains in the joints. Impurities were the problem. A major pharmaceutical company, Lederle Laboratories, made strenuous attempts to generate a pure product, but it proved too difficult even for them, and in 1960 they threw in the towel. Several other organisations, mainly in Europe and notably the Wellcome Laboratories, took up the chase, and eventually succeeded. Clinical trials gave ambiguous results, and not until 1985 was streptokinase saving large numbers of lives, especially in cases of heart attacks.*

Towards the beginning of the 1970s a rival to streptokinase, acting at a different point in the machinery of clot dispersal, was identified. When a blood clot has served its designated purpose of stopping a haemorrhage it has to be removed, an act performed by a proteolytic enzyme – one that breaks down proteins, often one particular protein. Such an enzyme, called plasmin, works selectively on fibrin. It is maintained when not needed in an inactive, as it were stoppered, state, a proenzyme, plasminogen. In 1947 a Swedish physiologist, Tage Astrup had discovered that plasminogen occurs in many tissues, not only blood, and in 1952 he had made an extract from pig hearts that displayed fibrinolytic (fibrin-dissolving) activity. It gradually became clear that plasminogen was inert – a proenzyme – and was turned on by an agent in blood or other tissues, a plasminogen activator. But this is an enzyme, a catalyst, and very little is needed suffices to turn over a lot of its substrate, plasminogen, and it was accordingly hard to prepare any useful amount for study. Then in the 1970s Edward Reich at Rockefeller University made a strange observation: many cancer cells, he found, secreted the tissue plasmin activator in quite high concentrations. By then researchers in the cardiovascular field were keeping an eye open for

---

* The mechanism of action of streptokinase had by then been sorted out. The plasmin is unleashed by a complex process. In the circulation it adopts a closed, tight structure, but when it encounters a blood clot it opens like a jacknife, exposing its interior to another specialised proteolytic enzyme, tissue plasminogen activator, tPA. This breaks the plasminogen's chain at one point, which turns the inactive plasminogen into active plasmin. The plasmin then proceeds to break down the clot. Streptokinase bypasses the last step, which normally requires the mobilisation of protein molecules from the liver, and is slow.

an alternative 'clot buster', as it was by then called, for after the introduction of streptokinase the mortality from acute heart attacks had dropped precipitately. It was in 1979 that Désiré Collet, professor in the Vascular Research Department of the University of Leuven in Belgium examined cells cultured from a patient with the deadly cancer, malignant melanoma and found that it secreted an unprecedented concentration of the tissue plasminogen activator (tPA for short), some hundred times greater than any seen before. The purified compound had powerful thrombolytic (blood-clot-dissolving) activity, and rescued rabbits with induced pulmonary embolisms (fatal blood clots in the lungs.) Animal tests undertaken in other centres were equally successful.

Collen gave an account of his data at a meeting in Sweden, but in a closed session for a group of experts. By chance a young researcher, Diane Pennica, recently recruited by the embryonic Californian biotechnology company, Genentech, accidentally stumbled into this discussion, and was not ejected because she was assumed to be the daughter of one of the participants. Genentech made a speciality of genetic manipulation, of cloning and expression of proteins, then still a somewhat arcane skill and not yet the commonplace it would shortly become. She proposed a collaboration to Collen, which resulted in the manufacture of recombinant tPA, made in bacteria. The success of this enterprise was reported in *Nature* in 1980, and clinical trials on patients with heart attacks followed in 1983. The product was pronounced effective, and was approved by the FDA. It was a great coup for Genentech, which quickly developed into a market giant. The company went on to produce a modified version of the protein, and then a large fragment that retained the full activity.* Streptokinase and recombinant tPA and (rtPA) were now in direct and bloody competition. It was argued that tPA had the edge because, as a human protein, unlike streptokinase, it could elicit no antigenic reaction, and because it also acted

---

* In the UK the patent application by Genentech was successfully opposed by Wellcome Laboratories, on the grounds that neither was tPA a new discovery, for it was a natural product, nor was the process of manufacturing the recombinant protein in any sense original. Another patent dispute, which rumbled on for nine years, was settled on payment by Genentech of a trifling $200 million to the University of California.

more quickly. Its cost, on the other hand, was ten times greater. Since the drug was launched there have been many comparative clinical trials, and in terms of the reduction in mortality from heart attacks there seems to be remarkably little difference. Larger trials appear still to be continuing, and different doctors have their own opinions. What is beyond doubt is that both drugs have saved many lives of victims of heart attacks and strokes, and that both have netted their inventors handsome profits.

Wheeze disease – relieving allergies and asthma

Allergies and asthma increased in prevalence at an alarming rate during the last four decades of the 20th century. Today, in the advanced countries, such as the U.S. and the U.K., about one in five of the population suffer from one or the other or both. The incidence of asthma in adults is about one in twelve, and in children slightly higher. It is estimated that in the U.K. more than a thousand people die of the condition each year. Worldwide there are an estimated 300 million asthmatics, of whom about a quarter of a million die of the disease each year. Asthma and allergies are therefore a primary concern in respiratory medicine, and of pressing interest to the pharmaceutical companies, the more so because there is no known cure, and dependence on medication can last a lifetime. Allergies and asthma are intertwined. An allergy is an anomalous reaction of the immune system to certain substances, such as pollen or dust-mite droppings, to which the victim has become sensitive. Allergies can lead to asthma, and indeed most cases of asthma stem from allergies. (A much less common form is exercise-induced asthma.) An asthma attack ensues when a surge of inflammatory substances is released from a special type of cell, the mast cells. This explosive event is a reaction to an encounter with an agent - perhaps a type of pollen – to which the individual has become sensitive. Histamine preponderates in the evil cocktail that the mast cell spews out, but the various substances work in different ways, causing spasms in the smooth muscle (p.) of the bronchia (the airways, or branches of the windpipe through which air passes into and out of the lungs); this and inflammation, with swelling, of the linings of the bronchia, causes constriction, which limits the access of the lungs to air.

Asthma has been known to physicians since ancient times. Many curious remedies were favoured, but there were some that did ease the symptoms. Among the best was stremonium, an extract of the toxic plant *Datura stremonium*, a member of the deadly nightshade family, and known as thorn apple, or in America as Jimson weed (p.). Atropine from the deadly nightshade, *Atropa belladonna* (p.), and more especially its accompanying compounds, acted in a similar way, as did henbane (*Hyoscyamus niger*), from which comes scopolamine (p.). All feature in Ayurvedic and ancient Egyptian traditions of medicine, and the Egyptians in fact valued the smoke from hot henbane as an inhalant. The idea spread to Europe, and from the early 19th century cigarettes containing one or other such plant preparation became popular. Among the most commercially successful were Asthmador, Potter's Asthma Cigarettes, and Dr J.D. Kellog's Asthma Remedy from the inventor of cornflakes. Opium or other narcotics sometimes formed a part of the patent remedies. Marcel Proust, an asthmatic, was one of many who found relief in anti-asthma cigarettes. Another widely touted nostrum was the alarming Carbolic Smoke Ball, conceived by an American inventor. It consisted of a rubber ball containing powdered carbolic acid, now called phenol, a highly corrosive substance, which must have inflicted terrible damage on the mucous surfaces. To avert any respiratory annoyance from asthma or from colds and flu one had only to blow the powder into one's nose by compressing the ball. It occasioned a minor *cause célèbre* in London when the husband of a woman who had sniffed the phenol and then contracted influenza took the inventor to court and won the case.

Through much of the 19th and early 20th century stramonium remained the respectable treatment for asthmatics. It was undoubtedly effective in easing the bronchial spasms, but it was highly dangerous because of the variable strengths of the preparations. A large proportion of hospital deaths from asthma resulted from a stramonium overdose. In the early part of the 20th century doctors began to experiment with some success, first with crude, and then purified adrenaline, to mitigate acute asthma attacks. Later ephedrine (p.) came into use for the same purpose. The last of the plant products that was prescribed from about 1920 for the treatment of acute asthma was theophylline, an alkaloid similar to caffeine, though found in tea, and first isolated in the 19th century. It has bronchodilator properties, but was apt to cause cardiac arrhythmia and diuresis (excessive urination). An overdose could kill, and theophylline soon became obsolete, except as a diuretic. The effects of all such natural products were transient, and accompanied by dangerous side-effects. There was little more comfort for asthmatics until the 1940s, when progress suddenly came from more than one direction. First the steroid hormones, with their remarkable anti-inflammatory properties, were discovered (p.). Cortisone and ACTH (adrenocorticotropic hormone) were isolated and later synthesised, and, taken orally, gave unprecedented relief from the paroxysms of asthma, but at a painful cost in terms of side-effects, both physical and psychological. By this time the search for expressly synthetic anti-allergic compounds was beginning to produce results. IG Farben in Germany and Rhône-Poulenc in France were in hot competition. Several drugs of limited value appeared on the market, until in 1942 IG Farben came up with fenpiprane, or Aspasan, an antispasmodic.

By then, with the tide of war flowing in their direction, the Germans had occupied the northern part of France, and IG Farben, with close links to the Nazi regime, were aiming to annexe the French pharmaceutical industry. This was fiercely resisted by Rhône-Poulenc, whose chemists, led by Ernest Fourneau and Daniel Bovet, had created the anti-histamine, Antergan (p.), which became available in the same year, 1942, and soon afterwards Neo-antergan. These were prescribed for allergies and asthma, but suffered from the disadvantage of a strong soporific action. Other companies joined the chase, and in 1943 a chemical engineer, George Rieveschl at the University of Cincinnati scored a notable success. Hoping apparently to synthesise an antispasmodic, he found an excellent antihistamine. This variant of Antergan was better than the precursor in that it induced less torpor. Rieveschl decamped to Parke Davis to exploit the pecuniary possibilities of his new compound, diphenylhydramine, and he grew rich from his royalties. Under its trade name of Benadryl it is still sold as an over-the-counter remedy for allergies, generally in formulations with other drugs. At about the same time the U.S. branch of the Swiss Ciba company produced the similar, and also successful mepyramine and especially tripelannamine, more familiar as Pyribenzamine.

In the early 1940s there had been one other development along different lines, when a chemist at another German company, C.H. Boehringer, prepared an adrenaline derivative, which was a stronger bronchodilator than adrenaline itself, and appeared to have fewer side-effects. This was isoprenaline (isoproterenol in the U.S.), which we have already encountered (p.). Side-effects in fact there were, but sadly, it was nearly two decades before they were recognised. The deaths due to asthma in Europe and America, as a proportion of the total number of asthmatics, was essentially unchanged from the time doctors began to keep records in the early years of the 20th century until the early 1960s. Even the rise of asthma incidence in the 1950s made little impact on the figures, but then in 1961 the death rate in Britain and a half-dozen other countries, notably Australia, New Zealand and Norway, began to rise sharply. It was an epidemic. In the U.S. and Canada, where the same drug was in equally wide use, there was no such phenomenon. What was going on? Epidemiological studies, notably one by three English researchers (one of them Richard Doll, who is commonly credited with demonstrating the causal link between smoking and lung cancer), established that the increase was genuine, and not a function of diagnostic methods or record keeping, and correlated it with the introduction of isoprenaline forte, a drug delivery system based on a high-pressure metered inhaler. The dose per puff was large, and there was nothing, besides warnings, to prevent users from repeated inhalations. Moreover, the drug, initially so highly effective, lost its potency as the users became habituated. The highest death rate, the epidemiologists determined, was in the 10 to 19 age-group – the age from which children become capable of dosing themselves at will to that at which they are least likely to take note of admonitions. When the 'Medihaler' was withdrawn the epidemic ended. Across the Atlantic the dosed had been better controlled and many deaths were averted. The fact was that the compound had broad, indiscriminate activity, exerting its effect not only on the bronchia but also on the heart, and inducing arrhythmias. The deaths fortunately did did not put an end to the search for adrenaline-related compounds with a more restricted action, and many were developed, some of which enjoyed better luck, as we shall shortly see.

But in 1942, when isoprenaline made its appearance in Germany, the war had severely cramped further research activities, other than those dictated by military needs, such as the mass production of penicillin. When peace came again the pharmaceutical companies returned to more profitable projects. Soon many variants on the existing anti-allergy and anti-asthma compounds emerged. This was a time of determined efforts to evade patent regulations by the creation of what became known as 'me too' drugs - compounds differing from established drugs only in an innocuous structural modification to justify a modest, most often probably specious claim to some kind of advantage. The 1960s, however, were a decade of great strides in the treatment of asthma. The adrenaline analogues were not a dead-end, but post-war progress really began with the work of Altounyan.

Roger Edward Collingwood Altounyan (1922-1987) was born in Aleppo in Syria to Armenian parents, who settled in England.* Altounyan began his medical studies after the, war, and, himself an asthmatic, developed an interest in the disease. This led him in 1956 to join the pharmaceutical company, Fisons, reinventing himself as a pharmacologist. He began searching for leads to an asthma therapy, and began with an ancient remedy, applied to a number of complaints. This was an extract from a ubiquitous flowering plant, *Ammi visnaga*, sometimes known as the toothpick plant, and in traditional medicine as khella. The extract, khellin diminished the response of a strip of animal intestine to an allergenic material to which the animal had been sensitised by injection. This appealed to Altounyan, for his plan was to try to impede the release of the inflammatory substances from mast cells, rather than to mitigate their actions when they had been released. He set about isolating the 'active principle' from khellin. Once he had determined its chemical structure he began the laborious task of synthesising derivatives of the compound, and assaying their effects on himself. This was a heroic and ultimately hazardous course. Two allergens – substances inducing an allergic attack – to which Altounyan

---

* He and two sisters are the thinly disguised heroes of the once-famous children's novel by Arthur Ransome, *Swallows and Amazons*. He had met the author while the family was on a visit to his maternal grand-parents in the English Lake District. Altounyan distinguished himself as a pilot and flying instructor in the war, and was decorated for introducing new techniques of night flying.

was highly sensitive were grass pollen (a very common allergen) and the skin cells, or dander, shed from guinea pigs. He exposed himself over and over to these preparations, well aware that repeated allergen challenge, as it is called, would lead to aggravation of his condition.

In all Altounyan inflicted this insult on his lungs more than 2000 times between 1957 and 1964, while observing any signs of alleviation by the khellin analogue under test of the resulting attack. With compound FPL 670 he struck luck. The effect of this compound, taken by inhalation, was instant and dramatic. Altounyan at once asked a doctor friend in Manchester to test the derivative on asthma patients in the university hospital. The clinical trial (double-blinded, so that neither patients nor doctors knew what the patients were given), was modest in scope, but conclusive. Ten patients were divided randomly into two equal groups; one group was treated for two weeks with disodium cromoglycate (as FPL 670 was now called), the other with a placebo. Then the groups were switched, the second receiving the drug, and the first the placebo. In both cases the symptoms of those who inhaled the drug were greatly alleviated. No side-effects were discovered in animal or human trials, and when it came into clinical use under the name of Intal, Altounyan's drug transformed the lives of many thousands of asthmatics. Altounyan continued with his research, and also devised a highly successful inhaling device, the 'Spinhaler', which is still in use. But the years of self-experimentation had taken their toll: he became dependent on oxygen cylinders to breathe, and in the end his heart failed and he died aged 65.

It is now time to meet one of the titans of 20th-century drug research. David Jack (1924-2011) was born, like James Black, in a mining village in East Fife in Scotland, and in the same year. He was the youngest of six children of a coal-miner father. He did well at school and was offered a place at Edinburgh University, which he turned down in favour of an apprenticeship at Boots the chemists. He recalled that disenchantment came in less than a week, for the task he was allocated was to dust all the many bottles on the pharmacy shelves. Before long he enrolled in the Royal College of Science and Technology (now the main constituent of the University of Strathclyde) in Glasgow for a degree in chemistry and pharmacy. His talents were recognised, for he won prizes, achieved a first-class honours degree, and was invited to proceed to a Ph.D., but once again he rejected the opportunity and took instead the humble position of assistant lecturer in pharmacology at Glasgow University. In 1951 he made his move into the pharmaceutical industry. At Glaxo his job was to formulate suspensions of antibiotics. It was boring, but he later maintained that the experience was of much value in his later career. After two years he moved on, this time to Smith, Kline and French, where, by now in his thirties, he had his first taste of research. He remained there until 1961, when he was appointed director of research at the small Glaxo subsidiary, Allen and Hanbury. He demanded a free hand and converted the manufacturer of fruit pastilles into a major centre of pharmacological research.

Jack never deviated in his determination to find compounds that would alleviate human suffering, and asthma was his first target. He started out from isoprenaline to look for a derivative without its devastating toxicity and with longer-lasting action. It was one of Jack's chemists, Larry Lunts, who divined which part of the molecule was responsible for its too rapid metabolic destruction, and modified it accordingly. The result was salbutamol, which became from 1969 the most important asthma treatment. At about this time evidence had accrued that the β-adrenergic receptors (p.) were of more than one kind: the β_1-adrenergic receptor was in the heart cells, whereas the bronchial cells exhibited the β_2 receptor. This explained at once why isoprenaline was so dangerous, for it attached itself indifferently to either, whence its undesired effect on the heart. Salbutamol, by contrast, picked out only the β_2 receptor. Yet Jack was not satisfied. The duration of action of the new drug, at 6-8 hours, was still too short, and would not guarantee the recipient a full night's rest. The work went on, and after more than another decade produced salmeterol, which supplanted salbutamol as the world's favourite asthma drug. It was sold under the name of Ventolin, and administered through an inhalant.

These were major advances, but David Jack had another concern. As long ago as 1900 some European doctors gave their asthma patients extracts of adrenal glands from abattoirs, which acted as bronchodilators. It is now thought that their effect was less due to adrenaline than corticosteroids – still unknown at the time – in this unwholesome soup. Soon after corticosteroids were isolated (p.), and their anti-inflammatory properties recognised, it was found that they constituted by far the most efficacious treatment for an acute asthma attack. So steroids were swallowed, perforce, by many asthmatics. Yet the side-effects were numerous and distressing, and patients strove to limit their intake. Jack pondered the matter, and knowing that one of Allen and Hanbury's products was a steroidal cream for the treatment of skin disorders, fell to wondering why a steroid might not equally well be applied to the lung tissue topically – in other words by inhalation. Many steroidal compounds were synthesised by Jack's team before beclomethasone dipropionate hit the mark. This compound gave relief from asthma attacks with greatly reduced side-effects, since other organs of the body were not exposed to the action of the steroid. It was sold by Allen and Hanbury in the form of Becotide, delivered through a pressurised inhaler. Many 'me too' variants appeared on the market, which differed little in their properties. The standard treatment now consists of beclomethasone dipropionate or a similar product, together with salmeterol or an equivalent. These drugs are equally favoured for another lung disease, commonly called COPD – chronic obstructive pulmonary disease, which is a manifestation of narrowed airways, caused most commonly by smoking, and sometimes by atmospheric pollution or occupational exposure to toxic particulate substances. It is also called emphysaemia, and is in general less tractable than asthma.

A later development in asthma therapy originated in 1996 in the laboratories of the British pharmaceutical company, AstraZeneca. This was zafirlukast (Accolade), an antagonist of a class of inflammatory agents, called leukotrienes, released from certain white blood cells. Leukotrienes are among the substances that engender asthma symptoms. Zafirlukast and some other related drugs differ in their action from all the previous asthma treatments, in that they are used to avert rather than treat attacks when they have already erupted. Zafirlukast was accidentally found to have useful properties for the prevention of certain problems in cosmetic breast surgery. Today great hopes repose in the treatment of asthma and allergic conditions (as so many other diseases) by 'humanised' monoclonal antibodies (p.). They may be directed against any one of the many natural cellular constituents that conspire to unloose the malign reaction. But asthma is a complex and varied disease, which can exert its symptoms by a number of different routes. So the problem in antibody therapy is first to establish the identities of the critical factors at work in the individual patient when the attack strikes. Several such antibodies have been commercially available for some years, and are often effective, This remains a busy area of research. As for David Jack, he had long before this found new fields to conquer. He was responsible for ranitidine (p.), the successor of James Black's Zantac, and for a drug to combat migraine. He received many honours, including, late in life, a knighthood.

Opening the sluice: the path to diuresis

The first essential step when grappling with dropsy, in other words, heart failure (p.), is to eliminate excess water and thus reduce the pressure on the heart. Other conditions, especially cirrhosis of the liver, demand the same treatment. The ancients had herbal medicines, which helped, and some, such as *infusum buchu*, an extract from the leaves of an African shrub, are still to be found in naturopathy shops. Caffeine and related alkaloids are also somewhat diuretic, especially theophylline from tea (which also found other medicinal uses [p.]). But these are generally feeble in their action, or at any rate too toxic in the concentrations at which they exert any worthwhile diuretic effect. Mercury and its compounds served as mild diuretics, though at no small cost to general health, since Paracelsus's time. The first vestiges of progress accompanied the introduction in the late 19th century of a new range ofof mercury compounds for the treatment of syphilis (Chapter). A breakthrough came in 1919, and, as ever, by chance.

This is how the story unfolded: Paul Saxl, a doctor in the cardiology clinic of the famous First Medical University of Vienna admitted a patient, a woman with advanced syphilis, and contingent heart disease and water retention. He instructed a third-year medical student, Arthur Vogl to administer a daily injection of 1 c.c. (a cubic centimetre, in modern usage 1 ml) of mercury salicylate. Vogl accordingly ordered a10% solution in water from the hospital dispensary. Only to be told that mercury salicylate, like most mercurials, had a very low solubility in water, and could be provided only as an oily suspension. Nonplussed, Vogl looked for an alternative, but then a chance encounter intervened. A retired army surgeon appeared in the clinic, and offered Vogl a cache that he no longer needed of Novasol, the trade name of merbaphen, an antisyphilitic mercurial, developed some years earlier by the Bayer company. It might, he thought, be of use to the hospital. Vogl accepted the gift, and immediately injected spme Novasol into Saxl's patient. Over the next day she passed a generous amount of urine, but the doctors were unimpressed. Vogl, though, persisted. By chance there was another patient with severe syphjlis in the ward, and Vogl seized the opportunity. Successive injections provoked first a doubling, then a quadrupling and finally a torrent of urine, which continued for a day and a night. By the next morning more than 10 litres (2.2 British or 2.3 U.S. gallons) had been collected. In giving this account of the discovery thirty years later in 1950, Vogl acknowledged its fortuitous nature, and allocated the greatest part of the credit to the nurses, who, unasked, had measured and reported the urine volumes.

The part that chance played in this episode became even greater when a survey of existing mercurial antisyphilitic compounds found none that displayed a diuretic potency remotely comparable with that of merbaphen. Saxl went on to study the action of merbaphen more extensively, and many patients with congestive heart failure were treated before it became clear that this was a dangerous drug, which could cause kidney damage and other lethal conditions. It was fortunate that these disasters did not put a stop to the search for related compounds with less catastrophic side-effects. Many mercurial had been synthesised in Ehrlich's time, among which was mersalyl. This had evidently been overlooked in the first study but was later found to be an effective diuretic, and less toxic than merbaphen. Used with caution, it did good service when it became in 1924 the diuretic of choice. It remained so for the next decade, although by no means devoid of toxicity.

A new departure came in the early 1940s. Mercury compounds were by then viewed with misgivings, while on the other hand the sulphonamides seemed to offer limitless promise in relation to all manner of maladies. A small team of chemists and pharmacologists at the American company of Sharp and Dohme (not yet allied with Merck) set up the 'Renal Project'. They based their strategy for creating a new kind of diuretic on a plausible (though incorrect) hypothesis of kidney function. The misconception was that the passage of urine was governed by a dehydrogenase. The dehydrogenases are a ubiquitous class of enzymes involved in many metabolic processes. (Among the most familiar are lactate dehydrogenase, the failure of which leads to difficulty in assimilating milk products, and liver alcohol dehydrogenase, which is responsible for breaking down alcohol into an innocuous product.) It had been shown that certain of the sulphonamides had the ability to bind to and inactivate dehydrogenases. It had also been remarked that patients given massive doses of a sulphonamide to overcome bacterial infections passed copious amounts of urine, and that this urine was appreciably alkaline (p.) by reason of a high content of sodium bicarbonate. The accretion of bicarbonate implies that the blood is failing to eliminate carbon dioxide, a metabolic waste product, normally exhaled from the lungs.

Some time before the Renal Project came into being, a well-known biochemist in Cambridge, David Keilin had shown that the breakdown of bicarbonate into carbon dioxide and water is driven by an enzyme, carbonic anhydrase. This enzyme, too, is inhibited by sulphonamides, which was the basis of their function as diuretics. Keilin had purified carbonic anhydrase, which made it possible to test new compounds for inhibitory activity. Several sulphonamides proved active, and were also diuretics, though mostly too weak or too toxic at the necessary concentrations to be of use. Some did reach the market but did not survive for long. At this point a highly accomplished chemist at the Lederle Laboratories, Richard Roblin (p.) chose to interest himself in the diuresis problem, and began to synthesise a series of sulphonamide analogues. It was not long before he had a compound with high diuretic potency and low toxicity. This was acetazolamide, which was tested on patients in 1954, and became famous under the trade name of Diamox. It did not in the event dominate the market for long, because in 1957 the Sharp and Dohme Renal Project struck gold with a molecule of a quite different nature, known to organic chemists as a thiazide. They had begun to explore the thiazide series some years before, and had indeed generated one, called ethacrynic acid (trade name, Edecrin) that showed promise. But the new one, introduced in 1958, swept all before it. Its name is chlorthiazide, or Diuril, and it gave rise to a succession of similar ('me too') compounds, but retains its clinical pre-eminence. Four of the Renal Project researchers shared the Lasker Prize (p.) in 1975 for its discovery. As for Diamox, it has by no means vanished, for it is used to treat glaucoma, a common source of impaired vision and blindness due to increased pressure of the fluid in the eye; it is equally favoured for countering epileptic seizures, and also altitude sickness. It is not without side-effects, and its application in the treatment of the serious hereditary disease, sickle cell anaemia did not have a good outcome.

Life savers: the control of blood pressure

High blood pressure, or hypertension, causes heart attacks and strokes. It has no symptoms, but is easily monitored, and was in fact first measured by the Revered Stephen Hales (on a horse) early in the 18th century. The control of high blood pressure became a major preoccupation in the latter part of the 19th century. Claude Bernard in Paris (Chapter), while studying the physiological effects of a variety of substances, discovered that a commonplace chemical, potassium thiocyanate, injected into the muscle, reduced the blood pressure of animals (apparently by relaxing the smooth muscle of the blood vessels) without killing them. The observation was published in 1857, but it was not until 1900 that a pair of German doctors tried it on patients. Potassium (and sodium) thiocyanate were known to be toxic, and as more doctors tried the treatment, debates broke out in the medical literature. Some found it effective and safe if used intelligently, others thought it too dangerous to justify, and others again thought it not only dangerous but also useless. Over the next decades the fashion came and went. The majority of reports in the journals concluded that thiocyanate did lower the blood pressure of many patients, although occasional deaths were also reported. Antiquated as it appeared, the treatment remained in use in some quarters until the 1950s. Another simple chemical, sodium nitroprusside was found in 1945 to possess a much more violent effect than thiocyanate on blood pressure. It is given by injection and also operates by relaxing smooth muscle, though by another route than thiocyanate. Called Nipride, it is still used despite high toxicity, though only in emergencies.

With the hazards of constitutionally high blood pressure firmly established, the demand for an anti-hypertensive agent, suitable for long-term – usually in fact lifelong – use, became increasingly insistent. In 1949 the wished-for drug seemed to have arrived. It was hydralazine, produced by the Ciba company. It was a vasodilator, that is to say dilated the blood vessels to reduce the pressure, and was also known to have some diuretic effect. It may still find a use as hypotensive, particularly in pregnancy, but its action is brief and variable. Almost immediately after its launch on the market, another pharmaceutical laboratory, the American branch of Schering, while in pursuit of thiazide diuretics, made a derivative of the same series, which proved to have only vestigial diuretic potency. The researchers knew that one of the sulphanilamides, which were precursors in the synthesis of the thiazines, had caused severe illness, and some deaths in patients treated for gastric infections in Montpellier, as already related (p.). They also knew that the cause was hypoglycaemia (a life-endangering drop in blood sugar. But they would probably have been impressed most of all was a further discovery by the physiologist, Auguste Loubatières, who had investigated the phenomenon in greater depth. He had found that different sulphanilamide derivatives affected the blood sugar level in different ways: some had indeed induced hypoglycaemia, but others had the contrary effect, and increased the blood sugar level –were hyperglycaemic. Some others again affected the blood sugar not at all. Starting from these findings the Schering pharmacologists and chemists arrived at several new diabetes drugs, such as torantil and chlorothiazide. It was perhaps not too surprising that the new thiazide that they had synthesised exerted a hyperglycaemic effect. It was first considered therefore as a likely treatment for conditions that cause low blood sugar levels. But it was also a strong vasodilator and an effective hypotensive agent (one that reduced blood pressure), and proved its value for both purposes.

All the diuretic compounds generated up to the mid-20th century were vasodilators. Was there then no other way to control evacuation of water? The complex process is ultimately regulated by the nervous system, which is itself driven by neurotransmitters. A possible target, therefore, is the encouragement of these neurotransmitters. In 1960 an inhibitor of an enzyme participating in the synthesis of noradrenaline and adrenaline, was evaluated at the U.S. National Institutes of Health. It had been prepared by chemists at Merck, Sharp and Dohme, and is known as methyldopa. It was a good diuretic, and was put on the market under various names, of which Aldomet was the most familiar, but tampering with the supply of adrenergic neurotransmitters is always apt to lead to complications. Aldomet was no exception to the rule, for it was found to have psychotropic effects, and has largely fallen out of use, although the discovery of better ways of controlling blood pressure was also a major factor. This began in the late 1960s.

Blood pressure is controlled by a number of hormones, all of them small molecules, and only one of which, adrenaline, had been recognised before the close of the 19th century. In 1898 two physiologists at the Karolinska Institute in Stockholm had found that a kidney extract exerted a hypertensive effect by constricting the blood vessels. It was not until nearly forty years later that an active natural peptide of eight amino acids was isolated in two laboratories independently, one in Buenos Aires, the other at the University of Indiana. The discovery of this peptide, which was given the name, angiotensin, excited relatively little interest, for physiologists were well enough satisfied with adrenaline as the controller of blood pressure, and it took long and exacting research to bring the role of angiotensin into focus. Illumination came from a totally unexpected direction. Mauricio Oscar Rocha e Silva (1910-1983) was a Brazilian physiologist, professor at University of São Paulo, with a longstanding interest in the action of snake and other venoms, but especially that of the fer de lance, or lancehead snake. In 1948 a colleague procured for him a sample of venom from one of the deadliest of snakes, the jararaca, *Bothrops jaracara*, a species of South American pit viper, also called the fer de lance, or lancehead snake (and even sometimes 'the mother-in-law snake' by reason of its tendency to strike without provocation). Rocha e Silva had noted that the bite of the jararaca killed by causing a catastrophic collapse in its victim's blood pressure. How, he wanted to know, did this happen. He injected a dog with venom, took a sample of its blood, and introduced it into a standard assay system, a strip of guinea pig intestine bathed in a physiological medium. An active substance might cause the strip to contract or relax, just as the smooth muscle in the artery wall would do. Initially there was no effect, but it was supposedly a student left guarding the experiment, who witnessed a relaxation slowly develop. There was thus indeed an active compound in the dog's blood, and Rocha e Silva coined for it the term, bradykinin, as usual from the Greek, meaning slow motion. It turned out to be another short peptide – a string of nine amino acids.

Investigation of the action of the jaracara venom was taken up by a young associate of Rocha e Silva's, Sérgio Ferreira. The venom contained, he discovered, several proteolytic (protein-destroying) enzymes (p.) and a profusion of small peptides. Ferreira isolated the bradykinin, and in 1960 its sequence, comprising nine amino acids, was determined at the National Institute for Medical Research in London. Soon after that it was synthesised (like the sequence determination, a laborious process at the time, whereas both would now be quite trivial). Bradykinin is a natural compound, which we all have in very low concentration in our bodies, but, Ferreira then made the first in a series of important discoveries when he found that the ynthetic peptide was much weaker in its action than the natural preparation from envenomed blood. The reason for this strange paradox was that the natural bradykinin was contaminated with another peptide, which when purified and added to the synthetic bradykinin elevated its physiological potency. Ferreira called it 'bradykinin potentiating factor', BPF. There was more: bradykinin has a physiologically inert precursor, a kind of storage form, which is trimmed down by a proteolytic enzyme to generate the active peptide. But the body must rid itself of the bradykinin when it has done what was required of it in the way of blood pressure adjustment; for this purpose we have yet another proteolytic enzyme, which destroys only bradykinin. The BPF works by inhibiting that protease, so that bradykinin accumulates, keeps working, and drives down the blood pressure. Evolution, then, has not only equipped the wily reptile with the means to generate a deadly excess of bradykinin in the envenomed blood, but also with an agent that will immobilise the victim's defence mechanism.

The subsequent course of Ferreira's career was largely determined by a happy opportunity: to escape the political turmoil overtaking his country at the time, but also no doubt to widen his experience. Seeking refuge in a laboratory abroad, he was offered the choice of two postdoctoral positions, one in Oxford, the other in John (later Sir John) Vane's laboratory at the Royal College of Surgeons in London. Ferreira chose the second, and his decision was again fortunate, and equally so for Vane, for their interests blended perfectly. Vane (1927-2004) was a chemist turned pharmacologist, and his interests lay in hormonal control of physiological processes. (He shared the Nobel Prize for Physiology or Medicine in 1982 for his work on prostaglandins [p.], which clarified the mechanism of action of anti-inflammatory drugs, especially aspirin.) Ferreira's BPF preparation was in reality a mixture of small peptides, and it concealed another activity of great interest to Vane. One of the preoccupations of his department at the Royal College of Surgeons was a second arm of the blood pressure control mechanism. This is the renin-angiotensin system. Renin is, once again, a proteolytic enzyme, first detected in kidney extracts, and its presence began to make sense when it emerged that the peptide hormone, angiotensin, which accompanied it in extract, had an active and an inert form. The layers of complexity in the renin-angiotensin system were gradually laid bare during the latter part of the last century by work in several laboratories. Angiotensin I, as the inactive form was termed, is converted into the active, artery-constricting (thus hypertension-promoting) state, angiotensin II, by a particular proteolytic enzyme, the angiotensin converting enzyme, or ACE. It, so to speak, uncorks the angiotensin I by snipping off a small piece – in fact two amino acids- from the end of its chain. But this enzyme, the ACE, has itself an inert precursor form, which must be cut ('uncorked') by yet another proteolytic enzyme, namely renin. The snake venom extract to which Ferreira introduced Vane and his colleagues was tested and found to contain not only the bradykinin potentiating peptide, BPF, but also one that did the same for angiotensin. The realisation now came to Vane that inhibition of ACE should result in dilation of the blood vessels, would therefore reduce the blood pressure, and might afford a means of treating people with high blood pressure, the curse that killed and disabled so many. The problem was that a peptide could only be injected; taken by mouth it would be digested in the stomach before it could do any good.

But animal studies did at least establish the principle that inhibiting ACE should be a highly attractive way to control blood pressure.

Vane was a consultant of Bristol-Myers Squibb, and evidently had little difficulty in persuading the directorate to take up the very alluring challenge. After many false starts, a group of workers at the Squibb Institute in New Jersey, led by David Cushman and Miguel Ondetti set about screening other types of compounds than peptides for ACE inhibitor capacity. They were guided by a conjecture. They knew that to convert angiotensin I to angiotensin II ACE breaks off the last two amino acids from the C-terminal (see p.) end of the chain end. The locat ion and identity of those two anino acids were reminiscent of the properties of a familiar proteolytic enzyme. This was was carboxypeptidase, which occurs in the pancreas, and nips off similar terminal fragments from other proteins. It had a known synthetic inhibitor, and the plan was to use this as the lead compound. More than 2000 variants of this molecule were synthesised before the sought-for inhibitor of ACE turned up. This compound became the first commercial ACE inhibitor, and an exceedingly successful drug for the treatment of high blood pressure. Calledm, and sold as Capoten, it was approved by the FDA in 1981 and instantly caught on. Cushman did not abandon the hunt for a peptide inhibitor, and in due time he found one. It consisted of only three amino acids (an isoleucine and two prolines, or IPP), was resistant to destruction by the digestive enzymes, and could therefore be taken by mouth.

There are now innumerable competing ACE inhibitors to be had, and they are reckoned to have saved many thousands of lives. More recently a new class of anti-hypertensive drugs, called calcium channel blockers, appeared and quickly became competitors of the ACE inhibitors in the immense market for blood pressure control. The principle was not new, for it had long been known that calcium ions were the trigger of the muscle contraction machinery. Calcium ions are released at the nerve terminals, and flow through regulated channels in the membranes surrounding the muscle cells (p.). If the channels remain closed and the calcium ions cannot pass, the muscle remains in its relaxed state. In the case of the smooth muscle that envelops the blood vessels, those vessels will stay flaccid. The trick was to find a compound that would act only, or at least primarily, on the channels in the smooth muscle membrane, and not elsewhere, as for instance in the heart muscle. A number of such drugs were developed, mainly members of the dihydropyridine class of compounds. The best known is probably Pfizer's amlodipine, also called Norvase, which became available in 1992, and within a short time the pills were being prescribed in huge numbers, to give long-lasting dilation of the arteries. The battery of anti-hypertensive drugs now on offer all have their advantages and disadvantages. Individual reactions vary, and doctors have to take account of such factors as age and even ethnic origins. The evidence is that these drugs have increased longevity of people with constitutionally high blood pressure, with relatively few adverse effects on their wellbeing.

The demon cholesterol

The late David Kritchevsky, nutritionist and sage, had this to say about cholesterol: 'In America, we no longer fear God or the communists, but we fear cholesterol.' Cholesterol is an essential body constituent, and it is transported in the blood as a complex with proteins, for the molecule itself is quite insoluble in water. In 1910 the great German physiological chemist, Adolf Windaus analysed the arterial plaques – deposits on the walls of coronary arteries - of people who had died of heart disease. He found them to contain large amounts of cholesterol, and so established a presumptive link between cholesterol and what was henceforth described as coronary artery disease. Then in 1939 a Norwegian study established a correlation between high blood cholesterol and the incidence of heart attacks in some families genetically predisposed to this condition. After World War II this line of inquiry was extended to random populations, most famously in the Framingham Heart Study. This began in 1948 when 5209 adults living in Framingham, Massachusetts were enrolled in a grand epidemiological design to relate heart disease to diet and other aspects of life-style. By now this encompasses three generations. It includes such factors as smoking (bad), obesity (also bad) and exercise (good), and makes clear the correlation of blood cholesterol level with heart disease and stroke. To what extent this is a matter of cause and effect is a more complex issue. Nevertheless, cholesterol had become associated in the American, and to a lesser extent the European psyche with premature death, and so the pharmaceutical companies took an interest on the not unreasonable supposition that a reduction in circulating cholesterol might decrease the risk of heart disease and stroke.

The development of the statins, as they came to be called, was based on the biochemistry of cholesterol synthesis in the human (or at least animal) body. A number of distinguished biochemists participated in the elucidation of this highly complex process, of whom three won the Nobel Prize. Thirty chemical steps are involved in the production of cholesterol, most of it in the liver, and the aim was to interrupt the sequence at any one of these points. There were, to be sure, earlier drugs, which had more empirical origins. The first of these was the vitamin, nicotinic acid, the effect of which on cholesterol biosynthesis was discerned in 1955. Around the same time chemists at Imperial Chemical Industries (I.C.I.), who had been concerned with plant hormones, examined the properties of a class of relatively simple organic compounds called fibrates. Some of them, and especially one, clofibrate reduced cholesterol levels in the blood of animals and people. (An effect that had actually been found shortly before by French chemists, who were looking to intervene in the course of steroid synthesis, on the grounds of sporadic reports that oestrogens lowered blood pressure.) Clofibrate entered clinical use as Atromid-S, and remained in currency for some years.

These compounds were of circumscribed value, and several pharmaceutical companies around the world were engaged in the search for something better. Akira Endo (b. 1933), a Japanese biochemist, had worked on moulds and on bacterial cell walls at the Sankyo Research Laboratories in Tokyo, and also for a period at the Einstein Medical College in New York. There his proximity to the hospital had brought to his attention the number of obese, and as he learned, hypercholesteraemic (that is cholesterol-loaded) patients were ferried in with heart attacks. This primed his interest in cholesterol biosynthesis, and on his return to Tokyo in 1968, he persuaded the company to allow him to strike out in that direction. To find an inhibitor of the enzymes catalysing one of the steps in the synthetic pathway he chose to start with antibiotics, for he had been impressed by the large number of biological reactions with which these compounds commonly interfered. The enzyme he chose as his first target was one of the most thoroughly studied, HMGCR (or in full for the pedantic, 3-hydroxy-3-methylglutaryl coenzyme A reductase), and his missile a *Penicillium* product. Even assaying the effect of trial compounds on the activity of the enzyme was not trivial, and required first of all an isotopically labelled* substrate on which the enzyme could work, and this required a difficult synthesis. Endo and his assistants set about screening many hundreds of *Penicillium* moulds for inhibitor activity, in fact they had reached 3800 strains before one with high activity surfaced. It was *Penicillium citrium*, recovered from a contaminated sample of rice, bought in a shop in Kyoto. The year was 1972, and after a further year of hard toil Endo and his team had purified three active compounds from a culture of the mould. One of them, to which they gave the name, mevastatin, was selected for commercial development.

Mevastatin was the first of the statins, but there was talk of toxicity, and in the event it was derivatives, subsequently generated, that captured the market. Mevastatin had in fact been simultaneously isolated from another mould of a similar kind, *Penicillium brevicompactum*, in England at Beecham Pharmaceuticals (a venerable company**, which later became, by way, of Smith, Kline and Beecham, GlaxoSmithKline, or GSK). There it received the name, compactin, but again was never developed commercially. The first statin to make an impact on the pharmaceutical market was the closely similar lovastatin (Mevacor), extracted in the Merck laboratories from a different species of mould, *Aspergillus terreum*. The first clinical trials, in 1982, threw up few, and quite innocuous side-

---

* See p. for an explanation of the isotopic labelling technique.

** It was a long-established family firm, which entered the so-called 'ethical' market late. A scion of the family was the celebrated conductor, Sir Thomas Beecham, whose musical studies and career were expedited by the family wealth. The most famous Beecham product was Beecham's Pills, a laxative invented by the founder in 1824, and claimed to possess a variety of curative properties. 'Worth a guinea a box' the advertising proclaimed, and when young Thomas brought his own opera company to the Royal Opera House at Covent Garden, wags urged the public to come to Beecham's opera – 'worth a guinea a box'.

effects. Endo persisted in the face of this competition, and of the series of mevaststain derivatives that his laboratory produced, one, (Mevalotin) became a commercial success for Sankyo, in association with Bristol-Myers-Squibb. Merck chemists isolated another, and somewhat more powerful compound from the same mould, and were able to produce it synthetically; this was simvastatin, or Zocor, and it is still in use. But 1985 saw the appearance of the first purely synthetic statin, not based on a natural product. It emerged from the Parke Davis laboratories (soon after absorbed by Pfizer), and largely displaced the natural, mould-derived compounds. It is called atorvastatin, trade name Lipitor. At much the same time AstraZeneca conjured up rosuvastatin, known as Crestor, which is the principal competitor of Lipitor.

Statins are big business, and they undoubtedly work, but exactly how is still uncertain. They all inhibit the enzyme, HMGCR, and reduce the amount of cholesterol in the blood, and more especially the fraction associated with LDL, the low-density lipoprotein, commonly referred to as the 'bad cholesterol'. A lipoprotein is a protein that is linked to lipids, (fats). The 'good cholesterol' is the part of the total blood cholesterol that is attached to another lipoprotein in the blood, the HDL, or high-density lipoprotein. (There is also another smaller component, the very-low-density lipoprotein or VLDL, which in this context can be subsumed in the LDL.) High levels of LDL are a statistical risk indicator, but not necessarily a cause, of cardiovascular disease. It has been argued that what statins do to preserve life is to stabilise the arterial plaques, and prevent them from breaking up and causing embolisms (obstructions in blood vessels caused by a blood clot, a lump of fatty substance, or even an air bubble, which in the wrong place can be fatal). The statins have the additional virtue of suppressing the release of inflammatory compounds into the blood, and also the concentration of triglycerides, metabolic fatty compounds. They thus have a multifarious action, not confined simply to reducing blood cholesterol.

A promising venture, which sadly came to grief, was initiated by Pfizer in 1990. The target was another enzyme engaged in the cholesterol synthesis cycle. CETP (cholesteryl ester transfer protein) shuffles the cholesterol burden between the high- and low-density lipoproteins (HDL and LDL) in the blood. Research during the preceding years had revealed that there are hereditary variants in the gene for the enzyme. The small proportion of the human population with an exceptionally high level of the enzyme in their blood develop atherosclerosis (the formation of arterial plaques) more quickly on average than the rest of us. On the contrary, those equally rare individuals with a genetic variant characterised by a very low levels of CETP are (again on average) exceptionally long-lived. Still more telling was the discovery that a sizeable proportion of the Japanese population possessed a reduced level of CETP, and a small proportion had none at all. The first had more HDL in the blood, and the second very much more. (These groups were respectively heterozygotes [p.], with a single copy of the gene, derived from one parent, instead of the normal two, and homozygotes, who had not inherited a functional CETP gene from either parent.) The idea, then, was that if an inhibitor of the CETP could be found it could be used to treat people with anomalously high cholesterol, and therefore at high risk of coronary heart disease. The drug, which would simulate the effect of the longevity gene would be given along with a statin (Lipitor, since the provider would be Pfizer). An inhibitor, torcetrapib, was indeed discovered, but animal tests were difficult, for mice have no CETP, and a strain containing the enzyme had to be genetically engineered and given atherosclerosis. The results on these mice and on rabbits (which do have CETP) were equivocal. Nevertheless the first small trials on patients in 1999 appeared encouraging. In 2006 a large-scale (Phase III) trial with 18,000 patients at risk of coronary heart disease was begun, but it lasted little more than a year, by which time 82 of the subjects given the drug were dead, and only51 in the control group. The proportion of patients who survived heart attacks and angina also rose. There were several lawsuits, and this was the sad end of torcetrapib.

There was still another route to the same objective that ended in a fiasco. Schering-Plough in America developed ezetimib, known as Zeita, which was meant to retard the absorption of cholesterol in the gut. It was never apparently seen as an independent drug, but was combined with simvastatin, a largely superseded statin, produced by Merck. The combination was called Vytorin, and it did not last long. It reduced the LDL and increased the HDL, but it did nothing to reduce arterial plaque formation. There were side-effects, and a minor flurry of lawsuits, which cost the two companies the derisory sum of $41 million, and in 2008 Vytorin faded into oblivion. It did, though, cause some cardiologists to question the veracity of the link between LDL and hear disease. This ignited an altercation about the quality of the clinical trial that had awoken the heresy, which seems unresolved still.

Viruses: the unyielding adversary

Viruses are an unceasing problem. They are not susceptible to antibiotics, and there are few effective drugs. There are many types of virus, but the one essential feature they all have in common is that they are not living organisms, for a virus cannot reproduce except by parasitising a living cell. Viruses are smaller than animal or plant cells, and smaller than bacteria. They have a coat of proteins, inside which lurks the genetic material, which may be DNA or RNA. We have already encountered the first RNA virus ever discovered, RSV, or Rous sarcoma virus (p.), To summarise: when the viral nucleic acid enters a cell it takes command of the reproductive machinery within, and uses it to translate the encoded virus components, which assemble into complete new viruses. They break out to host cell, killing it in the process, to attack more cells.

When the virus is of the kind that keeps its genome in the form of RNA, the host cell most often simply accepts this RNA as a messenger (p.), from which to make proteins. In some cases the mechanism is more complicated. Then there are viruses that store their RNA in the form of a 'negative' strand (like the non-coding strand of a DNA double helix [p.]). This has to be copied by an enzyme (a polymerase) into its complementary, coding, strand. A third type of RNA virus contains only double-stranded RNA, which resembles a DNA duplex. In 1970, as related above (p.), molecular biologists were startled by reports from two American laboratories of a quite different replication mechanism in certain tumour (cancer-inducing) viruses –startling because it violated Francis Cric. Their RNA is transcribed into DNA, which is assimilated into the DNA of the host cell. They are all then expressed in the normal way – host and viral genes, including of course the tumour inducer. There was initial scepticism about this discovery, for it violated what Francis Crick-s Central Dogma, a fundamental precept of biology, that genetic information flows from DNA to RNA, and never in the opposite direction. It was reminiscent of Oscar Wilde's response on being shown the Niagara Falls: he would have been more impressed had the water been flowing the other way. The retroviruses, as they are called, remain the only exception to the principle. HIV, human immunodeficiency virus, the cause of AIDS, is a retrovirus.

Until late in the 20th century there were no drugs to speak of for combatting viral infections. One impediment was (and is) that viruses, and particularly RNA viruses, mutate with bewildering frequency. Therefore any compound discovered by the traditional approach of culturing cells, infecting them with the virus, and trying hundreds, or even thousand of chemicals, is unlikely to produce anything that would work for long against that virus. No sooner has a compound found to disable an essential viral protein been tested against the virus, than a mutant emerges to make the target invulnerable once more. As in bacteria (p.), though far more swiftly, the random dice-throw that is evolution, ensures 'survival of the fittest'. A single virus or bacterium containing a target protein that a mutation has rendered resistant to the drug can divide and produce lethal progeny. The successful measures against viral diseases were vaccination - against smallpox, (invented in the late 18th century, and developed to eradicate the disease in the 20th), and poliomyelitis, which had almost disappeared by the end of the 20th century. But once a victim is infected, it is too late for vaccination. Few virologists in the first half of the 20th century were even trying, but two of those few had the tenacity to achieve at least a degree of success.

William Herman Prusoff (1920-2011), a pharmacologist at Yale University had been working for a decade and more, following the path of cancer chemotherapy first trodden by George Hitchings and Gertrude Elion at the Wellcome Research Laboratories (Chapter). Their scheme had been to find analogues of the four nucleotides that make up the nucleic acids, DNA and RNA, which of course are common to all cells in all life forms. An analogue of a nucleotide, a nucleoside or just its purine (A and G) or pyrimidine (C and T or U) base (p.) might subvert the replication machinery and bring it to a halt. It was modified nucleosides that worked for Hitchings and Elion, and also for Prusoff. He chose thymidine (or its equivalent in RNA, uridine) as the starting point, and in 1959 he found that one of the derivatives he had synthesised killed herpes virus (but no other) in culture. The compound was idoxyuridine (short for 5-iodo-2'-deoxyuridine), the chemical and generic drug name implying that the molecule contained an iodine atom. The substance was far too toxic to be taken by mouth, but applied superficially, it eliminated herpes sores. It is still sold in the guise orm of eye-drops (Herpex) to treat herpes keratinitis, the painful excrescences on the cornea caused by the virus. Idoxyuridine was the first antiviral agent approved by the FDA. Prusoff would have nothing to do with patents, and it was left to Bristol-Myers Squibb to manufacture and promote the drug.

At much the same time another researcher was travelling in the same direction. Frank Schabel (1918-1983) was the head of the chemotherapy division at the Southern Research Institute in Birmingham, Alabama, and a professor at the University of Alabama. His interests lay in cancer and in viruses, and he would undoubtedly have been influenced, as Prusoff was, by the work of Elion and Hitchings. Schabel and his team collected a large number of nucleoside analogues and others known to have an interesting effect in biological systems, added them to virus-infected cell cultures, and tested those that seemed promising by injecting them into infected mice. The strong group of researchers at the Wellcome laboratories were also starting to interest themselves in viruses, and supplied Schabel, who had the assay techniques finely honed, with a range of nucleoside analogues. Eleven of the compounds showed some degree of antiviral activity, and among them were adenosine and cytosine derivatives in which the natural sugar (ribose in RNA or deoxyribose in DNA) was replaced by another sugar, arabinose. This modification had its origin in a discovery made in 1950 by two chemists at Yale University, investigating the metabolites of sponges. From a Caribbean species of sponge they extracted two arabinosides (nucleosides in which arabinose was the sugar). They called these spongouridine and spongothymidine. These compounfd had weak activity against cancer cells, sufficient nonetheless to encourage further research. It led to the synthesis of adenine arabinoside, commonly known as ara-A or vidarabine. This was the compound that Schabel developed in 1968 into the first effective antiviral drug, which killed a range of DNA and RNA viruses in culture and in infected animals, and was well tolerated by patients. Like idoxyuridine, it can be bought over the counter, and still retains its place, especially against herpes infections (cold sores, genital herpes, and keratinitis of the eye).

There was suddenly a pressing incentive for the pharmaceutical industry to develop new antiviral agents, and innumerable nucleosides and their analogues were synthesised in a number of laboratories, many of them with just a vestigial sugar fragment at the normal site of attachment of the sugar to the base. It was Gertrude Elion at Wellcome once again, with a colleague, Howard Schaffer, who came up trumps with acycloguanosine. (The name implies that there is no intact sugar ring.) The compound, also known as aciclovir (or acyclovir), goes under various trade names, of which Zovirax is the best known. It has very low toxicity and remarkable efficacy against the above forms of herpes, and also shingles, chicken pox and viral encephalitis. It immediately established itself as the leading antiviral agent on the market, and harbinger of a new era in therapeutics. Its dominance has persisted despite the introduction of a plethora of new variants. But the true test of virologists' mettle came with the appearance of a new and terrifying plague, which initially struck only homosexual men. In 1981 the disease was given a name – acquired immunodeficiency syndrome, AIDS. It was hideous and deadly, and there was no treatment. The damage was caused by the failure of the immune system. In 1983 to 1984 a virus, human immunodeficiency virus, HIV*, was finally identified as the cause of the disease. The evidence that it was a retrovirus was widely disbelieved on the grounds that retroviruses were thought innocuous, and in any case had never been seen in humans. Yet it was indeed a retrovirus, and when this became clear it induced a wave of pessimism, and a reluctance on the part of the pharmaceutical industry to involve itself. It had been proved by the discoverers of retroviruses that the invader's genes were incorporated

---

* There are in fact two types of HIV, the common form in most of the world is HIV-1, whereas HIV-2 is found mainly in West Africa. It is less easily transmitted, and is slower to give place to the AIDS disease. Most often references to HIV can be taken to imply HIV-1.

into the DNA of the host cell. How then could any drug possibly gain access to the seat of the disease, short of destroying the cell? Moreover, studies of the reverse transcriptase, which copies the viral RNA into DNA, appeared to be a highly error-prone enzyme, that is to say it would all too frequently insert the wrong nucleotide at some point in the DNA, and thereby change the sequence of the protein that the mutated gene encodes. It would in other words ensure a high frequency of mutation, and an end to the commercial longevity of a drug.

Succour for the sick and enlightenment for the clinicians came from the public sector. The National Cancer Institute (NCI), one of the National Institutes of Health (NIH) in Bethesda near Washington, began its assault on the problem in 1984. The director of the programme was Samuel Broder. He assembled a strong team of virologists, immunologists and chemists, and considering the formidable obstacles that the system presented, success came with remarkable despatch. It stands now as one of the great achievements in medical science. The first priority was to establish an assay system for testing candidate drugs. The lethal damage wrought by the virus was to one of the essential elements of the immune system, a type of white blood cells, T lymphocytes, inseparable from an effective immune response to pathogens, and more specifically a subset of these cells, referred to as T helper, or $CD4^+$ cells. (The name implies that they display a protein, CD4 on their surface.) In victims of AIDS these cells are attacked by the virus and vanish from the circulation. The NCI workers cultured the $CD4^+$ cells to provide the assay target, isolated the virus (neither of them trivial accomplishment), and the testing of compounds, old and new, could now begin. As in earlier work on the development of anti-cancer drugs, and later acyclovir, the strategy at the outset was to find an inhibitor of DNA synthesis, but in this case it was the reverse transcriptase that was to be the target. Azidothymidine, a modified nucleoside, had been synthesised twenty years earlier by Jerome Horwitz (1919-2012), a chemist at the Michigan Cancer Foundation, who spent his long career in the pursuit of anti-cancer drugs. The derivative, containing an azide group ($-N_3$), attached to the ribose sugar, was only one of numerous compounds that Horwitz synthesised and tested on mice with leukaemia and other cancers. None were effective, and he could do no more than publish a paper detailing his negative results, and move on to other kinds of compound. Yet azidothymidine had shown promise in that it killed a type of leukaemia cells in culture, and ten years later a German researcher made the same observation on cells of a different leukaemia. But it remained a failure in animal tests, and was forgotten, along with hundreds of other such compounds.

Time passed, and in 1984, with the AIDS programme in full spate, Jean Rideout, one of Gertrude Elion's associates at Burroughs Wellcome picked out 14 of the many known nucleoside derivatives as possibly worth resurrecting. She synthesised them all, and sent samples to the NCI. Azidothymidine, AZT, was one of them, and its effect on the virus-infected cells was astonishing: replication of the virus came to a total halt. Tests on AIDS patients *in extremis* were at once initiated at NCI with equally dazzling results: the patients' T lymphocytes returned, and the disease symptoms receded. The next year, 1986 a full-scale placebo-controlled trial was organised. It was so successful that it had to be terminated after one of 145 patients given AZT died, and 17 of the 137 patients on a placebo. The next year the FDA, with exceptional celerity, approved zidovidine, as the drug was named when it was handed back to Burroughs Wellcome for manufacture as Retrovir. Toxicity assays had shown that AZT was well enough tolerated by patients at the doses required to keep the disease at bay. Research continued, and it emerged that AZT, and in fact all the nucleoside-based compounds were prodrugs (p.), for they were metabolically phosphorylated in the cell. They were, in other words, converted into the corresponding nucleotides, the immediate precursors of DNA. Where the DNA polymerase (the enzyme that copies the DNA chain), or in the case of the retrovirus, the reverse transcriptase, runs into the incorporated unnatural nucleotide, it stalls in its progress along the parent chain. It cannot extend the chain further, and so replication stops.

The hunt after more drugs like AZT now began. The most interesting were a class of nucleotide analogues, called dideoxynucleotides (deoxy twice over, lacking, that is, two hydroxyl (-OH) groups from what would otherwise be a ribose sugar). These are very effective terminators of DNA chain elongation, and treatments for AIDS (though to molecular biologists they are better known as the essential tools for the method of sequencing of DNA, devised by Frederick Sanger, and for which he was awarded the Nobel Prize). But a more urgent matter was to find a reagent that would act on a different part of the virus replication machinery. The need was to anticipate the development of resistance to any single drug, as we have already seen in relation to cancer chemotherapy. Again then, if one virus in a million (10^6) were to mutate to a form resistant to the drug, that single virus could multiply and quickly replace the million that are killed. But if the viruses are exposed to two drugs, each, for argument's aske, with the same chance that a resistant mutant will arise, the probability of the emergence of a mutant resistant to both drugs becomes 10^6 x 10^6, which is 10^{12}, or one thousand billion, which, one might hope, with luck, will make the emergence of resistance highly improbable. But emerge it still does.

As research workers, mainly in academic and government laboratories, delved ever deeper into the workings of retroviruses, new targets came to light. The most promising came from the discovery that the DNA of the infected host cell, with its incorporated viral genome, is translated (via messenger RNA), not into the individual proteins, but into one huge chain comprising all the proteins linked together head-to-tail. For these proteins to do their work they have first to be separated by a proteolytic enzyme. This and two other enzymes, and the reverse transcriptase are the only virus proteins expressed individually and ready for action, rather than strung together with the others as parts of the dormant chain. Kill the proteolytic enzyme then, and the virus is denied the tool-kit of proteins that it needs if it is to reproduce. The sequence of the entire protein string was determined by way of the DNA sequence (p.), and the protease was prepared in the laboratory by cloning, so that its properties could be examined, and the site of its action defined.* A new drug target was now in plain view, and a group of virologists at St. Mary's Hospital Medical School in London (the place at which the *Penicillium* spore had alighted on Fleming's Petri dish nearly half a century before [p.]) joined with the chemists of Roche Pharmaceuticals at Welwyn, north of London to develop such a compound. With AIDS now spreading at apocalyptic speed, especially in America, the FDA did not wait for the cumbersome ritual of Phase III trials to take its course, but approved the compound, sequinavir (formulated and sold as Invirase) in 1995. This was one of the first truly rational exercises in drug design.

The following year two more HIV protease inhibitors appeared. One, called indinavir or Virocept, sprang from the laboratories of Japan Tobacco Agouron, a part of Agrouron Pharmaceuticals in the U.S. (both now subsidiaries of the insatiable Pfizer). The other, ritonavir, was produced by Abbott Laboratories, but was viewed with suspicion by reason of gastrointestinal side-effects. A year later it was approved a second time, reformulated in a new delivery capsule, as Fortovase. By 2012 the FDA was listing 11 approved protease inhibitors, in addition to 19 reverse transcriptase inhibitors, 13 of them nucleoside derivatives, designed therefore along the lines laid down by Gertrude Elion and George Hitchings (p.). But reverse transcriptase and the viral protease were not the last of the targets for possible therapies of AIDS: there were three others. The first step in the attack of the virus on its host cell is fusion of the membranes of virus with

---

* There are many different proteolytic enzymes (proteases for short) in the natural world, and each type has a specificity, that is to say, will cut its substrate molecules (the proteins that it destroys) at particular sequence motifs in their amino acid chain. The HIV protease will strike only where the amino acid, proline occurs next to the amino acids tyrosine or phenylalanine. (Recall that proteins are made up of 20 species of amino acids, linked together). Two strategies for the creation of an inhibitor of the enzyme are then open to chemists. One way to proceed is to construct a kind of surrogate substrate, containing the two amino acids that the enzyme recognises, but joined by a modified link that the enzyme cannot cut, and further altered to strengthen the attachment. The other is to create an unrelated compound that will occupy the part of the enzyme molecule (generally a kind of cavity or pocket), into which the substrate normally fits – the 'active centre'. The inhibitor thus occludes the site at which the enzyme seizes and breaks down its substrate.

that of the cell. This requires an interlocking of surface proteins (or more precisely glycoproteins – proteins with attached sugar elements) interact. Covering, and thereby blocking the viral glycoprotein impedes the fusion process. A secondary receptor, also detected on the T cell surface turned out also to be a target for blocking agents, which appreciably reduced the likelihood of invasion. These surface blocking agents are 'entry inhibitors'. And finally there is another enzyme, one of only three that HIV produces in intact form, the task of which is to integrate the DNA, copied from the viral RNA by the reverse transcriptase, into the genome of the host cell. This enzyme is called an integrase, and for this too an inhibitor has been generated. People infected with HIV are now treated by combination therapies, as the best hope of overcoming the power of the virus to renew itself by mutation and acquire drug resistance. All the drugs combine to suppress invasion, and (so long as this is continued) can lead a symptom-free life. That is not all, for a course of zidovudine during pregnancy will prevent passage of the virus from mother to foetus. Such were the resources of the big pharmaceutical companies that, within five years of the reported success of zidovudine in 1985, clinicians could choose from more than thirty anti-AIDS drugs.

Among them were two that together opened a new vista, especially for those, wedded despite everything, to a promiscuous life style. In 1985 a chemist at the Czech Academy of Sciences in Prague synthesised a nucleoside analogue, which, because it was poorly absorbed, seemed to have few prospects as an antiviral drug. But some ten years later chemists at an American company, thalidomide Sciences looked again at the compound, and made a derivative with much better properties. Tenofovir was licensed by the FDA for the treatment of HIV infections, and received the name, Viread. In 2003 another nucleoside inhibitor of the viral reverse transcriptase, which had been synthesised by researchers at Emory University in Georgia, U.S.A., also reached the market. This was emtricilabine, or Emtriva. A remarkable development then followed, for Gilead Sciences announced that a combination of tenofovir and emtricilabine in a single pill was not only an effective treatment for HIV, but could actually prevent entry of the virus into the host cell. And so in 2012, named Truvada, it was licensed by the FDA as the first prophylactic pill against HIV. There are hopes that it will stem the spread of AIDS, but in lifting inhibitions it may yet bring unwanted social consequences. Problems remain: drug resistance is not easily conquered, cumulative side-effects are an ever-present fear, and so the search for more drugs, and with good fortune, an actual cure, continues. For the pharmaceutical companies AIDS drugs are a more attractive proposition than new antibiotics, for, whether used therapeutically or prophylactically, the consumers wil want to keep swallowing them.

Whither malaria?

Malaria was never the favourite disease of the big drug companies because it afflicted predominantly the people of the Third World, who couldn't afford drugs. Quinine was ever-present, at least in Europe and the Americas, as the means of quenching the fever, and the early dyes, such as Paul Ehrlich's Methylene Blue, and arsenicals had only limited value (p.). It was only in 1934 that an effective antimalarial was created, but even then it was not recognised as a useful therapy. Hans Andersag, a chemist in the Bayer laboratories synthesised chloroquine, which did indeed kill malaria parasites with high efficiency (and unlike the earlier drugs, without colouring the patients' skin), but was adjudged too toxic ever to be of use in human subjects. This verdict seems to have been reached on the basis of a clinical trial on four unfortunate syphilitics, confined to a psychiatric ward in Düsseldorf, and probably already dying. They were deliberately infected with the mildest human malaria parasite, *Plasmodium vivax*, and injected with a massive dose of Resochin, as the new compound was named by the Bayer company. The doses were presumably unrealistically high, for the compound certainly has considerable side-effects. Andersag continued to produce new derivatives, which he hoped might be less toxic, but the urgency imposed by the imminence of the Second World War led to a re-evaluation of the existing drug candidates. And so, in 1939, Resochin, or sontochin as it was also called, was rehabilitated after a proper trial on more than 1000 patients in a tropical diseases institute in Hamburg. Further Franco-German trials in Tunisia were equally positive in outcome, and chloroquine became forthwith the principal treatment for malaria (though not in the U.S. where it was introduced later by the Winthrop Chemical Company under an agreement with IG Farben, the owners of Bayer).

It was not long, alas, before, in 1957, drug resistance began to assert itself, and the search after new antimalarials gathered pace. One of the first was proguanil, which surfaced in a wartime search, conducted by Imperial Chemical Industries (ICI). They found in 1945 that it was more active than quinine in suppressing the symptoms of malaria in chickens. (Birds have their own species of malaria parasite.) Not long before, Lucy Wills (p.) had discovered folic acid, the cause of a form of anaemia. This revelation had given rise to the conjecture that leukaemia too might be bound up with folic acid, and therefore to a search for folic acid analogues that would inhibit its action. Among the interested parties were the scientists around George Hitchings and Gertrude Elion at Burroughs Wellcome, and it seems to have been the organic chemist, Elvira Falco who was struck by the similarity between the structure of a folic acid analogue that she had prepared and that of proguanil. The new compound, pyrimethamine, was indeed an antimalarial, and as it later turned out, an inhibitor of an enzyme essential for folic acid synthesis in the malaria parasite. So too was proguanil.

War was once again proving to be a spur to greater efforts. The Vietnam conflict was exposing American soldiers to malaria, and most troublingly its most deadly form, spread by the parasite, *Plasmodium falciparum*. The U.S. Government reacted by funding an unprecedented programme of antimalarial research at the Walter Reed Army Institute of Research in Washington. The Walter Reed was a venerable institution with a distinguished record in the study of tropical disease, which included the discovery of the yellow fever parasite, and the elucidation of its life-cycle. Over a period of fifteen years the Walter Reed researchers synthesised and tested more than a quarter of a million compounds for antimalarial properties, of which two, bearing the numbers, 142,490 and 171,669, were found in the 1960s to be highly active. They were licensed to collaborating pharmaceutical companies for manufacture and distribution for evaluation. The first, mefloquine, a quinine derivative, was marketed by Hoffmann-La Roche in Switzerland under the name of Lariam, the second, halofantine, or Halfan, by Smith Kline and Beecham (as it then was). Both, as now appears, were approved prematurely, and caused much grief, for mefloquine proved to be neurotoxic, and engendered psychiatric disturbances in many patients, while halofantine caused heart arrhythmias, which resulted in some deaths. All the same, both drugs are still used, though never prophylactically, and only in combination with other, less dangerous substances. There is now another class of drugs, notably atovaquone, which inhibit a different enzyme in the energy-generating centres (mitochondria) of the parasite's cells. These, like all the foregoing types, are prodrugs, converted into the active form by metabolic reactions in the parasite.

The discovery of compounds that blocked different reactions in the parasite metabolism was of great importance, for it meant that the all-important combination therapies could be devised. Chloroquine and its relatives disrupt the specialised process in the parasite that sequesters a toxic product of its digestion.* Almost all the antimalarial drugs are now given in combinations, except those used prophylactically before a malaria parasite has come on the scene. All are in greater or lesser degree toxic, and are used with great care. Despite all the advances, resistance has not been eliminated, and malaria, in particular that due to *Plasmodium falciparum*, kills by engendering anaemia through destruction of the red cells, and especially by blocking capillaries, worst of all in the brain. Cerebral malaria is indeed the greatest killer. In all, malaria even now takes about a million lives annually, a large proportion those of children. It was therefore a major event when something completely new, yet ancient, surfaced. *Artemisia annua*, the annual wormwood, is a plant used in Chinese traditional medicine for more than a thousand years, and, called *Qhinghaosu*, it ranked as a kind of panacea. A discussion of its explicit value for the treatment of malaria appeared in a therapeutic manual in about 400 A.D. In the 1960s the Chinese regime apparently became concerned at the toll that malaria was taking of its soldiers, set up a programme of research on

---

* The product is haem, the iron-containing part of the red protein, haemoglobin, of the blood. Haemoglobin is the food that the parasite digests when it infiltrates the red blood cell, leaving haem as the toxic waste product. The parasite rendersit harmless by converting it into an insoluble, inactive aggregate called haemozoin.

traditional therapeutics. Of some thousands of mainly plant preparations that were tested only one was found effective, but its potency was great. This occurred in 1971.

Little was heard of the discovery in the West, and indeed the Chinese were tight-lipped about this, as about everything other scientific advance at the time. It was only in 1979 that an article in English in a Chinese medical journal brought it to the attention of researchers in the outside world. Chinese scientists extracted the active substance from the leaves of the plant, and determined its structure. This structure was strange, and certainly unprecedented among the known natural products. Its validity was doubted by chemists in the West, for it contained a peroxide bridge (-O-O-) between two carbon atoms on a ring, and should, it was thought, have been too unstable to survive for long in a plant. The formula was correct nevertheless, and when parasitologists outside China were finally able to get their hands on the material, which was given the name, artemisinin, they found that it really was far quicker in eliminating malaria parasites from patients' bodies than any of the previously known drugs. Artemisinin is yet another prodrug, converted (reduced) in the parasite to the active dihydroartemisinin. The precise mode of its action is still not altogether clear, but it appears to involve the formation, by a sequence of chemical reactions, of oxygen radicals, highly reactive forms of oxygen, which can cause mayhem within the cell. A total synthesis of artemisinin was effected in 1984 by two German chemists, but their method did not lend itself to large-scale commercial production. Several semi-synthetic derivatives have been made, one of which is dihydroartesinin, the metabolically active form, known as artesunin. Another is artemether, a slightly modified version of the original (containing an added methyl ether group, $-OCH_3$). Both have the considerable advantage of better solubility in water, which means that they can be administered by injection, especially in acute cases. Artemisinin and its derivatives are a precious resource, and to avoid the build-up of resistant parasite strains are never to be given without a second drug. The pharmaceutical company, Novartis concocted the most widely used combination, sold as Riamet or Coartem, a mixture of artemether and a synthetic drug, synthesised by Chinese chemists, called lumefantin or benflumatol.

It is no surprise that artemisinin, like the other antimalarial compounds, has been tried out against other parasitic diseases, such as Chagas disease, which is caused by a species of trypanosome (p.), and is prevalent in South America. Like the malaria parasite, trypanosomes belong to a class of micro-organisms called protozoa, and are carried by insects. Other trypanosome species are responsible for the trypanosomiasis, also known as sleeping sickness, which afflicts a half-million or more sub-Saharan Africans, and great numbers of their cattle and other animals. Another protozoan, this one carried by the sand fly, is the cause of leishmaniasis. The disease causes unpleasant skin lesions, and can also penetrate into the internal organs. This visceral form is fatal if not expeditiously treated. Many drugs were tried for African trypanosomiasis, for the most part with limited success. For many years a toxic arsenical drug, melarsoprol was the best available, but resistance developed, and it was largely replaced by α-difluoromethylornithine, called eflornithine, or Ornidyl. This was not a new compound, but was developed by an American company in 1970 as an anti-cancer agent. It performed poorly in a clinical trial, but doctors observed an unsought activity: the compound strongly suppressed hair growth. This came to the notice of the Gillette razor company, which produced and patented a cream, Vaniqa, aimed not at rendering the razor obsolete, but at ridding women with hirsutism – an excess of facial hair – of the unwanted growth. That was in 1980 and eflornithine cream was approved in the U.S. and in Europe, and is still prescribed for the same purpose, but for whatever reason, the compound was also tested against tropical parasites. It was the first new drug against trypanosomiasis in sixty years. Introduced in 1990 by Aventis (as it then was), it was later abandoned on the grounds that selling to impoverished Africans yielded little profit. Under political pressure, the company entered into an agreement with the World Health Organization (WHO) to resume production, and the drug has been distributed to patients by Médecins sans Frontières.

As for leishmaniasis, this too received little attention from the drug industry. It was cautiously treated until quite recently with two highly toxic antimony compounds. Then, yet again, a compound intended for a quite different purpose, brought at least qualified help. Milteforine, or miltex was intended as a treatment for certain cancers by application to the skin, but was found startlingly effective against leishmaniasis. Marketed as Impavido, it was granted orphan drug (the term is defined on p.) approval by the FDA in 2006. Unhappily its popularity with patients waned rapidly when it was found to have teratogenic properties, of the kind associated with thalidomide (p.). More fortunately, interest revived in a much older compound, as a result once more of a chance observation. It was a largely forgotten antibiotic from a Streptomyces bacterium. Isolated by Parke Davis in 1950, paromomycin, also known as monomycin, found limited application for the treatment of a rare form of pneumonia, which suddenly became more widespread following the arrival of the AIDS epidemic. It also found some use in amoebic and other gut infections. It is now the treatment of choice for leishmaniasis in India and other Asian countries. Artemisinin, a much more expensive option, is also reported to inhibit the leishmania parasite. Schistosomiasis, a widespread parasitic disease in Africa and Asia, is the other great scourge, second only to malaria. Also known as bilharzia, it is caused by a microscopic worm, carried by water snails, and results in a wide range of unpleasant and chronic symptoms. There is only one satisfactory and accessible treatment: preziquantel is one of a long line of compounds developed by Bayer and Merck in Germany, where the traditional concern with tropical diseases, dating back to the days of Koch and Ehrlich (Chapter) still prevails.

Parkinson and the brain

Parkinson's disease is a progressive condition, marked by a stiffness in the limbs, tremors, and difficulties in controlling movement. It was recognised, and minutely described, by an English surgeon, James Parkinson in 1817, and held to be untreatable. The breakthrough came from Arvid Carlsson at the University of Lund in Sweden (p.). Carlsson hazarded a conjecture: might the brains of people with Parkinson's disease not be deficient in the neurotransmitter, dopamine (p.)? The speculation was borne out by a Polish pathologist, Oleh Hornykiewicz at the University of Vienna in 1960 from analyses of the brains of patients who had died of the disease. Thereupon a number of doctors tried dopamine on patients to generally minimal effect, although there were partial exceptions: George

Cotzias at Brookhaven National Laboratory in upstate New York dosed his patients with enormous quantities, as much as 16 grams (perhaps two tablespoonfulls) per day, and recorded modest improvements. So also did Hornykiewicz by way of intravenous injections. But it was Carlsson who realised that the dopamine precursor, which goes by the name of L-3,4-dihydrophenylalanine, would cross the blood-brain barrier – the structure that protects the brain against exposure to the many deleterious substances that could otherwise enter it. This led him to a critical experiment: he injected a solution into rats and rabbits with Parkinson symptoms, induced with reserpine (p.). The symptoms abated. The compound, more commonly known as,*, or generally now as levodopa (see p. for the meaning of L and *laevo*, or in American usage *levo*), was tried with spectacular success on patients. It became almost at once the most favoured treatment for the disease, with, as it appeared, few and generally tolerable side-effects.

But levodopa was not quite the perfect answer that it initially seemed to be. It brought on nausea, as Guggenheim had discovered, which could be

---

* To be precise, the original experiments were carried out with laboratory-synthesised dopa, which was a mixture of equal proportions of L- and D-dopa. It had first been synthesised in 1911 by a Polish biochemist, Casimir Funk (the man who coined the word *vitamine* from 'vital amine' – a misnomer, for Funk believed incorrectly that vitamins were all amines). Two years later, a chemist at Hoffmann-La Roche in Basel, Marcus Guggenheim got the pure L-dopa out of African fava beans. Guggenheim tasted some of the extract, which resulted in a violent vomiting fit, from which he concluded that the compound was toxic. In reality it was the dopamine to which it was converted jn his body that was responsible. It was only much later that L-dopa alone, and not the D-dopa, which accompanied it in the synthetic product, was found to be the active form. L-dopa entered public consciousness with the appearance in 1973 of *Awakenings*, a book by Oliver Sacks, later the basis of a film. It concerned the victims of a mysterious condition called encephalitis lethargica, which struck communities around the world during a brief period just before and after 1920. Its effects varied, but in many cases its victims entered a catatonic state; they were 'human statues', deprived of speech, movement or awareness of their surroundings. Sacks, a neurologist in New York, treated some of them with L-dopa, which induced a return to consciousness, though with no memory of the intervening decades. The effect, alas, was transient, and the outcome for the most part unhappy. A revised edition of Sacks's book appeared in 1976, and has been many times reprinted. The disease has not returned, at least in its academic form, and its cause is still debated.

dealt with, but in the longer term unpleasant manifestations appeared – involuntary movements of the limbs, known to doctors as dyskinesia, restlessness, psychiatric disturbances. Nor was it a very efficient drug, because a digestive enzyme destroyed all but about 1% of it before it reached the brain. The enzyme had in fact been discovered in 1939, and it converts levodopa into dopamine. This is the very same reaction that it provokes in the brain – turning the precursor into dopamine once more. But dopamine in the bloodstream does no good, since it cannot get to where it is needed, the brain cells. Two pharmaceutical companies set about finding a compound to inhibit the enzyme, guided as always by the chemical nature of the enzyme's normal target. So it came about that Hoffmann-La Roche in Switzerland created benserazide, and Merck in America carbidopa. Either is given to the patient along with levodopa, for by themselves they are therapeutically inert. The ready-made combinations are sold as Madopar and Sinemet (or Atamet or Co-careldopa) respectively.

Once the outlines of dopamine action had come into focus, other therapeutic targets swam nto view. Might there, for instance, be a dopamine agonist – probably a close analogue of dopamine that would react with the dopamine receptor? The answer came from a wholly unexpected quarter – the hallucinogenic and lethal ergot fungus (p.). In 1954 an endocrinologist at the Weizmann Institute in Israel, Moshe Shelesnyak, working on the control of ovulation, published a paper reporting that ergotoxin, a preparation from ergot, impeded the first step of pregnancy in rats. Implantation is the attachment of the newly-formed foetus to the wall of the uterus, and further study revealed that the seat of the toxin's action lay not in the uterus, but in the pituitary gland at the base of brain. Ergotoxin suppressed release of a protein hormone, prolactin. It later turned out that ergotoxin was not a pure compound, but a mixture of three related alkaloids, two of which Shelesnyak* found to be active. Prolactin, as its name implies, initiates milk production in the expectant mother, but it also exerts a range of other physiological effects, and when its secretion from the pituitary gland runs riot, a number of undesirable consequences ensue. Thus, oestrogen production rises and sexual activity is disturbed, ovulation and menstruation become less frequent or cease, and milk may be produced

---

* Shelesnyak was mysteriously murdered in California in 1994 at the age of 85.

when it is least wanted. The prevention of prolactin overproduction in such a case acquires some importance. Shelesnyak's observations may have been regarded as a mere physiological oddity, but at the Sandoz laboratories in Basel Edward Flückiger took note. He wanted to find a means of reducing the prolactin concentration in the blood, and began looking for a non-toxic analogue of ergoline, one of the two active ergot alkaloids tested by Shelesnyak, and one that could be taken orally. Flückiger found several, but all had a short life in the circulation, until in 1965, after some years of toil, he found what he was looking for. The compound contained a bromine atom, and was given the name bromocriptine. Five years later a group of workers in two Swedish laboratories reported that Flückiger's compound also acted as a dopamine agonist in rats. It was the first such ever used as a treatment for Parkinson's disease. Clinical trials exposed side-effects, especially in inducing psychiatric disturbances, but in properly regulated doses, and in combination with levodopa it became a valued treatment.

As the 20th century wore on new innovations appeared, but nothing supplanted levodopa. What they were all aimed at were intervention in the enzymic reactions that normally eliminate dopamine, once it has fulfilled its function at the synapse. One scheme is inactivation of the unwanted excess by monoamine oxidase (p.). It was discovered that in fact there are two monoamine oxidases, MAO-A and MAO-B for short, and the search was on for selective inhibitors. MAO-A inhibitors have found a place in the treatment of depression and like disturbances, while MAO-B inhibitors have been used to treat Parkinson's disease. Selegaline was the first such drug, acting largely on MAO-B, at least when given in moderate doses. By itself it has no more than a marginal effect on symptoms, but it does much better in combination with levodopa. A second MAO-B inhibitor, resagaline is more potent, both alone, when it can retard the onset of symptoms in the early stages of the disease, and again in combination with levodopa. Both drugs present hazards, not least because of their incompatibility with other drugs and with certain foods, which can have lethal consequences. (One to be specially avoided worst is grapefruit.) More important have been the inhibitors of another class of enzymes – an idea that sprang from the fertile mind of Julius Axelrod at the National Institutes of Health (p). The revelation that there are several enzymes which inactivate the neurotransmitters, the catecholamines came from several directions, but it was Axelrod who made the first critical incursions into this complex subject in the 1950s. First came monoamine oxidase, and then catechol-O-methyltransferase, or COMT, which Axelrod and his colleague, Raul Tomchick discovered in 1958.

COMT operates both in the brain and in the circulation. It works by inserting a methyl group ($-CH_3$) into the dopamine or levodopa structure, thereby blocking their attachment to the receptors. The design of inhibitors of the enzyme came only after its structure had been determined by X-ray crystallography in the University of Lund in Sweden. This is an exemplar of drug design as envisaged in the modern era. The three-dimensional lineaments of the substrate-binding site in the enzyme, laid bare by the crystallographic analysis, guided the search for a compound that would fit precisely into that site, taking account also of such factors as electrostatic charge distribution. The right molecule, a simulacrum of the natural substrate, would occlude the site and stop the enzyme from getting at its substrate. From two pharmaceutical companies, the Orion Corporation in Finland and Hoffmann-La Roche in Switzerland came compounds that were effective inhibitors of the enzyme with low toxicity, and encouraging therapeutic potency in animal tests. They were called entacapone and tolcapone, and both had the virtue of quenching the annihilation by COMT of dopamine as well as levodopa. The protection of the levodopa with which Parkinson's patients were treated was a critical advance. It meant that lower doses of levodopa would suffice, and with them a reduction of dyskinesia, the worst side-effect of prolonged levodopa treatment. These drugs, with the trade names of Comtan and Tasmar, came on stream in the early 1990s, but because of reported toxicity, tolcapone was withdrawn from the market. It was reinstated after a short interval by virtue of its superior performance in suppressing the symptoms of the disease. This was due to its ability to cross the blood-brain barrier (which its competitor could not do), and thus it could manifest its activity in the brain cells as well as in the circulation. It could therefore be prescribed at lower concentration, and proper management ensured that the toxicity was in general controlled. Both drugs are now most often used in combination with an MAO-B inhibitor, and of course levodopa.

The punishments of poverty

Obscure conditions have in general been worst served by the drug industry, but there are also many, too rare to merit space, for which effective therapies are available. The diseases that are for the most part confined to the impoverished countries of the south have also received little attention for the same obvious reasons. Prominent among them are many parasitic infestations, and also hereditary anaemias, which population migrations have brought to the advanced regions. Chief among these are sickle cell disease and the thalassaemias. Sickle cell disease originated in Africa, and it was the slave trade that took it to the United States and the Caribbean. In the 20th century African and Caribbean migrations ensured its appearance in Europe. Sickle cell disease is caused by a common mutation in a haemoglobin gene. It is in fact the commonest disease resulting from a single mutation (p.).* An offspring of two carriers of the disease who receives abnormal β chains from both parents will have sickle cell disease, whereas one endowed with an abnormal chain from one parent and a normal one from the other will have sickle cell trait, and will be a carrier. If both β chains in the haemoglobin have the sickle mutation the consequences are dire, for when it gives up its oxygen in the tissues of the body its properties are transformed. The molecules of this deoxygenated haemoglobin attach to each other, forming long stiff filaments that extend through the red cell, and cause it to become rigid.

---

* The haemoglobin molecule, which carries oxygen around the body in the red blood cells, is made up of four protein constituents bound together, a pair of α and a pair of β chains, the products of separate genes. The α protein chain is made up of 141 amino acids, and the β of 146. In the abnormal sickle cell haemoglobin a mutation in the β chain results in the substitution of a single amino acid for another. Sickle cell disease is one of the quite small minority of illnesses resulting from a mutation in a single gene. Our DNA is distributed between 23 chromosome pairs. We receive one member of each pair from our father, the other from our mother. Our parents, of course, also have 23 pairs of chromosomes, and either member of each pair can be copied to the offspring. This means that any of four possible parental chromosome combinations can pass at random to the offspring (AA, AB, BA, and BB). The β haemoglobin gene is on chromosome 11. Suppose now that there are many carriers of the mutant gene in a population, people, that is, with one normal (β^A) and one mutant (β^S) gene in their haemoglobin; then unions between two such carriers will lead to offspring with a 25% statistical probability of ending up with an $\alpha_2\beta^S_2$ haemoglobin, the same probability of possessing an $\alpha_2\beta^A_2$ haemoglobin, and a 50% probability of an $\alpha_2\beta^A\beta^S$ haemoglobin. In other words, the most unfortunate quarter of offspring will have a haemoglobin containing only the abnormal form of the β chain (β^S), the best-off will have only normal haemoglobin, and the remaining half will have a protein containing one mutant (β^S) and one normal (β^A) type of β chain. The individual with two abnormal chains is termed a homozygote, having been dealt the abnormal chain from both parents, whereas the one who has inherited one β chain of each kind is called a heterozygote. Clearly, in the case of a rare mutation, or of a mutation that is sparse in a particular population, the probability of a sexual encounter between two carriers is correspondingly improbable, and indeed any genetic trait is diluted through the generations. This is the basis of the famous principle enunciated by the great biologist, J.B.S. Haldane (given that evolutionary striving is to promote the individuals' gene pool), 'I will lay down my life for two brothers, and for more than eight first cousins'. This remark, said to have resulted from a calculation in the course of a pub conversation, encapsulates and predates by many years, Richard Dawkins's trope of 'The Selfish Gene'.

The cell acquires a curved elongated contour, which gives the disease its name. The cell membrane becomes irreversibly damaged, and the cells break, and also become trapped in the narrowest blood vessels. The victims of the disease are severely anaemic and suffer periodic painful 'crises'. In the past they did not live beyond puberty. Sickle cell trait, on the other hand, is a relatively mild disease, which does not in general preclude a normal lifestyle. The question why the disease retained its hold instead of vanishing by reason of its evolutionary disadvantage exercised geneticists for many years, until evidence accrued that the mutant haemoglobin afforded some modest defence against malaria. Thus the heterozygotes saved from death by malaria would have exceeded the heterozygotes who succumbed to their disease.

An early attempt at a therapy for sickle cell disease aimed at limiting the extent of oxygen release from the haemoglobin on the grounds that it is only the deoxygenated haemoglobin which forms the long filaments in the cell. Carbonic anhydrase, which we have already encountered (p.), is an enzyme found in the red blood cell. Its function is to convert the mildly alkaline bicarbonate (formed from exhaled carbon dioxide) back into carbon dioxide and water, thus rendering the cell contents more acidic. It is a well-known characteristic of haemoglobin that its affinity for oxygen is reduced in slightly acid conditions. (This property is known after the Bohr effect, after the Danish physiologist – father of the great physicist, Niels Bohr – who discovered it.) The therapy consisted of inhibiting the action of the enzyme, and itworked but the patients died, or at least fell seriously sick, for carbonic anhydrase is indispensable elsewhere in the body, and the treatment was hastily abandoned. (The inhibitor was acetazolamide, known as Diamox. It has legitimate uses, taken at low concentrations in the treatment of glaucoma, and of altitude sickness.)

And so, beyond giving blood transfusions, little remained by way of treatment for the victims of sickle cell disease until the 1980s, when the first, and still the only therapy appeared out of research at Harvard and other American medical schools. Illumination came from the discovery of mechanisms that control the expression of genes. An essential step is the introduction of methyl groups ($-CH_3$) into regions of DNA associated with gene regulation. Foetuses and newborn babies have a different haemoglobin from adults. This is called foetal haemoglobin, and differs from the adult version in that it has different β chains, called γ (gamma) chains. The switchover occurs before birth, and accompanies a reduction in methylation of the γ chain gene and an attendant rise in that of the (adult) β chain. Experimentation with nucleoside and nucleotide analogues of the kind first introduced by Gertrude Elion and George Hitchings (Chapter) produced an immediate result: a derivative called 5-azacytidine given to anaemic adult monkeys produced a surge of foetal haemoglobin synthesis, a protein never normally seen in the adult animal (or people). This was a promising phenomenon, for it was already known that in a genetic condition (see below) in which both foetal and sickle cell haemoglobin are produced, the disease symptoms are milder than in homozygous sickle cell disease. The presence in the red cell of the foetal haemoglobin reduces the formation of the destructive formation of filaments. There were brief trials in human patients, but azacytidine was feared to induce cancer, and was never widely used.

Soon afterwards another quite different substance was examined – hydroxyurea, a cheap and simple compound. It was known to inhibit an enzyme implicated in the production of nucleotides, and thus for the synthesis of DNA, and it had been used in earlier years to treat disorders of the bone marrow that cause overproduction of blood cells. Hydroxyurea, like azacytidine, provoked the reverse switch from adult to foetal haemoglobin in anaemic monkeys. Foetal haemoglobin does not have the sickling defect, and functions much like the normal adult protein, that healthy people all have. Clinical trials were a great success: the toxicity of hydroxyurea is low and it can be taken by mouth. The distressing symptoms of patients treated in this manner were much alleviated, the crises declined in frequency and severity, other manifestations of the disease receded, and the patients survived into adulthood, and were enabled to lead a fairly tolerable life. Hydroxyurea appears to have a number of other benign effects, including stimulation of metabolic signalling processes, and a diminution of the stickiness of the red cells, and therefore of the occlusion of blood vessels. It is still the only treatment for sickle cell disease.

The term thalassaemia (from the Greek for the sea) embraces a collection of genetic defects, all of them resulting in an abnormality in haemoglobin synthesis. They comprise failure of either α or β chain synthesis, and the contingent formation of red cells containing unstable incomplete haemoglobins. The cells break down, causing anaemia and occlusion of blood vessels as in sickle cell disease. There are homo- and heterozygous forms, known as thalassaemia major and minor, which differ greatly in severity. The thalassaemias are widespread in their occurrence, though as the name implies, they tend to be most concentrated in maritime regions, mainly in Africa and Asia. Again, like the sickle cell gene, those for thalassaemias appear to give some degree of protection against malaria. There are no drugs known to ameliorate these diseases. The only treatment is periodic blood transfusions, but these cause their own problems (aside from their limited feasibility in poor communities), in particular the accumulation of iron (ferric) ions in the circulation. This 'iron overload' inflicts serious damage on the heart and other organs, and if not treated is ultimately fatal. But in the 1970s iron-specific chelating agents were introduced. Chelators are compounds with the property of taking up, and clutching tightly particular metal ions. A high degree of specificity is clearly necessary, for otherwise the calcium, and more especially magnesium ions, which abound in the body, would saturate them.

An excellent iron chelator with reasonably low toxicity, which also found other applications, especially in treating cases of serious iron poisoning, came out of a series of chance observations, beginning at the Ciba laboratories in Switzerland in 1959. Hans Bickel was investigating a family of iron-containing antibiotics, called ferrimycins. In the course of purifying one of these compounds Bickel discovered that they were accompanied by several iron-containing impurities, which counteracted the antibiotic activity. The ferrimycins appeared promising antibiotics, but bacteria developed resistance very quickly, and so they were discarded. Bickel, though, was interested enough in the curious properties of the impurities to study them further. He prepared enough of one, which was given the name, desferrioxamine B (or deferrioxamine), to allow determination of its structure. The task was entrusted to Vladimir Prelog, one of the leading organic chemists of the time (and a Nobel Laureate) at the Swiss Federal

Research Institute, the ETH, in Zurich. Prelog did as he was asked, and also then carried out a complete synthesis. Interest in the compound spread, and the head of clinical research at Ciba thought it worth trying it as a source of iron in cases of iron deficiency anaemia. He arranged for a trial at the University Clinic in Freiburg in Germany. The compound was given to a patient who was startled to find his urine turned to a rich reddish brown: it was the desferrioxamine, which had been repaidly eliminated by the kidneys without giving up its iron. It would clearly therefore not function as an iron donor, but it was more remarkable in the eyes of the clinicians that the compound could pass through the body and still retain its iron. No known iron compound had ever been seen to do this. From there it was a short step to test its capacity to prevent iron overload (as well as to treat cases of iron poisoning.) It was later found to possess some toxicity, but it could be tolerated in modest doses. Desferrioxamine revolutionised the treatment of thalassaemia patients, and others requiring frequent blood transfusions. It cannot usefully be taken by mouth, as the experiment in Freiburg had indicated, and is normally administered by an implanted pump. Since that time other iron chelators that can be taken orally have been developed, most notably deferasirox (Exjade), but are more toxic than desferrioxamine. Indeed Exjade, introduced in 2005, has been responsible for deaths from kidney and liver failure, and is apt to cause gastric and intenstinal bleeding, so has to be treated with great respect. It seems nevertheless to be better tolerated than desferrioxamine, pumped into a vein.

Bad sex and the most popular pill of all

Until well into the 20th century male impotence, or as it is now called, erectile dysfunction, could be treated only by essentially ineffective injections of extracts from animal testes, or by mechanical devices. The vogue for testis implants (Chapter) faded when their futility was finally demonstrated. In 1977 a French surgeon injected his anaesthetised patient with papaverine in the genital area. Papaverine is an opium alkaloid, used, like several similar compounds, to dilate blood vessels, and arrest gut spasms, by relaxing the smooth muscle surrounding the tissue. He probably got closer to the penis than he intended, but the consequence was a very apparent erection, to the dismay apparently of the operating theatre staff. When the observation was reported it excited a certain interest, but the prospect of an injection in a tender area did not have wide appeal. There was moreover the danger of a side-effect in the form of priapism, the term for an erection that could endure (painfully) for a day or more.

Nevertheless, some research was initiated*, but It was not until about 1990 that the prospect of a pill to overcome sexual impotence became a reality. It happened, inevitably, by accident. In the late 1980s the researchers in

---

* An outlandish episode, meant to demonstrate the feasibility of the papaverine treatment caused a greater stir. It took place at a meeting in Las Vegas in 1983 of the Urodynamics Society. The occasion was an evening lecture, preceding the conference banquet, and the speaker was Giles Brindley, a professor at the Institute of Psychiatry in London. Brindley achieved high distinction in physiology. His name is associated with major advances in the understanding of colour vision, and with other areas of his discipline. At the Institute of Psychiatry he concerned himself mainly with the development of prosthetic devices for the handicapped, most notably for the blind. As a musician of professional calibre he invented 'the logical bassoon', with stops operated by a keyboard. The title of Brindley\s notorious lecture in Las Vegas promised little, but when he arrived on the podium in a tracksuit he announced that he had injected himself with papaverine in his hotel room. Assuring his audience that a public lecture was not an erotogenic occasion, he proceeded to demonstrate that the papaverine had done its work. For an eyewitness account of the occasion, published in a learned journal, we have a Canadian urologist, Laurence Klotz, to thank. Brindley began by showing a series of slides, testifying to the efficacy of various compounds in producing the desired effect. He had, he said, chosen the loose-fitting clothing so as to be able to present the audience with proof. 'He pulled his loose pants tight around his genitalia in an attempt to demonstrate his erection', Klotz relates. Brindley was not satisfied and shook his head, and announced that this did not adequately reveal the effect. 'He then summarily dropped his trousers and shorts, revealing a long, thin, clearly erect penis. There was not a sound in the room. Everyone had stopped breathing.' This was still not enough. As Klotz remembered it, Brindley paused, and then spoke again: '"I'd like to give some of the audience the opportunity to confirm the degree of tumescence". With trousers round his knees, the lecturer descended from the podium and advanced awkwardly towards the front row of the audience, preceded by his erection, which he invited them to inspect that they might reassure themselves there was no deception. The seats were occupied by eminent urologists and some of their wives, who had come dressed for the formal banquet. As the apparition drew near, some of the women threw up their arms and screamed. Brindley, apparently discomposed, pulled up his trousers, returned to the podium, and quickly ended his lecture. Klotz concludes: 'Professor Brindley belongs in the pantheon of famous British eccentrics who have made spectacular contributions to science. The story of his lecture deserves a place in the urological history books'. It is only fair to add that some of the other witnesses gave accounts of the lecture differing in some details, but it drew attention, at all events, to the possibility of help for the desperate human male.

the Pfizer laboratories at Sandwich on the English south coast were on the trail of a blood-vessel dilator for angina sufferers, when their human guinea pigs reported an unexpected phenomenon. The drug was proving a disappointment, at least in terms of its intended purpose. By then much was known about the control of arterial tension, including the important part playes by the class of natural compounds, the prostaglandins (p.) in constricting the vessels. The process also requires an enzyme of a widely distributed type known as a phosphodiesterase. The plan of the Pfizer group was therefore to find an inhibitor of this and no other member of the class. A moderately promising candidate duly emerged, entered as UK-92480 in the laboratory log. It worked in laboratory animals, and reasonably well in the human volunteers, but it was rapidly degraded in the body, and would therefore have to be taken at frequent intervals to do any good. Moreover it appeared incompatible with the nitrogenous chemicals generally taken by angina sufferers, because the combination caused an alarming drop in blood pressure. UK-92480 seemed to have no future. But then came reports from several of the trial subjects that they had experienced unsought erections over a period of a few days after taking the drug.

This was seen as a curiosity and evoked little interest, but then, as more such reports came in, a few chemists, led by Ian Osterloh decided to look into the matter further. The next step was to find volunteers with erectile dysfunction. They were wired up to an apparatus that measured the circumference and rigidity of the penis, and were confronted with erotic videos, having first been administered a dose of UK-92480 or a placebo. `The results were dramatic, and led to further trials on some 300 subjects in three countries, several with diabetes, an organic source of dysfunction. In this trial 90% of the subjects responded very satisfactorily to the drug. In 1997, after four years of trials sildenafil citrate – the generic name of the compound – broke on the market. Viagra became almost immediately the fastest-selling drug ever produced. Since that time other similar products have appeared, but none have replaced the original, the name of which quickly found a place in contemporary social discourse.

The orphans

An 'orphan disease' is nothing more than an ailment too rare to catch the attention of the pharmaceutical industry. For a major company to concern itself with such a commercial trifle and develop an 'orphan drug' some form of pecuniary incentive is needed. This commonly takes the form of a Government guarantee of exclusive ownership of the rights for an extended period, a direct subvention or assistance from a Government research institution. Certainly easing of the requirements in Phase III trials would be taken for granted (often inevitable in any case, because the usual number of patients simply cannot be found). In the U.S. all this has been enshrined in the Orphan Drug Act of 1983, and in the Rare Diseases Act of 2002. (This legislation brought vociferous accusations of violation of the free-market principle.) The European Union introduced a similar law in 2000. The concept of rarity is not defined: there is at least one disease with only one known sufferer on the planet, but there are others that vary widely in their incidence between different parts of the world. The commonest rare disease may be cystic fibrosis, which afflicts about 30,000 Americans and 20,000 Europeans. These are still small numbers in commercial terms, and it is very likely that without government assistance effective treatments would not have been developed, so that children with the disease would still be barely reaching puberty*. They now receive Pulmozyme, together with an antibiotic, tobramycin, derived from a Streptomyces species (*Streptomyces tenebrarius*), which is effective against the airborne bacterium, *Pseudomonas aeruginosa*, a common source of infection in immunologically weakened victims. This treatment helps sufferers from cystic fibrosis to live longer and better lives.

The striking aspect of orphan diseases is that they are largely hereditary, and due to single-nucleotide (p.) mutations. This means in general that the protein specified by the gene has the wrong amino acid at one point in its sequence. Most often the protein in question is an enzyme, and the mutation may render it inactive or sometimes missing altogether**. Therefore some essential metabolic reaction does not occur, and a substance that is required for normal life is not made, or a metabolic product that does harm if not eliminated remains in place. The first such diseases to be discovered, about a century ago, were nutritional anomalies, such

---

* The development of the drug was in fact a rather simple matter. In cystic fibrosis the primary defect leads in turn to an inflammatory reaction, and a surge of white blood cells into the respiratory system. The cells burst open, spilling out their contents, including the DNA. The DNA molecules are very long filaments, which form an extremely viscous, tacky solution, which clogs the lungs and airways. Animals and humans possess enzymes (nucleases) that break down nucleic acids (p.) into small pieces. One of these is a pancreatic enzyme, deoxyribonuclease 1 (DNase 1). When DNase 1 from cow pancreas was tried on cystic fibrosis patients, it worked very well, but as an alien protein it generated an immune reaction. The answer therefore was to use human DNas 1, which the famous Californian biotechnology company, Genentech was able to produce by cloning and expression in bacteria. There was one further problem: the action of DNase 1 is inhibited by a widespread cellular protein, actin, and actin also spills out of the ruptured white cells. The Genentech scientists therefore produced a modified human DNase 1 deprived of its capacity to bind actin. This product, called domase-α, is marketed as Pulmozyme, and is given to the patient in an aerosol spray.

** Most mutations, it should be said, are harmless, or 'silent', and have no or little effect on the workings of the enzyme. If the enzyme is missing there are two possible explanations. One is that the mutation prevents the protein chain from folding – from assuming, that is, its active and stable conformation - and it is then eliminated by enzymic processes in the cell. The other possible reason is that the mutation is not in the gene itself, but in a segment of the DNA that directs the gene to be switched on and start the process of making (expressing) the protein.

as phenylketonuria. This disorder is due to the lack on an enzyme that degrades phenylalanine, one of the 20 amino acids that make up proteins. Phenylalanine accumulates in the nervous system with dire results. The defect can be detected in a newborn baby by a simple test of its urine. The condition is then treated by means of a diet low in phenylalanine content. The child can then expect to lead a normal and satisfactory life, except for the need to endure a monotonous and unpalatable diet. Phenylketonuria, like many such diseases is recessive, meaning that it reveals itself only when both parents are 'carriers', or heterozygotes (p.). The number of known single-gene diseases in the world's population is estimated as about 7,000, but new ones are turning up all the time. There are only some 350 drugs for orphan diseases. Thus for the great majority there is no cure or often even treatment, and an estimated third of babies with an orphan disease die before the age of five. On the other hand, the symptoms of many orphan diseases are mild, or at least tolerable, so for a large proportion of the survivors – about 55 million in America and Western Europe – the outlook is not as bleak as may appear.

The search for treatments for rare diseases have on occasion led to valuable advances in knowledge, and to new drugs of broader application. So for instance, Wilson's disease is a rare defect in copper metabolism. Copper is a constituent of certain proteins, but by itself it is neurotoxic, so must not be permitted to accumulate in the body, as it does in Wilson's disease if left untreated. In 1956 a London doctor found a metabolite of penicillin in the urine of patients given the antibiotic. This was penicillamine, which he found to be a chelator (a compound that takes up a metal ion with high avidity) of copper. Just as the excess of toxic iron in people dependent on frequent blood transfusions is taken up by an iron chelator (p...), and eliminated in the urine, so copper is removed by penicillinamine. There are side-effects, but Wilson's disease is no longer deadly. Moreover, penicillamine, or Cupramine to give it its commercial name, has other benign attributes. It will dissolve the 'cystine stones' in the urinary tract of people plagued by the rare but unpleasant disease, cystinuria, and it has also been used to treat the auto-immune (p.) condition, rheumatoid arthritis.

But why, you may ask, can one not simply supply someone troubled by a dud or missing enzyme with the enzyme from an external source, just as type 1 diabetics are provided with the missing hormone, insulin? The reason is that it is seldom possible to direct the enzyme to the right place. A protein given by mouth will be destroyed by the digestive enzymes in the stomach, and if injected it is apt to do damage before it is destroyed by the digestive enzymes in the stomach or excreted by the kidneys. *Enzyme replacement therapy*, as it is called, has been successful in only one class of rare genetic conditions, the lysosomal storage diseases. Lysosomes are organelles (small structures inside cells), which have the essential function of eliminating metabolic detritus. Their interior is quite acidic and contains a battery of enzymes, which break down protein, fatty and especially carbohydrate matter. In the lysosomal storage diseases (of which there are many, even though their combined incidence in the world's population is no more than one in 100,000) one or other enzyme in the lysosome does not function. The consequences vary from the relatively mild to the lethal, with symptoms that may comprise retarded development, immobility, blindness, deafness, dementia and early death. One of the most notorious is Tay-Sachs disease, which afflicts only Jews, but the most common (though still rare) is probably Gaucher's disease. This is caused by the lack of an enzyme that digests a glycolipid (a fatty molecule attached to a sugar). When this substance is allowed to accumulate it enters the macrophages – blood cells, which engulf and destroy intruders, and constitute an indispensable part of the immune system – and ends in bone damage, brain impairment, an enlarged liver, defective clotting of the blood, and anaemia. In another form, the disease may manifest only in old age, and in a less aggressive form.

Until the advent of enzyme replacement therapy all that could be done was to treat the symptoms. In the 1970s a means was found of purifying the missing enzyme in Gaucher's disease from placentas, and preparations were tried on patients. Success was only marginal until the idea arose of chemically coupling the enzyme to a sugar, mannose, for which there is a receptor on the surfaces of macrophages. The enzyme homed in on the macrophages, was engulfed and digested the errant glycolipid, just as in the normal cell. Soon thereafter the enzyme was prepared by expression in bacteria and became at least marginally less expensive. There was now a very effective treatment for the disease, which could be given intravenously at suitable intervals. It has given the victims of Gaucher's disease a relatively normal life, though at no small expense. There have been similar developments in research on therapies for at least two other lysosomal storage diseases, but concerns remain over the costs of treating a small number of patients*,

---

* For some three decades now a body of enthusiasts have proclaimed the need to cure, and not merely treat the symptoms of single-gene diseases, and possibly others, by gene therapy. This means introducing into the patient's cells (and of course the right cells) a piece of DNA containing the gene that will express the missing or defective enzyme. It is done generally with the aid of a virus, modified so as to render it harmless, which acts as a vehicle to carry the therapeutic DNA into the cell. This is a complex and demanding technique, which has so far been carried out only experimentally, with modest success and some deaths. It will no doubt be accomplished in time. There has been much investment of time, skill and effort in a plan to supply an enzyme to the cells of failing hearts in the hope that it will boost the inadequate entry of calcium into the muscle. Whether and to what extent gene therapy will evolve into a widely available and affordable technique is hard to predict.

Chapter 17

DISASTERS: SOME MALIGN EPISODES IN THE HISTORY OF DRUGS

Drugs are dangerous chemicals, and the fear is never banished of an unforeseen malign effect. In earlier times, before clinical trials were thought of, physicians commonly based their treatments on theoretical concepts that appear ludicrous to their successors. They killed with compounds of mercury, arsenic and antimony (although not in such numbers as the bleeders and purgers, who dominated the profession over the centuries). Often adulteration has brought death and disease. A tragic example in the 20th century was the 'Elixir Sulfanilamide' with its ethylene glycol solvent, released onto the American market in 1937 (p.). A later, and much worse case was the disaster of diethylstilboestrol (DES), the synthetic steroidal compound that exposed mainly women, their offspring, and possibly even a third generation, to the risk of otherwise rare cancers (p.). The consequences are still being studied. An insidious cause of damage to health may be an unpredictable interaction of one drug with another, or with something in a food, such as the common fermentation product, tyramine. This compound is found in a number of foods, but especially in strong cheeses, and is responsible for the 'cheese effect', the violent surge in blood pressure when the cheese is eaten by a patient on a monoamine oxidase inhibitor (p.). Rare metabolic traits have also on occasion exposed an untoward drug reaction. The first recorded example was probably discovered during World War II, when doctors found that a few soldiers experienced a haemolytic crisis – rupture of the red cells of the blood, causing their contents(nearly all haemoglobin) to spill into the bloodstream – when given the antimalarial drug, primaquine. This was fortunately a transient phenomenon, which receded if there were no further doses of the drug. In 1956 the reason for this susceptibility to primaquine (and other related antimalarials) was tracked down: the affected individuals all had G6PD deficiency. G6PD – glucose-6-phosphate dehydrogenase – is a metabolic enzyme, and its hereditary insufficiency is the commonest of all the many known human enzyme defects.*

The condition renders some of those affected sensitive to several common drugs, some individuals even to aspirin. Since then many such links between an enzyme mutation and an adverse response to a drug have reported. That has resulted in the withdrawal of a number of otherwise satisfactory drugs in cases of serious or even lethal reactions. The drug companies could scarcely have been blamed for such unforseeable mishaps, but the worst disasters have come about by negligence, when those responsible for testing new compounds have cut corners, even if at times sheer ill-luck has played its part.

Thalidomide

Thalidomide, a derivative of piperidine, which is the core structural element of a variety of drugs, was first synthesised in 1953, or so it was always asserted, by chemists at Chemie Grünenthal, a German company based near Aachen. Recent quarrying in the company archives has come up with a different story, namely that the compound originated during World War II at I.G. Farben, and that the man responsible was a chemist,

---

* About 4 billion people in the world have one of the forms of this condition, and they mainly live in regions in which malaria is, or was endemic. This is because red blood cells deficient in G6PD are relatively resistant to attack by the malaria parasite. The condition was once commonly known as favism because a minority of the possessors of the mutation have a severe haemolytic reaction to the ingestion of broad beans (fava beans).

Otto Ambros.* At all events Grünenthal made and tested the compound as part of a programme to develop psychotropic drugs, and observed a strange phenomenon: animals dosed with the substance lapsed into a sleep from which they could not be aroused until the effect wore off. Volunteers tried it also and found it to have a powerful hypnotic, sedative effect. Animal tests revealed no toxicity, even at high doses. Small scattered human trials gave wholly pleasing results, and in 1957 the company introduced the drug with much fanfare as a sedative and sleeping pill in what was then West Germany. Its virtues, the advertising proclaimed, were its total safety, even in huge doses, so that it could not cause death by accidental or deliberate overdosing. The drug was sold over the counter under the market name. Contergan. It was much favoured in hospitals, and in mental clinics to soothe the inmates, and a liquid formulation was meant for children, and became indeed the country's 'baby-sitter'. Unfortunately it also relieved morning sickness in pregnant women.

Thalidomide spread around the world. In Britain it was taken up by the Distillers Company, an old-established Scottish producer of whiskeys, which in 1942 had formed Distillers Company (Biochemicals) for the purpose initially of manufacturing penicillin. Distillers (Biochemicals) entered into an agreement to produce thalidomide, having first procured from Grünenthal a quantity of the chemical for clinical testing. Distillers gave it the trade name of Distaval, and supplied it to many countries, and especially to Australia, where it was first tried in 1961 on pregnant women in two hospitals in Sydney. Meanwhile, in 1960 the William S. Merrell

---

* Ambros, a highly-placed member of the Nazi party, had worked on the development of nerve gases, especially the most lethal, sarin. (The name is derived from the initials of the four principal scientists involved.) Ambros admitted to performing experiments on captives in concentration camps (a practice which he later sought to justify). At a war-crimes trial in 1948 he received an eight-year prison sentence, but was released after serving only three. On his release he was engaged as a consultant on chemical weapons to the American army, and also lent his services to the American chemical industry. In Germany he became an adviser to President Adenauer, and also joined the board of Chemie Grünenthal, owned at the time by a family that had been much involved with the Nazi regime. Chemie Grünenthal also benefited from the services of other war criminals, who had participated in experimentation on prisoners in concentration camps.

Company of Cincinnati had entered into a licensing agreement to make and distribute the drug in the United States. The application for approval of the drug came before the FDA in September of 1960. It was assigned for evaluation to Frances Oldham Kelsey, a Canadian pharmacologist, who had qualified in medicine at the University of Chicago, and had been at the FDA only a month. Thalidomide came with strong assertions of its efficacy and assurances of its safety, but Frances Kelsey was unimpressed: she found the testing by Grünenthal dismayingly shoddy, and opined that the claims made for the drug were 'too good to be true'. She was backed by two colleagues, with whom she shared the responsibility, a pharmacologist and a chemist. So it was that she turned her thumbs down on the grounds of insufficient evidence of long-term safety. The company in the shape of its executive, Dr Joseph Murray objected strenuously to the judgement, for had thalidomide not emerged from many months of continuous use in several European countries with nothing to impugn its safety? Frances Kelsey stood firm, and a year-long tussle developed, in which Murray argued and bullied, and tried also to bypass his adversary by appealing to the FDA directorate.

Then on the last day of 1960 a letter appeared in the *British Medical Journal* from a Scottish GP. Four of his patients, he reported, had developed a distressing condition called peripheral neuritis, marked by pains in the extremities, cramps, numbness and muscle weakness. All four, he discovered, had been taking thalidomide for some time. When Frances Kelsey read the letter it strengthened her concerns, and especially with respect to the developing human foetus. Murray took the warnings seriously to the extent of arranging some tests, but only in late-stage pregnancy. There were no effects, and he decided that the peripheral neuritis must have been trivial and the nerve damage reversible. But he was willing, he told the FDA, to mention the toxic symptoms on the labels of the pill bottles. Then suddenly everything changed. Murray called Frances Kelsey and told her that the company was withdrawing the drug. There had been the first reports of birth defects. A leading expert on the subject, Helen Taussig, a professor at Johns Hopkins Medical School, had seen thalidomide-induced defects on a visit to Europe, and had communicated with Murray. So confident had the William S. Merrell Company been of rapid approval of thalidomide by the FDA that they had sent samples of the drug to some thousand doctors to try out. Among the patients were 80 pregnant women, taking the drug mainly for insomnia, and for the most part in the late stage of pregnancy. But there were three recorded instances of birth malformations, and nor could Merrell trace all the pills that had been sent out. It became known that the director of medical research at Merrell had indulged in a disreputable practice, which we will encounter again: he wrote a paper giving a favourable report on the outcome of thalidomide trials, to which he persuaded a compliant doctor to lend his name as the ostensible author. Some cases came to court, and the affair led to a revision of the laws governing the licensing and use of new drugs. Frances Kelsey became, deservedly, a national heroine, and received an award for Distinguished Federal Civilian Service at the hands of President Kennedy.

In other countries the outcome was altogether less satisfactory. In Germany, where the evil originated, thalidomide, or Contergan, broke over the market in 1957 after a round of clinical trials. It was touted as the safe sleeping pill, which could be taken in high doses, because it was non-addictive and devoid of depressant properties. It could be bought without prescription, and was favoured by many hospital doctors. So pleased were suppliers and consumers alike that Contergan not only displaced a large proportion of the available barbiturates, but also entered into use against all manner of complaints for which it was never intended – for coughs, for diarrhoea and for inflammatory conditions. It appeared in East and West Germany, as in other countries, in combinations with other drugs, and under a variety of names. The first murmurs of alarm became audible in 1960, although a few months earlier a solitary neurologist had expressed unease about possible nerve damage. Indications that this might actually be a widespread problem now came from several university clinics in West Germany, and then in late 1961 the blow fell. Widukind Lenz*, professor of paediatrics at Hamburg University, informed Chemie Grünenthal by telephone that thalidomide, taken in the early stages of pregnancy, was associated with birth malformations. The condition was termed phocomelia, meaning limbs like the flippers of a seal. Lenz had been consulted by the parents of a baby born with vestigial arms, and he had sought out the medicines that the mother, and later the mothers of other malformed babies, had been taking during pregnancy. He recognised thalidomide as the common factor, and also established that it was generally only in the first fifty or so days of development that the effect occurred. Grünenthal apparently would not hear of it, having carried out some tests on pregnant animals, and it was only when corroborating reports began to arrive from other quarters that they accepted Lenz's advice to withdraw the drug from the market.

Lenz's observations were in fact anticipated by an Australian gynaecologist and obstetrician a few months earlier. Thalidomide had been strongly promoted in Australia by Distillers, until in 1961 a letter from Dr William McBride, working in one of the major Sydney hospitals, appeared in *The Lancet*. Congenital malformations, he began, occurred statistically in about 1.5% of births, but 'In recent months I have observed that the incidence of multiple severe abnormalities in babies delivered of women who were given the drug thalidomide ("Distaval") during pregnancy, as an anti-emetic, to be almost 20%.' On another page of the journal the managing director of Distillers (Biochemicals) Ltd states that reports from 'two overseas sources', though not from Great Britain, had reached the company of 'harmful effects on the foetus in early pregnancy', 'possibly

* Lenz (1919-1995) was a highly-regarded paediatrician and clinical geneticist. He was the son of Fritz Lenz, one of the first and most unpleasant proponents of 'racial hygiene', the racist theory that was so congenial to the Nazis. The son followed in his father's footsteps. As a student, he was a group leader in the Hitler Youth, and then a member of the National Socialist Students' League, and an enthusiastic member of the SA, the paramilitary 'Brownshirts', who helped to bring Hitler to power. He was for a period a prisoner of war, but thereafter his career thrived, and he became a leader in his field, continuing until his death to make contributions to the study of genetic defects – the kinds of stigmata that would have attracted a mandatory death sentence for children during the Third Reich.

associated with thalidomide', and that therefore Distaval and other products containing thalidomide, had been withdrawn from the market as a precaution. McBride had in fact written twice to Distillers before sending his letter to *The Lancet* about his observations, but to no effect. Indeed the management was still instructing its sales force that while thalidomide 'almost certainly does cross the placental barrier', no harmful effects on the foetus had been reported. It was not long before enraged victims brought legal actions against Grünenthal and Distillers. Investigations revealed that rather perfunctory tests had been performed on pregnant animals by both companies, but that no account had been taken of the stage of foetal development. It appeared that in one series the drug dose was so large that the foetuses had died at an early stage, presumably unnoticed. Too late, Distillers did carry out proper animal tests, and found a high frequency of malformations and stillbirths.

The number of babies born with severe malformations – short or missing arms or legs, abnormal digits, no ears, defective digestive tracts – has been variously estimated as around 10,000, or as twice that, in Europe and Africa alone. To this must be added the large number of foetuses that died before birth. The Australian population was probably the worst affected because the first field tests of the drug had been carried out in Sydney hospitals. Chemie Grünenthal refused to accept liability, and took fifty years to express regret and acknowledge responsibility. Distillers acted more promptly and honourably. Large amounts of compensation were paid out, but many legal actions are unresolved even now. Fifty years after the event, in 2012, Chemie Grünenthal finally came through with an apology to the victims and compensation for those who survived. The heroes in the lamentable tale – Frances Kelsey, Wedukind Lenz and William McBride – were showered with well-merited acclaim. In Britain the *Sunday Times* 'Insight' team and the editor, Harold Evans played an admirable part in bringing the facts of the scandal to light.

In McBride's case there is a sad postscript, for in 1982 he convinced himself that another anti-emetic drug, which had become popular as a treatment for morning sickness in pregnant women, was similarly teratogenic (engendering malformations). This was Debendox (or Bendeclin in the

U.S.), developed in the U.S. by Merrell-Dow, the organisation formed by a merger of Walter S. Merrell (the company that had tried so hard to push thalidomide onto the American market, with the mighty Dow Chemical Company. In 1982 McBride had published a paper with his conclusions, based on experiments with pregnant rabbits. Merrell-Dow had at once withdrawn the product, but this was insufficient to forestall a series of lawsuits by women who had taken Debendox during pregnancy. Debendox contained two substances, pyridoxine, which is vitamin B_6, and doxylamine, a familiar anti-histamine. It was this last that, McBride asserted, was the teratogenic component. The ensuing inquiry by the New South Wales Health Department turned into a bad-tempered debate, with conflicting opinions voiced by the many witnesses, and it continued for a decade. McBride eventually conceded that he had 'cut corners', and in 1993 he was found guilty of scientific fraud, and was struck off the medical register. He never accepted the verdict, claiming to be a victim of a conspiracy by the pharmaceutical industry. But in 1981 a study by a group of Scottish doctors on a large cohort of pregnancies in Scotland and beyond had been published in the *British Medical Journal*. It concluded convincingly that Debendox engendered no birth defects. McBride was forgiven and his name was restored to the medical register in 1998.

The rehabilitation of thalidomide

The dark cloud of thalidomide proved in time to have a silver lining. The mode of its teratogenic action was studied, and some valuable information was gleaned. The synthetic compound was in fact a mixture of two enantiomers – a left- and a right-handed form (p.), only one of which had physiological activity. It has multiple actions, of which the most significant may be its capacity to bind to and inactivate an enzyme with an essential role in limb development. It also impedes the spread of blood vessels into a developing tissue. So it is perhaps not surprising that pharmacologists and others should have sought to find a more benign function for this compound, despite its evil reputation. As early as 1964, long before this knowledge had accrued, Jacob Sheskin, a doctor at a leper hospital in Israel had the idea of trying thalidomide on a patient, desperately ill with a painful skin condition, erythema nodosus leprosy. The patient, who had been crippled and unable to stand, slept and was able, when he awoke, to walk for the first time in many months. Sheskin arranged a clinical trial, which bore out the dramatic effect.

Yet interest in the compound and its broader potential lapsed. Three decades later, though, thalidomide was circulating among AIDS sufferers in America as a cure for mouth ulcers. Then came a remarkable advance. In 1994 a young ophthalmologist, Robert D'Amato in the Massachusetts Eye and Ear Hospital in Boston attended a seminar by one of the luminaries of the Harvard Medical School, Judah Folkman, who was searching for a cancer treatment based on the inhibition of angiogenesis - the development of blood vessels in proliferating tissues, such as tumours. Folkman, exuberant and charismatic, was fixated on angiogenesis, and believed that it was equally relevant to eye conditions, such as macular degeneration. D'Amato was inspired, and managed to insinuate himself into Folkman's laboratory with the plan of finding an angiogenesis inhibitor. The idea of thalidomide, which terminated limb üowth in the developing foetus, came to him as a possible candidate. Thalidomide indeed proved a powerful inhibitor of angiogenesis. This not only gave an indication of the mechanism by which it did its damage to the developing foetus, but also encouraged an exploration of possible uses in treating malignant conditions*. One of these indeed proved to be highly susceptible to repression by thalidomide. This was multiple myeloma, a type of cancer of the bone marrow, in which certain white blood cells proliferate uncontrollably. Thalidomide turned out to outdo all other available drugs in reversing the process, and it reappeared in the clinic, with the blessing of the FDA, in 1998 as Thalomid. Used in association with a conventional chemotherapeutic agent, it changed the

---

* Later work in several laboratories has uncovered other üowth-restricting mechanisms of action of this multifarious, and once infamous molecule: thalidomide suppresses the activity of members of a family of small proteins called growth factors, which are abundant in tumours and promote proliferation of the malignant cells. Secondly it switches off synthesis of adhesion molecules - proteins on the cell surface, which in certain malignancies anchor the malignant cell to cells in the bone marrow. If the cells cannot cohere they die.

outlook for many patients, and it has driven the industry to search for new analogues, which are also being examined for activity against other cancers and HIV, as well as inflammatory agents, like thalidomide itself. An American biotechnology company, the Celgene Corporation produced an analogue of thalidomide, lemalidomide, trade name Revlimid, hiding the unwholesome name of its parent. Lemalidomide has fewer side-effects, and hugely exceeds thalidomide in potency, but even more so (by perhaps a thousandfold) in cost. Ravlimid is also effective against other, rarer blood diseases, and there are prospects of additional uses to treat diseases in which a ubiquitous growth factor that it suppresses (tumour necrosis factor-α) plays a part. The rehabilitation of thalidomide continues, for its action against various cancers has been generating interest. Prominent among these appear to be forms of prostate cancer. There have been reports of success in treating 'castration-refractory prostate cancer'*, and also a very aggressive form of the disease, but in any event the drug that was an irreparable disaster for so many thousands may yet turn out a blessing for a much larger number.

Vioxx, the lethal miracle

In purely numerical terms, Vioxx, a non-steroidal anti-inflammatory drug, or NSAID (p.), was the cause of a catastrophe, which far exceeded that of thalidomide. Rofecoxib was to be the ultimate relief for victims of arthritis and many other painful ailments. The drug's life on the market was relatively brief – from its approval by the FDA in 1999 to its obliteration in September of 2004. An estimated 80 million people took the drug at some time during that period. The principle of rofecoxib was a new one. Inflammation and its associated pain is activated by prostaglandins – important natural molecules that act like hormones, and which we have

---

* The growth of prostate cancer cells is stimulated by male sex hormones (androgens), the supply of which can be turned off by castration. Some prostate cancers are, or become, resistant to the loss of the hormone, and begin to grow again after an interval. These are the androgen-independent, or castration-refractory form of the disease. The aggressive form develops rapidly, and was discovered in the U.S. to afflict African Americans disproportionately (though whether this is a true genetically based phenomenon must be uncertain).

already encountered (pp.). Suppress the generation of prostaglandins and you suppress inflammation and pain. In 1990 exploration of the inflammation pathway brought to light an enzyme involved in the synthesis of prostaglandins, and therefore in the generation of inflammation and in protecting the stomach linings against ulceration. The enzyme was given the name cyclooxygenase, or COX for short, and the conjecture at the time was that the common painkillers, such as aspirin, which was already known from the work of the English pharmacologist (and Nobel Laureate), John Vane to act by blocking prostaglandin synthesis, could cause stomach ulcers for the same reason. Then came a further revelation: it turned out that there are in reality two closely related cyclooxygenases, COX-1 and COX-2, which are responsible for the formation of different prostaglandins. The pain-inducing member of the family is made with the help of COX-2, while the COX-1-dependent species has the benign property of protecting the stomach linings. So an inhibitor of COX-2 that does not trouble COX-1 might reasonably be expected to suppress pain without risk of damage to the stomach. But nature proved, as so often, to be more complicated.

In 1994 the pharmaceutical giant, Merck and Co. plunged into a programme of developing a specific COX-2 inhibitor that would sweep all the other analgesics from the market. But they did not have the field to themselves, for the directors of another company, G.D. Searle had the same idea. It seemed in fact so good an idea that yet another American giant, Pfizer bought the project from Searle, and then the company. It was to be war. Both organisations had famously ambitious and determined heads of research, and the stakes were high. There are differing versions of the sequence of events that led up to the creation of the two drugs; who merited plaudits and who blame was equally a matter of debate, at least until both undertakings were engulfed in scandal and obloquy. Even before any compound had been synthesised an unseemly patent dispute had arisen: Philip Needleman, the Head of Research at Searle, and at the time a professor at Washington University in St Louis, who had been working on biosynthesis of prostaglandins, had guessed that there were two COX enzymes. and if this were so then there would be the prospect of a selective enzyme inhibitor to control pain without the risk of stomach ulcers. Needleman thought the idea good enough to merit a patent application. But was he the first to entertain this notion? It seemed not, for research groups in three other universities – the University of Rochester, the University of California in Los Angeles, and Brigham Young University in Utah - had actual evidence that there really were two COX enzymes with different functions, and all three had begun to study their properties. The researchers in Rochester had taken legal advice on whether the concept of an analgesic based on a COX-2 inhibitor could be patented. The University, on the basis presumably of a positive answer, sued Searle, though to no avail.

Rofecoxib, which was to be marketed by Merck as Vioxx, and the Pfizer equivalent, celecoxib, or Celebrex were apparently rational drugs, the design guided by the function and structure of a specific physiological target. These were the drugs of the future, and their attraction was obvious. But optimism could not negate the first principle of pharmacology, that ultimately there is no completely safe drug (and in fact Vioxx was not really as rational as all that, having apparently been generated by minor tinkering with a compound of uncertain action, synthesised by Japanese researchers). A counterpoint of muted cautions accompanied the extravagant hype that preceded even the clinical trials, and they grew louder as the trials progressed. The first signs of trouble appeared during the Phase II trials of Vioxx – the initial tests on a small group of actual arthritis patients, late in 1996. The doses were large, for the proclaimed total safety of the drug eliminated, it was thought, the need for restraint. Some patients reported chest pains, while in some, blood tests pointed to incipient disorders, and in others disturbances of heart function. The limits for doses in cases of severe arthritic pain were therefore set at a level several times lower and continuous treatment was restricted to five days at a time; apart from issuing this caveat the Merck management appeared unperturbed. When the drug was eventually marketed the concerns were stated on the label or mentioned in the sales literature. There was worse: animal tests for effects on the kidneys had been contracted out to experts at the University of Pennsylvania, who reported that the drug caused kidney damage, not seen in controls with an older analgesic, commonly used in the management of arthritis pain. Yet, despite the angry protestations of the professor who had supervised the animal assays, the data were suppressed, and came to light only some years later. Warnings that the COX-2-dependent prostaglandins exerted a protective action on the heart, planned cardiology tests of rofecoxib were abandoned. At this point the FDA stepped in, and issued a stern warning to Merck, directing that the hazards of taking Vioxx be clearly set out on the label, but did not demand withdrawal of the drug. Merck countered the FDA's strictures with the assertion that the drug would not only spare sufferes from arthritis and other painful conditions much distress, but that any complications from its side-effects would be offset by the reduced number of deaths from gastrointestinal effects sometimes occasioned by all the other available analgesics.

The statistical data, however, were inadequate, and prodded by the FDA, Merck set up a study at the beginning of 1999 aimed at vindicating their claims. This was called the Vioxx Gastrointestinal Outcome Research, or VIGOR. In an attempt to ensure success Merck chose the least effective of the many NSAID (p.) products on the market, with the greatest record of gastrointestinal episodes. Members, including the chairman, of the supposedly independent committee charged with overseeing the trial, were consultants of Merck, or were generously compensated in other ways, and it later emerged that the procedure was flawed in important respects. Almost from the outset heart attacks were recorded; five of the participants taking Vioxx died, and only one in the control group on the old drug. The FDA stated afterwards that the trial should have been aborted at the first indications. The head of research at Merck, Edward Scolnick then engaged in a dispute with the statisticians charged with analysing the data. The statisticians stood firm, and refused to alter their conclusions, and the VIGOR study ended in disarray. Nor had it shown that the incidence of gastrointestinal incidents, such as ulceration or perforation of the stomach or the duodenum, was significantly reduced when the patient took Vioxx rather than naproxen (an older NSAID) or indeed aspirin. All this was rather opaquely presented in a report in the *New England Journal of Medicine*, but the authors stopped short of condemning the drug, on account of the small number of patients in the trial, suggesting instead that the higher number of heart attacks *might* be the result of chance. A few months later an indignant editorial statement appeared in the journal:

Merck had been in possession of data far less favourable to the performance of Vioxx, which they had not disclosed. The FDA issued another stern warning to Merck, but the drug remained on the market for another two years, though with a discreet caution on the label that it could kill.

Merck reached the pinnacle of duplicity with a further trial, the ADVANTAGE trial (another laboured acronym, standing for Difference between Vioxx and Naproxen to Ascertain Gastrointestinal Tolerability and Effectiveness), begun in 1999, but published only in 2003. This was acknowledged, though never by Merck, to be what was known as a 'seeding trial', or as one physician called it, 'marketing disguised as science'. The objective was to produce a glittering outcome, which could be disseminated among prospective prescribers around the country – to 'seed the field'. Unfortunately the results were by no means what Merck had hoped, and so they had to be given cosmetic improvements before they were fit for exposure in a respectable, peer-reviewed journal. The first author, a university doctor, admitted afterwards that he had had no hand in writing the paper: that had all been done by the Merck staff, as court papers revealed after the downfall.

Arguments about use of Vioxx arose in other countries besides the U.S. The FDA communicated their grave reservations about the safety of the drug to medical authorities around the world, but these were for the most part disregarded. In Britain the issue came before the Committee on the Safety of Medicines, on which sat an eminent gastroenterologist, professor and dean of the medical school of the University of Birmingham. He based his advice on the hundreds of deaths that, he averred, resulted annually from the use of NSAIDs. His research had also been supported by Merck, and he was therefore asked to leave the room while the committee discussed the evidence. The upshot was that doctors should be apprised of the dangers to patients at risk of cardiovascular episodes, but that the drug should still be prescribed. Merck had meanwhile published evidence that Vioxx might have off-label uses (be of value, that is, for the treatment of conditions for which it was not licensed). Merck claimed that there were indications the drug could retard the progress of Alzheimer's disease. More especially, animal tests suggested that it might have the power to avert

701

the formation of intestinal polyps, which are commonly precancerous, and prevent cancer of the colon. A large international trial was organised under the name, Vioxx Colorectal Cancer Therapy (VICTOR), and with the approval of the committee, volunteers were recruited in 2002. The trial was cut short after two and a half years and a number of heart attacks in September of 2004, when Merck threw in the towel and withdrew Vioxx from the market.

The news that Vioxx had indeed been withdrawn, and the estimates that now appeared of the deaths that it had caused, elicited a storm of recriminations and lawsuits. Merck set aside the sum of $950 million for compensation settlements (though, seen against the background of $100 million annual outlay for advertising the drug, and several billion in sales, this does not appear excessive). Incriminating documents and e-mails were revealed to the press during the investigation that followed, and criminal charges were brought. The claim by the Merck management that the discovery of the cardiotoxicity of Vioxx was 'unexpected' was proved false. Even after the calamitous trial results Merck had issued a press release, headed with the legend, 'Merck confirms cardiovascular safety profile of Vioxx'. This had drawn an exasperated response from the FDA, who had found it 'simply incomprehensible', and branded it 'misrepresentation'. One of Scolnick's colleagues, Alise Reicin, had proposed that subjects considered vulnerable should be excluded from trials, so that the risk to such as them 'would not be evident'. Scolnick had agreed, and Reicin was later rewarded for her loyalty by elevation to the post of vice-president for clinical research. There was much more evidence of concealment of the dangers to patients. Even before the large-scale trials there had been several disregarded warnings from experts. A group of American doctors, led by David Graham, drug safety officer at the FDA, published in *The Lancet* in February 2005 an analysis of the numbers of heart attacks attributable to Vioxx during its five years as a market leader. In America, they calculated, it had caused 140,000 heart attacks, 55,000 of them fatal. Worldwide, according to best estimates, at least 165,000 of the 80 million or so people who took Vioxx had died of it. To these should be added cases of kidney damage and of stomach perforation. Dr Graham had been dismayed by the indecisiveness of his employer, the FDA, and had voiced his concerns publicly, suggesting that the organisation, as constituted, was unequal to the task of protecting the American public against such disasters. Giving evidence before a Federal committee, he described the Vioxx scandal as 'the single greatest drug safety catastrophe in the history of [the United States] or the history of the world'. It could, and should have been prevented, '[b] ut it wasn't, and over 100,000 Americans have paid dearly for the failure'.

As for Celebrex, it had fared little better. It had reached the market only a few months after Vioxx, and not before questions about its safety had been raised. Philip Needleman, head of research at Pfizer introduced it to an audience of his confreres at a conference at the end of 1998. The number of deaths in the country, occasioned by NSAIDs, could, he affirmed, be estimated at 16,000 annually, and the number of hospital admissions at no less than 100,000. Celecoxib would put an end to all that, for tests had shown that it was 'supersafe'. Yet there were sceptics, among whom was a highly respected professor at the University of Calgary in Canada, John Wallace. He warned of the possibility of damage to heart, kidneys and stomach. His arguments were vociferously dismissed and ridiculed by the representatives of Merck and Pfizer, and especially by Needleman, who was adamant that he and his myrmidons had considered each argument that had been raised, and had covered all possibilities of ill-effects. One fervent advocate was a doctor at the Beth Israel Medical Center in Boston and professor at Harvard Medical School. He lauded Celebra, as it was first called, in a widely read and quoted article in the *New Yorker* magazine, with the title, Superaspirin. It presaged a revolution in medicine, readers were assured. The FDA approved celecoxib in a fast-track procedure. It was launched in June of 1999, manufactured by another company, Pharmacia under an agreement with Pfizer, and like Vioxx, it was ruthlessly promoted. Also like Vioxx it performed no better than many other NSAIDs, and by some criteria less well than aspirin.

With Celebrex already well-entrenched on the market, a so-called Phase 4 trial was undertaken at the FDA's urging to make up for the rather scant evaluation that had preceded approval. This so-called CLASS trial (for Celebrex Long-Term Arthritis Safety Study) was intended to determine the safety of the drug in respect of gastrointestinal injuries. It was to be compared to three older NSAIDs and aspirin, and involved 8000 arthritis patients. The results were not all Pfizer expected, but this was not apparent from the published article. The deception was not long concealed. The trial was to have lasted one year, but the data in the paper pertained only to the first six months. When FDA discovered the infraction they made their displeasure plain, and sent a threatening letter to Pfizer. The fate of Celebrex paralleled that of Vioxx. It was found to have little or no advantage in respect of gastrointestinal safety, nor was it significantly more effective than naproxen, ibuprofen and the rest as an analgesic. It presented the same dangers of cardiovascular crises as Vioxx, and when Vioxx was withdrawn from the market in 2004, Pfizer ceased to advertise their product, or a similar COX-2 inhibitor that they had developed, valdecoxib, or Bextra, but did not withdraw Celebrex from the market for some more months. The company set aside $894 million for the impending compensation claims, and were fined $2.3 billion for violating the Federal False Claims Act, and other forms of chicanery, including bribery. Many legal actions against Pfizer (as against Merck) are far from concluded. The story sits uncomfortably with Pfizer's advertised slogan of always putting patients' safety first. Celebrex still has FDA's endorsement, with warnings and provisos, for treating some rare inflammatory conditions.

The banishment of pain

A growing belief in man's entitlement to a wholly pain-free life has brought with it an ever-increasing demand for pain-killers, and with it the return of opioids. We have seen (Chapter) how in the early part of the 20th century Bayer especially strove to find an opium analogue that was not addictive. The pharmacologists believed they had found one in heroin, which was advertised as a sure and safe cure for coughs and other minor troubles, and the consequences were tragic. Morphine, despite all hazards, remained in use, perforce, for the treatment of severe pain, for there were no better options. In the U.S. in 1914 the use of narcotic drugs without prescription was made a criminal offence by an Act of Congress. The growing social problems that accompanied drug addiction, including smuggling of drugs on a massive scale, led finally to a publicly-funded search for safer analgesics. In 1928 the Bureau of Social Hygiene, supported by the Rockefeller Foundation, issued an influential report, which led the following year to the establishment by National Research Council of the Committee on Drug Addiction and Narcotics. With the participation of the U.S. Public Health Service a decision was taken to establish two hospitals-cum-prisons, or as they were called Narcotic Farms, one in Lexington, Kentucky, which was opened in 1935, the other, which opened in 1938, at Fort Worth, Kansas. They were designed to shelter both felons and voluntary patients seeking treatment. A pharmacologist at the University of Michigan, Nathan Eddy, and a chemist, Lyndon Small at the University of Virginia, were appointed to develop a research programme on the discovery of non-addictive analgesic compounds. Small had gained experience of opioid chemistry in the laboratory of the great German chemist, Heinrich Wieland, and set to work synthesising an enormous number of new compounds, which Eddy then tested, first on monkeys and then on inmates of the Lexington Narcotics Farm. But despite a huge investment of labour and money, no useful new analgesics came to light, with the arguable exception of the morphine analogue, metopon, which was a powerful and longer-lasting analgesic than morphine. It found some use in alleviation of chronic pain, but was never commercially exploited. The best outcome of the work of Eddy and Small was that it established relationships between structures and function of opioid compounds for future investigations.

A seemingly limitless number of opioid drugs came and went over the ensuing decades, and were for the most part displaced by codeine (also a morphine derivative [p.]) and paracetamol in its various guises (p.), while aspirin went serenely on. Yet such was the demand for pain-killers that the pharmaceutical companies began to resurrect forgotten remedies. OxyContin, also known as Percocet, and by many other names, was first made in Germany in 1916 by modification of a minor opium poppy constituent, thebaine. It was taken up by Bayer during their search for a less habit-forming substance, but soon abandoned. It is weaker and shorter-acting than many other opioids, and appeared less addictive. It was brought to America by Merck in 1939, and thrived. It is now manufactured as OxyNeo by Purdue Pharma, and in 2007 some 80% of the drug's sales

705

were in the U.S. But that year Purdue was charged with misleading the public by concealing the drug's true addictive character. The company admitted guilt, and was fined $600 million. The president and two other executives were also found guilty of the crime of 'misbranding' and made to pay $34.5 million in fines.

Hydrocodone is another related compound, which originated in Germany as a semi-synthetic opioid in 1920, and was approved by the FDA in 1943. It has numerous trade-names, such as Vicodin. A third widely used (and abused) semi-synthetic opioid pain-killer, first prepared in 1914, once again by German chemists, is oxymorphone, otherwise Opama or Numorphen. The Japanese company, Endo Pharmaceuticals brought it to the American market in 1959, and also to several other countries. It is about as effective as morphine, with less severe side-effects, but this drug too has supported the habits of many addicts. The prevalence of opioid addiction is a matter of no little concern. The American suppliers of morphine-related analgesics, which are an essential element in the treatment of patients suffering from cancers and other painful illnesses, are perpetually begged to make their preparations unsuitable for use by addicts. The attempts mainly focus on formulating them in pills that are hard to crush or to dissolve, or in the form of gels that cannot be drawn into a syringe.

Wasp waist or death: fen-phen and worse

With the change in the mid-20th century in women's body-contour fashions from pneumatic to anorectic, followed by the dismaying rise in obesity during the following decades, the market in weight-loss preparations expanded inexorably. In England in the 19th century some pharmacists sold an effective slimming pill, containing a tapeworm egg as the active ingredient. But the first synthetic anorectic (to give the slimming medicine its technical name) was amphetamine. This compound, well-known for its capacity to increase alertness and combat fatigue, and also for other uses (p.), was found to be an excellent appetite suppressant. But it was also addictive, and because it was available without prescription, did no little harm. The obesity epidemic that struck the United States, and spread to European countries in the later years of the 20th century brought with it an

First Do No Harm

unprecedented incidence of type 2 diabetes, with its attendant woes. The condition is marked by hyperglycaemia – an elevated level of circulating glucose – which leads in turn to a destruction of the insulin receptors. The body's cells can no longer respond to the insulin-dependent signal, which normally regulates the sugar level, and a vicious cycle ensues. Weight-loss was now a clinical and not merely a social or cosmetic imperative, and the pharmaceutical industry reacted.

Amphetamine and its analogues act in the brain: they are SSRIs – serotonin reuptake inhibitors (p.) - but little of this was known when the appetite-suppressing activity was first noted in the 1960s. Nor was there any indication of the damage that many of the compounds inflict on the controlling neurones. In 1960 chemists in the French pharmaceutical company, Servier synthesised a close relative of amphetamine, which was more potent. It was called fenfluramine, and was introduced as a slimming aid, Ponderal. At almost the same time Smith Kline and French (SKF) created norfenfluramine. (It later turned out that fenfluramine, a mixture of left- and right-handed enantiomers [p.], was a prodrug, one of the enantiomers of which was metabolically converted into norfenfluramine.) SKF also gave birth to another amphetamine-like appetite-suppressant, phentermine, known as Fastin, which the FDA approved in 1975. None of these had had had any great immediate success when they became available from 1973 onwards, until the American company, Wyeth Ayerst Laboratories had the idea of combining fenfluramine, or its right-handed enantiomer, dextro- or dexfenfluramine, with phentermine. The phentermine admixture was said to eliminate some trivial but annoying side-effects. Approved for short-term use as a diet aid, it was forcefully promoted, and, known as fen-phen, became highly popular. It was in fact a rather poor treatment for obesity, and was moreover used by many dieters for far longer periods, and in larger doses, than had originally been specified. Wyeth and the FDA were blamed in the aftermath for not ensuring that proper warnings were issued.

It was in 1994 that evidence began to accrue of serious side-effects, starting with cardiac arrhythmias of an unusual kind, found later to arise from damaged heart valves. Worse was to follow. The serious, often fatal and essentially untreatable condition, pulmonary hypertension is caused by an abnormally high pressure in the narrow arteries of the lungs, putting a high strain on the heart. That same year, patients with this condition were appearing in hospitals; they had been swallowing fen-phen for months and years. In late 1995 the drug was withdrawn. A high proportion, perhaps one in three, long-term fen-phen users had damaged heart valves. Similar problems attached to Wyeth's dexfenfluramine, approved by the FDA in 1994 on the supposition that it was safer than the original racemic (left- and right-handed mixture) in fenfluramine, despite warnings by a member of Wyeth's staff. Some six million Americans took one or the other of the two preparations at some time, and many apparently paid the price. There have been some 50,000 court actions in the U.S., where the overwhelming majority of users were based. Nevertheless, there is still debate in the learned journals about the extent of the damage caused by fen-phen. The lawyers were busy, and Wyeth reserved $2.1 billion for compensation claims.

A slimming aid, also marketed as a cure for smoking, eagerly awaited in the U.S., reached the market in 2004. Two years later it was approved in Britain, and it was soon licensed in more than fifty other countries. It is called rimonabant, known as Acomplin, and by other trade names, and was invented by the French company, Sanofi (at the time Sanofi-Aventis). Like other such drugs it acts in the brain, which may be an uncomfortable consideration to at least some prospective users. It is in fact an inhibitor of one of two cannabinoid receptors, on which cannabis and related substances exert their effect. Rimonabant worked in clinical trials, but it was clearly viewed with unease by the regulatory agencies. The obese participants in clinical trials lost appetite, and consequently also weight and girth, and the proportion of 'bad' cholesterol, LDL (p.) in the blood dropped sharply, in favour of the 'good' (HDL). And yet the arterial plaques did not diminish, so that the danger of a heart attack or stroke did not recede. Side-effects appeared, especially depression and thoughts of suicide. The European Medicines Agency, EMEA (an EU-regulated body), which had decided that the benefits of weight loss outweighed the risks, cooled, and in 2009 the sale of rimonabant was suspended in the countries of the European Union.

Servier, a French company, which entered the chase after weight-loss pills over a half century ago, received approval in France in 1976 for the sale of their latest product as a diet adjuvant – an aid but not an independent treatment for weight loss. It was yet another amphetamine analogue, very similar chemically to fenfluramine, but the company claimed that it was something completely new. It was called benfluorex, and given the trade name of Mediator. Two small trials suggested that it could control blood sugar levels, and thus prevent or retard the progress of diabetes. As with fenfluramine and the rest, evidence began to seep out of a link to heart valve disease. For a long time no action was taken, and Mediator was increasingly used 'off-label' in a way that the regulatory agency had not intended – for long-term weight control, and for treating clinical obesity. It was often prescribed together with the anti-diabetes compound, sulphonylurea, another French discovery, but one that dated back to the 1940s (p.). The auguries, especially after the withdrawal of fen-phen and its relatives in America in 1995, were plain, but for another decade, as reports of heart disease cases and deaths came in, Mediator sailed serenely on. Nor was it even a particularly good weight-loss treatment. Finally in December of 2009 the EMEA urged that all products containing benfluorex be withdrawn. Accusations against Servier for its claims, contrary to the known activity of the drug, came from a French government office, IGAS (Inspection Générale des Affaires Sociales), and much ordure descended on the drug regulatory body, AFSSAPS, which IGAS accused of being 'inexplicably tolerant of a drug with no real therapeutic value'. Excuses of understaffing, overwork, and impenetrable state bureaucracy were made, but in the end the director resigned. One of the main agitators against Mediator, a doctor in Brest, Irène Frachon, wrote papers and a book about the affair, which during the 33 years of the life of Mediator on the French market, resulted in deaths, estimated to be between 500 and 2,000, and many more serious illnesses. Mediator was banished from the market in 2009, and litigation has begun. The ninety-year old foun der and former head of the company may be charged with manslaughter.

Anti-obesity drugs have not, on the whole, fared well on the market. One that came close was Contravan, a mixture of an antidepressant of shaky reputation, bupropion or Wellbutrin (see below), and naltrexone, which has been used to treat alcohol addiction. The FDA's advisory panel voted by a small majority to recommend approval, but in 2012 the FDA demurred on the grounds that possible heart damage could not be excluded. A further clinical trial to confront this question would have been too expensive for the manufacturer, a company of modest size, to contemplate. A few months before, the FDA had rejected two other anti-obesity candidates, neither of which appeared to have been highly effective. The *New York Times* quoted the words of an outraged anti-obesity campaigner: 'In the current environment, tap water would not be approved'. There are good reasons for the FDA's caution, considering the disasters of the recent past. But there would be serious money in an effective anti-obesity drug, and it does not seem that the drug companies are abandoning the chase. The only available drug, expressly designated a treatment for obesity can be bought over the counter. It was approved by the FDA in 1999, and is used by 6 million Americans, and many Europeans. It was developed by Roche, and is called orlistat (trade name, Xenical). It is a derivative of a compound isolated from bacteria, and it blocks the action of fat-processing enzymes in the pancreas, thereby reducing the metabolic uptake of fats. Other drugs are in preparation, and some are in use.

The pursuit of happiness: antidepressants

Reboxetine, which presents itself in the guise of Edronix, Norebox or any of a variety of other trade names, was launched with exuberant publicity in 2005 by Pharmacia (soon afterwards annexed by Pfizer). It was to be the sovereign treatment for clinical depression, for panic states and for ADHD. It was something relatively new – not an SSRI, but an NRI, a noradrenaline reuptake inhibitor. The drug was approved in Britain, where it originated, and in many European countries, but not in the U.S. Pharmacia made extravagant claims for the efficacy of reboxetine in treating clinical depression, and glossing over the drug's side-effects. These were not serious, but enough of the patients experienced insomnia, disturbances of the ears, causing vertigo, and other manifestations that persuaded an appreciable proportion of volunteers to withdrew from trials. A German Government health organisation performed a meta-analysis of trial data and concluded that Pfizer had grossly overstated the efficacy of their drug (by 115% - optimistically precise to be sure - in relation to placebos), and understated the incidence of side-effects by 75%. In 2010 came what ought to have been the death blow to reboxetine in the form especially of a devastating publication in the *British Medical Journal* by nine authors from six German specialist centres. This relentlessly thorough study, drawing on all available data, concluded: 'Reboxetine is, overall, an ineffective and potentially harmful antidepressant.' And, the authors continue, 'Published evidence [from the producers of the drug] is affected by publication bias, underlining the urgent need for mandatory publication of trial data'. It is a cry emanating from many quarters today, and still partly unanswered. Reboxetin has not been withdrawn from the market, but at least there is no evidence of lasting damage to any patients, though quite a lot, if not to their bank accounts, then to European tax-payers. There will be more about placebos later, but the likelihood is that there were patients who felt better after taking the drug, as they would have done from sugar pills.

Bupropion is another presumptive noradrenaline reuptake inhibitor, first synthesised before these things were properly understood in the Burroughs Wellcome laboratories (later part of GlaxoSmithKline) in 1969. It was thought to be a safe and effective antidepressant, and was approved for the purpose by the FDA in 1985. It appeared under many names, but was most widely sold as Wellbutrin or Zyban. After only a year it was withdrawn because it induced epileptic seizures in mice, and also in some patients when taken in sufficient doses. But bupropion had also come into use for combatting nicotine addiction, for it was found to suppress the craving for tobacco. In 1996 the drug returned to favour, approved in a slow-release form to limit concentrations in the body to harmless levels. But in 2012 GSK were adjudged to have erred by selling the drug for purposes not approved by the FDA - for loss of sexual function, for weight control, for drug addiction and for ADHD (p.). These were not the only misdemeanours of which federal prosecutors had accused GSK: the company had also recommended the administration of Paxil (p.) to children, even though it was not approved for anyone under the age of 18, of concealing the outcome of two clinical trials of the diabetes drug,

Avandia, and of bribing doctors in the U.S. to prescribe a range of the company's products. The company had no option but to admit guilt and pay a hefty fine of $3 billion, the largest ever imposed on a pharmaceutical concern. If it seems a large penalty it should be viewed against the $11.7 billion profit from sales of Paxil alone, and in the U.S. alone, over about the same period.

A similar fate to that of Wellbutrin befell a product from the second-largest British pharmaceutical organisation, AstraZeneca. Also an 'atypical' antidepressant – that is to say a compound chemically unrelated to any of the major approved chemical classes – called quetiapine, known as Seroquel, or Xeroquel. It was first approved by the FDA for the treatment of schizophrenia and bipolar disorder (known in less jargon-ridden days as manic depression). Five years later it was pressed into service against serious clinical depression (mania), to be given together with an SSRI, and was also prescribed for Alzheimer disease until adjudged ineffective. The annual sales rose to nearly $6 billion, the greater part in the U.S. Trouble began soon after, when the company was deluged with legal actions, mostly from users who had developed diabetes as a result apparently of taking the drug. There were also distressing withdrawal effects. Internal documents demanded by a court brought to light evidence of deliberate concealment of trial results, and worst of all, exaggeration of the therapeutic value of quetiapine by a highly placed academic pharmacologist. In 2009 AstraZeneca settled with the plaintiffs for a total of $520 million. Immediately the share price rose steeply, for shareholders had expected worse. The drug remains on the market, but is accompanied by warnings, and may well be on its way out.

Unforeseeable or just unforeseen?

Extraneous intervention in a system as complex as a living being is inevitably fraught with risks, and one can demand no more of those who work in this taxing profession than that they should be vigilant and open when the unexpected occurs. Benoxaprofen was a promising anti-inflammatory drug, an NSAID, developed in the British laboratories of Eli Lilley in 1966. Phase III trials began in 1976 on 2,000 patients, conducted by more than 100 doctors in different centres. It was approved and put on the market in 1980 in Britain, and two years later in the U.S. In May of 1982 a paper appeared in the *British Medical Journal* in which the authors voiced the suspicion that twelve deaths from kidney or liver failure might have been associated with the drug. There had also been some cases of gastrointestinal disorders and skin rashes. A few months later the National Health Service imposed a temporary suspension on Benoxaprofen. The British Committee on Safety of Medicines informed the FDA by telegram that some 3,500 reports had been received of unpleasant side-effects, and that there were 61 deaths, tentatively attributed to the drug, nearly all of old people. Almost simultaneously the FDA announced that 11 deaths had been reported from the same causes. That same day Eli Lilley stopped sales and withdrew the drug. Here was a case in which everyone appeared to have acted responsibly.

Breathe easy: asthma problems

The 'Practolol Disaster', as it became known, coming quite soon after the thalidomide tragedy, shook the British pharmaceutical establishment and the Government of the day, and brought about changes in the regulation of drugs in Britain. The pharmaceutical division of ICI (Imperial Chemical Industries) under James Black (p.) had enjoyed great success with β-receptor blockers (p.) for the treatment of angina pectoris, asthma and high blood pressure. The first was pronethanol, which showed high promise, but was abandoned after a year on the market in 1963, when it was found to cause thyroid cancer in mice. Then in 1964 came the most famous of ICI's pharmaceutical products, propranalol (Inderal). From a slow start in it became the preferred treatment for angina, and maintained its supremacy on the market for 30 years in the face of a profusion of 'me-too' competitors. But propranalol had a small drawback: it could induce bronchial spasms in asthmatics taking it for angina, because it acted not only on the β-adrenergic receptors of the heart (the β_1 receptors), but also on the receptors of the smooth muscle of the airways (the β_2 receptors). So the search for something more selective continued, and, as it appeared, bore fruit in 1964, when a derivative was synthesised, which caused no significant bronchial perturbations in animals, while still acting like propranolol on the heart. This was the ill-starred practolol, which was given the trade name, Eraldin, and hit the pharmacies in 1970.

Practolol was considered especially suitable for asthmatics with heart disorders, but was vigorously promoted in addition as a major advance on propranolol in the treatment of angina. – a 'breakthrough'. But neither animal tests, nor a trial on 127 patients over varying periods seemed to bear out this optimistic assessment. Indeed some doctors around the country generally found it no better in treating angina than propranolol, and even inferior. But the Committee on Safety of Medicines did not dissent from ICI's view, and Eraldin was rapturously received, and by 1974 it was the leading angina drug in Britain. The FDA was more cautious. ICI had entered into a licensing agreement with Wyeth-Ayerst Laboratories to make and distribute the drug in the U.S., but the FDA demurred because of some indications of carcinogenicity in mice - an uncomfortable reminder of the very similar ICI compound, the ill-fated pronethanol. Wyeth-Ayerst had started a trial on a small number of patients, but after some debate about the risk-benefit balance, this was aborted. In Britain, where practolol was in wide use, evidence began to turn up as early as 1970, the year of the launch, of ill-effects. It was difficult initially to associate the stray reports with the drug, but by 1972 the writing was on the wall. The side-effects were alarming. Practolol was engendering a rare auto-immune disease - one in which the immune system makes antibodies against one or more of the body's own constituents, as though they were alien intruders. It is called optomucocutaneous syndrome, also known as Kawasaki syndrome. This is a serious condition, fatal in a minority of cases. It affects the skin, the conjunctiva, which covers the cornea, tissues of the ear, and the thin membranes that coat the interior of the lungs and the gut. It can lead to skin eruptions, to scarring of the cornea, culminating often in loss of sight, to deafness, and to a form of peritonitis, inflammation of the abdominal walls. In some cases the patients made a good recovery, in others severe handicaps persisted, or death supervened.

ICI stopped the oral version of the drug in 1975, but practolol could still be prescribed for brief use. As the lawsuits began to mount ICI insisted that the disaster could not have been predicted on the basis of clinical trials, but in retrospect skin rashes and dry eyes, recorded during the trials, which presaged the eruption of Kawasaki syndrome, ought perhaps to have attracted more attention. A doctor reported in middle of 1974 a succession of cases of serious injury to patients on practolol, which he had collected since the previous year. After the event the famous epidemiologist, Richard Doll (the man generally credited with placing the link between smoking and lung cancer on a firm basis), and his colleague Richard Skeggs opined in a publication that the effects on the eye could easily have been detected, but that there had been no deliberate deception on the part of ICI. Practolol limped on – permitted in small doses for patients who failed to respond to other β-blockers, until finally withdrawn in late 1975. By then there had been 40 recorded deaths, and some 8000 cases of more or less serious injury, including more than 1100 of severe eye damage, and 300 of deafness. These must be reckoned as large underestimates because of diagnostic uncertainty. ICI showed little remorse, but the episode did lead to a fairly rigorous revision of drug safety legislation. The other fortunate aspect of the tragedy was that practolol never penetrated beyond the British Isles.

The demon cholesterol bites back

Cerivastatin was to have been Bayer's answer to Pfizer's Lipitor (atorvastatin), the world's favourite statin (p.). Bayer AG launched it in 1997 as Baycol, and withdrew it four years later in 2001, after 52 people died, 31 of them in the U.S. In those patients, and in others who recovered, it had induced rhabdomyolysis, the destruction of muscles, such as is sometimes seen in athletes who have trained too violently and too long. This is a serious condition, for the muscles simply break down, spilling their proteins into the blood. The high concentrations of proteins, and especially of myoglobin, an oxygen-carrying protein closely related to haemoglobin, overtaxes the kidneys. The most unlucky users died of kidney failure. A curious property of cerivastatin was that it also interfered with the metabolic elimination (as was later proved) of another fat-controlling drug, gemfibrozil. Of the 31 users who died in America 12 fell into this group – conclusive evidence linking cause and effect, because only a very small proportion of all cerivastatin consumers were also taking gemfibrozil. In the course of the litigation that ensued, it emerged that Bayer had had some evidence before the drug was approved of a propensity to damage muscles. It took Bayer more than 18 months to add a warning of the genfibrozil effect on the label.

Temafloxacin syndrome, after the antibiotic of that name, consisted of violent allergic reactions, and the onset in some people of haemolytic anaemia, the rupture of the red blood cells with release of their contents into the plasma. It was the result of taking a new synthetic quinolone antibiotic. The antibiotics of this chemical class (p.) were an important innovation at a time at which resistance of pathogenic bacteria to the older, mainly mould- and soil-derived types was spreading alarmingly. Temafloxacin was synthesised by the chemists of Abbott Laboratories in Illinois, and was found to be highly effective against a broad range of especially respiratory pathogens. Abbott supplied the American market, and ICI the European, under the names respectively of Omni and Teflex. It lasted on;y five months from its introduction at the beginning of 1992, by which time three deaths, and some fifty cases of haemolytic anaemia had been linked to the drug.

An interesting case, which illustrates the varying attitudes to risk is that of terfenadine, known as Seldane in the U.S. and Triludan in Britain. It was a highly efficient anti-histamine, an H1 receptor antagonist (p.), in Britain the most widely used drug against hay fever and similar troubles, and could be bought over the counter. It was created by what was at the time (1985) Hoechst Marion Roussel*, and had the great merit of lacking sedative properties. As time went on, cases of a rare kind of cardiac arrhythmia that could lead to heart attacks were recorded, and were eventually traced to

---

* The august German firm of Hoechst has gone through a bewildering succession of mergers, takeovers and name changes in recent decades. In 1985 it absorbed the American company of Marion Merrell Dow, itself the product of a series of mergers; four years later Hoechst swallowed the French Roussel-Uclaf, and in 1999 merged with the mighty French Rhône-Poulenc, and rose again as Aventis. That was acquired by the giant Sanofi organisation, so the drugs are now made by Sanofi-Aventis.

the drug. But this occurred only when the users had at the same time(as the FDA established) been taking other drugs, specifically macrolide antibiotics – a class of compounds based on a structure known to chemists as a macrolide ring, of which the most familiar is erythromycin – or an anti-fungal drug, ketonazole (trade name, Nizoral). People with liver damage were also at risk. There were apparently no deaths, but there was a good deal of alarm, and in late 1997 terfenadine was forbidden in the U.S. But all was not lost, for terfenadine is a prodrug, and the active metabolite to which it gives rise was synthesised in the laborratory, and found, not surprisingly, to be at least as effective a hay fever remedy as the parent compound, though without the unfortunate interaction with other drugs. It is called fexofenadine, and has replaced terfenadine in America. In Britain the Committee on Safety of Medicines took another course: it merely made Teludan a prescription-only drug, with abundant warnings of the circumstances in which it must not be taken. It is presumably cheaper than fexofenadine, and no mishaps seem to have been reported.

Whither diabetes?

The history of the chemical family of drugs designed to treat type 2 diabetes (p.), all closely related, and known as azolidinediones (sometimes also called glitazones) is a sordid tale of over-confidence, negligence and duplicity. It began promisingly enough with a new drug target – a receptor, discovered not long before, for fatty substances that circulate in the blood (fatty acids and certain of their derivatives). When these compounds bind to the receptors various metabolic reactions are set in train. For those with type 2 diabetics who have lost most of their insulin receptors, the important effect of occupancy of the fatty-acid receptors by an azolidinedione drug, is to relieve the resultant resistance to insulin. The idea was a good one, and it has had one qualified success. Pioglitazone was introduced by the Takeda Pharmaceutical Company of Osaka in Japan. It received the FDA's blessing in 1999, and arrived on the market under the name of Atos. All went well for a time, but there were reports of cardiovascular episodes, and a warning was issued that patients with a history of heart problems were not to take the drug. There followed another alarm, this time from France, where pioglitazone was manufactured by Laboratoires Takeda, a subsidiary of the Japanese company: there was an increased risk of bladder cancer. The French regulatory agency demanded immediate withdrawal. Other European countries soon followed suit. The increased bladder cancer risk was in truth extremely small, and pioglitazone is still prescribed, although with warnings against extended use. In America and elsewhere. Takeda appeared to have acted in good faith throughout.

Such openness did not accompany the travails of the competing glitazone drugs. The first was troglitazone, which became infamous as Resulin (also Rezulin, Romozin and Noscal). It was created by another Japanese organisation, the Daiichi Sankyo Company, and was offered as a treatment for type 2 diabetes and also as an anti-inflammatory. The compound was licensed to Parke Davis for manufacture in the U.S., and their application went before the FDA in 1996. There had indeed been concerns about a possible link to hepatitis, and the FDA officer directed to evaluate the drug argued firmly against approval on grounds of possible liver and cardiovascular damage. The actions of the FDA later came in for much criticism, for Parke Davis objected to the report, and the panel overruled their officer's recommendation, removed him from the case and in 1997 approved the drug. It lasted on the market for only two years. Parke Davis allocated production to their subsidiary company, Warner-Lambert, which began turning out Resulin in the same year, 1997. In Britain troglitazone was licensed to Glaxo Wellcome, and approved by the regulatory agency. All too soon reports began to arrive of acute liver failure linked to the drug. The FDA reacted by recommending doctors to monitor the liver function of patients on troglitazone, but before this measure could be introduced in the country a patient in a trial of the drug on diabetics at the National Institutes of Health died of liver failure, even though she had been closely monitored, like all the others. The trial was at once stopped. David Graham, the FDA epidemiologist (who was later to distinguish himself by his work on Vioxx [p.]), was called in, and concluded that troglitazone had been responsible for a minimum of 430 cases of liver failure, and that the drug increased the risk of such an event by a factor of 1,200. Resulin had done well during its brief life before the FDA ordered its withdrawal in early 2000, with annual sales of some $2.1 billion, but now the cost to Pfizer, which had swallowed Parke Davis in the interim, was considerable. A congressional committee, investigating the 63 known deaths from liver failure, and many cases of serious liver damage, found that the pre-approval clinical trials had given abundant evidence of the danger, and the chairman, Senator Edward Kennedy declared that the manufacturers had deliberately concealed the high toxicity, and had misrepresented the results of the clinical trials. Pfizer were compelled to pay compensations amounting to about $500 million, and in 2004 the company reserved a sum of nearly $1 billion for future settlements.

A greater disaster, or so it appears, was bubbled up from the rise and fall of rosiglitazone, or Avandia, another azolidinedione compound, developed, in this case by GlaxoSmithKline (GSK) as a successor to pioglitazone and troglitazone, for the treatment of type 2 diabetes. It was let loose on the American public in 1999 as a huge improvement on its predecessors in terms of potency and safety. At its peak, five years later, it was netting GSK $3 billion per year, mainly in the form of Avandamet, a combination with the well-tried metformin (p.), sometimes also, when combined with another anti-diabetic drug, glimepiride, as Avandaryl. Two years on, its popularity had dwindled, and for good reasons. Rumours of heart attacks, apparently linked to the drug, became increasingly insistent. By mid-2010 the rumours had become fact, GSK had a series of legal actions on its hands, and agreed to 11,500 out-of-court settlements. The number of strokes and heart attacks occasioned by rosiglitazone in the U.S. between 1999 and 2007 was estimated as 83,000. The risk of cardiovascular damage had in fact first been raised almost as soon as the drug was approved, on the grounds of the changes that it engendered in the blood lipids (fats), and the warnings of what these disturbances portended. A leading specialist, soon to become President of the American Diabetes Association, John Buse, a professor at the University of North Carolina first articulated his concerns before the FDA in 2000. This provoked a fierce reaction from GSK, who communicated their displeasure to Buse, and tried to stifle his objections. Buse complained of intimidation by the company, a complaint borne out by evidence given at a congressional investigation. The committee also noted that there were no data to suggest that rosiglitazone had any advantages over its competitors in respect of the control of diabetes. David

Graham was again at the forefront in compiling a meta-analysis, and extracting an estimate of the risk of strokes, heart attacks and deaths from the drug. Analyses of data continue still. A miasma of doubt has shrouded the suppression by the FDA of a publication by Graham and a colleague, and there has been further conflict over the results of a new clinical trial. It concluded that rosiglitazone did not in fact increase the probability of strokes and heart attacks. This was challenged on the grounds that the statistics were not based on a comparison with other available anti-diabetics. The FDA did not ask that the drug be withdrawn, but rather that information about possible hazards be made known to doctors and included in the packaging. (This measure is known as a 'boxed' or 'black box' warning.) In 2012 GSK were accused of (among other misdeeds [p.]) concealing the results of two clinical trials that had revealed cardiovascular effects. By then the company had paid out $700 million in compensation in actions brought by users of Avandia.

If there was one redeeming outcome of the rosiglitazone debacle it was the fresh light that it cast on the mephitic atmosphere of conflicting interests that engulfed all too many clinical trials. An article in the *British Medical Journal* in 2010 analysed all publications which alluded to published observations pertinent to the rosiglitazone affair. According to an analysis that appeared twelve years earlier, only 3% of authors had admitted to a conflict of interest. But what now emerged was that of 27 relevant articles published before the FDA imposed the 'black box' warning on the drug eight gave the drug a thumbs-up and nine a thumbs-down, while the remaining ten were undecided. The shocking results was that authors of six of the eight articles in the first group had financially profitable links to the manufacturers of the drug, compared with only two of the nine in the second group. There were similar results when papers published after the FDA's 'black box' warning took effect, with 24 out of 27 authors with conflicting interests in the first group, and 9 out of 38 in the second. This was not the only study of bias rather obviously the result of financial advantage (see p.), but its influence was considerable. Now all authors in medical (and indeed scientific) journals are required to state any such interests in their publication.

CAST a pearl

Cardiac arrhythmias, an alarming accelerated or irregular heartbeat, can have several distinct origins, and some forms are more dangerous than others. Two heavily advertised drugs, encainide and flecainide (trade name Tambocor, among others) were developed to treat arrhythmias. There was unease in some clinical circles from the time of a small pilot trial of the two drugs, and so a much larger trial, spread over several clinical centres, was organised by the U.S. National Institute of Heart, Lung and Blood Institute (one of the National Institutes of Health near Washington), and began in 1986. This was called the Cardiac Arrhythmia Suppression Trial, or CAST. It took place in two phases, CAST 1 and CAST 2. The outcome was dismal: the subjects, with an 'asymptomatic' arrhythmia – one that is not accompanied by cardiac distress – on either drug did indeed experience some relief from their disorder, but now had a much increased chance - by a factor of 3.6 - of sudden death from an arrhythmia attack. The trial was stopped as soon as the high risk became apparent. There was still more bad news: the trial also showed that taking the drugs carried the risk of serious liver, kidney or lung damage.

Even before these disclosures there had been unease about anti-arrhythmia drugs generally, and a great reappraisal of received cardiological lore now ensued. It had been known for some years that one common form of arrhythmia, called 'ventricular premature depolarisation', or VPD, is most often harmless, except in people who have had heart attacks (myocardial infarcts). VPD is perceptible in the electrocardiogram (ECG) in the form of a premature contraction of the heart muscle, causing a delayed beat. Death from VPD is very rare, but the probability increases when a cardiologist makes the decision to treat the patient with an anti-arrhythmic drug. Given that deaths from arrhythmias overall have been variously estimated as 3 to 6 per hundred per year, that proportion of patients might be saved by the drugs at the expense of a far higher number of needless deaths among the rest. A major objective of CAST was in fact to determine whether survivors of heart attacks would benefit from treatment with anti-arrhythmics. When the great mass of data thrown up by the extensive trials was published some cardiologists and physiologists undertook a rigorous statistical analysis. A major outcome was the rebuttal of the widely held belief that the prospects of people who had suffered heart attacks were improved by drug-induced suppression of arrhythmias. Another change of direction was the return to favour of β-blockers for treatment of heart attacks, which was explored in another trial. And so the lives lost through encainide and flecainide – no small number – may have been offset by the saving of lives through the re-evaluation that the results of the trials provoked. Flecainide has survived, and is still sometimes used, though with caution, to treat patients with forms of arrhythmia but no record of heart disease.

An episode with an unhappy, if less dramatic outcome, concerned a drug developed by Pfizer in the 1990s for the treatment of high blood pressure. Doxazosin, alias Cardura or Carduran. Was an α-receptor blocker (p.), approved by the FDA in 2005. By virtue of its muscle relaxant property, it turned out also to relieve urine retention in men with enlarged prostate glands. But initially the drug did not fare well. In 2000 the part relating to doxazosin of a trial under the rubric, ALLHAT (the Antihypertensive and Lipid Lowering Treatment to prevent Heart Attack Trial), was terminated early. The reason was that the drug performed poorly, causing a 25% higher incidence of cardiovascular disease, compared to an old and much cheaper product, the diuretic, chlorthalidone, and also twice the risk of congestive heart failure (p.). Nor was it any better than the control diuretic in promoting urine flow. The report in the *Journal of the American Medical Association* concluded that 'thiazide-type diuretics are superior in preventing one or more major forms of CVD [cardiovascular disease] and are less expensive. They should be preferred for first-step antihypertensive therapy'. Pfizer got wind of this message, and launched an energetic advertising campaign to counteract the evidence. Advertising of pharmaceuticals is a highly refined business, confided to specialist public relations firms with offices in such patrician locations as New York's Madison Avenue. The result was that the sales of Carduran did not fall, despite the objurgations in the medical press. The *British Medical Journal* carried an article by a medical journalist under the heading 'Marketing spin doctors soft pedal data on antihypertensives'. Jeanne Lenzer, the author had discovered that the Pfizer representatives had been instructed not to allude to the ALLHAT trial when speaking to doctors, unless asked, in the expectation presumably that most doctors did not read the medical literature too closely. She also unearthed an exchange between Pfizer and the American College of Cardiologists, which the company subsidised to the extent of $500,000 per year. The College had reacted to the report by recommending to the readers of their literature to cease prescribing doxazosin in favour of a diuretic. Pfizer applied discreet pressure, and suggested the College 'clarify' the statement, diluting the too-explicit wording. The College acceded to the suggestion. Lenzer found that little was made of the virtues of diuretics in treating hypertension, and to find the reason for the shift in emphasis she spoke to the executive of a company created to give marketing advice to pharmaceutical concerns. His answer was blunt: 'because diuretics aren't promoted'. He was therefore not at all surprised when the conclusions of ALLHAT made no impact on sales. Doxazosin was, though, reported to have other and quite unforeseen activities, such as repressing the symptoms of post-traumatic stress disorder (PTSD) - nightmares and panic attacks and such - and is now prescribed for those, as well of course as hypertension, ALLHAT notwithstanding.

Chapter 18

WHITHER DRUG RESEARCH?

Where are the new ideas?

Economic and technological developments have wrought great changes in recent years in the ways of drug research. It now costs – or so the drug companies seek to persuade us - around £2 billion to bring a genuinely new drug to market, and takes perhaps 10 or 15 years. This is in large part partly due to the nature of the clinical trials process, allied to the costs of research. Worse yet, the majority of new drugs fail at the final stage, the large, expensive Phase III clinical trial. One consequence of all this is the increasingly lustful gaze that the industry has turned on university and government laboratories, for these harbour the largest reserve of highly skilled, yet relatively money-starved labour. And so the industry now supports many research projects with generous sums, but with provisos. Thus the company reserves the right to forbid publication of the results, at least until such time (which can be years) as it judges commercially safe. The company will waive this right whenever it decides that the discovery is of no commercial interest. This conflicts with the age-old principle of free dissemination of knowledge, and publications are, of course, the currency of a scientific career. But academics will put up with that when times are hard, and also if they can see a practical and socially desirable, or in some cases lucrative outcome of their work as a priority. (We have already seen the additional advantages that companies have too often gained a spurious credibility for their products by suborning academic scientists, and mainly, it seems, doctors – the 'companies' whores', as one respected researcher has described them.) The large companies also often derive their new products from the work of the biotechnology industry, which is now a huge international resource, although few of these companies have the means to develop a new drug commercially on their own. The pharmaceutical giants, which from their inception built up research operations of legendary quality, and invented so many new drugs, are now gradually withdrawing from this traditional activity, closing down their research arms, and increasingly cultivating links with - sometimes to the extent of colonising - academic and state-funded research centres.

The pharmaceutical companies do though continuously develop 'me-too' drugs, an activity for which there is limitless scope, but limited prospects of a blockbusting end-product. A growing interest is the re-examination of shelved compounds, the numbers of which may run into millions. It seems scarcely likely that a careful search among these discards will not uncover compounds of interest. There have also been efforts for some time to examine the possible virtues of traditional Chinese, Indian and South American traditional remedies, but these have so far produced remarkably little of consequence. Much greater promise has sprung from the renewed interest in toxins and venoms.

Bugs, plants and animals: lead compounds new and old

Our most valuable drugs stem in large measure, whether directly or indirectly, from nature. Among the most obvious and enduring examples in the first category are digitalis, aspirin, opium, quinine and penicillin, and there are many more. But the great majority are of indirect provenance – synthetic or semisynthetic variants of the natural compounds, commonly at several removes. In recent years, partly no doubt because of the ravaging of the natural environment, and the threat to the survival of so many species of plants and animals, there has been an upsurge of interest in what rare species, especially from the rain forests and the sea, have to offer. It is new chemical classes of lead compounds that are wanted. So far the animal kingdom has provided more numerous and more propitious leads. The most important of the new plant products in the last half-century, new antibiotics aside, is the antimalarial drug from China, artemisinin (p.). A few jungle plants have held out promise, among them the Areca palm. It produces oil and a fruit, which the local people chew as a stimulant, like betel leaves. The active constituent, arecoline is a weak agonist of a set of acetylcholine receptors (p.), and causes constriction of the bronchi and the pupils. It was reported in addition to have the more interesting effect of enhancing learning and retention, and was therefore seen as a prospective treatment for Alzheimer disease, but at working concentrations it proved to be carcinogenic, and so has never so far been taken further. Fungi and algae have proved rather more fruitful. Numerous antibiotics (p.), and immunosuppressants, such as cyclosporin A (p.), an indispensable aid to organ transplantation, have sprung from fungi, and with the need for new antibiotics now critical, there will be more intensive searches for new, and re-evaluation of old, disregarded fungal compounds.

Evolutionary pressures have provided animal species with a vast and wildly varied range of compounds for defence or aggression. A major proportion are proteins or peptides (in effect small proteins). It is striking that protein toxins are vastly more potent than the substances the famous Roman and Victorian poisoners had to hand – arsenic, cyanides, strychnine – by a factor of commonly a million. (This is quantitatively expressed in terms of the LD_{50} value (LD for lethal dose) – the weight of the substance per kilogram of bodyweight of a laboratory animal (including a human) needed to kill half the individuals that received it. One of the most familiar and deadly proteins is botulinum toxin, which comes from the bacterium, *Clostridium botulinum*. The word derives from the Latin, *botulus*, a little bag, otherwise a sausage, for it was first recognised in infected sausages, but is more often found in spoiled tinned food. (Botulism, as the resulting illness is called, is fortunately rare, but another related bacterium, *Clostridium perfringens*, which is unpleasant, but much less dangerous, is a common source of food poisoning.) Botulinum toxin consists, as many protein toxins do, of two parts, really two conjoined molecules, one of which has evolved to attach itself to receptors on a nerve cell surface; this allows the other protein to penetrate into the cell, where it stops the release of the neurotransmitter, acetylcholine. The muscles normally supplied by the acetylcholine cannot contract, become slack, and paralysis supervenes. Botulinum toxin has found many clinical uses, as in the treatment of myasthaenia gravis (p.) and of hyperactivity of the sweat-glands and eyelids, and of course cosmetically as Botox, to turn the skin from prune into plum. Other bacterial toxins – cholera, diphtheria, tetanus toxins and more – have been extensively studied, and their modes of action analysed. Even if they have found no application in therapeutics, they become important research tools.

The estimated number of species of insects runs into millions. Close on a half-million species of beetles alone have been identified and named. When the great biologist, J.B.S. Haldane was asked what his studies had revealed to him about the nature of God, he replied that the deity (if such a one existed, for Haldane was well-known to be an atheist) must have had 'an inordinate fondness for beetles'. Without doubt these species, with their widely varied habitats, prey, predators and lifestyles, harbour multitudes of New Chemical Entities (NCIs), as the drug agencies term them (p.). The number of animal products with remarkable physiological activities, a number of of which have already come into clinical use, is too long to enumerate, but let us at least contemplate a few that have obvious interest. Among terrestrial creatures, worms, insects, snakes, frogs and mammals have thrown up a plenitude of analgesics and dispersers of blood clots. The venoms of tarantulas and other species of spider and the secretions of vampire bats and of leeches have been found to contain types of molecules new to chemistry. Among them are powerful analgesics, which act on the various kinds of ion channels (p.) and receptors in the nervous system, and may therefore find uses individually or in combinations.

Other compounds found in the secretions of blood-sucking creatures prevent clotting of the blood or dissolve the clot. These activities are directed at different components of the highly complicated clotting cascade (p.). So the many species of leeches all inject an anticoagulant of their own into their victims, but these anticoagulants differ in the ways in which they act. The clinical choice of anticoagulant depends on the cause of the clot, or the degree of danger of clot formation. In cases of stroke the speed with which the clot is made to dissolve is critical, and this will vary with the identity of the target of the drug. The common European leech, *Hirudo officinalis* has given us two types of anticoagulant, both of which found application in the clinic, and one is now regarded as indispensable (p.). The giant Amazonian jawed leech of nightmare – sometimes called the banana leech, it is about 18 inches or up to 50 centimetres long - secretes a compound that acts on the specialised platelet cells, and will dissolve the most refractory blood clots. The Mexican leech has an anticoagulant of its own, antistasin, which acts on a different clotting component. A common tick has another chemical weapon, called TAP (tick anticoagulant peptide), prevents a protease, or proteolytic enzyme (one that breaks down other proteins) from performing a critical step in clot formation. Different again is the vampire bat, which has in its saliva a highly selective protease, desmoteplase, which attacks only the preponderant clot component, fibrin. Desmoteplase showed itself to possess some very desirable properties, which seem to give it every advantage over the drugs in current use for dealing with strokes, pulmonary embolisms, and other mishaps demanding rapid treatment. The enzyme has been cloned and expressed in bulk, and has been given the pleasingly apposite commercial name, Draculin. A comparison with tissue plasminogen activator (tPA), which together with streptokinase has dominated the market for two decades (both discussed earlier [pp.]) shows it to be more specific in its action and more potent, some fifty times longer-lasting in the bloodstream, and devoid apparently of significant side-effects.

Venoms from reptiles and other creatures all contain formidable arrays of biologically active compounds, some with clinical uses, actual or potential. Snake venoms have yielded leads for a wide range of anticoagulant and anti-hypertensive agents. The latter are for the most part ACE inhibitors (p.), and the first of them, captopril, which has saved many lives, we have already encountered. A common side-effect of this drug is a skin rash, and another is loss of taste acuity. It is also a less than ideal drug in that its persistence in the body is brief. These shortcomings encouraged other drug companies to tinker with the captopril structure in the hope of producing something that would supersede it. This was largely achieved by Merck with their Enalapril, and there are now many other related products. The other major contribution that snakes have made to human well-being is through anticoagulants, which are abundant in venoms. The Malaysian pit viper provided one of the earliest 'clot-busters' from its venom, a proteolytic enzyme, arvin, which found clinical use for some years. Of greater interest are more recently studied anticoagulants belonging for the most part to a class of small proteins called disintegrins.

Blood platelets are central players in the clotting process. They are induced by a chemical signal to cluster together in clumps, to which the clotting protein, fibrin then binds. The platelets interact with one another through glycoproteins (proteins carrying attached sugar moieties), which protrude from the surface. These glycoproteins are called integrins. (The integrins are a ubiquitous family of proteins, largely responsible for attaching cells to other cells or to elements of the body's architecture.) The disintegrins are integrin receptor antagonists; they bind like the integrins themselves to the integrin receptors on the cell surfaces, and so block access to the integrins. The platelets can then no longer form clusters and the clotting process is interrupted. There are dozens of these disintegrins, falling into several structural classes. Many new compounds have been developed from snake toxins. The most therapeutically successful in preventing or reversing pathological clot formation, as in pulmonary embolism or deep-vein thrombosis, appears to be eptifibalide, trade name Integrilin, from the pigmy rattlesnake, common in Florida. A drug with similar action, designed by Merck chemists on the basis of a compound found in the venom of the saw-scaled viper, found in Africa and parts of Asia, is tirofiban, known as Aggracan and by other trade names. It is administered by injection in acute cardiovascular conditions. Among other reptiles, the Gila monster, a large venomous lizard, living in the western U.S.-Mexican border region, has yielded from its saliva a peptide hormone resembling the animal (including human) peptide, glucagon, which counterbalances the activity of insulin. Exenatide was approved by the FDA in a synthetic version of the natural compound (first isolated in 1992) as a treatment for type 2 diabetes. Such new options are much needed, as the Avandia disaster and the growing incidence of the disease make clear.

Venom products that have stirred up serious interest are the analgesics. Here again, there are numerous compounds, previously unknown to chemists. Each acts on one of the ion channels and receptors in brain and nerves that play their parts in the perception of pain. The arrow-poison frogs of South America have provided the indigenous hunters with the perfect means to kill their prey. The frogs secrete toxins in their skin, which make them lethal to predators, and a drop smeared on the tip of an arrow or dart will kill or paralyse an animal, and the anointed dart can generally be used many times. The frogs are small and brilliantly coloured - an evolutionary survival advantage, for it warns off would-be predators. All are now endangered species. The best-studied, which lives in a few locations in Ecuador, is the phantasmal poison frog, *Epipedobates tricolor*. It is no more than about a centimetre long and so dangerous that the tribesmen will capture it only on the surface of a sticky leaf before picking up a drop of the exudate from its skin on the tip of their dart. In 1974 John Daly, a pharmacologist at the National Institutes of Health in Maryland, who had been studying poison frogs in the jungles of South America for more than ten years, isolated the toxin, which he named epibatidine. He was unable to collect sufficient of the substance to determine its structure with the means available at the time, but he showed that it was an analgesic, more powerful than any previously known, some 200 times more effective than morphine. Daly also found that another species of miniature frog, the golden poison frog, *Phyllobates terribilis*, about a half-centimetre long, produces an even more lethal secretion.

These creatures derive their toxins by metabolising chemicals in the insects on which they feed, and therefore become harmless if deprived on their specialised food. Many species of poison frogs from several genuses (families) are now known, and more than 100 toxins have been isolated. Batrachotoxin (from the Greek for frog) is the most widespread; it is an alkaloid with the structure of a steroid. The toxins have the common effect of preventing the operation of a particular type of ion channel in the membranes of nerves and muscle, including that of the heart. The channels are in effect wedged in the open state, and the most violent result is cardiac arrhythmia, fibrillation, or quivering of the heart muscle, and finally cessation of the heartbeat. Epibatidine, a compound of a quite different structure, exerts its pain-killing effects by binding to two kinds of acetylcholine receptors in nerves. Not only does it so greatly exceed the potency of morphine, but it seems also to be devoid of addictive properties and of the unpleasant gastrointestinal side-effects of the opioids, especially constipation. Its discoverers had high hopes of its clinical possibilities, but the knife-edge on which the compound is poised, between its analgesic effect and its lethal toxicity, has precluded its practical use. It is no surprise, at the same time, that there should have been attempts to modify the structure to eliminate the toxicity. This objective was eventually achieved by the chemists of Abbott Laboratories in Chicago. Their compound, ABT 594 is said to retain the high analgesic potency of its precursor with none of its toxicity, and is presumably in clinical trials.

The sea, which is home to a large proportion of the Earth's species, is probably also the greatest repository of New Chemical Entities, and therefore drugs. Even that most ancient of life-forms, the blue-green algae, or cyanobacteria, contain unusual chemicals. Among them is an anti-fungal compound, evolved presumably to protect the algae from fungal competitors. This compound, cryptophycin binds to, and inactivates tubulin, the protein of the microtubules, central elements in the machinery of cell division. Though quite different in structure[*], the substance resembles in its action such compounds as paclitaxel (Taxol), and colchicine, and thus arrests the proliferation of cancer cells. It has the advantage, apparently, of acting preferentially on rapidly dividing cells. A total synthesis of the compound was effected in 1995. Three other microtubule inhibitors have emerged from the sea, one of which, eleutherobin was extracted from a species of coral, and found to be 100 times more effective than Taxol in killing breast, ovary and lung cancer cells in culture, and apparently better in respect of likely side-effects. Its quantity in the corral is small, and although it has been synthesised in

---

[*] It belongs to a class of compounds known to chemists as a depsipeptides, in which the peptide linkages that join the constituent amino acids in proteins, are replaced by ether linkages. This means that successive pairs of carbon atoms in a chain are linked by an oxygen atom. As in peptides and proteins, the carbon atoms carry side chains that distinguish the different amino acids (of which there are twenty kinds in proteins) from each other.

the laboratory, commercial production may still be a remote prospect. A similar compound from a Caribbean coral has been found effective against Taxol-resistant cancer cells, and yet another anti-cancer candidate was extracted from a sponge.

The list goes on, and indeed back, because for a period beginning in the 1950s the National Cancer Institute in the U.S., as related previously (p.), began a trawl through the natural world for new curative compounds. Besides Taxol, little of enduring value came of it, although there was no lack of promise. Some of the leads were pursued in academic and government laboratories, and some by small commercial organisations. But natural materials cannot be patented, and in any case, the techniques then available for isolating plant and animal extracts in quantity were much more limited than they now are. An example was the anti-cancer activity discerned in 1969 in extracts of the sea squirt, *Ecteinascidia turbinata*, found among reefs in the Caribbean. An intrepid biochemist at the University of Illinois spent much time diving for the creatures, and prepared and assayed preparations. By 1984 he had determined it structure, but a laboratory synthesis must have seemed too formidable a prospect to contemplate, and there was never enough material for clinical testing. Eventually the patent rights to the procedures were surrendered to a Spanish pharmaceutical company, PharmaMar. Attempts to farm the sea squirts were unsuccessful, but in time the company's scientists managed to collect one gram of pure active compound from a ton (one-thousand kilograms) of sea squirts. It was still insufficient for clinical trials, and help was sought from an eminent Harvard University chemist, E.J. Corey (who was to win the Nobel Prize for chemistry in 1990). Corey found a route to a synthesis in 1996, and with later improvements this formed the basis of a commercial process. Ectinasceidin 743, also known as trabectedin and by its trade name, Yondelis, was approved by the EMAA in 2007, and by the FDA for the treatment of a particularly unpleasant type of cancer, soft-tissue sarcoma, and for ovarian cancer, to be used in conjunction with a traditional drug, doxorubicin (Adriamycin or Doxyl). The interval of nearly 40 years between the discovery of the activity in a sea squirt extract and the appearance of the drug on the market illustrates the difficulties that commonly attend the transformation of a sparse natural material into a useful product. Advances in chemical analysis, synthesis and purification methods have wrought great changes in the efficiency of the drug development process, and made the technology, at least, less intimidating.

Of all the therapeutic riches that nature seems to hold out it is the conotoxins that have created the greatest stir in recent years. The cone snails are marine predators. They have been valued in the past for the beauty of their brightly coloured shells, but their remarkable chemical armoury first caught the attention of scientists barely fifty years ago. The snails, which live on rocks, mainly in the Pacific, vary in size from two inches or so down, and are carnivores. At the approach of a fish, worm or mollusc the snail throws out a harpoon with a spear point, which injects the prey with a cocktail of toxins, paralysing it instantly. The snail then shuffles towards its prize and engulfs it. The venom is powerful enough to kill people, as occasionally happens. The cone snails have been objects of intense research, and it is now estimated that the genus *Conus* embraces some 500 species. The venom of each one may contain 100 components, and therefore, with upwards of 50,000 physiologically active compounds waiting to be isolated, the scope for investigation is unlikely soon to be exhausted. The first sporadic publications about the properties of the venom appeared in the early 1960s, but the first systematic exploration was undertaken some 20 years later by a Philippino biochemist, Baldomero Olivera, working at the University of Utah in Salt Lake City. Olivera has related that the early breakthroughs were due to undergraduates, engaged in research projects in his laboratory. Craig Clark was 18 when he had the idea of injecting fractions of a cone snail venom that he had separated into the central nervous system of mice. The results were startling: some constituents of the venom induced a trance-like state, and others a ceaseless hyperactivity. More students found more such phenomena, and one, Michael McIntosh, who had not even begun his undergraduate course, purified a 'shaker' toxin, which caused tremors in the animals.

All these active compounds were peptides (made up of strings of amino acids). The conotoxins are in fact all peptides, varying in length from 10 to 35 amino acids, with up to four internal cross-links, called disulphide bridges*. Such short chains of amino acids can these days be synthesised by standard routines, although there can still be a problem in ensuring that the disulphide bridges are formed in the correct positions. Of the many families of cone snail toxins there are mainly six that have been studied in some depth. These are designated by the Greek letters, alpha (α), delta (δ), mu (μ), iota (ι), kappa (κ) and omega (ω), and they are all neurotoxins, acting on one or other of the many ion channels** or on neurotransmitter receptors (p.), by which the nervous system operates. So the α-conotoxins are antagonists that prevent one type of receptor in the nervous system from functioning, and serve the snail by paralysing its prey. The δ-conotoxins act on a type of sodium ion channel in the membrane of nerve cells, but do not affect heart or muscle, whereas μ-conotoxins find their way to sodium ion channels in the membranes of muscles, but not of nerves. The ι- and κ-conotoxins act on different subtypes of potassium ion channels in the membranes of many tissues, and ω-conotoxins block calcium ion channels in nerve membranes. Despite the intensive scrutiny to which conotoxins from many species of snail have been subjected over the last twenty years or more, and their undoubted promise, there appears to be only one product that has yet entered into clinical use. This is zicocotide, an ω-toxin from the snail, *Conus magus*, which is a powerful analgesic. Its very considerable disadvantage is that it has to be injected into the cerebrospinal fluid (generally by an implanted pump), and so is used, under its trade name, Prialt, to treat refractory pain. No doubt more will

---

* One of the 20 amino acids from which protein chains are built contains a sulphydryl (or thiol) group (-SH, where S is a sulphur and H a hydrogen atom). This amino acid is called cysteine. Under oxidising conditions, two such groups can lose their hydrogen atom and bond together to form a disulphide bridge (-S-S-). Disulphide bridges occur in proteins that are free outside cells, for instance in the blood plasma or the stomach fluid, or in the venom of the cone snails and other creatures. For such a protein to enter its active form the disulphide bridges must be in the correct positions, that is between designated cysteines, not between any other pairs.
** The ion channels are 'gated', which means that each type of channel will open as required, to let through the ions of the kind that it recognises. There are channels for sodium, for potassium and for calcium. Within these types there are many subtypes, each with its special function. The specificity of each of the various conotoxins is what gives them their special pharmacological interest, for it holds out the hope that a toxin may be capable of selectively treating one single type of disorder.

be heard about conotoxin-derived products when chemical modifications have been found that overcome the toxicity problems.

The soil is another source of unexplored life-forms and hidden compounds. We have seen (Chapter) how the majority of antibiotics now in use were discovered in soil micro-organisms or derivd from them, but only a minute proportion of those micro-organisms have been studied. Indeed, it has been estimated that the soil's eco-system contains a third of our planet's species, so every shovelfull of earth must contain many thousands, if not millions of different kinds of living bacteria, fungi, microscopic worms, and even archaea*. These organisms live in a highly hostile environment, competing with one another for the limited supply of nutrients. They have therefore evolved a defence mechanism in the form of compounds that will repel or kill their competitors. These include antibiotics, antifungal agents, compounds that will kill parasitic nematode worms or insects, and some archaea even make immunosuppressants. The problem for researchers in this area has been the reluctance of all but a few of these micro-organisms to allow themselves to be cultured. Their natural environment is so different from anything that can be easily simulated in the laboratory that they have not been made to grow *in vitro*, and certainly not in the standard nutrient media. It is only with the advent of the molecular cloning techniques developed in the last three or so decades that it has become possible to generate some of the proteins of these species in appreciable quantity. This is done by isolating and amplifying DNA (p.) from the mixture of species in what has been termed the soil 'metagenome', stitching pieces of DNA containing genes at random into a bacterial DNA, which can then be put back into the bacterium (in practice *E. coli*). By this means proteins of the soil micro-organisms are expressed by 'tame' bacteria furnished with the alien genes. This is now the basis of a major research programme, still in its early stages. So far a pharmaceutical company collaborating with the university researchers who developed the procedures, has produced a pair

---

* The archaea, previously thought to be a category of bacteria, are now recognised as a third evolutionary 'domain' of life, in addition to the bacteria and the eukaryota (the last of which are those like ourselves which pack their cellular DNA into a nucleus). The archaea were first found in the thermal vents under the Pacific Ocean, thriving at temperatures close to boiling.

of antibiotics with activity against a wide range of pathogenic bacteria, called turbomycin *a* and *b*, but so far there is no indication of their clinical potential.* A source of concern now is the rapid erosion of soil through ruthless agricultural practices, leading to the loss of large swathes of the eco-system, and its myriad flora.

Antibodies: magic bullet finds target

Paul Ehrlich prefigured it all. When, at the start of the 20th century, the unique specificity and versatility of antibodies became apparent he conceived the idea of treating a disease, such as an infection, with an antibody directed against the agent of the disease, to which would be attached to a toxic chemical. The antibody – the missile - would attach itself to the target, and the warhead would destroy it. It was not for another eighty or so years that the means to realise Ehrlich's vision became a reality. Antibodies can be generated against almost any substance alien to the body. An animal, immunised with a chosen antigen, such as a protein or a whole virus or bacterium, will produce antibodies, which circulate in the blood, and can be isolated from the plasma. There are several types of antibody, but the most abundant, and most relevant here is immunoglobulin G, or IgG. All IgG antibodies are built up of two pairs of protein chains (p.) assembled in the shape of a Y, and are all identical in overall structure. The

---

* So far the most interesting outcome of this line of investigation does not relate directly to drug discovery, but to a matter of no lesser urgency. The idea arose in the minds of some researchers that the enormously competitive nature of the eco-system in the soil might lead not only to the appearance of antibiotic compounds, but also of resistance to those same compounds. A group of researchers at Washington University Medical School in St. Louis isolated DNA from soil samples taken at eleven sites around the U.S., and found a large number of gene sequences with close similarity to those in antibiotic-resistant strains of human pathogenic bacteria, and 18 out of 252 which were precisely identical. Now it is known that bacteria engage in a kind of sexual activity, transferring DNA from one to another with which it is in contact. The startling identity proves that such exchange has taken place between a soil bacterium and a pathogen, although it does not tell us in which direction. Nevertheless, this amounts to a strong suspicion that antibiotic resistance may have derived from a blameless soil bacterium. The main reason that this discovery is so important is that it opens a new route into the mechanism of antibiotic resistance.

specificity resides in small regions at the two tips of the Y, which recognise and bind to the antigen. The problem with using an antibody to target, for example, a tumour – for it has long been known that tumours make antigens of their own - is first that the antibodies are heterogeneous, and will recognise different parts of an antigen, such as a protein, and some of the different members of the mixed antibody population may also bind to similar parts of other molecules in the body that resemble the target in the original antigen. Secondly, the immunoglobulins of different animals, while all similar in structure, differ in the amino acid sequences of the predominating parts beyond the antigen-binding sites. Thus a rabbit or horse antibody will be recognised by the human immune system as an interloper, and will itself then be treated as an antigen. The consequences of these shortcomings are apt to be serious.

The turning point in the hunt for a therapeutic antibody came in the 1980s. Two researchers in Cambridge, César Milstein (1927-2002) and Georges Köhler (1946-1995) were searching for a way to isolate and replicate a single antibody-producing cell. One cell would make only a single form of antibody molecule, and thus solve the heterogeneity problem. The idea was not new, but it was Milstein and Köhler who hit on the solution to its implementation (and were rewarded in 1984 with the Nobel Prize* for Physiology or Medicine, shared with the, Danish immunologist, Niels Kaj Jerne). Ten years or so previously an American worker had discovered a remarkable phenomenon. Multiple myeloma is a cancer of the B-lymphocytes, which are important elementpart of the immune system. The B-cells reside mainly in the spleen and in bodies called lymph nodes. When activated in the last of a chain of steps initiated by the arrival in

---

* Milstein foresaw the implications of the discovery, and asked the British Government body then charged with the exploitation of scientific discoveries, the National Research and Development Corporation, to take out a patent. In later years he liked to begin his lectures on monoclonal antibodies by showing a slide of the letter he had received in reply. It read: 'It is certainly difficult for us to identify any immediate practical application which could be pursued as a commercial venture'. What the decision cost the Government and Milstein's employer, the Medical Research Council, not to mention Milstein and Köhler themselves, is hard to calculate, but their discovery gave rise in very short order to a multi-billion dollar industry.

the body of an antigen, they make antibodies and display them on their outer surfaces. The cancerous B-cells in multiple myeloma all produce a single antibody. Being cancerous, they proliferate furiously when cultured in the laboratory.*

Milstein and Köhler found a cell line - that is a culture of cells from some source that has been kept growing in the laboratory – in this case of myeloma cells that had lost the capacity to produce the antibody, but simply kept reproducing. This was the key: Milstein and Köhler now took B-cells from the spleen of an immunised mouse and fused them with the unproductive myeloma cells – easily done with certain chemicals that bring the cells into close contact by squeezing out the water between them, thus allowing the surface membranes to coalesce. They called the resulting compound cell a *hybridoma*, and its constituent B-cell was now – to use another jargon term - immortalised. Deposited on a Petri dish (p.), single cells would settle on the agar and divide, forming little clumps of growing cells, called colonies, each started by a single parent cell. An individual colony could then be grown up in a culture medium to produce billions of identical cells, all producing a population of identical antibodies.

The problem of heterogeneity was now overcome, but since what the system generated was a mouse antibody, the other problem, that of antigenicity, had still to be solved. What was needed was a human antibody with the desired specificity. There were several approaches to the problem, but the method now favoured is to perform the entire operation with B-cells from a transgenic mouse, bred to express human, not mouse antibodies. (This is essentially the same process as is used commercially to produce drugs and other substances in the milk of genetically modified cows or in genetically modified plant crops.) These 'humanised' monoclonal antibodies are now a commonplace in the drug industry. They are by no means totally proof against an immune or allergic reaction in the patient, because some vestiges of mouse protein inevitably remain, and so some un-humanised antibodies

---

* Cells taken from an organ or tissue and maintained in culture will keep on dividing for about 50 generations and will then die (see p.). Cancer cells are an exception to this rule, and keep dividing indefinitely if properly looked after and supplied with nutrients: they are immortal.

have also found therapeutic use. The antibody may also be coupled to a toxin, as described above (and envisaged by Ehrlich), and carry it to the target cell. Or the antibody may carry a radioactive isotope, and destroy its target by irradiation, without (in principle) damaging the surrounding healthy tissue – a refinement of the crude process of radiotherapy.

Monoclonal antibodies have been developed for treating several diseases, rheumatoid arthritis and asthma among them, but especially cancer. Rheumatoid arthritis is one of the autoimmune conditions (p.), in which a natural protein, tumour necrosis factor (TNF-α) is implicated. TNF-α is a cytokine, one of the signalling molecules, which control many metabolic processes. It has, amongst its beneficent activities, an inflammatory action. Its elimination suppresses the symptoms of rheumatoid arthritis and other inflammatory conditions, among which are Crohn's disease, and inflammatory affliction of the bowel, and psoriasis, which could previously only be treated by corticosteroids, with all their attendant side-effects. Within a short period three inhibitors of TNF-α, active against these conditions, came from biotechnology companies. Each was the outcome of great ingenuity, but it was the last to arrive that proved most successful: adalimumab was the product of a collaborative effort by three companies, and is unusual in that it is not a chimaeric (a mouse-human hybrid), but a fully human antibody, originating in a human serum. First approved by the FDA for the treatment of rheumatoid arthritis in 2002, and subsequently for other inflammatory diseases, it appears under the name of HUMIRA (Human Monoclonal Antibody in Rheumatoid Arthritis), and in 2012 its worldwide sales amounted to $9.3 billion.

Yet the majority of monoclonal antibodies so far are aimed at cancers, including leukaemias. Many mysteries remain about their exact mode of action, and their efficacy is hugely variable. A dozen or more antibodies are in common use, and probably hundreds more are in various stages of development; a minority of those will prove valuable. There are three identifiable modes of action. The largest proportion work by binding to and thereby disabling a particular receptor on the outer surface of the malignant cell. There are many kinds of surface receptors on cells. When occupied by a ligand – a molecule that fits into the receptor like a key into a lock - a signal passes to the interior of the cell and initiates a chain of events culminating in the activation of a metabolic switch. It may set off, or shut off, the synthesus of a particular substance, such as glucose when insulin binds to its receptor, or it may release the restraints on growth and proliferation of the cells. The ligands for that are called growth factors, and cancer cells generally over-express – that is, make in excess – growth factor receptors. The antibody, then, against a particular cancer cell receptor (for different cancers have different receptors) may impede cell division, or it may prevent the formation of new blood vessels that nourish the tumour (angiogenesis – see p.). A second possible mechanism operates when the antibody encourages the body's immune system to mount a defence against the tumour by making its complex with the tumour simulate a foreign intruder.

There is now a wide range of monoclonal antibodies, each directed at a particular kind of cancer. The most striking success was scored by rituximab (Rituxan or Mabthera), which was invented by scientists at Biogen IDEC Pharmaceuticals, a biotechnology company in California. The objective was to kill B cells, which go wrong in many variety of blood cancers, including B cell lymphoma, Hodgkin's and non-Hodgkin's lymphoma, several types of leukaemia, and some autoimmune diseases. It had long been known known that B cells expose on their surface a protein of uncertain function, called CD20, and the reasoning behind rituximab was that an antibody binding specifically to this protein might encompass the destruction of the cells. The conjecture proved correct. The antibody was first tried, with success, on a patient in 1993, and in 1997, after a strikingly successful trial on 50 patients with malignant lymphomas, it gained FDA approval, and some time thereafter it was accepted in the European Union and elsewhere. The action of the antibody is complex, but what it certainly does is collect into clusters the CD20 proteins, which float in the (essentially fluid) outer cell membrane. The distorted structure of the cell surface makes it appear as a foreign body, which is then attacked and destroyed by another class of white blood cells, called natural killer (NK) cells. There were several remarkable features to this happy outcome. One was that the rituximab was effective against such a range of blood cancers – multiple myeloma was an exception – and another that the destruction of the normal B cells in the circulation seemed to do no harm. And in addition, it was found that several autoimmune conditions, such as rheumatoid arthritis, also responded to the treatment. The drug has even been used to prevent rejection of grafts. Retuximab is supplied to the U.S. market by two of the country's most prominent biotechnology companies, Biogen IDEC and Genentech, and to European countries by Hoffmann-La Roche.

Monoclonal antibodies carrying a lethal payload to destroy the target cell are still relatively few. One that has been used successfully against a form of leukaemia (acute myelogenous leukaemia) is gemtuzumab. (The ending, *mab* denotes a therapeutic monoclonal antibody.) This is a humanised antibody, sold under the name of Myelotarg, in which the antibody is coupled to calicheamicin, an antibiotic produced by a species of bacteria discovered in chalk pits in Texas, which is enormously toxic to all cells – it breaks the DNA chains – and therefore to the leukaemia cells. Other monoclonal antibodies on the market directed at particular cancers carry lethal radioactive isotopes of iodine, and in one case of the metal, yttrium. But the best-known of the monoclonal antibodies are all of the first kind – those that obstruct the receptors to which they bind. The first to make a major commercial impact, and therefore the most famous, was trastuzumab, Herceptin, developed by Genentech from research carried out at the University of California in Los Angeles, licensed by the FDA in 1998 for the treatment of breast cancer. It has also been used to treat stomach and some other cancers, but its high cost has been a source of contention. Another monoclonal antibody, which became famous for the wrong reasons was cetuximab, or Erbitux. It was developed by a biotechnology company, ImClone for the treatment of bowel cancer, but towards the end of 2001 it was rejected by the FDA. It later transpired that before the outcome of the application had been announced, the chairman of the company and his family and friends had unburdened themselves of many million dollarsworth of stock. When this came to light, several people were found guilty of insider trading and served prison sentences. However, in 2004 a new clinical trial was organised, and this time FDA approved the drug. Even so, its performance appeared less than impressive: 11% of the patients in the trial evinced a favourable response, amounting to a retardation of tumour growth by 1.5 months. When the Erbitux was administered together with a conventional chemotherapeutic drug this rose to 23%, with an extension of 4.1 months. Such results are not atypical of the performance of monoclonal antibodies.

Better fortune has accompanied bevacisumab, best known as Avastin, which is different again in its action. It came once more from the prodigious Genentech, and is manufactured in association with Roche Products. It is a humanised antibody, designed to bind to a growth factor, required for the reproduction of the cells in many cancers. This growth factor VEGF (vascular endothelial growth factor) directs off the development of blood vessels in the tumour, and bevacisumab associates with it in a tight complex, which can no longer recognise its receptor. It therefore stops the formation of blood vessels and thus growth of the tumour (more or less). In 2004 the FDA licensed it for the treatment of metastatic (that is, spreading) colon cancer, with the proviso that it must be given together with chemotherapy. The license was later extended to any bowel cancer, whether metastatic or not, and ovarian, lung and kidney cancers. It was briefly approved for breast cancer, but a committee of experts judged that the benefit was minimal and outweighed by the side-effects, mainly a large rise in blood pressure and periodic haemorrhages. That decision was more recently again reversed, though provisionally, on appeal from Genentech. In European countries Avastin was approved for breast cancer, but seems to have been little used. In Britain NICE (the National Institute for Health and Care Excellence), the body responsible for recommendations of treatments in the National Health Service, ruled against Avastin even for colon cancer on grounds of excessive cost and limited efficacy. An American trial concluded that bevacizumab, given with chemotherapy drugs, extended life by an average of 21.3 months, whereas chemotherapy alone gave the patients an average of 19.9 months. The additional six weeks or so of life would cost some £21,000, which was held to be poor value for money. There have also recently been concerns about possible damage to the blood vessels of the heart.

There was to be an interesting sequel however. It occurred to some eye specialists that since age-dependent 'wet' macular degeneration, the main cause of blindness in the old, was the result of anomalous growth of blood vessels behind the retina (leading to accumulation of fluid and separation of the retina from its support), bevacizumab might be used to arrest the condition. When it was tried (by injection into the eye) the result was remarkable: not only did it arrest progress in the great majority of cases, but the deterioration in sight was actually reversed. Moreover, the quantities required for treatment were minute: a standard vial of the antibody solution could yield dozens of doses for injection. This quintessential off-label use did not please Genentech, and threats of legal action mounted. The company also responded by developing a version of the drug explicitly for use against macular degeneration. It is caked ranibizumab, or Lucentis, and it consists of a fragment – one arm of the Y with a single growth factor binding site – of the same antibody. One difference is that its duration in the tissue is one-hundred times shorter than that of the parent bevacizumab. Long exposure to the antibody is an advantage for the treatment of cancer, but might conceivably have been a disadvantage for long residence in the eye. Genentech also warned against the dangers of infection from inexpert manipulation of Avastin taken out of its sterile vial. A trial in a large number of eye clinics in the U.S. found no difference in efficacy between Avastin and Lucentis, which after all comes from the same antibody generated by the selfsame cell culture derived from the one original mouse. The legal situation seems uncertain still, and meanwhile the use of Avastin for the treatment of macular degeneration presumably continues in many hospitals and clinics on the quiet.

There is no doubt that monoclonal antibodies will wax increasingly large in the treatment of many diseases, most of all cancers of various kinds. But so far it seems that all the ones now in use are treated as adjuncts to conventional chemotherapy agents. Their attraction as magic bullets is alluring nevertheless, and hopes for their future are still enormous. The question remains when - or indeed whether - they will become cheap enough for mass use in any but the rich countries. To take only one example, the annual cost of treating one patient with adalimumab (HUMIRA) in Europe has been estimated as 10,800 – 14,400 euros (thus about $14,000 – 19,000, or £9,000 – 12,000). This will no doubt fall when the patent eventually expires, but for most of the world's population in will remain prohibitive, failing some large and unforeseen technological advance in cell culture.

743

Which drug for you?

'Personalised medicine' is a catch-phrase in drug research today. The human genome is made up of about 3 billion nucleotides, distributed between 23 diploid (that is, paired) chromosomes (or twice that number if one includes both the maternally and paternally-derived partners). Only about 1% of all this DNA is made up of genes. Humans have something over 20,000 genes, but these give rise to several times that number of proteins, because in the course of expression (translation into proteins) a large proportion of these genes are broken into several pieces, which can then be assembled in different combinations to yield different proteins. These different protein forms arising from one gene are called 'splice variants'. There is yet another level of complexity, for the expressed proteins are subject to chemical modifications, most importantly the introduction of phosphate ($-PO_3$) groups, but also others, which affect their functions. Altogether, then, the total number of protein variants in our bodies exceeds one million. In 2000 the first genome sequence of an anonymous individual (actually a 'draft', and so still therefore far from complete) was exposed to view. The international effort had taken a decade and cost some $3 bn, but. sequencing technology has evolved at bewildering speed, and in the ensuing years the target of $1,000 is within sight. Consequently the genomes of a large number of people of widely different origins have been decoded. What has become even easier is the sequencing of single genes, so that mutations, both harmless (polymorphisms, as such are called), and pathological, can be identified. Moreover, these can now be matched by automated procedures against a standard 'normal' version, so that any difference can be detected. This matching is now done for hundreds of genes at the same time against standards deposited on a microchip (a gene array). Genetic anomalies, in other words, can be easily spotted.

It has long been clear that different people may respond differently to a given drug. A familiar example is the reaction to the commonest drug of all, alcohol. Most people have a reasonable tolerance for alcohol because an enzyme called liver alcohol dehydrogenase (LADH) will destroy it within a relatively short time. Others have low levels of LADH and react badly to alcohol. This trait is most common in Asian populations and in many

Jews. If so simple a compound as alcohol can have such disparate effects one would surely expect many of the complex, highly active substances, typical of modern drugs, to behave in similarly uncertain ways. Such notions gave rise to the elusive concept of 'race-specific' drugs'. The first substance so designated, and approved by the FDA on that basis, was isosorbide dinitrate, known as BiDil, a vasodilator, combined with an old compound of similar action, hydralazine hydrochloride. The product was developed by a U.S. company, NitroMed for the treatment of congestive heart failure (p.). In 1997 the FDA declined to approve the drug on the grounds of a poor showing in a clinical trial. In 2005 the company tried again, this time for the treatment solely of African Americans, who were reportedly particularly liable to the condition, and resistant to the drugs in common use. This time the drug won FDA approval as a 'race-specific' treatment, based on a new clinical trial, conducted on patients who identified themselves as black. The result appeared to be a triumph, with a 40% reduction in deaths. But given the objections to the first trial, which, it was asserted, was ill-designed, the exclusion of Caucasians from the second left a curious question hanging in the air.

The result was variously greeted - with enthusiasm as the first triumph of personalised medicine, and a portent of things to come, or with apprehension as the thin end of a dangerous racial wedge. The selection of patients had, however, been inadequate. There is no racial purity among African Americans (nor in most other racial groups), and self-proclamation as black is no answer. Moreover, both constituent drugs of BiDil were not new and had been in use to treat some patients with heart disease regardless of colour, Therefore one might envisage a situation in which this or other medicines, licensed exclusively as race-specific, might be denied to a large section of the population.* But in any event, doubts arose about BiDil, sufficient to cause NitroMed to cease producing the drug after two years, and the first 'race-specific' therapy faded into oblivion.

Race, since then, has not featured strongly in personalised medicine, but the number of individual traits that are now known to be responsible for major differences in the response to drugs has been growing apace. The incidence of serious conditions resulting from bad reactions to even the most common drugs is substantial. According to a recent estimate, a thousand or so hospital patients in Britain at any time are there for this reason. The amount of the anticoagulant ('blood thinner'), warfarin (Coumadin), prescribed for people who have had strokes or thromboses (and generally take for the rest of their lives) has to be carefully adapted to the response of the individual. The commonplace opiate analgesic (p.), Codeine (in the U.S. a constituent of Co-codamol and versions of Tylenol) is another, and more extreme example. The drug acts on an enzyme, which is mutated in about one in ten of the population, and those individuals are wholly unresponsive to the drug; they could thus be driven to swallow dangerous quantities of tablets in vain hope of relief.

---

* Like most racial issues, race-specific drugs are a minefield, and in 2006 one American pharmaceutical company, Schering-Plough trod on a mine. A Phase II clinical trial of a drug aimed at the suppression of hepatitis C infections, which were particularly prevalent in sufferers from AIDS because of the sharing of needles, explicitly excluded African Americans. The reason imputed to Schering-Plough by protesters was that confining the trial to the less widely infected white population might ensure a better statistical outcome. In response, the company enrolled 15 African Americans, though not as part of the randomised complement of subjects. This small group was to be given the highest of the doses allocated to the different cohorts in the dose-dependent study (customary in Phase II trials). In 2012 the drug, now called boceprivir, or Victrelis, and the similar compound, telaprevir (Incivek), produced by Vertex Pharmaceuticals, were licensed. But either was to be given only as part of a triple therapy, in combination with an antiviral, ribavirin, and a chemically modified interferon (p.).

Again, trastuzumab (Herceptin) acts on a receptor for a growth factor that only one in five of breast-cancer patients possess* - and of those, as of the rest, fewer than one-third respond.

Another reported case of genetic variation in drug response pertains to gefitinib, a growth-factor receptor blocker, created by Astra-Zeneca, and sold as Iressa for the treatment of a type of lung cancer. The FDA approved the drug in 2003, but reversed its decision two years later, except for continuation of treatment of patients already receiving it, and who were deemed by their doctors to be benefitting. Evidence, the FDA decided, that gefitinib prolonged life was wanting. In Europe it appears to be still in use. Evidence has in fact been offered that patients with one particular mutation in the gene overexpressed in this type of cancer do benefit, while all the others do not. More examples of the bearing that genetic traits have on drug reactions are constantly coming to light, and the means are now available for recording the individual's genotypes by the analytical methods described earlier.

Cancer is in fact a special case, for it is in all its forms determined by mutations, and, as we have seen (p.), the tumour cells mutate all the time. This should make it a particularly apt target for the personalised approach, but it is also the most difficult. In the leading advanced treatment centres patients are now routinely screened for an increasing number, currently about 200, gene variants related to cancers, and a similar number of mutations in a range of tumours, to determine which drugs might work and which not. Screening has brought to light a number of curious relationships. In 2006, for instance, a group of cancer researchers at Johns Hopkins University found a mutation in a gene coding for a seemingly innocuous metabolic enzyme in one of 35 patients with colon cancer. It was an isolated case, and probably, the investigators thought, of no consequence. The mutation did not turn up again in any of the patients

---

* The notorious BRCA-1 and BRCA-2 genes are unrelated to this phenotype (see p. for definition). These genotypes predispose to breast cancer, but are linked to no more than one in ten cases. Screenung for the BRCA genes can dissuade women from taking drastic prophylactic measures, in particular surgical removale of healthy breasts.

in a much larger study. But two years later, there it was in a sizeable minority (12%) if people suffering from a glioblastoma, a type of brain cancer, and also in 8% of patients in a form of leukaemia. The mutant enzyme, it turned out, was responsible for the accretion of a carcinogenic metabolic reaction product. Here was a clear target for a new drug. This was a good outcome for genetic screening, and oncologists must be hoping for more such results from a worldwide screening programme now aimed at sequencing the genomes of thousands of tumours. But most tumours so far sequenced display not one, but many mutations, and therefore the data that will accrue from such surveys will be overwhelming in its volume and complexity. It will thus present a correspondingly intimidating problem for those hoping to use it as a basis for treatment.

How (disregarding for the moment the special case of cancer) do individual differences in response to drugs come about? Many are as we have seen, genetic, inherited from one or other parent, or both. They can occasionally arise from a spontaneous mutation, a first, which the victim – the founder - will pass on to the next generation. But they may also be acquired from lifestyle or environment, from diet, alcohol, tobacco, past drug treatments, illnesses, toxins in the atmosphere, and so on. They may even stem at second-hand from life forms in the gut and elsewhere. The gut microbiota are estimated to comprise somewhere between 100 and 500 different species of bacteria, and many viruses and single-celled creatures, such as protozoa and fungi. The assembled microbiota are plentiful: they make up, by one measure, some 60% of the dry-weight of our faeces, and exert a strong effect on many of our metabolic processes. They are important in repelling parasites and other intruders (including *Clostridium difficile*, as we have already seen [p.]), and produce compounds of their own, which also participate in metabolism in the intestines and below. Micro-organisms also thrive in the urinary and respiratory tracts, though clearly in much smaller numbers. Much is now known about the microbiota, about how they interact with their host, and their state and composition has to be taken into account in any comprehensive evaluation of personalised drug treatments. All this considered, it is clear that there are formidable problems to be solved as drug research enters, as many believe, a brave new future. Some visionaries believe that we will all of us in time carry on our persons a chip bearing a complete catalogue of our genotypes to ensure that we will, when needed, receive optimal treatments for whatever disorders nature may inflict on us. There are clearly legal issues in allowing doctors and researchers to pry into the genomes of their patients, and gaze into the future – perhaps a likely early death from a deadly disease, or dementia - that it may reveal. Yet in some decades from now it may appear that we have been living in the dark ages of medicine.

Epigenetics: new headaches

Epigenetics adds another layer of complexity to visions of personalised drug treatment, The word, literally 'above genetics', has changed its connotation several times since it was coined seventy years ago, and just what it ought to mean is still a matter of (sometimes angry) debate. A recent definition will do for our purpose: an epigenetic (as opposed to genetic) trait is 'a stable heritable phenotype resulting from changes in a chromosome without alteration in the DNA sequence'. When deconstructed, this means a change in some physical characteristic, that is transmitted from parent to offspring (just like a gene), but has not arisen from a change in the sequence of nucleotides that defines a gene. What sort of change might this be? It is a chemical modification of nucleotides or of a protein attached to DNA in the chromosome, imposed by something in the environment or a metabolic malfunction. 'Stable' implies that the altered phenotype will pass down through the generations, and to the pedant this means 'the inheritance of an acquired characteristic', also known as Lamarckian inheritance (after Darwin's adversary, Jean-Baptiste Pierre Antoine de Monet, Chevalier de Lamarck), and a heresy in modern biology.

The most frequent of the chemical changes that affect our genetic material is methylation – the introduction of a methyl ($-CH_3$) group into a cytosine or adenine base (a C or A) by an enzyme, DNA methylase. It is the methylation of cytosines next to a guanine (G) that is of particular significance. Methylation in parts of the DNA that are not actually genes, but control the activity of their neighbouring genes are a normal and essential part of the life of the cell. It is when this process goes wrong, usually, but not always, in the direction of excessive methylation – hypermethylation - that trouble ensues. Regulation of gene expression breaks down, and one common consequence is a failure of the system that searches out and repairs errors in DNA that inevitably accompany replication of cells. Cancer is then the most likely result. Methylation also occurs in proteins, in particular on the histones, the small proteins that package the DNA into compact modules disposed at intervals along its length, and this too can affects gene expression. Because epigenetic changes are so prevalent and all so similar they present a formidable challenge for drug design. So far it seems to have been met only once. Myelodisplastic syndrome (MDS) comprises a set of leukaemia-like conditions, cancers of the bone marrow, which prevent the production of essential blood cells. It is treated by bone-marrow transplants or by injections of stem cells that will turn into blood cells. In victims of this disease hypermethylation has run riot, in fact some 600 genes in all are affected. In 2004 an American company, Celgene produced a new drug, 5-azacytidine, a modified nucleoside of the kind developed long before by George Hitchings and Gertrude Elion (p.). It was given the trade name, Vidaza, and its target was the enzyme, DNA methylase. To this was added another similar compound in which the ribose (the sugar in the nucleotide units of RNA) was replaced by deoxyribose, the sugar of DNA. The compound, which had actually first been synthesised by a Czech chemist thirty years before, 5-azadeoxycytidine was called decitabine. It was approved by the FDA for the treatment of MDS on the basis of total or partial improvement in 16% of the patients in a clinical trial. The European agency, the EMEA followed suit, and recommended Vidaza for patients who do not qualify for a stem-cell transplant. According to the European trial, the average survival compared to that with 'conventional treatment' rose from15.0 to 24.5 months; this amounted to a doubling of the proportion of patients surviving for two years – less than dramatic, it may appear, but an encouraging landmark in the long haul towards epigenetic drug therapy.

The mighty micro: miRNA

In 1993 a small research group at Dartmouth College in New Hampshire, led by Victor Ambros, made a strange discovery. They were studying embryo development in one of the favourite creatures of developmental biologists, a tiny worm, called *Caenorhabditis elegans*, and they found a very small piece of RNA, consisting of only 22 nucleotides, in the cells of the larvae, without which maturation could not proceed. This was thought initially to be a curious idiosyncrasy of the worm, but early in the next decade identical RNA molecules came to light in higher organisms, including mammals. Thus the small RNAs with their characteristic nucleotide sequences had been preserved through the evolutionary millennia, a sure indication that they are essential for life. These miRNAs, as they are now called, are transcribed like messenger RNA (p.) from the DNA, but unlike the messenger they do not carry a message coding for a protein. The human genome appears to encode more than a thousand miRNAs. They have been found to exert a regulatory effect, both positive and negative, on the expression of genes. They do this by attaching to complementary regions of messenger RNA or DNA, in other words all or a sizeable stretch of their nucleotides pair off with a sequence on their target nucleic acid (C with G, and A with T in DNA or with U in RNA). This association can most obviously be used to silence a target gene. Or it may stifle the function of the messenger for a particular gene by impeding its attachment to the ribosome – the reading-head on which translation into protein occurs (p.) – or preventing the message carried by the messenger from being read off.

Studies with genetically engineered mice - deprived of a gene of interest, or been given instead an abnormal, or a human version of that gene, or have had the segment of DNA coding for an miRNAof choice artificially disabled - have yielded an abundance of information on miRNA function. The first such experiment showed that mice lacking just one of the many miRNA genes died young from a hole in the heart. Many diseases have by now been linked to mutant miRNAs, and since miRNAs are estimated to interact with about 60% of all genes, this has opened a large new field of research. An RNA of the size of any natural miRNA with an identical or complementary sequence is easily synthesised by automated methods, and procedures can in principle be designed to suppress an injurious gene or increase the production of a desired protein. But the problems of developing therapies on this basis are nonetheless far from trivial. Much needs to be known about the range of possible activities of an miRNA to ensure that a complementary polynucleotide does not cause mayhem in the cell. And of course the means have to be found to induce the molecule to pass reliably into cells. An industry has arisen around miRNAs, and hopes are high. So far only one compound appears to have secured FDA approval as an orphan drug. This has been marketed by a biotechnology company, and is intended as a therapy for a genetic condition (polycythaemia rubra vera), which causes overproduction of red blood cells and some white cells. (This normally requires the bearer of the disease to be bled at about monthly intervals.) Many more miRNA remedies* are being pursued, and aficionados hold that they will bring About a huge range of new therapeutic options.

---

* This line of research is not to be confused with a much earlier, and now largely abandoned route of RNA therapy, known as *antisense*. DNA contains the genes in one of its two strands, called the coding, or sense strand, whereas the nucleotide sequence of the complementary strand carries no message, and is termed the antisense strand. If one constructs a piece of RNA with a sequence complementary to the coding sequence for a gene, it will bind to the gene sequence to form a piece of double helix. When a gene is expressed its sequence in the DNA is copied into an RNA, the messenger (p.), which is read off on the protein synthesising machinery, and the encoded protein is produced. In principle a piece of antisense RNA introduced into the cell can thus prevent production of the protein by sequestering the messenger RNA in the double helical state. This of course can only succeed in curing a disease that is caused by a single aberrant gene, or prevent the replication of a virus. Attempts were therefore made to develop antisense therapies against viruses, but only one such drug was ever approved. This was called formivirsen (trade name Vitravene), and was designed to combat cytomegalovirus, a herpes-like virus, which is generally quite harmless, except in immunologically compromised patients, whom it can dosome damage, especially to the eyes. Antisense therapy is of limited effectiveness, because it does not prevent more messenger RNA from being produced, and formivirsen, which was introduced in 1995, was withdrawn ten years later.

Chapter 19

THE CONDUCT OF DRUG RESEARCH: THE SHAPE OF THINGS TO COME

What goes in and what comes out

An attendant at a crematorium reportedly confessed that it was for him an eternal source of fascination how much went in and how little came out. It has often been said that the pharmaceutical industry is in crisis for exactly this reason. The investment in research and development has risen relentlessly in recent years, unmatched by any rise in the emergence of genuinely novel drugs - those defined as 'new chemical entities' (NCEs), and not mere derivatives of the old (comprising, 'me-too' compounds and reformulated versions and mixtures of two or more established drugs). The *true* cost of bringing a new drug to market is a subject of controversy. The figure given by the industry in the U.S. has for some time hovered around $1.3 billion, and a little less in Europe. In 1995 the sum was about $125 million, so it rose a hundredfold in less than three decades. A different, and some say more meaningful way to compute the cost is to factor in the lost investment in drugs that failed, for the success rate is no more than 7%. The cost extracted on this basis rises to a staggering $4.5 billion. But there are also quite different opinions, most trenchantly articulated by Marcia Angell, former editor of the foremost American medical journal, the *New England Journal of Medicine*, and by the English doctor and writer,

Ben Goldacre. The case for an effectively much lower average cost to the company rests on the undoubted fact that in the vast majority of cases the research that points the way to a conceptually new treatment comes from research done in a state- or sometimes charity-funded project, based in a university department or a national research institute or foundation. (Prominent institutions are the National Institutes of Health in the U.S., the Medical Research Council and the Wellcome Foundation in Britain, INSERM (the Institut National de la Santé et de la Recherche Médicale) in France, The Max-Planck Society in Germany, and so on.)

This has been true since the birth of Big Pharma, but a different kind of relation with academic researchers has developed more recently, to the point that many university laboratories are now financially dependent on a pharmaceutical company. Governments have sought to foster such arrangements, partly because economically 'relevant', or 'translational' research is the current mantra, and partly also to reduce the pressure on public funds. The company thereby acquires skilled research at modest cost, but for the scientists there are disadvantages, especially constraints on the choice of research topics, and as already mentioned (p.), restrictions imposed by the company on publication of results. Nevertheless, the system has operated reasonably smoothly. All the same, there is no denying that the industry, for all its huge profits, is in crisis. Despite the continuing growth in spending (however measured), the rate of invention of new drugs has remained practically unchanged throughout the years of the new millennium onwards. So between 2003 and 2008, for instance, the global annual expenditure on research and development rose by a third, while the rate of discovery of genuinely new drugs ('new molecular entities') remained about the same. (The number has fluctuated between 20 and 25 per year, lower than in the mid-20th century.) Nor has the quality of the new drugs in terms of efficacy and extent of side-effects changed a great deal. The expected benefits from the information flooding in out of research on human genes, and on the function and the structure of proteins have not yet eventuated to any great extent. (That, though, must surely come.)

Among the suggested explanations for the relative stagnation of pharmaceutical discovery is the possibility that the bulk of the 'low-hanging fruit'(to use the current cliché) has been plucked, and what remains is hard to reach. Another theory attributes the problem to the changes that have overtaken the structure of the industry, beginning in the latter part of the last century. The enormously productive pharmaceutical companies of modest size from which the modern industry sprang, directed by visionary scientists, are long gone. The smallest were absorbed by the larger, which then merged with others, or were swallowed in their turn, until today there are only gigantic, bloated global concerns. These are directed not by scientists but by moguls from the financial sector, whose duty is to the shareholders. This stifles originality and the willingness to take risks. Consequently innovation now comes increasingly from biotechnology companies, all but a few quite small, all run by scientists, who foster an adventurous and collegial spirit. It is striking that, whereas only half a century earlier it was the larger companies that produced the great major majority of genuinely new drugs, the NMEs, they have now been equalled or overtaken by the smallest ones.

Old friends in new clothes: drug 'repurposing'

This barbaric word has recently crept into the drug-trade vocabulary. The history of drugs, as the alert reader may have noticed, is shot through with accidental discoveries, here an anti-diabetes drug that cures a bacterial infection, there an antidepressant that finds an application in urology. Especially in hard times, a re-examination of current or superseded products for unforeseen virtues is at least as attractive as the creation of more 'me-too' compounds. And what of all the compounds that proved a failure in clinical trials, but were never explicitly tried for uses never envisaged? Sir James Black, one of the luminaries of 20th-century pharmacology (p.), opined that 'the most fruitful basis for the discovery of a new drug is to start with an old drug', and he adhered to this principle to no little effect. It is a course that the drug companies are beginning to take, and will no doubt pursue further. For one thing, no more than one-tenth or so of the 10,000 compounds that have ever undergone a clinical trial are protected by a patent, and for another, they will have been subjected to toxicity testing, duration in the body, and so on, at least in animals. There may even be evidence of successful off-label use by doctors. In general then, if the compound has been approved by the FDA or equivalent body for use against one disorder, it will much more easily gain approval against another. Drug companies all have immense collections of compounds held in limbo; some estimates suggest that, between them all, there may be at least 100,000. Procuring an existing compound for testing is easy if it is stored in-house, but to re-synthesise one or a set of substances would be expensive. There have therefore been moves to establish collections, ot 'libraries' of compounds by commercial or governmentally-funded organisations. Some such indeed already exist, but their collections are small compared to those belonging to the pharmaceutical companies. There is a, perhaps utopian, vision of an all-encompassing global resource, to which the companies will contribute for the common good.

What's wrong with the clinical trial?

Clinical trials form a major part of the drug development process, in terms of time, skill and especu=ially cost. The costs of trials were rising until the drug companies hit on a stratagem. According to Marcia Angell, writing in 2002, the proportion of the expenditure by a typical pharmaceutical company on Research and Development was 15%, while twice that amount went into marketing and advertising, to be set against a profit margin of some 20%. Clinical trials, though certainly expensive, are most often left to specialist companies, which have proliferated in many parts of the world. These 'contract research organisations' perform the work more cheaply and often less fastidiously than the researchers in academic institutions, who used to be the backbone of the system. The contract research bodies take instructions, relating to the organisation of the trials and the selection of patients, from the client company, and their pecuniary interest will tend to make them more tractable than the academics. Nor do they have any interest in publishing the data. As we have seen, the results of the trials, at least in the U.S., are often unavailable to all but the FDA, which treats them as confidential. This situation shows signs of changing, due to pressure from academic and political sources. To an extent, indeed, the secrecy has already been breached by investigative journalists and academics by recourse to Freedom of Information legislation.

A large proportion of the clinical trials are actually now quite small affairs, not aimed at evaluating new drugs. 'Phase IV' trials were originally intended as investigations, sometimes demanded by the FDA or an equivalent regulatory agency, into the performance of a drug that had been in use for some time. In many cases the instigation has been a concern about previously undetected side-effects. But in the last two decades the purpose has more commonly been profit than illumination. The producers want their drug to be prescribed for a wider range of conditions than that for which it was originally licensed, and the trial will thus not be confined to patients with that condition. Such trials can be quite perfunctory because, after all, the critical matter of side-effects would have been settled when the drug was approved the first time round. And of course publication of the drug's extended reach, and lavish advertisements cab impress themselves on the minds of doctors, and keep the contract contract research organisations profitably occupied.

The fundamental structure of the clinical trial has not changed since the concept was first introduced. The idea has taken root in some circles that it is too expensive, too cumbersome, and no longer meets modern demands. A number of innovations have been seriously discussed. One common concern is that the rigid nature of the current procedure, which results in the rejection of the great majority of the compounds subjected to drug trials (50% even in Phase III, and a far greater proportion in the earlier stages), may mean that valuable drugs are discarded. A proposed measure to reduce such waste is the so-called 'Phase 0 trial'. The proposal is to give a small number of volunteers minute amounts of the compound – one-hundredth or less of the presumptive therapeutic dose. The number of subjects put at risk of side-effects would be very small, and toxicity at such concentrations would in general be minimal, but modern analytical techniques would allow determination of essential features, such as the lifetime of the substance in the body, its metabolic transformations, and whether, or to what extent, it reaches its intended target. Another route to more effective trials would depend on the prospects of personalised therapy for the condition in question. If it is known that the ailment is associated with particular genetic forms (genotypes) of a protein – as, for instance, is breast cancer, then the participants in a drug trial could be selected according to genotype. In this way a clear result would emerge, supposing that, as is often the case, the drug is more effective, or is only effective, against the condition in the one class of patients. This of course would require a genetic test to be performed on all potential recruits. Pharmaceutical companies are beginning now to provide genetic testing kits with certain drugs, so the approach is undoubtedly feasible, but the gain in efficiency could be offset by the cost of such stringent selection of trial participants. A widely discussed innovation is the so-called adaptive trial. This embodies the seemingly heretical option of a change of direction in mid-trial, that is to say switching subjects between the groups. So if a new drug appears clearly more effective than a control drug or placebo, patients could be moved without their knowledge into the drug group to increase the statistical strength of the ultimate conclusion, and also possibly help to identify genetic differences that may be associated with an altered result. This scheme has drawn opposition from some experts, but is apparently being increasingly tried. One further proposal is to streamline recruitment for trials by establishing networks of centres, mainly hospitals, which maintain records of genetic and other tests, and can contribute participants.

There have been second thoughts even about the pre-trial stages of drug development, such as animal testing. One proposition that has been aired is to treat the animals more like human patients, in the sense that the seriously ill often do not receive a drug, and especially a drug 'of last resort', until other medications have failed. The metabolism of a drug is often changed by exposure of a patient to another drug, or more often several drugs. The suggestion is that drugs should be tested in such a regime, rather than only in isolation. Drug researchers are increasingly forced to listen to the dictates of epidemiologists and statisticians, and it is they who are mainly now formulating new strategies of drug testing.

Better placebos!

Placebo is a curious word, which reached its present meaning by an uncertain route. The Latin word, *placebo* means I shall please. It occurs, in the Roman Catholic Latin rite, in the Office of the Dead, and translates as, "I shall please the Lord in the land of the living". Then in medieval times it attracted another connotation, that of servility or sycophancy, therefore 'intending to flatter or please'. And so it entered medicine as something given to the patient, not as a cure but as a comfort. The idea that such an offering can do more than console and lift the morale a little, and can can ease suffering or help recovery goes back to ancient times, foreshadows, in a sense, the modern concept. The great 16th-century physician and surgeon, Ambroise Paré (p.) wrote, with elegant concision, that a doctor's function was *'guérir quelquefois, soulager souvent, consoler toujours'* – cure sometimes, relieve often, console always. 'Placebo' was used in this sense of consoling until well into the 20th century, and attained its present meaning as a control in a clinical trial only in the 1930s.

The double-blind placebo-controlled randomised clinical trial has held sway for half a century, but its deficiencies have become clear only in the last decade. The introduction of the procedure owed much to a publication in 1955 in the *New England Journal of Medicine* by a professor of anaesthetics at one of the major clinical centres associated with Harvard University, the Massachusetts General Hospital in Boston. Henry Beecher (*né* Unangst in Kansas in 1904) had been responsible for the codification of ethical principles of human experimentation, including that of 'informed consent' by the subjects.[*] His publication did much to convince doctors in America and around the world of the power of the placebo, although later work showed Beecher's trials to have been badly designed, for he had omitted to consider the number of patients who would have got better during the period of the trial, whose symptoms might have varied from day to day, and so on. But this did not diminish the influence of Beecher's paper, which became for the most part the accepted wisdom and also stimulated

---

[*] The irony was that after his death in 1976 historical documents were discovered that exposed Beecher as a collaboraord with the CIA in some highly questionable experiments on prisoners in Germany after World War II.

much research on the nature and reach of the placebo effect. It was only in 2001 that two Danish scientists breached the general consensus with a paper published, once again in the *New England Journal of Medicine*, with the provocative title, 'Is the Placebo Powerless?' The answer, according to Asbjørn Hróbjartsson and Peter Gøtzsche, was essentially 'yes', insofar as they saw 'little evidence in general that placebos had powerful effects'. They based their conclusion on a meta-analysis of a range of clinical trials. The paper appears to have caused some consternation, but later scrutiny revealed the expected weaknesses. The study confined itself to trials in which the results for the patients on the placebo were compared with those of patients who received nothing at all. The only (modest) positive result was for trials in which there was only a subjective estimate of benefit – patients feeling better or judged by doctors to *appear* better, but with no measurable criterion, such as reduced blood pressure or red blood cell count. This of course eliminates the important psychological element. For a simple yes-and-no test (better or not better) there was no placebo effect. But the survey reveals that there was more of a placebo effect in small than in large trials, which can be explained only by biased assessment of the subjects.

By the time Hróbtartsson and Gøtzsch's paper was published the evidence for the potency of placebos was in fact already overwhelming, as will appear, and indeed proof had been available for more than two centuries from the continuing survival of homeopathy, which treats the sick by giving them a little water to swallow (p.). The placebo control will remain an inseparable part of drug development, but the subtlety and complexity of the phenomenon has only recently been recognised, and is starting to change the form of clinical trials. One innovation that is now taking root is the concept of the active placebo. We have seen that in conventional placebo-controlled trials of SSRI antidepressants, the placebo effect accounts for about 80% of the perceived benefit (p.). The psychologist, Irving Kirsch extracted this result from published and previously unpublished clinical trials, but he went further: he discovered that none of these trials were properly blinded, for the participants, though not told whether they would be receiving the drug or the placebo, were warned that the drug had side-effects, which might cause then to experience headaches, stomach upsets, or other bearable forms of discomfort. If, then, they were not troubled by such an effect they could deduce that they had been given the placebo (whereas of course, the onset of a head- or stomach-ache would raise the patients' expectation that the pill would be doing them good). The remedy was obvious: ensure that the placebo would contain a harmless substance that would provoke the same kind of symptom. When the patients in the control groups in SSRI trials were given such an 'active', or 'powerful' placebo the residual 20% of the therapeutic effect, thought to have been exerted by the drug, vanished almost completely. This raises the important question of how much more value people taking the drug are getting for their considerable outlay of money than they would get from a sugar pill. That naturally leads to an ethical dilemma: can people properly not be sold sugar pills masquerading as drugs if they alleviate suffering? If the answer is yes, might we not then find ourselves returning to the (perhaps then, not so evil) days of the itinerant quacks. Then again, there have been many recorded cases of placebos working for patients even after they have been told that they are taking nothing but tiny amounts of sugar, and demanding, after learning the truth, that the 'medication' be continued. The fact is that, according to a study by American researchers, published in 2008, 58% of U.S. GPs and rheumatologists routinely prescribed placebos.

But there is more. The effect of a placebo, whether it is the shadow of a drug against pain, stomach acid, asthma, or some other affliction, depends acutely on how it is administered. It is known from many trials that a large pill is generally more effective than a small, two pills than one, a capsule than a pill, and the colour of a pill also counts. As far back as 1972, a group of researchers tested the effects of sugar pills on the concentration of medical students attending a (presumably tedious) lecture. They were told that they would receive either a stimulant or a sedative. Some were then given a single pill, and some two, and some, moreover, were pink and others blue. The outcome was that two sugar pills were better than one, that red sugar pills were most often identified as stimulants, and the blue as sedatives.*

Packaging, as the industry is fully aware, and as the breakdown of its expenditure shows, is an important part of the placebo effect, and so too is novelty. Dr Ben Goldacre has unearthed the interesting fact that the reported effectiveness of the first rational stomach-ulcer remedy, cimetidine (p.) fell over five years from 80% at its inception to 50%. The drop appeared largely to coincide with the introduction of a new drug, ranitidine (although such factors as more colourful advertising could have had something to do with it). Even the greatest minds can be snared by the placebo effect. Linus Pauling, who changed the face of chemistry in the 20th century, and won the Nobel Prize for his many seminal contributions (and the Nobel Peace Prize as well, for good measure) was one. Pauling persuaded himself that vitamin C, consumed in gargantuan doses, lifted his spirits, his health and his strength, and in particular banished the common colds that had plagued him for most of his life. He published a book on the subject in 1970, and soon much of the American populace was buying vitamin C from pharmacies and supermarkets. Pauling then became deranged and proclaimed that vitamin C, taken with equally excessive amounts of vitamin E, β-carotene (which is converted in the body to vitamin A) and the trace element, selenium would encompass the conquest of cancer, diabetes, cardiovascular disease,

---

* There are other examples of how the mind can be deceived in this way. In 2001 a neurobiologist at the University of Bordeaux, Frédéric Brochet assembled a group of fifty-seven wine experts and subjected them to a series of tests of taste acuity. In the first he placed before each a glass of high-quality white and a glass of fake red wine, which was nothing more than the same white wine coloured with a red dye. The tasting reports adhered precisely to the terminology that wine writers use to describe white and to red wines (steely dry, gooseberry on the nose and so on for on the one hand, full-bodied, with good depth and well-balanced tannin and the like, on the other). Brochet conducted a similar faked trial of a single wine from two bottles, one with a label proclaiming it to be a *grand cru*, the other a *gros rouge*. Again the experts came up with descriptions apposite to the label, rather than the wine. It would be absurd to conclude that wine experts were all charlatans, nor did Brochet do so. The lesson to be drawn is that the senses do not function in isolation, and are all too easily misled, most treacherously perhaps by the accompanying visual impressions - colour, label, ambience and so on in the case of the wine – and fail to overcome the spurious evidence of the first powerful impact.

arthritis, asthma, and a long litany of other afflictions, great and small, and stop the ravages of age.* He was unperturbed by the results of full clinical trials conducted in several medical schools – for Pauling's name carried great authority showed that this exacting regime had no effect on the incidence or relief of the common cold or cancer. Some trials even continued after his own death in 1994 (from cancer), with the same outcome. It is likely that his wife's death from cancer was hastened by her husband's insistence that she be treated with nothing but his vitamin remedy. Several clinical trials have now established that, so far from lengthening life and reducing illness, ingestion of vitamins much beyond the range of concentrations found in the normal diet, actually increased the risk of cancers and other diseases. (An exception has been made for the anti-rickettsial vitamin D, which is recommended for post-menopausal women to keep osteoporosis at bay. Folic acid deficiency is also to be avoided in pregnancy.) What is most striking is that, despite warnings to this effect by health agencies, and the pointlessness, at best, of taking vitamin supplements, their consumption has risen rather than diminished since Pauling's time, and it is now a billion-dollar business in the developed world, most of all in the U.S. In the 1990s a long struggle developed between the FDA, attempting to curb the extravagant advertising claims for diet supplements, and Congress, which largely took the side of the industry. It seems, the with public is still in thrall to Pauling and to vitamins generally, that the FDA has never fully got its way. There is no shortage of testimonials to the health-giving virtues of diet supplements. The placebo rules.

---

* Pauling, the great chemist, naturally had a rationale for ingesting all this: vitamin C (ascorbic acid) and vitamin E, namely that they are both reducing agents. Oxidative reactions in the metabolism, in particular in the mitochondria, the energy-generating bodies in our cells (p.) produce *free radicals*, molcules containing a surplus electron. Free radicals (primarily, so far as living organisms are concerned, oxygen radicals) are highly reactive, and can do damage to substances that they encounter. They can, for instance, induce mutations in DNA. Pauling came to believe that deterioration due to age and disease was due to ravages caused by free radicals. The two vitamins fall into the class of free-radical 'scavengers'. The action of anti-oxidants, in practice free-radical scavengers, was a preoccupation of many biochemists and medical researchers in the latter part of the 20th century, and the nature and extent of their activity jn nature is still a subject of debate, but for several good reasons interest in the subject has waned in recent years.

These effects are not restricted to the mind, for physiological responses can also often be detected. Functional magnetic resonance imaging (fMRI) gives physiologists the means, for example, of observing biochemical changes in the brain and spinal cord engendered by pain. In 2009 German researchers induced pain by applying heat to the arms of volunteers, telling them that the purpose was evaluation of a local anaesthetic. Some volunteers were told that the cream smeared on the site of the heat was the anaesthetic, and others that it was a control. It was the same inert cream in all cases, but the nerve response in the pain receptors of the spine was reduced only in those subjects who believed they had been protected by an active painkilling cream. This kind of phenomenon clearly has its limits, for a placebo will not cure a cancer, mend a broken leg, or even reduce blood pressure in the long term, but there are innumerable indications that it will often help to mobilise the body's own defensive mechanisms.

All the foregoing does still not exhaust the ramifications of the placebo effect, for it also acts in another way – by raising the expectation of relief. Thus the doctor standing over the patient with a syringe creates hope, which trials have shown to exert a physiological effect: 1995, for illustration, saw the appearance of a landmark paper from the laboratory of one of the pioneers in the field, Fabrizio Benedetti in the medical school of the University of Turin. Proglumide is, among other things, an agonist of a receptor in the brain on which the body's opioid compounds react in response to pain. The drug's intended use is to treat gastric disturbances, but it has a secondary action in stimulating the activity of an opioid receptor in the brain, thereby enhancing the effect of substances such as morphine or of the body's own pain-relieving secretions. What Benedetti and his colleagues examined the efficacy of proglumide for the relief of pain experienced by patients recovering from surgery, and found that it performed markedly better than a placebo. An effective painkiller, then? Actually, no. The drug had been delivered by injection in full view of the patient, but then Benedetti and his team tried injecting it surreptitiously, so that the patients were unaware of what was happening, and then the difference between drug and placebo vanished. So proglumide is not a painkiller, but exerted its placebo effect in the first trial by exciting the patients' expectation of the verbally promised analgesia. Opioid release is only one of the known pathways by which pain arises, and Benedetti and others have used an established analgesic, naloxone, which is known to block the opioid pathway, to study how other pathways respond to a placebo. It turns out that the expectation of analgesia allows a placebo to work both with and without the intervention of naloxone. If, on the other hand, the subject, treated with naloxone and given pain, is led by the doctor not to expect relief from the placebo, then the placebo will not work. This means that the expectation effect operates on both opioid-dependent and independent pathways. The placebo effect in such circumstances is a genuinely physiological, and not merely psychological phenomenon, for opioids, whether extraneous or endogenous, do more than suppress pain: they also lower respiration and heartbeat, and this is also occasioned by the placebo. It is worth noting finally that real drugs are also placebos: morphine is more effective in stilling pain when openly injected into the patient than when given surreptitiously. All these considerations do not of course apply only to analgesia; so for instance, movement control in people with Parkinson's disease has been found to improve due to expectation when they receive a placebo, and at the same time dopamine activity in the brain increases.

This kind of informative comparison between an overt and a concealed administration of drugs is remarkably powerful, and can be exploited in a particularly economical way. Trial patients are divided into two groups, both of which are given the same dose of the drug; the first group receives it by an unconcealed injection, while the second are infused by a physiological saline solution to which, at an undisclosed time, the drug is added. These patients know therefore that they will be receiving the drug, which will work – relieve their pain, say – but not when it will be administered. Both groups will know the real time interval between injection and subsidence of the pain, but this will not help the second group. The patients in the first group will experience a placebo effect, to which the second group is not subject. These patients will report the alleviation of pain only when the drug enters the vein. The greater the difference in pain relief between the two groups, regardless of the time at which the effect is reported, is then a measure of the extent of the placebo effect, despite the absence of any pure placebo from the trial. This device eliminates many of the problems attaching to the conventional placebo-controlled trial. There can be little doubt that it will influence the future evolution of the clinical trial.

New means to an old end

It will be obvious from the foregoing chapters that, until relatively recently, the creation of new drugs was a rather haphazard affair. Even with the advent of target-directed drug design, it has still required the synthesis of often thousands of derivatives of a lead compound, and innumerable animal assays, to arrive at a useful compound. The main concern now is to make the whole process more efficient and economical. One important direction is the use of cultured cells for the evaluation of new derivatives. This is not new in principle, but the methods of manipulating cells in culture have been evolving rapidly. Mammalian (and other) cells have been cultured in the laboratory since the early decades of the last century, thanks to early research into the nutrient substances that must be included in the culture medium if the cells are to grow and divide. Even so, cell culture was an uncertain and rather arcane area of biology, which required skill, experience and much patience. Moreover, different cultures from the same type of cell showed differences, and worse, the cells in culture would divide only 40 to 60 times before the culture died – the so-called Hayflick limit after the researcher who established the effect in 1962. The reason for this is now understood, and stems from a kind of molecular clock, the telomere, which is a part of the cell's DNA. The telomeres shorten by one base-pair at each cell division, and when they have been totally eroded the cell dies. The Hayflick limit can now be overcome by introducing into the cell a virus gene, which disrupts the cell cycle - the process of growth, maturation and finally division into a pair of daughter cells. Or the telomeres can be protected by adding an inhibitor of the enzyme that trims them down. Either method of beating the Hayflick limit leads to what is termed as immortalisation. This is in practice done, starting from a single cell, which becomes the progenitor of an endless succession of generations of identical cells (clones). These can then be maintained indefinitely in culture, and are called a cell line.

First Do No Harm

Such a limitless supply of essentially identical copies of cells from human brain, liver, kidney or any other source, makes up a very reliable base on which to test the action of a new compound. But this still leaves the problem of presenting the drug to its target. The great majority of drug targets are proteins, generally enzymes or receptors (p.). An enzyme known to be implicated in a disease, or the gene encoding that enzyme can be introduced into the cell by the standard methods of molecular genetics. The enzyme can also be modified by attachment of a fluorescent marker, which will cause a cell containing that enzyme to light up under ultraviolet light. This allows the fate of the enzyme to be followed in the cell, and it also enables a population of such cells to be isolated in an instrument that separates fluorescent from dark cells. The health of the cell, or various of its properties before and after exposure to a possible drug can then be examined. Similarly fluorescence detection can allow the extent of expression of the enzyme by the alien gene to be followed. This is an immensely powerful and sensitive way to identify compounds of possible interest. The sensitivity comes from the 'high-throughput' screening (HTS) methods now in routine use and being continually refined further. These methods owe much to robotics and nanotechnology, but one common factor has been a simple standard item of equipment in use for at least 25 years now. This is the microtitre, or micro-well plate. It is nothing more than a transparent plastic plate with a square grid of small wells moulded into its surface. There may be 96 wells in each plate, or multiples of 96, up to 9600, each serving as a reaction vessel, holding a small volume of a test solution or cell suspension. The volume may be as little as some nanolitres (ten billionths of a litre), or even now picolitres (a thousand times smaller yet); this is important when many samples of a precious compound, synthesised with difficulty, is the test substance. The liquid is dispensed by a robotic device, capable of metering such minuscule volumes. (There is even a special nanotechnology devoted to the handling of the minute volumes of liquids, called microfluidics [see below].) A test compound to be studied at a series of concentrations or over periods of time, or both, is introduced into the wells, or a number of compounds can be tested and compared on a single plate. The intensity of fluorescence, which reflects the extent or course of a reaction between the test compound and the enzyme or receptors in or on the cells, say, is measured in each of the wells, aligned automatically one at a time beneath the detector of the fluorescence. By this means, standard equipment allows millions of samples to be measured in a matter of hours, and the results processed by an integrated computer. This of course is incomparably faster and cheaper than the drug assays of old, in test-tubes or in animals, and the identification of a lead compound – something with at least a measurable effect - is correspondingly accelerated. There are many technological variants of microtitre analysis, which is widely applied, not only in research, but most of all in diagnosis, as performed in many hospital laboratories. (Here the wells, or chips, may contain a range of normal and mutant gene fragments or proteins [p.].) In drug research the methods of nanotechnology are also entering into the synthesis of new compounds.

A mirror for Caliban

Yet the heady power and scope of this technology, and the speed with which it produces results carries a certain danger. The sheer volume of new data can create an illusory sense of achievement. The increased pace of discovery, as reflected at least in the vast output of publications in learned journals, has not been matched, as we have seen, and as many have remarked, by the emergence of valuable new drugs. There have been critical analyses of the reliability of published data with, in many cases, embarrassing results. The situation, according to two cancer researchers, writing in 2012, is worst in their own field. They have taken 53 'landmark' papers in cancer research, and determined the proportion that have stood up to the cardinal criterion of reproducibility. The answer was a shameful 13%. A similar German study on a selected set of papers came up with a proportion of 25%. Moreover, the majority of reported research that proved irreproducible, and therefore generally valueless, had led to a secondary tier of scientific literature reporting results based on the previous incorrect, or at least seriously flawed conclusions. This is clearly an intolerable situation. The authors of the American study note that cancer research is one of the most difficult subject for biomedical inquiry because of the complexity of the systems. They suggest that many of the problems stem from the use of too few, and sometimes poorly defined, cell lines, and others from putting excessive faith in animal assays, while disregarding the special environment of a tumour in a human organ. They make a number of recommendations, among which are that no research making use of cell lines, should be regarded as complete unless the experiments have been conducted on several different cell lines. There should be more extensive collaboration between different laboratories, with cross-checking of observations and exchanges of materials. Experiments should be performed by 'blinded' researchers, just as clinical trials routinely are. And in addition editors of journals should be more discriminating.

The power of structure

The best starting point for the invention of a drug that will work by blocking the action of a protein - an enzyme or receptor - is its structure. Determination of a protein structure by X-ray crystallography was a formidable, indeed as many experts thought, impossible proposition. In 1961 two chemists in Cambridge, John Kendrew and Max Perutz succeeded. They and their teams solved the structures of two closely related proteins, myoglobin, the oxygen-carrying protein of muscle, and haemoglobin, the four times larger protein, haemoglobin, which transports oxygen in the blood and gives it its red colour. Perutz had begun on the quest nearly twenty years earlier, and Kendrew soon after. Theirs had been a heroic undertaking, and it won them the Nobel Prize in 1962. Like all heroic pioneering endeavours, protein structure determination, while never easy, became a commonplace. Better methods of growing good crystals, improving instrumentation, and above all, the modern computer, brought about an astonishing surge in the number of protein structures solved, which ran into tens of thousands. In addition another technique entered the field; this was nuclear magnetic resonance spectroscopy, which allowed, equally laboriously at the start, structures of at least the smaller proteins to be solved, without the need of crystallisation. To date, this accounts for about 10% of the known structures, but because it delivers the structures in free solution, it often has advantages. In any case, examination of a protein structure, assisted by biochemical evidence, generally allows the site of its action to be identified. In an enzyme this is called the active centre (p.), and it is the part of the structure, most often a cavity, at which the substrate – the substance that the enzyme destroys or alters – offers itself. Knowing the precise structure of the active centre, and the amino acid side chains (p.) of which it is constructed, a chemist can now try to devise a compound that will fit tightly into the active site, and so block the enzyme's action. The same principle will hold true for a receptor that can usefully be blocked. It is also now evident that the great majority of processes in the cell involve interactions between different proteins. Work is therefore proceeding to compile a map (the 'interactome') of the vast number of such interactions, often transient and sometimes involving several different protein molecules at a time, happening at the different stages of the cell's life. To understand how these work the interfaces between two proteins need to be defined, just like enzyme-substrate interactions. Structure determination may therefore often be the best starting point for the design of many types of drugs, meant to impede these associations. There are nevertheless many situations in which it cannot be applied, as when the target is unknown, beyond the organ in which it is located, or is not an enzyme or a single receptor. Nevertheless, about 300 proteins and some RNAs have so far been defined as possible therapeutic targets.

The march of chemistry

The other respect in which the craft of drug development is changing is that synthetic chemistry has become vastly easier and more versatile in the last two decades. There is a widely held belief that the great majority of future drugs will be small molecules, as opposed to macromolecules (proteins, nucleic acids or carbohydrates). Monoclonal antibodies are a clear exception, likely to remain with us for many years to come, and similarly some short peptides of a few amino acids and micro RNAs (miRNAs), too short to count as macromolecules. The scope for the creation of new 'molecular entities' is almost limitless. In 2007 two chemists calculated how many possible compounds could in principle be made, consisting of 11 atoms in any combinations of carbon, nitrogen, oxygen and fluorine, the constituents elements of the greatest proportion of known drugs. The answer was more than 26 million. But the number of currently known compounds, at least as listed in accessible databases, is a mere 0.24% of that. Eleven atoms make quite a small compound, so the space for chemists to bustle in is boundless. The drug companies have probably already screened between them for various purposes a range of of compounds running into millions. Chemists' task in generating compounds of altogether new classes to keep pace with high-throughput screening is made easier by new synthetic methods, allied to fast techniques for validating the structures of the products. Nuclear magnetic resonance (NMR) is a technique that has changed the face of chemistry. Most often it is proton magnetic resonance that is used for the identification of small molecules[*]

The second and equally important method of identifying a compound is mass spectrometry, which in its modern guise uses a minute amount of the material to deliver its precise molecular weight. The molecular weight of the compound supposedly synthesised is merely the sum of the atomic weights of the constituent atoms (carbon, nitrogen, hydrogen, and whatever others may be present). If this agrees with the measured value then the chances are high that it is indeed the right compound. If it does not, then the chemist can calculate the molecular weights of possible alternative products that his attempted synthesis may have created to find one that matches. The limitation of mass spectrometry is that it will not distinguish between isomers – compounds with the same atomic composition but different structures. It is thus a more restricted technique than NMR, but the two are often used in tandem.

Chemists now have many aids, undreamed of a few decades ago, to synthesis. One is the lab-on-a-chip, which is increasingly encroaching on conventional chemistry in drug research. The lab-on-a-chip is a micro-fabricated device, generally a centimetre or two in size, in which, with

---

[*] The proton is the nucleus of the hydrogen atom, and the method discriminates between hydrogen atoms in different environments in the structure. The spectrum is thus a kind of fingerprint of the structure, as reflected by the hydrogen atoms that it contains. NMR, as indicated above, is used not only to identify, but also to determine structures, even of large molecules, such as proteins, although this is a much more complex and demanding application. At this level spectra can also be generated by other atomic nuclei, in particular carbon and nitrogen, and these also give structural information, important for structure determination.

the aid of microfluidics (the manipulation of fluid volumes down to the picolitre level. (1 pl = 10^{-12} litre, or a million millionth of a litre), serial chemical operations (steps in a synthesis, separations of intermediate products and so on) can proceed. The advantages are economy of materials and labour, and greatly enhanced speed of reactions because of the small volumes within which the reactants are allowed to diffuse, and the possibility of running many such chips in parallel. Another option open to chemists is *combinatorial chemistry*. This is a method of producing thousands, even millions of compounds by successive synthetic steps, in which the chemical building blocks are joined together in an endless variety of permutations. There are several routes towards this end, but they all have in common their reliance on what is called solid-phase synthesis. In a typical procedure each of the possible starting components, commonly about five, is chemically attached to a patterned reactive surface, each to its own little compartment. Then robots deliver a new reactive building-block, from the same selection of five, to each tethered starting component, and the process is repeated. Very soon the surface will display a huge range of compounds, each comprising a unique combination and sequence of the five components. The products can then be assayed on the chip for binding to a biologically interesting target compound, a protein, say, exactly as on an analytical microarray (p.).

A strategy for the discovery of new drugs has come into vogue as an alternative to high-throughput screening of a vast multitude of essentially randomly generated compounds. This is the fragment-based method. It will be clear from what has gone before that the structures of nearly all drugs embody several chemical groups. To take a simple example, an aminophenol would be defined by a hydroxyl (-OH) attached to a benzene ring of six carbon atoms, with an amino group ($-NH_2$) at another corner of the ring. The therapeutic properties of the compound will vary according to what groups it contains, and where in these structures they are located. Assuming that each group makes a contribution, a starting point might be to look for binding, which will probably be very weak of a piece of a potential drug of a drug to the therapeutic target compound. The next step would be to search for a quite different small compound with a like effect, and then to try both of these small fragments chemically bound together. The reasoning is that a two-point binding is vastly stronger, commonly by a million times or so, than binding at only one point, for the weakly bound end of the compound is prevented from escaping by the (weak) interaction at the other end. Very weak interactions were in earlier days very difficult to detect, but now by NMR, the change in the spectrum when there is only vestigial binding (that is to say, when only a very small proportion of the small molecule in solution is bound at any moment) is more easily discerned and measured. An offshoot of the fragment-based approach is 'click chemistry'. Here the two compounds to be explored are modified to contain a highly reactive group. When both are added to the target a chemical bearing at both ends a group with high reactivity towards a reactive group on each of the bound fragments. If both have alighted, even in passing, on the target they will become linked to each other by the third reagent, forming a bridge, and by this means the new lead compound candidate will be captured. [THE ABOVE SECTION REALLY DEMANDS TWO DIAGRAMS TO MAKE IT COMPREHENSIBLE.]

Fragment-based explorations have given rise to several new drugs. Of course the choice of the initial fragments is not random, for their geometry can be calculated with reasonable accuracy; or if the compound is already available, its structure can be determined by NMR or X-ray crystallography (easily done since it is small). Now, if as is commonly the case, the structure of the target, perhaps an enzyme or receptor, is known, computer modelling will divulge the likelihood of a fit. Other considerations also enter, such as the size of the molecule and its hydrophobicity (p.), which determines to what extent it will pass through the cell membrane into the cell's interior of the cell. Some pharmacologists would also ask whether the structure complies with the empirical 'rule-of-three' or 'rule-of-five' (three or five attributes according to whose precepts you follow) of fragments to give the best prospect of a strong interaction).

Yet there are deeper questions of principle that drug researchers have been debating in the last decade or so. Given that such a small proportion of diseases result from the malfunction of a single gene, how secure can the choice of a drug target ever be? All too often a new compound has been successfully designed to inactivate a primary target, such as a surface receptor of a cancer cell, say, and yet worked feebly, erratically between patients, or not at all. The new hope and catchword is 'systems biology'. This signifies a way of confronting the bewilderingly complex systems that characterise the workings of the cell. The huge advances in cell biology, molecular biology and genetics during the last few decades have generated an unimaginable mass of information – a veritable data glut – about the molecules of life and their manifold interactions, which form networks of interdependent processes, all with their positive and negative feedback loops. Drawn out in the form of circuit diagrams, they resemble vast electrical switching circuits. The aim of systems biology is to make sense of these networks, relying to no small extent on mathematical modelling. A realistic model must simulate the actual function of the network; it must correctly predict, for example, the effect of a perturbation, such as introducing a mutation that weakens or strengthens an interaction and thereby perhaps changes the amount of a metabolic product. The model may thus identify a new drug target or indicate the genotypes (p.) - expressed for instance in the properties of a particular enzyme - of the patients who will benefit from a drug and those who will not. There seem so far to have been only a few examples of successful applications of systems biology in drug development, but many drug researchers believe that this is where the future of the science lies.

However this ultimately turns out, it seems unlikely that all the problems that have plagued drug research through the ages – the unforeseeable emergence of side effects and toxicity, and more – will all go away. It is hard to imagine that, despite all the victories past and to come, drug discovery will not retain, at least in part, its historic character as a dark art.

GLOSSARY

Alkaloid A type of natural chemical found in many plants, characterised by their content of nitrogen atoms. The compounds are in general weakly basic (as opposed to acidic).

Antibody A protein that recognises and binds to a substance identified by the body as foreign (not-self); the first line of defence mounted by the immune system.

Antigen A substance that is recognised by an antibody and binds to it.

Black-box In the U.S. an explicit warning of severe side-effects that a drug may produce, which the FDA (q.v.) demands to be set out on the label.

Branded medicine/brand name A drug product protected by a patent/ the trade name given to that product by the company holding the patent. The name is capitalised.

Double-blind The condition in a clinical trial that neither those who administer the drug or placebo, nor the patients, may know who gets which.ww

European Medicines Agency (EMEA) The body responsible for the approval of drugs in the countries of the European Union (EU).

Federal Drug Administration (FDA) The all-powerful body responsible for the approval of drugs for use in the U.S.A.

Galenicals Named after the influential Roman physician, they are extracts of [lants, and sometimes animals, held to have specific curative propertes

Generic medicine/ name A medicine copied from a branded medicine the patent of which has expired/ the name given to that medicine by the company marketing it. The name is not capitalised.

Hormone Any one of the many natural compounds, secreted by endocrine (hormone-producing) gland into the bloodstream, which conveys it to a target organ on which it exerts a physiological effect.

Meta-analysis An analysis of the results of many clinical trials taken together.

'Me-too' drug A drug developed with a structure just different enough from an existing and successful drug to be patentable.

New chemical entity (NCE) A new drug with a new type of structure, or developed according to a new concept, as distinct from a 'me-too' drug.

Off-label Prescription of a drug for a use for which it is not licensed by a regulatory agency, such as the FDA (q.v.) in the U.S.A.

Orphan drug A drug developed to treat a rare disease, not subject to the same rigorous approval criteria as other new drugs.

Placebo An inert substance ("sugar pill") given to the control group of subjects in a clinical trial to provide a baseline for the efficacy of a compound beingtested.

Polypharmacy The use for medicinal purposes of complex mixtures of natural substances.

Prodrug A substance in itself inactive, but converted into an active drug by a metabolic reaction.

Signatures, doctrine of The belief that cures for conditions of particular organs could be found in plants supposed to resemble that organ (e.g. plants with kidney- or ear-shaped leaves would cure kidney or ear complaints).

Simple Simples were single medicinal herbs or their extracts.

Steroid Any of a class of compounds made in the body or sometimes by a plant, including cholesterol and the sex hormones, characterised by a structure containing four fused carbon rings.

Syndrome The symptoms and signs that together characterise a given disease.

Vitamin A natural substance required in small amounts to allow the metabolism to function normally, and therefore for health.

BIBLIOGRAPHY

This is not a textbook, and the references listed below are not in the main to primary scholarly sources. A few such have been included on grounds, as it seems to me, of a particular historical interest. A large proportion of the total are nonetheless taken from the scientific literature, for many of these journals feature every so often accounts of past achievements, or sometimes noteworthy failures, often also the reflections of participants. I have tried to avoid listing works in foreign languages, but a very few in French and in German have insinuated themselves, where I could find no English equivalent, or any of equal cogency. The list includes a good number of books. None of them are highly technical, and some are not merely informative, but offer the reader an illuminating tour of the social, medical or scientific milieu in which the events that fill the foregoing pages unfolded. For general background reading I would recommend *The Greatest Benefit to Mankind – A Medical History of Humanity from Antiquity to the Present* by Roy Porter (HarperCollins, London, 1997); *Science and the Practice of Medicine in the Nineteenth Century* by W.F. Bynum (Cambridge University Press, Cambridge, 1994); *Therapeutics from the Primitives to the 20th Century* by Erwin H. Ackerknecht (Hafner Press, New York, 1973); and, for the more ambitious, the indispensable, more technical treatise, *Drug Discovery: a History* by Walter Sneader (Wiley, Chichester, and Hoboken, NJ, N.J., 2005), and see also *Drug Discovery from Nature* (S. Grabley and R.Thiericke, ed., Springer, Berlin 1999).

Internet search engines will of course disgorge a seemingly limitless amount of information (not all of it necessarily reliable). As I have indicted, I have not felt it necessary to list anything approaching the mass of primary references pertaining to the contents of this book. That material is readily found on the invaluable Pubmed site of the U.S. National Institutes of Health of the U.S.A. (www.ncbi.nlm.nih.gov/pubmed).

REFERENCES

An asterisk denotes a book of interest beyond its immediate bearing on the section of text to which the page reference relates, or a work of scholarly and literary lustre that repays reading for pleasure.

Page

1 – *Drugs – A Very Short Introduction* – Leslie Iversen (Oxford University Press, Oxford, 2001).

5 *Alchemy* – E.J. Holmyard (Penguin, London, 1957).

6 *The Ebers Papyrus: a New English Translation with Commentaries and Glossary* – Paul Ghalioungui (Cairo Academy of Scientific Research and Technology, 1987).

   The Medical Features of the Papyrus Ebers – Carl Christoph von Klein (Isha Press, New Delhi, 2010).

   Natural diseases and rational treatments in primitive medicine – Akerknecht, E.H. (1946) *Bulletin of the History of Medicine* **19**, 467-497.

   The Medical Features of the Papyrus Ebers – Carl Christian von Klein (Isha Press, New Delhi, 2010).

10 *Hippocratic Writings* – Geoffrey, E.R. Lloyd, ed. (Penguin Classics, London, 1984).

Nymphaea cult in ancient Egypt and the New World: a lesson in empirical pharmacology – Bertol, E. *et al.* (2004) *Journal of the Royal Society of Medicine* **97**, 84-85.

12 The doctrine of signatures – Pearce, J.M.S. (2008) *European Neurology* **60**, 51-52.

13 *Dioscorides on Pharmacy and Medicine* – John M. Riddle (University of Texas Press, Austin, Texas, 1985).

17 *Pliny the Elder – Natural History: A Selection* – John Healy (translation and introduction – Penguin, London, 2004).

19 *Contraception and Abortion from the Ancient World to the Renaissance* – John M. Riddle (Harvard University Press, Cambridge, Massachusetts, 1992).

20 Therapeutics – Debru, A. in *The Cambridge Companion to Galen* (Hankinson, R.J. ed., Cambridge University Press, Cambridge, 2008).

21 Venetian theriac and the foundation of medicines regulation – Griffin J.P. (2004) *Journal of Clinical Pharmacology* **58**,317-325.

25 *Medieval Islamic medicine* – Peter E. Pomann and Emmilie Savage-Smith (Edinburgh University Press, Edinburgh, 2007).

30 Ancient and medieval chemotherapy for cancer – Riddle, J.M. (1985) *ISIS* **76**, 319-330.

31 *The Devil's Doctor: Paracelsus and the World of Renaissance Magic and Society* – Phillip Ball (Heinemann, London, 2006).

33 What is there that is not poison? A study of the *Third Defense* by Paracelsus – Deichmann, W.B. *et al.* (1986) *Archives of Toxicology* **58**, 207-213.

34 The last alchemist – the first biochemist: J.B. van Helmont – Rosenfeld, L. (1985) *Clinical Chemistry* **31**, 1755-1760.

35 *The Fever Tree – In Search of the Cure for Malaria* – Mark Honigsbaum (Macmillan, London, 2001).

40 Lapidary medicine – Loomis, C.G. (1944) *Bulletin of the History of Medicine* **16**, 319-324.

42 English translation of Pierre Pomet – *A Complaet History of Druggs written in French by Monsieur Pomet, chief druggist to the late French King Lewis XIV....* 4th corrected edition (printed for J and J. Borwicke *et al.*, London, 1748).

The exotic world of Pierre Pomet's *A Compleat History of Druggs* – Sherman, S. (2004) *Endeavour* **28**, 156-160.

Pharmacopoeia Lemeriana Contracta – Lemery's Universal pharmacopoeia abridg'd in a collection of recepe's and observations compar'd with the London and with the Bates's dispensatories, and also with Charas's Royal pharmacy: to which are added some remedies recommended by the members of the French Royal Academy of Science, most collected out of the history of that society lately published by John Baptista Hamel. By Nicolas Lémery (printed for Walter Kettilby, 1700).

English translation of Nicolas Lémery – *A course of chymistry. Containing an easie method of preparing those chymocal medicines which are used in physic, with curious remarks and useful discourses... .....* (printed for Walter Kettilby, London, 1698).

43 Treatments for bubonic plague: reports from seventeenth century British epidemics – Holland, B.K. (2000) *Journal of the Royal Society of Medicine* **93**, 322-324.

45 *Anglo-Saxon* Medicine – M.L. Cameron (Cambridge University Press, Cambridge, 1993).

Man as medicine: pharmacological and ritual aspects of traditional therapy using drugs derived from the human body – Cooper, W.C. in *Chinese Science: an Exploration of an Ancient Tradition* (S.Nakayama and N. Silvin, ed., MIT Press, Cambridge, Massachusetts, 1973).

Heal Thyself – Nicholas Culpeper and the Seventeenth Century Struggle to Bring Medicine to the People – Benjamin Woolley (Harper Collins, New York, 2004)

The English Physitian, enlarged with three hundred, sixty and nine Medicines, made of English Herbs that were not in any impression before this, being of the vulgar Herbs of this Nation - Nicholas Culpeper (Proquest Ebo Editions, U.S.A., 2010).

46 *The Herball or Generall Historie of Plantes* –John Gerard – *The complete 1633 editio, revised and enlarged by Thomas Johnso n* (Dover Publications, New York, 1975).

The Folk-lore of Plants – T.H. Thiselton Dyer (1888, published by The Echo Library, Teddington, Middlesex).

54 *Heilsame Dreck-Apotheke: wie nämlich mit Koth und Urin meiste Krankheiten und Schäden glück;ich geheilt werden* – Christian Franz Paullini (Verlag des Herausgeber, 1847).

Die Heilsame Dreck-Apotheke – A. Leegaard (Kreisselmeier, Icking/ München, 1968).

60 The folk-lore of pulmonary tuberculosis – Rolleston, J.D. (1941) *Tubercle* **21**, 55-65.

64 William Cullen – Johnstone, R.W. (1959) *Medical History* **3**, 33-46.

65 *Considerations on the Medicinal Use and on the Production of Factitious Airs* – Thomas Beddoes and James Watt (Bulgin and Rosser, Bristol, 1795).

Thomas Beddoes, M.D., 1760-1808: Chemist, Physician, Democrat –
Dorothy A. Stansfield (D. Riedel, Dordrecht, Holland, 1984).

66 The medical reputation of Benjamin Rush: contrasts over two centuries –
Shryock, R.H. (1971) *Bulletin of the History of Medicine* **45**, 507-552.

Benjamin Rush, MD: assassin or beloved healer? – North, R.L.
(2000) *Baylor University Medical Center Proceedings* **13**, 45-49.

67 William Cobbett, Benjamin Rush, and the death of General
Washington – Davies, N.E. *et al.* (1983) *Journal of the American Medical
Association* **249**, 912-915.

70 The renaissance of bloodletting: a chapter in modern therapeutics –
Risse, G. (1979) *Journal of the History of Medicine* **34**, 1-22.

Decline of bloodletting: A study in 19th-century ratiocinations –
Haller, J.S. (1986) *Southern Medical Journal* **79**, 469-474.

The early chemical and pharmaceutical history of calomel –
Urdang, G. (1948) *Chymia* **1**, 93-108.

71 Samson of the materia medica: Therapy and use and abuse of calomel –
Haller, J.S. (1971) *Pharmacy History* **13**, 67-76.

72 The rise and fall of Pink Disease – Dally, A. (1997) *Social History of
Medicine* **10**, *291-304.*

73 Notes on Dr. Thomas Goulard's Treatise on the Effects and Various
Preparations of Lead – particularly of the Extract of Saturn – for different
Chirurgical Disorders – Thompson, J.H. (1938) *Proceedings of the Royal
Society of Medicine* **31**, 27-31.

Lead exposure from lead crystal – Graziano, J.H. and Blum, C.
(1991) *The Lancet* **327**, 141-142.

75 A cure for the ague: the contribution of Robert Talbor (1642-81) – Keeble, T.W. (1997) *Journal of the Royal Society of Medicine* **90**, 285-289.

78 Notoriety to respectability: a short history of arsenic prior to its present day use in haematology – Doyle, D. (2009) *British Journal of Haematology* **145**, 309-317.

Arsenic curiosa and humanity – Bentley, R. and Chasteen, T.G. (2002) *Chemical Educator* **7**, 51-60.

79 The introduction of hydrocyanic acid into medicine – a study in the history of clinical pharmacology – Earles, M.P. (1967) *Medical History* **11**, 305-313.

81 *The Natural History of Quackery* – Eric Jameson (Michael Joseph, London, 1961.

83 Quackery – Comment (1829) *The Lancet* **11**, 783.

Quackery extraordinary – Comment (1846) *The Lancet* **48**, 2016.

84 From the grave …. Rest in Peace without comment – Boyle, M. (2003) *The Lancet* **362**, 2125.

The Natural History of Quackery – Eric Jameson (Michael Joseph, London, 1961).

Religion and quackery – Comment (1896) *The Lancet* **148**, 1401.

86 *An Account of the Foxglove and its Medical Uses 1785-1985* – James K. Aronson (Oxford University Press, Oxford, 1985).

William Withering and digitalis – Moore, D.A. (1985) *British Medical Journal* **290**, 324.

William Withering (1741-1799): A Birmingham Lunatic – Lee, M.R. (2009) *Proceedings of the College of Physicians Edinburgh* **31**, 77-83.

The Lunar Men: The Friends who Made the Future – Jenny Uglow (Faber, London,2002).

88 The historical development of therapeutic trials – Bull, J.P. (1959) *Journal of Chronic Diseases* **10**, 218-148.

89 Comparing like with like: some historical milestones in the evolution of methods to create unbiased comparison groups in therapeutic experiments – Chalmers, I (2001) *International Journal of Epidemiology* **30**, 1156-1164.

Intentional ignorance: a history of blind assessment and placebo controls in medicine – Kaptchuk, T.I. (1998) *Bulletin of the History of Medicine and Allied Sciences* **72**, 389-433.

90 Unbiased divination, unbiased evidence, and the patulin clinical trial – Kaptchuk, T.J. and Kerr, C.E. (2004) *Journal of Epidemiology* **33**, 17-25.

91 *A Treatise on the Scurvy in Three Parts. Containing an Inquiry into the Nature, Causes, and Cure of the Disease. Together with a Critical and Chronological View of what has been Published on the Subject* (Printed by Sands, Murray and Cochran for Kincaid and Donaldson, Edinburgh, 1753). Edinburgh, 1753).

The History of Scurvy and Vitamin C – Kenneth J. Carpenter, (Cambridge University Press, Cambridge, 1988).

Limeys: the true History of one Man's War against Ignorance, the Establishment and the deadly Scurvy – David Harvie (Sutton, Stroud, 2002).

James Lind and the cure of scurvy: an experimental approach – Hughes, R.E. (1975) *Medicine History* **51**, 342-351.

92 Apothecaries and chemists in the 17th century – Hall, M.B. (1967) *Pharmaceutical* (**23 Oct**), **33-36.**

93 Sir Gilbert Blane, Bt. (1749-1834) – Beasley, A.W. (1985) *Annals of the Royal College of Surgeons of England* **67**, 332-333.

96 In a time of cholera – Grace, P.A. (2014) *Irish Journal of Medical Science* **183**, 133-137.

98 Homeopathy and its kindred delusions – in *Medical Essays: 1842-1882* – Oliver Wendell Holmes (Houghton Mifflin, Boston, 1888).

99 *Bad Science* – Ben Goldacre (Fourth Estate, London, 2008).

101 *The White Death: A History of Tuberculosis* – Thomas Dormandy (New Yirk University Press, New York, 2000).

102 Vitamin D, cod-liver oil, and rickets: a historical perspective – Rajkumar, K. ((2003) *Pediatrics* **112**, e132-e135.

103 *Development of Inhalation Anaesthesia* – Barbara M. Duncum (Royal Society of Medicine Press, London, 1947).

104 *Chloroform: the Quest for Oblivion* – Linda Stratmann (History Press, Stroud, UK, 2003).

106 'Yankee dodge': the first British public demonstration of anaesthesia – Usher, S.M. and Chieveley-Williams, S. (2002) *Grand Rounds* **4**, L12-L14.

107 Surgery between Hunter and Lister as exemplified by the life and works of Robert Liston (1794-1847) – Coltart, D.J. (1996) *Proceedings of the Royal Society of Medicine* **65**, 556-560.

108 Sir James Young Simpson (1811-1870) and obstetric anaesthesia – Dunn, P.M. (2002) *Archives of Disease in Childhood – Fetal and Neonatal Edition* **86**, F207-F209;

111 The isolation of morphine – first principles in science and ethics – Huxtable, R.J. and Schwarz, S.K.W. (2001) *Molecular Interventions* **1**, 189-191.

Über das Morphium, eine salzfähige Grundlage, und die Mekonsäure als Hauptbestandtheile des Opiums – Sertürner, F. (1817) *Annalen der Physik* **55**, 56-89.

113 Friedrich Wilhelm Sertürner and the discovery of morphine – Schmitz, R. (1985) *Pharmacy in History* **27**, 61-67.

115 A short history of alkaloids –Wink, M. in *Alkaloids: Biochemistry, Ecology, and Medical Applications* (Roberts, M.F. and Wink, M., ed; Plenum Press, New York, 1998).

116 Pierre-Jean Robiquet – Rennes 14 janvier 1780- Paris 29 avril 1840 – Warolin, C. (1999) *Revue d'Histoire de la Pharmacie* **87** (321), 97-110.

117 Les travaux scientifiques de Joseph Pelletier – Dillmann, G. (1989) *Revue d'Histoire de la Pharmacie* **77**, 128-134.

121 Research on iodine and goiter in the nineteenth and early twentieth centuries – Zimmermann, M.B. (2008) *Journal of Nutrition* **138**, 2060-2063.

125 History of anaethesia: early forms of local anaesthesia – Zimmer, M.(2014) *European Journal of Anaesthesiology* **31**, 1-12.

126 Vassily von Anrep, forgotten pioneer of regional anesthesia – Yentid, S.M. and Vlassakov, K.V. (1999) *Anesthesiology* **90**, 890-895.

127 *Freud and Cocaine: the Freudian Fallacy* - Thomson, E.M. (Blond and Briggs, London, 1983).

(f.n.) *Der Totale Rausch: Drogen im Dritten Reich* – Norman Ohler (Kiepenheuer & Witsch, Cologne 2015).

128 From cocaine to ropivacaine: the history of local anesthesia - Ruetsch, Y.A. *et al.* (2001) *Current Topics in Medicinal Chemnistry* **1**, 175-182.

Carl Koller: The man and the drug – McAuley, J.E. (1985) *British Dental Journal* **158**, 339-342.

Carl Koller: mankind's greatest benefactor? The story of local anesthaesia - Leonard, M. (1998) *Journal of Dental Research* **77**, 535-538.

Cocaine's use in ophthalmology – our 100-year heritage – Altman, A.J. *et al.* ((1985) *Surveys of Ophthalmology* **29**, 300-306.

130 Leaves and needles: the introduction of surgical local anesthesia – Fink, R. (1985) *Anesthesiology* **63**, 77-83.

132 *François Magendie, Pioneer of Experimental Physiology and Scientific Medicine in XIX Century France* – J.B. Olmstead (Schuman, New York, 1944).

134 *Claude Bernard and Animal Chemistry. The Emergence of a Science* – Frederick L. Holmes (Harvard University Press, Boston,. U.S.A., 1974).

135 Medical components in Cabanis's science of man – Staum, M.S. (1978) *Studies in the History of Biology* **2**, 1-31.

136 F.J.V. Broussais (1772-18380): his life and doctrines – Rolleston, D.J. (1939) *Proceedings of the Royal Society of Medicine* **32**, 27-33.

Pierre-Charles-Alexandre Louis and the evaluation of bloodletting – Morabia, A. (2006) *Proceedibgs of the Royal Society of Medicine* **99**, 158-160.

Recherche sur les effets de la seignée dans plusieurs maladies inflammatoires – Louis, P.C.A. (1828) *Archieves Generals de Médecine* **18**, 321-336.

138 *Louis Pasteur, Free Lance of Science* – René Dubos (Plenum Publishing Corp., New York, 1950).

141 *The Private Science of Louis Pasteur* – Gerald L. Geison (Princeton University Press, Princeton, NJ, 1995).

144 *Robert Koch – A Life in Medicine and Bacteriology* – Thomas D. Brock (Science Tech PubLications, Madison, WI, 1988).

147 The Koch-Pasteur dispute on establishing the cause of anthrax – Carter, K.C. (1988) *Bulletin of the History of Medicine and Allied Sciences* **62**. 42-57.

148 *The Greatest Story Never Tojd: The Human Story of the Search for the Cure for Tuberculosis and the New Global Threat* – Frank Ryan (Swift Publishers, U.K., 1992).

151 Koch's postulates then and now – Grimes, D.J. (2006) *Microbe* **1**, 223-228.

155 Use of amyl nitrite in angina – Lauder Brunton, T. (1867) *The Lancet* **90**. 97-98.

156 *A Short History of Cardiology* – Peter Fleming (Rodopi, Amsterdam, Holland, 1997).

William Murrell, physician and practical therapist – Smith, E. and Dudley Hart, F. (1971) *British Medical Journal* **ii**, 632-633.

157 Nitro-glycerine as a remedy for angina pectoris – Murrell, W. (1879) *The Lancet* **141**, 86-87; 113-115;151-152; 225-227.

159 *Paul Ehrlich, Scientist for Life* – Ernst Bäumler (trans. Grant Edwards; Holme and Meier, New York, 1984).

166 *Paul Ehrlich* – Maria Marquardt, mit einer Einleitung von Sir Henry H. Dale (Springer, Berlin, 1951).

167 The search for a chemical cure for cancer – MacGregor, A.B. (1966) *Medical History* **10**, 374-385.

173 *Opium: A History* – Martin Booth (Doubleday, New York, 1998).

174 Old beliefs concerning tobacco – Editorial comment (1920) *The Lancet* **196**, 909-910.

The germicidal properties of tobacco smoke – Editorial comment (1913) – *The Lancet* **181**, 406.

A history of the medical uses of tobacco 1492-1860 – Stewart, G.G. (1967) *Medical History* **11**, 228-268.'

176 An Account of the Success of the Bark of the Willow in a Cure of Ague (a Letter to the Right Honourable George Earl of Macclesfield, President of the R.S. from the Rev. Mr. Edmund Stone of Chipping Norton in Oxfordshire. *Philosophical Transactions of the Royal Society of London,* (1763), p. 7.

Edward Stone (1702-1768) and Edmund Stone (1700-1768). Confused identities resolved – Pierpoint, W. (1997) *Notes and Records of the Royal Society of London* **51**, 211-217.

181 *Mauve: How one man invented the colour that changed the world* – Simon Garfield (Faber and Faber, London, 2000).

183 The discovery of aspirin: a reappraisal - Sneader, W. (2000) *British Medical Journal* **321**, 1591.

Aspirin – the Remarkable Story of a Wonder Drug – Jeffrey Diarmuid (Bloomsbury Publishing Plc, London, 2004).

188 *The Demon under the Microscope – From Battlefield Hosppital to Nazi Labs, one Doctor's Heroic Search for the World's First Miracle Drug* – Thomas Hager (Harmony Books, New York, 2006).

Die Geschichte der Sulfonamidforschung – Robert Behnisch (Medizinische unde Pharmazeutische Studiengesellschaft Verlag, Mainz, Germany, 1986).

189 From methylene blue to chloroquine: a brief review of the development of an antimalarial therapy – Kraft, K. *et al.* (2012) *Parasitology Research* **111**, 1-6.

190 *The First Miracle Drugs – How the Sulfa Drugs Transformed Medicine* – Lesch, J.E. (Oxford University Press, New York 2007).

191 Treatment of human puerperal infections and experimental infections in mice with Prontosil – Colebrook, L. and Kenny, M. (1936) *The Lancet* **228**. 1279-1286.

Leonard Colebrook: the chemotherapy and control of streptococcal infections – Turk, J.L. (1994) *Journal of the Royal Society of Medicine* **87**, 727-728.

192 Daniel Bovet (23 March 1907- 8 April 1992) – Olivario, A. (1994) *Biographical Memoirs of Fellows of the Royal Society* **39**, 60-70.

193 News of Dr Gelmo, discoverer of sulphanilamide – Notes and Queries (1950) *Journal of the History of Medicine* **5**, 213-214.

195 Chemists and biologists during the National Socialist era – Deichmann, U. (2002) *Angewandte Chemie International Edition* **41**, 00001310-1328.

196 *The Crime and Punishment of IG Farben* – Joseph Borken (Pocket Books, New York, 1979).

200 The relation of *p*-aminobenzoic acid to the mechanism of action of sulphanilamide – Woods, D.D. (1940) *British Journa; of Experimental Pathology* **21**, 74-90.

201 **Alexander Fleming: the Man and the Myth* – Gwyn Macfarlane (Chatto and Windus, London, 1984).

203 On the antibacterial action of cultures of a penicillium, with special reference to the use in isolation of B. influenza – Fleming, A. (1929) *British Journal of Experomental Pathology* **10**, 226-236.

Almroth Wright: Founder of Modern Vaccine-Therapy – Cope, Z. (Thomas Nelson, London, 1966).

207 *Howard Florey – the Making of a Great Scientist – Gwyn Macfarlane (Oxford University Press, Oxford, 1979).

209 The Birth of Penicillin – Ronald Hare (Allen and Unwin, London, 1970).

212 Penicillin: its development for medical uses – Florey, H.W. (1944) Nature 153, 40-42.

213 Norman Heatley: Obituary – Ruth Evans The Guardian 8 January, 2004.

Dr Norman Heatley – Hamilton-Miller, J.M.T. (2004) Journal of Microbial Chemotherapy 53, 691-692.

214 *The Yougest Science – Lewis Thomas (Viking Books, New York, 1983).

219 Streptomycin, Schatz, Waksman and the balance of credit for discovery – Kingston, W. (2004) Journal of the History of Medicine and Allied Sciences 59, 441-462. *Leaps in the Dark – the Making of Scientific Reputations – John Waller (Oxford University Press, Oxfor2004).

220 My Life with the Microbes – Waksman, S. (The Scientific Book Club, London, 1958).

222 Mycobacterium tuberculosis and the cause of consumption from discovery to fact – Murray, J.F. (2004) American Journal of Respiratory and Critical Care Medicine 169, 1086-1088.

227 Carbapenems: Past, present and future – Wallace, K.M. et al. (2011) Antimicrobial Agents and Chemotherapy 52, 4943-4960.

228 Fecal microbiota transplant – an old therapy comes of age – Kelly, C.P. (2013) New England Journal of Medicine 368, 474-475.

FDA gets to grips with faeces – Mole, B. (2013 *Nature* **498**, 47-48.

230 Peptides from frog skin – Bevin, C. and Zasloff, M. (1990) *Annul Reviews of Biochemistry* **59**, 395-414.

231 An Investigation on the nature of ultra-microscopic viruses – Twort, F.W. (1915) *The Lancet* **186**, 1213-1214.

The bacteriophage: the breaking down of bacteria by associated filter-passing lysins – Twort, F.W. (1922) *British Medical Journal* **ii**, 291-296.

232 *Félix d'Herelle and the Origin of Molecular Biology* – William C. Summers (Yale University Press, New Haven, CT and London, 1999)

Sur un microbe invisible antagoniste des bacilles dysentériques – d'Herelle, F. (1917) *Comptes rendus de l'Académie des Sciences Paris* **165**, 173-175.

Identité du phénomène de Twort et du phénomène de d'Herelle - Gratia, A. and Jaumain, D. (1921) *Comptes rendus de la Société de Biologie Paris* **85**, 880-881.

Cholera and plague in Indochina: The bacteriophage inquiry of 1927-1936 – Summers, W.C. (1996) *Journal of the Hisyory of Medicine and Allied Sciences* **48**, 275-301.

233 Bacteriophage therapy for bacterial infections – Ho, K. (2001) *Perspectives in Biology and Medicine* **44**, 133-141.

234 Smaller fleas ad infinitum – therapeutic bacteriophage redux – Thiel, K. (1996) *Proceedings of the National Academy of Sciences of the United States* **93**, 3167-3168.

239 Antiviral drugs – a short history of their discovery and development – Field, H. and De Clenca, E. (2004) *Microbiology* **31**, 58-61.

240 *Agostino Bassi (1773-1856)* – Geoffrey C. Ainsworth (Fisher, Knight & Co., St. Albans, UK, 1956).

Agostino Bassi bicentennial (1773-1973) – Porter, J.R. (1973) *Bacteriological Reviews* **37**, 284-288.

242 Nystatin – Elizabeth Lee Hazen and Rachel Brown – Introduction, Maramoreck, K. (1960) *Annals of the New York Academy of Sciences* **89**, 253-266.

243 Chemical regulation of the secretory process (Croonian Lecture) – Bayliss, W.M. and Starling, E.H. (1904) *Proceedings of the Royal Society of London* **73**, 310-322.

Ernest Starling and 'hormones': an historical commentary – Henderson, J. (2005) *Endocrinology* **184**, 5-10.

246 David Marine and the problem of goiter – Carpenter, K.J. (2005) *Journal of Nutrition* **135**, 675-680.

249 **Discovery of Insulin* – Michael Bliss (Faber and Faber, London, 1988).

254 Drug discovery: metformin and the control of diabetes – Drondfield, A. and Ellis, P. *Education in Chemistry* (November 2011).

Charles-Édouard Brown-Séquard: A Nineteenth Century Neurologist and Endocrinologist – J.M.D. Olmsted (Johns Hopkins University Press, Baltimore, MD, 1946).

255 The effects produced on man by subcutaneous injection of a liquid obtained from the testicles of animals – Brown-Séquard, C. E. (1899) *The Lancet* **137**, 105-107.

Brown-Séquard's organotherapy and its appearance in America at the end of the nineteenth century – Borell, M. (1976) *Bulletin of the History of Medicine and Allied Sciences* **50**, 309-320.

258 *The Monkey Gland Affair* – David Hamilton (Chatto and Windus, London, 1986).

Regaining lost youth: The controversial and colorful beginnings of hormone replacement therapy – Kahn, A. (2005) *Journals of Gerontology, Series A: Biological Science and Medical Science* **60**, 142-147.

263 The great radium scandal – Macklis, R. (1993) *Scientific American* **269**, 94-99.

267 Better prepared than synthesized. Adolf Butenandt, Schering Ag and the transformation of steroids into drugs (1930-1946) – Gandilière, J.E. (2005) *Studies in the History and Philosophy of the Biological and Biomedical Sciences* **36**, 612-644.

269 *Toxic Bodies: Hormone Disruptors and the Legacy of DES* – Nancy Langston (Yale University Press, New Haven, CT, 2010).

Worse than the Disease – Pitfalls of Medical Progress – Diana B. Dutton (Cambridge University Press, New York, 1988).

270 The discovery and early use of cortisone – Glyn, J (1998) *Journal of the Royal Society of Medicine* **91**,513-517.

Diamonds are forever: the cortisone legacy – Hillier, S.G. (2007) *Journal of Endocrinology* **195**, 1-6.

276 Ludwig Haberlandt – "Grandfather of the Pill" – Djerassi, C. (2009) *Wiener Klinische Wochenschrift* **121**, 727-728.

Ludwig Haberlandt – pioneer in hormonal contraception – Haberlandt, E. (2009) *Wiener Klinische Wochenschrift* **121**, 746-749.

277 *The Pill, Pygmy Chimps and Degas' Horse* – Carl Djerassi (Basic Books, New York, 1992).

History of oral contraception – Dhont, M. (2010) *European Journal of Contraception and Reproductive Health Care* 15, Suppl 2, S12-S18.

The Pill – Bernard Asbell (Random House, New York, 1995).

282 *A Commotion in the Blood – Life, Death and the Immune System* – Stephen S. Hall (Little, Brown and Company, London, 1997).

283 The treatment of malignant tumors by repeated inoculations of erysipelas: with a report of ten original cases – Coley, W.B. (1893) *American Journal of Medicl Science* **105**, 487-511.

The failure of the erysipelas toxins – Editorial (1894) *Journal of the American Medical Association* **24**, 919.

Coley's toxins in perspective – Starnes, C.O. (1992) *Nature* **357**, 11-12.

285 *The Cure – A Story of Cancer and Politics from the Annals of the Cold War* – Nikolai Krementsov (University of Chicago Press, Chicago, 2002).

2.091 From basic research to cancer drug: the story of cisplatin – Lewis, R.)1999) *The Scientist* **13**, 11-13.

304 Ethnobotany and drug discovery: the experience of the National Cancer Institute – Cragg, G.M. *et al.* (1994) *Ciba Foundation Symposia* **185**, 178-190.

305 *The Story of Taxol: Nature and Politics in the Pursuit of an Anti-Cancer Drug* – Jordan Goodman and Vivien Walsh (Cambridge University Press, Cambridge, 2001).

309 *The Cancer Treatment Revolution: How Smart Drugs and Other New Therapies are Reneweing our Hopes and Changing the Face of Medicine* – David Nathan (John Wiley, New York, 2007).

313 Schmiedeberg in Strassburg (1872-1919): The making of modern pharmacology – Kochweser, J. and Schechter, P.J. (1978) *Life Sciences* **22**, 13-15.

315 The history of barbiturates a century after their clinical introduction – López-Muñoz, F. *et al.* (2005) *Neuropsychiatric Disease and Treatment* **1**, 329-344.

318 *Ten Years that Changed the Face of Mental Illness* – Jean Thuillier (Martin Dunitz, London, 1999) [translation of *Les Dix Ans qui ont Changé la Folie, la Dépression et l'Angoisse* (Erès, Paris, 1921)]

321 Neurosyphilis, malaria, and the discovery of antipsychotic agents – Frankenburg, F.R. and Baldessarum, R.J. (2008) *Harvard Review of Psychiatry* **16**, 299-307.

322 Lithium and bipolar disorder – Fyfe, I. (2009) *The Biochemist* **31**, 2-4.

327 Brain Gain – the underground world of "neuroenhancing" drugs – Talbot, M. *The New Yorker* (27 April, 2009).

The age of enhancement – Edmonds, D. *Prospect* (3 September 2009).

333 *Pharmageddon* – David Healy (University of California Press, Berkeley, CA, 2012)

334 *Unhinged: The Trouble with Psychiatry – A Doctor's Revelations About a Profession in Crisis* – Daniel Carlat (Free Press, New York, 2009).

Anatomy of an Epidemic: Magic Bullets, Psychiatric Drugs, and the Astonishing Rise of Mental Illness in America – Robert Whitaker (Broadway Books, New York, 2011).

Happy Pills in America: from Miltown to Prozac – David Herzberg (Johns Hopkins Universoty Press, Baltimore, MD, 2010).

Bitter pills – Check, E. (2004) *Nature* **431**, 122-124.

335 *Protecting America's Health: The FDA, Business and One Hundred Years of Regulation* – Philip J. Hilts (Alfred A. Knopf, New York, 2004).

Outcome reporting industry-sponsored trials of Gabapentin for off-label use – Vedula, S.S. *et al.* (2009) *New England Journal of Medicine* **361**, 1963-1971.

Huge penalty in drug fraud. Pfizer settles felony case for Neurentin off-label promotion – Bernadette Tansey – *San Francisco Chronicle*, 14 May 2004.

336 Paxil study under fire - Wadman, M. (2011) *Nature* **475**, 153.

Levodopa: the story so far – Abbott, A.(2010) *Nature* **466**, 56-57.

337 Stacking the deck – Studies of the medical literature confirm what many suspected – reporters of clinical trials do not always play straight – Giles, J. (2006) *Nature* **440**, 270-272.

339 **The Emperor's New Drugs: Exploding the Antidepressant Myth* – Irving Kirsch (Bodley Head, Oxford, 2009).

*Let Them Ear Prozac: the Unhealthy Relationship Between the Pharmaceutical Industry and Depression – David Healy (New York University Press, New York, 2004).

343 *Cannabis: A History* – Martin Booth (St. Martin's Press, London, 2003).

The history of the ergot of rye (*Claviceps purpurea*) III: 1940-80 – Lee, M.R. (2010) *Journal of the Royal College of Physicians of Edinburgh* **40**, 277-280.

344 Lysergic acid diethylamide: its effect on a male Asian elephant – West, L.J. *et al. (1962) Science* **138**, 1100-1102.

345 Comfortably numb – it started as anaesthetic, then became a psychedelic club drug. Now researchers think ketamine could hold the key to understanding and treating depression – Check, E. (2006) *Nature* **443**, 629-631.

348 *The War of the Soups and the Sparks: The Discovery of Neurotransmitters and the Dispute over How Nerves Communicate* – Elliot Valenstein (Columbia Unversity Press, New York, 2005).

352 Ernest Fourneau (1872-1949) – Tréfouël, J. (1949) *Bulletin de l'Académie Nationale de Médecine* **31**, 589.

354 *A Modern History of the Stomach: Gastric Illness, Medicine and British Society, 1800-1950* – Ian Miller (Pickering and Chatto, London, 2011).

Gutted – Shapin, S. (2011) *London Review of Books,* **13**, 30 June.

356 Cimetidine – Ganellin, C.R. (1982) in *Chronicles of Drug Discovery*, J.Bindra and D. Lednicer, ed. (Wiley-Interscience, New York) **1**, 1-38.

Reminiscences of the development of cimetidine – Duncan, W.M. and Parsons, M.E. (1980)*Gastroenterology* **78**, 620-622.

357 Unidentified curved bacilli in the stomach of patients with gastritis and peptic ulceration – Marshall, B.J. and Warren, J.R. (1983) *The Lancet* **321**,1311-1315.

Helicobacter pylori twenty years on – Marshall, B.J. (2002) *Clinical Medicine* **21**, 147-152.

359 History of leeching and hirudin – Fields, W.S. (1991) *Haemostasis* **21**, Suppl. 1, 3-10.

360 The discovery of heparin – McLean, J. (1959) *Circulation* **19**, 75-78.

361 The discovery of dicoumarol and its sequels – Link, K. (159) *Circulation* **19**, 97-107.

364 Battle of the clotbusters – O'Donnell, M. (1991) *British Medical Journal* **302**, 1259-1261.

366 *Asthma: the Biography* – Mark Jackson (Oxford University Press, Oxford, 2009).

368 Roger Altounyan and the discovery of cromolyn (sodium cromoglycate) – Howell, J. (2005) *Journal of Asthma and Clinical Immunology* **115**, 882-885.

371 Developing diuretics – Pizzi, R.A. (2003) *Modern Drug Discovery* February, 2003.

372 From blood pressure to hypertension: the history of research – Esunge, P.M. (1991) *Journal of the Royal Society of Medicine* **84**, 621.

Controlling hypertension, a research success story – Dustan, H.P. (1996) *Archives of Internal Medicine* **156**, 1925-1935.

377 A historical perspective on the discovery of statins – Endo, A. (2010) *Proceedings of the Japan Academy Series B Physical and Biological Sciences* **86**,484-493.

378 When good cholesterol turns bad – Pearson, H. (2006) *Nature* **444**, 794-796.

Cholesterol veers off script – Couzin, J. (2008) *Science* **322**, 220-223

Off-target effects of torcetrapib – Osório, J. (2010) *Nature Reviews Cardiology* **7**, 541.

380 The antiviral activity of 9-β-D-arabinofurosyladenine (ARA-A) – Schabel, F.M. (1968) *Chemotherapy* **13**, 321-328.

381 On high alert – in Outlook: HIV/AIDS (2010) – Marris, E. *Nature* **466**, S2-S3.

382 The outlook for a cure – in Outlook: HIV/AIDS – Hughes, V. (2010) *Nature* **466**, S11-S13.

383 Thalidomide and its analogues – Cooper, C.R. (2010) *The Biochemist* **32**, 36-39.

Thalidomide therapy – Filmore, D. (2004) *Modern Drug Discovery*, November 2004, 35-36.

384 Pitfalls in a discovery: the chronicle of chloroquine – Coatney, G.R. (1963) *American Journal of Tropical Medicine and Hygiene* **12**, 121-128.

385 A lesson learnt: the rise and fall of Lariam and Halfan – Croft, A.M. (2007) *Journal of the Royal Society of Edinburgh* **100**, 170-174.

387 Carlsson and the discovery of dopamine – Benes, M. (2001) *Trends in Pharmacological Sciences* **22**, 46-47.

Experimental treatment of parkinsonism with L-Dopa – Cotzias, G.C. *et al.* (1968) *Neurology* **18**, 267-277.

Distribution of noradrenaline and dopamine (3-hydroxytyramine) in the human brain, and their behaviour in diseases of the extrapyramidal system [translated from the German] – Ehringer, H. and Hornykiewicz, O. (1960) *Wiener Klinische Wochenschrift* **38**, 1236-1239.

390 Bromocriptine in parkinsonism – Calne, D.B. *et al.* (1974) *British Medical Journal* **4**, 444-446.

393 (f.n.) How (not) to communicate new scientific information: a memoir of the famous Brindley lecture – Klotz, L. (2005) *British Journal of Urology International* **96**, 956-957.

396 The history of erectile dysfunction management – Jonas, D. (2001) *International Journal of Impotence Research* **13**, Supplement 3, S3-S7.

399 sqq. *Suffer the Children: TheStory of Thalidomide* – The Insight eam of the *Sunday Times* (André Deutsch, London, 1979).*Bovet*

Thalidomide and the Power of the Drug Companies – Henning Sjöström and Robert Nilsson ((Harmondsworth, Penguin, London1972).

Dark Remedy: The Impact of Thalidomide and its Survival as a Vital Medicine – Trevor Stephens and Rock Brynner (Perseus, Cambridge, MA, 2001).

400 Thalidomide in America: a brush with tragedy – McFadyen, R.E. (1976) *Clio Medicina* **11**, 79-93.

401 A personal perspective on the thalidomide tragedy – Lenz, W. (1992) *Teratology* **46**, 417-418.

Medikamentskandal: Contergan Firma droht Förderung von Milliardenhöhe – *Der Spiegel* 10 November, 2007.

403 Generic HIV drugs will widen US treatment net – Maxmen, A. (2012) *Nature* **488**, 267.

404 Risk of acute myocardial infarction and sudden cardiac death in patients treated with cyclooxygenase 2 selective and non-selective anti-inflammatory drugs: nested case comtrol studies – Graham, D.J. *et al.* (2005) *The Lancet* **365**, 475-481.

Fever pitch – Ledford, H. (2006) *Nature* **450**, 600-601.

408 *The Worst of Evils – The Fight against Pain* – Thomas Dormandy (Yale University Press, New Haven, CT, 2006).

Opioids in anesthesia – Berger, J.M. (2005) *Seminars in Anesthesiology, Perioperative Medicine and Pain* **24**, 108-119.

409 Appetite suppressants and valvular heart disease – Weissman, N.J. (2001) *American Journal of Medicine Science* **321**, 285-289.

Making the first antidepressant: Amphetamine in American medicine, 1920-1959 – Rasmussen, N. (2006) *Journal of the History of Medicine and Allied Sciences* **61**, 288-323.

America's first amphetamine epidemic 1929-1971 – Rasmussen, N. (2008) *American Journal of Public Health* **98**, 974-985. -

410 Mediator scandal rocks French medical community – Mullard, A. (2011) *The Lancet* **377**, 890-892.

Valvular heart disease associated with fenfluramine-phentermine – Connolly, H.M. *et al.* (1997) *New England Journal of Medicine* **337**, 581-588.

411 Medicinal strategies in the treatment of obesity – Bray, G.A. and Tartaglia, L.A. (2000) *Nature* – Insight (Obesity) **404**, 672-677.

412 The brain: A mindless obsession – Barber, C. (2008) *he Wilson Quarterly* winter, 32-39.

Glaxo agree to pay $3 billion in fraud settlement – Katie Thomas and Michael Schmidt, *New York Times*, 2 July, 2012.

GlaxoSmithKline fined $3 bn after bribing doctors to increase drug sales – Simon Neville, *The Guardian*, 3 July 2012.

413 Drugs for asthma – Barnes, P.J. (2006) *British Journal of Pharmacology* **147**, S297-S303.

416 Association between industry affiliation and position on cardiovascular risk with rosiglitazone: cross sectional systematic review – Wang, A. *et al.* (2010).

British Medical Journal **340**, c1344.

Setting the record straight – Nissen, S. (2010) *Journal of the American Medical Association* **303**, 1194-1195.

Drug company push on doctors is disclosed – Liz Kowalczyk, *Boston Globe*, 19 May 2002.

418 *The Truth about Drug Companies: How they Deceive Us and What to Do About It* – Marcia Angell (Random House, New York, 2004).

Bad Pharma: how Drug Companies Mislead Doctors and Harm Patients – Ben Goldacre (Fourth Estate, London, 2012).

423 New uses for old drugs – Chong, C.R. and Sullivan, D.J. (2007) *Nature* **448**, 645-646.

In vivo antiviral properties of biologically active compounds. II. Studies with influenza and vaccinia viruses – Sidwell, R.M. *et al.* (1968) *Applied Microbiology* **16**, 370-392.

Therapeutic potential of venom peptides – Lewis, R.J. and Garcia, M.L. (2003) *Nature Reviews Drug Discovery* **2**, 790-802.

420 Techniques: Bioprospecting historical herbal texts by hunting for new leads in old tomes – Buenz, E.J. *et al.* (2004) *Trends in Pharmacological Science* **25**, 494-498.

A culture in the balance – Qiu, J. (2007) *Nature* **448**, 126-128.

425 The influence of natural products on drug discovery – Newman, D.J. *et al.* (2000) *Natural Products Reports* **17**, 215-234.

Natural products as sources of new drugs over the period 1981-2003 – Newman, D.J. *et al.* (2003) *Journal of Natural Products* **66**, 1022-1037.

423 Venom-based medicines – Shaw, C. (2009) *The Biochemist* **5**, 34-39.

421 Drugs from the deep – Marris, E. (2006) *Nature* **443**, 904-906.

424 The secrets of voracious killer snails – Barinaga, M. (1990) *Science* 249, 250-251

Conus venoms: a rich source of novel ion-channel targets – Terlau, H. and Olivera, B.M. (2004) *Physiological Reviews*60, 52-60.

Pruning nature: Biodiversity-derived discovery of novel sodium channel blocking conotoxins from *Conus bullatus* – Olivera, B.M. (2008) *Toxicon* **53**, 90-98.

426 Isolation of antibiotics turbomycin A and B from a metagenomic library of soil microbial DNA – Gillespie, D.M. *et al.* (2002) *Applied Environmental Microbiology* **68**, 4301-4306.

425 Therapeutic antibodies – Cochlovius, B. *et al.* (2003) *Modern Drug Discovery* **33**, 33-38.

428 When good drugs go bad – Giacomini, K. *et al.* (2007) *Nature* **446**, 975-977.

Drugs, bugs and personalized medicine: pharmacometabolomics enters the ring – Wilson, I.D. (2009) *Proceedings of the National Academy of Science of the U.S.A.* **106**, 14187-14188.

431 An agenda for Personalized medicine – Ng, P.C. *et al.* (2009) *Nature* **461**, 724-726.

434 Race-specific drugs: regulatory trends and public policy – Winickoff, D.E. and Obasogie, O.K. (2008) *Trends in Pharmacological Sciences*29, 277-279.

The short life of a race drug – Krimsky, S. (2012) *The Lancet* **379**, 114-115.

435 MicroRNAs make big impression in disease after disease – Couzin, J. (2008) *Science* **319**, 1782-1781784.

Challenges for academic drug discovery – Jorgensen, W. (2012) *Angewandte Chemie, International Edition* **51**, 11680=11684.

436 Repurposing with a difference – Boguski, M.S. *et al.* (2009) *Science* **324**, 1394-1395.

439 Power of the placebo – Beecher, H.K. (1955) *Journal of the American Medical Association* **159**, 1602-1606.

Powerful placebo: The dark side of the randomized controlled trial – Kaptchuk, T.J. (1998) *The Lancet* **351**, 1722-1725.

441 Prescribing "placebo treatments": Results of a national survey of U.S. internists and rheumatologists – Tilburn, L.C. *et al.* (2008) *British Medical Journal* **337**, a1938.

Ways to fix clinical trial – Ledford, H. (2011) *Nature* **477**, 526-531.

446 Does chemistry have a future in therapeutic innovation – Meunier, B. (2012) *A5gewandte Chemie International Edition* **51**, 8702-8706.

The importance of chemistry for the future of the pharma industry – Wild, H. (2011) *Angewandtw Chemie International Edition* **50**, 7452-7453.

446 The rise, fall and reinvention of combinatorial chemistry – Kodadad, T. (2011) *Chemical Communications (Cambridge, England)* **47**, 9957-9963.

450 A decade of fragment-based drug design: strategic advances and lessons learned – Hajduk, P.J. and Greer, J. (2007) *Nature Reviews Drug Discovery* **6**, 211-219.

A fiendish puzzle – Abbott, A. (2008) *Nature* **452**, 1165-1167.

In situ click chemistry: probing the binding landscape of biological molecules – Seeeman, K. *et al.* (2010) *Chemical Society Reviews* **39**, 1252-1261.

Printed in the United States
By Bookmasters

Printed in the United States
By Bookmasters